THE COMPLETE
CALORIE
fat & carb
COUNTER

Includes Fiber & Protein!

OVER 500
Fast-Food Chains, Restaurants & Popular Brands

By Alex A. Lluch
Health & Fitness Expert
Author of Over 3 Million Books Sold!

WS Publishing Group
San Diego, California

THE COMPLETE CALORIE, FAT & CARB COUNTER

By Alex A. Lluch

Published by WS Publishing Group
San Diego, California 92119
Copyright © 2009 by WS Publishing Group

Nutritional and fitness guidelines based on information provided by the United States Food and Drug Administration, Food and Nutrition Information Center, National Agricultural Library, Agricultural Research Service, and the U.S. Department of Agriculture.

Designed by: David Defenbaugh, WS Publishing Group

Photo Credits:
Front cover image: © iStockphoto/Fuat Kose
Back cover image: © Stockbyte Royalty Free Photos
Food icons: © iStockphoto/stdemi (dairy, meats, bread, grains, seafood, etc.)
Food icons: © iStockphoto/Jane Norton (condiments)
Food icons: © iStockphoto/Viviyan (fast foods, donuts, coffee, cupcakes, pizza)
Food icons: © iStockphoto/Kristina Smirnova (alcoholic beverages)
Food icons: © iStockphoto/RoccoMontoya (jam)
Food icons: © iStockphoto/totallyjamie (ice cream, candy and dounut)
Food icons: © iStockphoto/DimensionsDesigns (taco and burrito)

For inquiries:
Log on to www.WSPublishingGroup.com
E-mail info@WSPublishingGroup.com

ISBN-13: 978-1-934386-34-7

Printed in China

Table of Contents

Table of Contents

RESTAURANTS & FAST-FOOD CHAINS   41

Table of Contents

Table of Contents

RESTAURANTS & FAST-FOOD CHAINS (CONT.)

Table of Contents

RESTAURANTS & FAST-FOOD CHAINS (CONT.)

Table of Contents

FOOD ITEMS BY CATEGORY

Table of Contents

Table of Contents

COMPLETE LIST OF NAME BRANDS

Table of Contents

COMPLETE LIST OF NAME BRANDS (CONT.)

Table of Contents

COMPLETE LIST OF NAME BRANDS (CONT.)

Table of Contents

COMPLETE LIST OF NAME BRANDS (CONT.)

Table of Contents

COMPLETE LIST OF NAME BRANDS (CONT.)

Table of Contents

COMPLETE LIST OF NAME BRANDS (CONT.)

 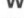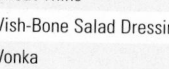

Introduction

By purchasing this book you have taken the first and most important step to lose weight, stay in shape, feel better, and have more energy than you ever thought possible. Research has shown, again and again, that the best way to accomplish your health and weight-loss goals is to track the calories, fat, carbs, protein, and fiber in the foods you eat on a daily basis.

THE BENEFITS OF LOSING WEIGHT

Losing weight has major benefits that can improve your way of life. Weight loss can lower the risk of numerous diseases, including heart disease, stroke, cancer, and diabetes.

However, it is difficult in today's society to make the right choices regarding your health and diet. Our jobs promote sedentary lifestyles, our days are busier than ever, and fast-food, while usually unhealthy, is convenient and inexpensive. Many food companies use larger portions as a selling point, making the claim that bigger is better. It then becomes the consumer's responsibility to monitor what and how much he or she eats.

INTRODUCTION

We know how difficult it can be to choose wisely when you are eating out, dining with friends, and planning meals at home. Portions at restaurants are larger than ever, and meals are often cooked with unhealthy sauces, dressings, and breading. It is extremely hard to locate a healthy option on many restaurant menus. Additionally, it has been scientifically proven that most people will consume hundreds of extra calories when dining in a group or social setting.

Think back to the last dinner you attended with a group of friends: Did you order an extra cocktail, partake in a fatty appetizer, or share a large dessert? The answer is probably yes. But have you ever thought about how many extra calories you are consuming during these get-togethers?

What about when you plan meals at home or make a grocery list? Do you know which are the most nutritious options? When you aren't sure of the nutritional content of different foods, it can be difficult to plan meals and grocery shop for healthy items. Perhaps you never realized that eating a seemingly healthy salad with vegetables can actually contain more calories and fat and less fiber and protein than a cheeseburger, if you coat the salad in ranch dressing!

The wonderful thing about *The Complete Fat & Carb Counter* is that it takes the guesswork out of ordering or preparing a healthy meal. The book's portable size makes it easy to put in your purse or car so you can quickly and conveniently look up the nutritional values for any food item.

The Complete Fat & Carb Counter is the most comprehensive book on the market, providing nutritional information and serving sizes for over 300 national brands and over 200 restaurants and fast-food chains. Better still, this book highlights the most healthy and least healthy food choices in every category.

USING THIS BOOK WHEN DINING OUT

Refer to this book when planning to eat out, and you will be able to determine the restaurant that best suits your needs. For instance, if you are in the mood for a hamburger, you can browse this book and choose a restaurant that has the healthiest burger choices.

If you have decided where to go, you can use the information provided in this book to choose the best options from the restaurant's menu. For example, you may find that the steak and potato entrée has fewer calories than a chicken salad made with high-fat mayonnaise-based dressing. Wouldn't it be nice to enjoy the steak dish you crave, knowing that you're making the healthy choice?

Or, perhaps you will refer to the section on mixed drinks, wine, and spirits and learn that one piña colada contains 440 calories. This knowledge can help you decide between having the piña colada or a dessert at the end of your meal.

As you can see, this book allows you to plan ahead and make tradeoffs when dining out, so you eat and drink within your daily limits.

USING THIS BOOK WHEN MAKING A GROCERY LIST AND PLANNING MEALS AT HOME

Use this book when writing your grocery list. You will be able to plan healthy, hearty meals and buy only items or national brands that contribute to eating smart, losing weight, and feeling better.

For instance, while using this book, you may realize that the muffin you usually eat for breakfast has a whopping 500 calories, 24 grams of fat, and 60 grams of carbs! An alternative meal might be an omelet with 1 large egg, ½ ounce of cheese, and ½ ounce of ham, as well as a whole wheat english muffin. The nutritional totals for this hearty breakfast option come to only 284 calories, 12 grams of fat, and 26 grams of carbohydrates. Although a ham-and-cheese omelet and english muffin may sound like more food than the muffin, that meal is actually better for you. Throw in an apple for good measure— it has just 55 calories, no fat, and all-natural carbs!

The omelet and english muffin breakfast contains more healthy nutrients, fewer grams of sugar, and less calories from fat. Before reading this book, you may have been under the mistaken impression that a muffin is actually the healthier option! This is just one example of how using *The Complete Fat & Carb Counter* can help you make better meal choices.

So, next time you go shopping, you might skip the bakery aisle and, instead, buy healthy breakfast items like low-fat cheese, low-fat yogurt, fresh fruit, and eggs. With these types of ingredients, you will be able to make delicious, filling meals, with much less fat and many healthy nutrients, such as natural fiber and protein. When you plan your meals with this book, you will be able to buy healthy ingredients and cook better meals.

By using *The Complete Fat & Carb Counter* you can stop relying on fad diets or depriving yourself of the things you love to eat. With this handy book, you can easily compare and contrast foods to make the best selections, even while dining out or on-the-go. You will find that by monitoring what you eat on a daily basis, you will lose weight and feel great, almost effortlessly.

Congratulations, and happy eating!

Your Weight & Health Status

The most important reasons to start a weight-loss program are to look and feel great, and to reduce the risk of health complications such as heart disease and diabetes. Before you start, however, it is important to assess your health status. There are three methods to determine your overall physical condition: your height and weight measurements, waist size, and Body Mass Index (BMI). Another consideration is your family history.

For adults 18 years and older, the first step is to measure your height and weight. Use those two numbers to find your BMI on the following page. If your BMI falls within the range of 19 to 24, you are considered healthy. If your BMI lands from 25 to 29, then you have an increased risk of developing health problems. If your BMI is 30 or above, you could be considered obese. If you fall into the last two categories, it is essential to plan and manage your weight-loss program.

The second factor in evaluating your weight is your waist size. Use a tape measure to calculate your waist circumference below your rib cage and above your belly button. You have an increased health risk for developing serious chronic illness if your waist size is more than 35 inches for women and 40 inches for men.

INTRODUCTION

Your personal history and family background can shed additional light on possible health risks. Be aware of increased potential problems if your family history includes arthritis, high blood pressure, high cholesterol, high blood sugar, death at a young age, heart problems, cancer, or respiratory illness. A history of family illness doesn't mean these conditions are destined to be a part of your future, but it is yet another reason to get started on the road to good health and physical fitness.

BODY MASS INDEX - BMI

The most common way to determine whether or not a person is obese is through Body Mass Index, or BMI. This is a ratio of a person's height and weight. When a person's BMI is over 25, he or she can be considered overweight. Unfortunately, BMIs over 25 are an increasing trend in America's health statistics. We are a nation whose waistline is expanding and will continue to grow unless we take control of our eating habits.

Body composition can vary greatly from individual to individual. Two people who possess the same height and weight can have different bone structure and varying percentages of muscle and fat. Therefore, your weight alone is not the only factor in assessing your risk for weight-related health issues. Your BMI can help indicate whether or not your health is at risk.

Calculating your BMI: Locate your height in the left-hand column of the chart. Then move across the row to your weight. The number at the very top of the column is your BMI.

BMI	19	20	21	22	23	24	25	26	27	28	29	30	31	32	33	34	35
Height							**Weight in pounds**										
4'10"	91	96	100	105	110	115	119	124	129	134	138	143	148	153	158	162	167
4'11"	94	99	104	109	114	119	124	128	133	138	143	148	153	158	163	168	173
5'	97	102	107	112	118	123	128	133	138	143	148	153	158	163	158	174	179
5'1"	100	106	111	116	122	127	132	137	143	148	153	158	164	169	174	180	185
5'2"	104	109	115	120	126	131	136	142	147	153	158	164	169	175	180	186	191
5'3"	107	113	118	124	130	135	141	146	152	158	163	169	175	180	186	191	197
5'4"	110	116	122	128	134	140	145	151	157	163	169	174	180	186	192	197	204
5'5"	114	120	126	132	138	144	150	156	162	168	174	180	186	192	198	204	210
5'6"	118	124	130	136	142	148	155	161	167	173	179	186	192	198	204	210	216
5'7"	121	127	134	140	146	153	159	166	172	178	185	191	198	204	211	217	223
5'8"	125	131	138	144	151	158	164	171	177	184	190	197	203	210	216	223	230
5'9"	128	135	142	149	155	162	169	176	182	189	196	203	209	216	223	230	236
5'10"	132	139	146	153	160	167	174	181	188	195	202	209	216	222	229	236	243
5'11"	136	143	150	157	165	172	179	186	193	200	208	215	222	229	236	243	250
6'	140	147	154	162	169	177	184	191	199	206	213	221	228	235	242	250	258
6'1"	144	151	159	166	174	182	189	197	204	212	219	227	235	242	250	257	265
6'2"	148	155	163	171	179	186	194	202	210	218	225	233	241	249	256	264	272
6'3"	152	160	168	176	184	192	200	208	216	224	232	240	248	256	264	272	279

Healthy	Overweight	Obese

HEALTH RISKS AND YOUR WEIGHT

For most adults, BMI and waist size are fairly reliable indicators of whether or not you are overweight. These two indicators are also effective in assessing your risk of weight-related health issues.

Your waist measurement determines whether or not you have the tendency to carry fat around your midsection. A higher waist size may indicate a greater risk for weight-related health issues such as high blood pressure, type-2 diabetes and coronary artery disease. Typically, the higher your Body Mass Index, the greater risk to your health. This risk also increases if your waist is greater than 35 inches for women or 40 inches for men.

If your weight indicates that you are at a higher risk for health problems, consult your primary care physician to determine safe and effective ways to improve your health. Even moderate amounts of weight loss, around 5 to 10 percent of your weight, can have long-lasting health benefits.

Risk of Associated Disease According to BMI and Waist Size

Body Mass Index		Waist less than or equal to 40" Men 35" Women	Waist greater than 40" Men 35" Women
18 or less	Underweight	N/A	N/A
19-24	Normal	N/A	N/A
25-29	Overweight	Increased	High
30-35	Obese	High	Very High
over 35	Obese	Very High	Very High

IDENTIFY YOUR EATING PATTERNS

Changing your eating habits requires adjusting your attitude toward food. Begin by understanding the situations and emotional triggers that lead to overeating. Let's take a look at some common behaviors:

Are you compelled to eat as an emotional response to your thoughts and feelings? If you eat when you're upset, frustrated, angry, lonely, or tired, the answer most likely is yes. Food feels like the perfect temporary solution that is, until it is finished, and then guilt sets in because the food choice may not have been healthy. Try to choose other behaviors as an emotional response, such as taking a walk or calling a friend.

Do you eat when you are not hungry because you think you should? Sometimes the time of day is enough encouragement to eat a meal or a quick snack, despite a lack of actual physical hunger. Instead, learn to listen to your body. If you are not hungry, you shouldn't eat.

Do you feel guilty leaving food on your plate? Perhaps when you were a child, you were told to finish all of the food on your plate. This sense of guilt should no longer gauge how much food you should eat. It is acceptable to stop eating when you feel full.

Do you make poor food choices because of peer pressure? It is far easier to go with the flow when those around you are eating unhealthy foods. It takes self-control and determination to follow your weight-loss plan at social gatherings or all-you-can-eat buffets. Congratulate yourself when you stick to your plan and successfully fend off unhealthy snacking urges.

Do you eat out of boredom? Food can become a time-filler when you are bored. Don't fall into this trap! Try to motivate yourself and choose a fun and interesting activity as an alternative to snacking. If you are otherwise occupied with an activity where food is not involved, it will be easier to wait for your regularly scheduled meal.

PERSONAL SUCCESS

Reaching your personal goals for weight-loss and health starts with the desire for success. You've started on the path to success by buying this book and honestly assessing your eating habits.

Motivation: Your journey takes on a new challenge as you look at the reasons behind your desire for personal success. The first component is to discover your source of motivation. What are your top three reasons for pursuing your weight-loss goal? Write them down in a journal and read them often as a reminder and a source of inspiration. They will help you stay focused on your future goals.

Realistic Timelines: The second component is to set realistic goals for yourself. Using this book to monitor what you eat is the best way to lose weight and stay healthy. However, promises of instant weight loss are too good to be true and are most likely unhealthy and even dangerous. Just keep track of what you eat, make healthy decisions, and stick to a realistic timeline. General guidelines for healthy weight loss suggest losing 1 to 2 pounds per week.

Celebrating Success: The third component is to focus on the positive aspects of your weight loss. Try to celebrate small achievements along the way to keep yourself motivated toward your long-term goal. These personal achievements will help you keep a positive attitude. For instance, if you turned down a caloric dessert in favor of a fiber-filled piece of fruit, pat yourself on the back! Acknowledge your accomplishments, no matter if they are baby steps or huge leaps of progress.

Visualization: A mental picture is worth a thousand words. In your mind's eye, envision your weight loss before it happens. Visualize all aspects of the new you, from your appearance to your improved health. Remember, if you can see it, chances are very good that you can make that healthy visual a reality.

Maintenance: The fifth and final component is maintaining your weight loss long after you have achieved your goal. Remember to stick with the healthy behaviors, habits, and attitudes that led you to your goal. Refer to this book each time you join go out for dinner, attend a party, write a grocery list, or make a meal at home. Keep up the good work, for there is nothing more gratifying than maintaining an ideal weight and a healthy lifestyle!

Secrets to Losing Weight

SUGGESTED DAILY CALORIES FOR WEIGHT MAINTENANCE

Your total daily calories should be based on your age, gender, body type, and level of physical activity. Active men should consume approximately 2,800 calories per day to maintain their ideal weight. Active women and sedentary men should eat 2,200 calories. Sedentary women and older adults should strive for 1,600 calories. If you are not sure of how many daily calories you should consume, consult your primary care physician for a recommendation.

Suggested Daily Calories for Weight Maintenance

Sedentary women and older adults should consume approximately 1,600 calories daily.	Most children, teenage girls, active women and sedentary men should consume approximately 2,200 calories daily. Pregnant or breast-feeding women may need to consume more.	Most teenage boys and active men and some very active women should consume approximately 2,800 calories daily.

SUGGESTED DAILY CALORIES FOR WEIGHT LOSS

The total number of daily calories for a weight-loss plan will depend on the number of pounds you wish to lose. Once you have determined the daily number of calories that you should eat to maintain your weight (based on the chart above), you should decrease your total caloric intake by an average of 500 calories per day for a moderate weight loss. To proceed in a safe and healthy manner, you can eliminate those 500 calories simply by decreasing the amount of sugars, refined carbohydrates, and alcohol in your diet, most of which provide calories with little nutritional value.

RECOMMENDED DAILY AMOUNT
FROM EACH FOOD GROUP

The United States Department of Agriculture is known for its Food Guide, which is a nutritional reference for many health groups and dietary plans. The USDA Food Guide separates the foods you should eat into six different categories: 1) grains, 2) vegetables, 3) fruits, 4) fats and oils, 5) milk and dairy products, and 6) meat, beans, fish, eggs, and nuts. The suggested amounts have been developed to help you select the proper amount of food to eat from each group on a daily basis. Each group provides you with a different set of essential nutrients. By following the recommended serving sizes, you can be assured that you are getting the proper amounts of protein, fats, carbohydrates, fiber, vitamins, and minerals. This guide can be adjusted to suit your personal needs.

The USDA Food Guide separates the foods you should eat into six different categories:

1. **GRAINS**
(6-11 SERVINGS)

2. **VEGETABLES**
(3-5 SERVINGS)

3. **FRUITS**
(2-4 SERVINGS)

4. **MILK & DAIRY PRODUCTS**
(2-3 SERVINGS)

5. **MEAT, BEANS, FISH, EGGS & NUTS**
(2-3 SERVINGS)

6. **FATS & OILS**
(USE SPARINGLY)

DAILY AMOUNT OF FOOD FROM EACH GROUP

Daily Calorie Level	1,200	1,400	1,600	1,800	2,000	2,200	2,400	2,600	2,800	3,000
Grains	4 oz.	5 oz.	5 oz.	6 oz.	6 oz.	7 oz.	8 oz.	9 oz.	10 oz.	10 oz.
Vegetables	1.5 C (3 srv)	1.5 C (2 srv)	2 C (4 srv)	2.5 C (5 srv)	2.5 C (5 srv)	3 C (6 srv)	3 C (6 srv)	3.5 C (7 srv)	3.5 C (7 srv)	4 C (8 srv)
Fruits	1 C (2 srv)	1.5 C (3 srv)	1.5 C (3 srv)	1.5 C (3 srv)	2 C (4 srv)	2 C (4 srv)	2 C (4 srv)	2 C (4 srv)	2.5 C (5 srv)	2.5 C (5 srv)
Milk	2 C	2 C	3 C	3 C	3 C	3 C	3 C	3 C	3 C	3 C
Meat, Beans, Fish & Nuts	3 oz.	4 oz.	5 oz.	5 oz.	5.5 oz.	6 oz.	6.5 oz.	6.5 oz.	7 oz.	7 oz.
Fats & Oils	17 g	17 g	22 g	24 g	27 g	29 g	31 g	34 g	36 g	44 g

Food group amounts shown in cups (C) or ounces (oz.), with number of servings (srv) in parentheses. Oils are shown in grams.

THE NUTRITION FACTS LABEL

Most packaged foods have a nutrition facts label. Use this information to make healthy choices quickly and easily.

Nutrition Facts

Serving Size 1 cup (228g)
Servings Per Container 2

Amount per Serving	
Calories 250	Calories from Fat 110

	% Daily Value*
Total Fat 12g	**18%**
Saturated Fat 3g	**15%**
Trans Fat 3g	
Cholesterol 30mg	**10%**
Sodium 470mg	**20%**
Total Carbohydrate 31g	**10%**
Dietary Fiber 0g	**0%**
Sugars 5g	
Protein 5g	

Vitamin A	4%
Vitamin C	2%
Calcium	20%
Iron	4%

* Percent Daily Values are based on a 2,000 calorie diet. Your Daily Values may be higher or lower depending on your calorie needs.

	Calories:	2,000	2,500
Total Fat	Less than	65g	80g
Sat Fat	Less than	20g	25g
Cholesterol	Less than	300mg	300mg
Sodium	Less than	2,400mg	2,400mg
Total Carbohydrate		300g	375g
Dietary Fiber		25g	30g

LABEL AT A GLANCE

Start Here: Check the serving size and servings per container.

Calories: 400 or more calories per serving is considered high. Note the calories from fat.

Daily Values: 5%=low, 20%=high.

Limit These Nutrients: Eating too much fat, saturated fat, trans fat, cholesterol, or sodium may put you at an increased health risk for diseases such as heart disease, some cancers, or high blood pressure.

Get Enough of These Nutrients: Most Americans do not receive the proper amount of fiber, vitamins A and C, calcium or iron from their diets. Eating enough of these nutrients can limit your risk of diseases such as osteoporosis and heart disease.

Daily Values Footnote: This footnote makes recommendations for key nutrients based on diets of 2,000 and 2,500 daily calories.

A BREAKDOWN OF THE NUTRITION FACTS LABEL

The first place to look when selecting foods at the market is the product label. Check out the Nutrition Facts for the ingredient list, serving size, calories, amounts, nutrients, portions, and percentage of daily nutritional values. Often you will see "enriched" food sources for wheat or pasta. This is an indication that vitamins or minerals have been added for nutrition. Commonly added nutrients are calcium, thiamin, riboflavin, niacin, iron, and folic acid. The ingredient list tells you exactly what is in the food, including nutrients and whether fat or sugar have been added. The ingredients are also listed in descending order by weight.

What is a Serving Size?: When hunger strikes and a type of food calls out to you, it is important to look at the label for serving size information. The Nutrition Facts label indicates the quantity of food per portion and the number of servings in the package. Serving sizes are now standardized to make it easier to compare foods in familiar units like cups, pieces, grams, or metric amounts. According to the sample label on the previous page, 1 serving of food equals 1 cup containing 250 calories. If you ate the whole package, you would have consumed 2 cups or 500 calories.

All Calories Are Not Created Equal: Calories provide a concrete measure of how much energy you receive from a serving size of a selected food. If you are overweight, chances are you consume more calories than your body needs on a daily basis. You should also be aware of how many calories per serving come from fat. In the sample label, there are 250 calories in a serving, and 110 of those come from fat. That means almost half of the calories are from fat. If you ate 2 servings or 500 calories, 220 would come from fat, which is 44 percent. To lose weight, select foods with 20 percent or less of its calories per serving coming from fat. These can be from proteins, dairy products, and whole grain breads, cereals, and pasta. Most fresh fruits and vegetables are naturally low in fat.

Keep Tabs on Cholesterol: Cholesterol is a fat-like substance present in all animal foods, such as meat, poultry, fish, milk and milk products, and egg yolks. It's a good idea to select lean meats, avoid eating the skin of poultry, and use low-fat milk products. Egg yolks and organ meats, like liver, are high in cholesterol. Plant foods, such as fruit and vegetables, do not contain cholesterol. Why is this important information? Eating foods high in dietary cholesterol increases blood cholesterol in many people, which increases their risk for heart disease. Most health authorities suggest dietary cholesterol should be limited to 300 mg or less per day.

Salt and Sodium: It's important to include some salt in your diet, but it should be limited to 2,400 mg per day. You can keep track of your daily intake by looking at the Nutrition Facts label. Go easy on luncheon and cured meats, cheeses, canned soups and vegetables, and soy sauce. Look for no-salt-added products at your supermarket. Be cautious and avoid adding table salt to your food. Each teaspoon of salt adds 2,000 mg of sodium to your diet. So put down the salt shaker and retrain your taste buds.

Sugar – How Sweet It Isn't: Sugar is an ingredient that is found in almost every food product. If you are counting calories, it is important to look at the list of ingredients to identify all sources of sugar. Obvious foods that add sugar are jams, ice cream, canned fruit and chocolate milk. You will also find it in cereals, sauces, frozen foods, and salad dressings. Here's a list of common sweeteners that are essentially sugar: white sugar, honey, sucrose, fructose, maltose, lactose, syrup, corn syrup, high fructose corn syrup, molasses, and fruit juice concentrate. If these terms are found in the first four listings on the label, that food is likely to be very high in sugar. Hint: labels are listed in grams. Consider 4 grams to equal 1 teaspoon of sugar. The total daily intake for all added sugar sources not found naturally in the food itself should be a maximum 6 teaspoons a day.

Carbohydrates: Breads, cereals, rice, and pasta provide carbohydrates, which are excellent sources of energy. If you are on a weight-loss plan, it is important to include them in your diet because they provide vitamins, minerals, and fiber. One serving of carbohydrates equals one slice of bread, one ounce of ready-to-eat cereal, or 1/2 cup cooked cereal, rice or pasta. Focus on complex carbohydrates, such as whole grain breads, cereals, and brown rice. Keep these foods healthy by not adding additional butter, margarine, cream, cheese, sugar, oils, and fat. Limit refined carbohydrates, such as white flour and sugar, as well as processed foods like prepackaged candy, cookies, cakes, and chips.

Fruits & Vegetables: Fruits and vegetables can be works of art if you select a rainbow of nine colorful choices throughout your day. For example, eat a yellow banana, green broccoli, orange carrots, a red apple, purple cabbage, and blueberries. Rotate your selections to get the most from your foods. Fruits and vegetables provide vitamins A and C, and folate. They also contain minerals like iron, potassium, and magnesium. Keep in mind that it is important to eat these foods as fresh as possible, preferably raw, and avoid adding butter, salt, and high-fat salad dressings. When possible, choose the actual piece of fruit, like an apple, over juice.

Protein: The USDA Food Guide suggests eating cooked lean meat as a source of protein for optimum health. Protein provides an essential supply of B vitamins, zinc, and iron. Make sure you get enough of these nutrients by combining a variety of choices, such as lean cuts of beef, pork, veal, lamb, chicken, turkey, fish, and shellfish. Other protein possibilities are eggs, beans, nut butters, tofu, dried nuts, and seeds. Try to choose lean cuts of meat, remove the skin from poultry, trim away all visible fat, go easy on egg yolks, and eat nuts and seeds sparingly.

Fat: As a food source, fat supplies energy and essential fatty acids to your body. Fat-soluble vitamins like A, D, E and K and carotenoids need fat to be absorbed into the body. Not all types of fat are healthy, however, especially saturated fats found in whole milk, butter, ice cream, poultry skin, and palm oil. Unsaturated fats, found mainly in vegetable oils, do not increase blood cholesterol.

A third category called trans fat is formed when liquid oils are made into solid fats, like shortening and hard margarine. This type of fat is dangerous because it raises blood cholesterol and increases the risk of coronary heart disease, which is one of the leading causes of death in the United States. Foods high in trans fat are processed foods made with partially hydrogenated vegetable oils, such as vegetable shortenings. These oils can be found in crackers, cookies, candies, snack foods, fried foods, and baked goods. It is difficult to avoid all foods with trans fat, so the ideal goal would be to limit your intake of processed foods as much as possible.

Foods With Healthy Sources of Fat: Try choosing vegetable oils like olive, canola, soybean, sunflower, and corn. Avoid coconut and palm kernel oils. Consider adding fish to your menu twice a week. Salmon and mackerel have omega-3 fatty acids, which offer protection against heart disease. Choose lean meats like skinless chicken, lean beef, and pork. Avoid all fried foods. Watch your fat calories because they contain 9 calories per gram, compared to carbohydrates and protein, which have only 4 calories per gram.

THE DIFFERENT TYPES OF FATS

FATS & THEIR SOURCES

Saturated Fats: Limit these fats. Saturated fats tend to raise blood cholesterol. Foods that contain higher amounts of saturated fats include high fat dairy products (like cheese, whole milk, cream, and regular ice cream), butter, fatty meats, lard, palm oil, and coconut oil.

Trans fatty acids: Limit these fats. Foods that are high

in trans fatty acids tend to raise blood cholesterol as well. These foods include those high in partially hydrogenated vegetable oils, such as hard margarine and shortenings. Foods with a high amount of this type of fat include some commercially fried foods and some baked goods.

Dietary Cholesterol: Limit cholesterol. Foods that are high in cholesterol also tend to raise blood cholesterol. These foods include liver and other organ meats, egg yolks, and dairy fat.

Unsaturated Fats: Unsaturated fats and oils do not raise blood cholesterol. These types of fats occur in vegetable oils such as olive, canola and corn oils, most nuts, avocados, and fatty fish like salmon. Some fish, such as salmon, tuna, and mackerel, contain omega-3 fatty acids that may offer protection against heart disease. This is the best type of fat to include in your diet. Just be sure to avoid excess calories.

EXERCISE AND WEIGHT CONTROL

Carrying around too much body fat is a nuisance. Many people fight the "battle of the bulge" through diet alone because exercise is not always convenient. Few of today's occupations require physical activity, and many people spend hours behind desks and computers. In addition, much of our leisure time is spent in sedentary pursuits. To reverse this trend, it is important to adjust your attitude and find time to exercise each day. Some of the most common reasons people use to avoid physical activity include:

1. "I don't have the time."
2. "I'm too tired and I don't feel like it."
3. "I'm not very good at exercising."
4. "It's not convenient to get to my workout place."
5. "I'm afraid and embarrassed."

Overweight or Overfat?: Being overweight and being overfat are two different dilemmas. Some people, such as athletes, have a muscular physique and weigh more than average for their age and height. But their body composition, which is the amount of fat versus lean body mass (muscle, bone, organs and tissue), is within an acceptable range. Others can weigh within the range of U.S. guidelines, yet they can carry around too much fat. Use exercise as a way to balance your body fat percentage. An easy self-test is to pinch the thickness of fat at your waist and abdomen. If you can pinch more than an inch of fat, excluding muscles, chances are you have too much body fat.

Energy Balance and Counting Calories: Losing weight boils down to a simple mathematical formula: consume fewer calories than you burn. Learn how to balance energy intake (food) with energy output (calories burned through physical activity). If you take in more calories than your body needs to perform your day's activities, it will be stored as fat. Therefore, the only solution is to consume the proper amount of calories that your body needs to maintain good health. Then exercise so that your body can utilize the stored fat. The end result will be your desired weight loss.

CALORIES BURNED BY
TYPICAL PHYSICAL ACTIVITIES

LIGHT ACTIVITIES: 150 or less	CAL/HR.
Billiards	140
Lying down/sleeping	60
Office work	140
Sitting	80
Standing	100

MODERATE ACTIVITIES: 150-350	CAL/HR.
Aerobic dancing	340
Ballroom dancing	210
Bicycling (5 mph)	170
Bowling	160
Canoeing (2.5 mph)	170
Dancing (social)	210
Gardening (moderate)	270
Golf (with cart)	180
Golf (without cart)	320
Grocery shopping	180
Horseback riding (sitting trot)	250
Light housework/cleaning, etc.	250
Ping-pong	270
Swimming (20 yards/min)	290
Tennis (recreational doubles)	310
Vacuuming	220
Volleyball (recreational)	260
Walking (2 mph)	200
Walking (3 mph)	240
Walking (4 mph)	300

SECRETS TO LOSING WEIGHT

VIGOROUS ACTIVITIES: 350 or MORE	CAL/HR.
Aerobics (step)	440
Backpacking (10 lb load)	540
Badminton	450
Basketball (competitive)	660
Basketball (leisure)	390
Bicycling (10 mph)	375
Bicycling (13 mph)	600
Cross country skiing (leisurely)	460
Cross country skiing (moderate)	660
Hiking	460
Ice skating (9 mph)	384
Jogging (5 mph)	550
Jogging (6 mph)	690
Racquetball	620
Rollerblading	384
Rowing machine	540
Running (8 mph)	900
Scuba diving	570
Shoveling snow	580
Soccer	580
Spinning	650
Stair climber machine	480
Swimming (50 yards/min.)	680
Water aerobics	400
Water skiing	480
Weight training (30 sec. between sets)	760
Weight training (60 sec. between sets)	570

FAVORITE ALCOHOLIC DRINKS

Beers

Beers	Cal	Fat	Cbs	Fbr	Prtn
Light					
Amstel Light, 1 bottle	100	0	5	0	1
Bud Light, 12 fl oz	110	0	7	0	1
Coors Light, 12 fl oz	102	0	5	0	1
Corona Light, 1 bottle	105	0	5	0	1
Kirin Light, 12.2 fl oz	100	0	7	0	1
• Michelob Ultra, 1 bottle	73	0	2	0	1
Miller Lite, 12 fl oz	96	0	3	0	1
Milwaukee's Best Light, 12.2 fl oz	98	0	4	0	1
Natural Light, 12 fl oz	95	0	3	0	1
• Samuel Adams Light, 12 fl oz	119	0	10	0	1
Regular					
Blue Moon, 12 fl oz	171	0	14	0	3
Budweiser , 12 fl oz	145	0	11	0	1
Corona Extra, 1 bottle	148	0	13	0	1
Guinness, Stout, 1 pint	170	0	6	0	1
• Heineken, 1 bottle	140	0	11	0	2
Kirin,12.2 fl oz	145	0	10	0	2
Miller Genuine Draft,12 fl oz	143	0	13	0	1
Newcastle, 12 fl oz	140	0	12	0	1
• Samuel Adams, 12 fl oz	180	0	18	0	2
Stella Artois, 11.2 fl oz	154	0	6	0	1
Non-Alcoholic					
Beck's Non-Alcoholic, 12 fl oz	90	0	20	0	2
• Coors Non-Alcoholic, 1 bottle	65	0	14	0	1
O'Douls, 12 fl oz	70	0	15	0	1
Old Milwaukee NA, 1 can	71	0	15	0	0
• St. Pauli Girl NA, 12 fl oz	95	0	22	0	0

Cocktails

Cocktails	Cal	Fat	Cbs	Fbr	Prtn
Alexander, 1 cocktail	170	2	8	0	0
Black Russian, 1 cocktail	240	0	16	0	0
Bloody Mary, 1 cocktail	115	0	5	0	0
Bourbon & Soda, 1 cocktail	105	0	0	0	0
Daiquiri, 1 cocktail	113	0	4	0	1
Gin & Tonic, 1 cocktail	197	0	16	0	0
Grasshopper, 1 cocktail	222	4	22	0	0
High Ball, 1 cocktail	107	0	2	0	0
Lemon Drop Martini, 1 cocktail	150	0	32	0	0
Long Island Ice Tea, 1 cocktail	140	0	11	0	0
Mai Tai, 1 cocktail	264	0	23	0	0
Manhattan, 1 cocktail	136	0	2	0	0
Margarita, 1 cocktail	159	0	6	0	0
Mint Julep, 1 cocktail	188	0	4	0	0
• Mojito, 1 cocktail	100	0	21	0	0
• Piña Colada, 1 cocktail	440	9	26	0	1
Rum and Coke , 1 cocktail	150	0	15	0	0
Sangria, 1 cocktail	165	0	23	0	0
Screwdriver, 1 cocktail	171	0	18	0	1
Seabreeze, 1 cocktail	170	0	20	0	0
Seven and Seven , 1 cocktail	180	0	16	0	0
Singapore Sling, 1 cocktail	230	0	12	0	0

FAVORITE ALCOHOLIC DRINKS

FAVORITE ALCOHOLIC DRINKS

Cocktails (cont.)

	Cal	Fat	Cbs	Fbr	Prtn
Tequila Sunrise, 1 cocktail	175	0	15	0	1
Tom Collins, 1 cocktail	156	0	3	0	0
Whiskey Sour, 1 cocktail	139	0	5	0	0
White Russian, 1 cocktail	253	1	17	0	0

Liqueurs

	Cal	Fat	Cbs	Fbr	Prtn
99 Apples - 49.5% (99 prf), 1 oz.	72	0	8	0	0
Alize - 16.0% (32 prf), 1 oz.	103	0	11	0	0
• Amaretto - 28.0% (56 prf), 1 oz.	110	0	17	0	0
Barenfang - 40.0% (80 prf), 1 oz.	103	0	11	0	0
Continental - 17.5% (35 proof), 1 oz.	85	2	0	0	1
Crème de Cassis - 20.0% (40 proof), 1 oz.	80	0	11	0	0
Crème de Coconut - 17.0% (34 proof), 1 oz.	103	0	11	0	0
DeKuyper Grape Schnapps, 1 oz.	70	0	10	0	0
Forbidden Fruit - 50.0% (100 proof), 1 oz.	103	0	11	0	0
Godiva - 17.0% (34 proof), 1 oz.	103	0	11	0	0
Hypnotiq - 17.5% (35 proof), 1 oz.	103	0	11	0	0
Jagermeister - 35.0% (70 proof), 1 oz.	103	0	11	0	0
Jubilee - 24.0% (48 proof), 1 oz.	72	0	6	0	0
• Kahlua- 26.5% (53 proof), 1 oz.	53	0	11	0	0
Maui Blue Hawaiian - 15.0% (30 proof), 1 oz.	72	0	10	0	0
Midori - 23.0% (46 proof), 1 oz.	79	0	11	0	0
Sour Puss - 15.5% (31 proof), 1 oz.	103	0	11	0	0
Tequila Rose - 17.0% (34 proof), 1 oz.	69	0	7	0	0
Tia Maria - 27.0% (54 proof), 1 oz.	92	0	10	0	0
Zwack - 43.0% (86 proof), 1 oz.	87	12	9	0	0

Liquors

	Cal	Fat	Cbs	Fbr	Prtn
Brandy - 40.0% (80 proof), 1 oz.	69	0	2	0	0
Gin - 40.0% (80 proof), 1 oz.	69	0	0	0	0
Rum - 40.0% (80 proof), 1 oz.	69	0	0	0	0
Tequila - 40.0% (80 proof), 1 oz.	69	0	0	0	0
Vodka - 40.0% (80 proof), 1 oz.	69	0	0	0	0
Whiskey - 40.0% (80 proof), 1 oz.	69	0	0	0	0

Shooters

	Cal	Fat	Cbs	Fbr	Prtn
Buttery Nipple, 1.5 fl oz	130	2	14	0	0
Chocolate Cake Shot, 1 shot	85	0	6	0	0
Fuzzy Navel, 1.5 fl oz	120	0	7	0	0
Kamikazi, 1.5 fl oz	150	0	2	0	0
Purple Hooter, 1.5 fl oz	90	0	6	0	0
Red-Headed Slut, 2 oz	164	0	18	0	0
• Soco Lime, 2 oz	167	0	15	0	0
• Vodka Lemon Drop, 1 oz	38	0	2	0	0
Washington Apple, 3 oz	140	0	10	0	0

Wine

	Cal	Fat	Cbs	Fbr	Prtn
Dry Dessert Wine, 1 fl. oz.	45	0	3	0	0
Red Table Wine, 1 fl. oz.	25	0	1	0	0
• Sweet Dessert Wine, 1 fl. oz.	47	0	4	0	0
• White Table Wine, 1 fl. oz.	25	0	1	0	0

A&W Restaurant

	Cal	Fat	Cbs	Fbr	Prtn
Dipping Sauces					
• BBQ, 28 g	40	0	10	0	0
Honey Mustard, 28 g	100	6	12	0	0
• Ranch, 28 g	160	17	2	0	0
Sweet & Sour, 28 g	45	0	12	0	0
Hot Dogs					
Cheese Dog, 126 g	320	20	25	0	11
• Coney (Chili) Cheese Dog, 154 g	350	21	27	0	13
Coney (Chili) Dog, 126 g	310	18	24	0	13
• Dog (plain), 90 g	280	17	22	0	11
Root Beer					
A&W Diet Root Beer, 20 fl.oz.	0	0	0	0	0
A&W Regular Root Beer, 20 fl.oz.	290	0	76	0	0
Root Beer Floats					
A&W Root Beer Float, 468 g	350	5	77	0	2
A&W Diet Root Beer Float, 468 g	170	5	30	0	2
Sandwiches & Strips					
Chicken Strips (3 pieces), 159 g	500	29	32	2	28
Crispy Chicken Sandwich, 219 g	590	29	54	3	31
Grilled Chicken Sandwich, 213 g	440	19	34	2	36
Kids Cheeseburger, 175 g	460	24	39	2	23
• Kids Hamburger, 161 g	420	22	35	2	21
Original Bacon Cheeseburger, 223 g	570	33	41	2	27
• Original Bacon Double Chzburger, 303 g	800	48	47	2	45
Original Double Cheeseburger, 288 g	720	42	46	2	41
Papa Burger, 288 g	720	42	46	2	41
Sides					
• Cheese Curds, 142 g	570	40	27	2	27
Cheese Fries, 170 g	380	19	50	4	4
• Chili Bowl, 225 g	190	6	22	5	12
Chili Cheese Fries, 198 g	400	19	51	5	8
Chili Fries, 170 g	370	16	49	5	8
Kids Fries, 113 g	310	13	45	4	3
• Large Fries, 156 g	430	18	61	6	5
Onion Rings, 113 g	350	16	45	2	5
Sweets & Treats - Medium					
A&W Root Beer Freeze, 510 g	480	10	89	0	10
Caramel Sundae, 189 g	340	9	57	0	8
Chocolate Milkshake, 475 g	700	29	100	2	11
Chocolate Sundae, 189 g	320	8	53	0	8
Hot Fudge Sundae, 189 g	350	11	54	1	8
M&M Polar Swirl, 340 g	710	25	107	2	15
Oreo Polar Swirl, 340 g	690	24	107	3	14
• Reese's Polar Swirl, 340 g	740	31	97	3	18
Strawberry Milkshake, 475 g	670	29	90	0	11
Strawberry Sundae, 189 g	300	8	47	0	7
• Vanilla Cone, 157 g	260	7	41	0	7
Vanilla Milkshake, 475 g	720	31	97	0	12
Vanilla Sundae, 189 g	310	8	52	0	7

Amazon Café

	Cal	Fat	Cbs	Fbr	Prtn
Smoothie					
Amazon Power Boost, 16 oz.	229	1	68	5	2
Bananarama, 16 oz.	239	1	65	2	3

(• = most healthy • = least healthy) **RESTAURANTS & FAST-FOOD • 41**

RESTAURANTS & FAST-FOOD CHAINS

Amazon Café (cont.)

	Cal	Fat	Cbs	Fbr	Prtn
Smoothie (cont.)					
Chocolate Nirvana, 16 oz.	225	1	76	2	12
Citrus Sunrise, 16 oz.	254	2	88	3	3
Coffee Utopia, 16 oz.	251	0	43	2	10
Coldblaster, 16 oz.	247	1	65	3	3
Orange Outrage, 16 oz.	215	1	65	2	6
Orange Sensation, 16 oz.	242	2	63	3	2
Paradise Lust, 16 oz.	265	3	60	3	3
• Piña Colada, 16 oz.	320	4	63	4	4
Raspberry Rage, 16 oz.	234	1	69	2	2
Raspberry Razzle, 16 oz.	207	1	62	3	5
• Skinny Delight, 16 oz.	186	1	44	3	1
Soy Smoothie, 16 oz.	191	0	50	3	9
Strawberry Supreme, 16 oz.	221	0	55	3	3
Tropical Passion, 16 oz.	236	1	71	3	2
Soup					
Broccoli & Cheese, 8 oz.	110	6	10	2	3
Chicken & Sausage Gumbo, 8 oz.	100	3	12	1	7
Chicken & Wild Rice, 8 oz.	120	3	17	1	6
• Chili Con Carne, 8 oz.	250	7	29	8	16
Chipotle Black Bean, 8 oz.	130	1	21	8	8
Classic Chicken Noodle, 8 oz.	80	2	9	2	6
Corn Chowder, 8 oz.	110	4	19	1	3
Cream of Broccoli, 8 oz.	110	5	14	6	3
Cream of Potato with Bacon, 8 oz.	120	4	18	2	4
Hearty Vegetable, 8 oz.	70	1	15	3	2
Italian Wedding, 8 oz.	130	4	16	1	6
Mushroom Barley, 8 oz.	80	2	14	2	2
New England Clam Chowder, 8 oz.	90	2	15	1	3
Rosemary Chicken Dumpling, 8 oz.	80	1	12	1	5
Rustic Beef & Mushroom, 8 oz.	70	2	6	1	7
Split Pea with Ham, 8 oz.	160	5	22	8	9
Sweet Pepper & Beef, 8 oz.	90	2	14	3	6
Three Bean Chili, 8 oz.	130	0	47	28	9
• Tomato & Three Cheese, 8 oz.	60	2	7	3	4

Applebee's

	Cal	Fat	Cbs	Fbr	Prtn
Angus Burgers or Chicken Sandwiches					
Bruschetta	780	N/A	N/A	N/A	N/A
• Chicken Bruschetta	600	N/A	N/A	N/A	N/A
Chicken Cowboy	950	N/A	N/A	N/A	N/A
Chicken Quesadilla	1240	N/A	N/A	N/A	N/A
Cowboy	1140	N/A	N/A	N/A	N/A
• Quesadilla	1420	N/A	N/A	N/A	N/A
Appetizers					
• Appetizer Sampler	2540	N/A	N/A	N/A	N/A
Boneless Buffalo Wings	1460	N/A	N/A	N/A	N/A
Buffalo Chicken Wings	1130	N/A	N/A	N/A	N/A
Chicken Quesadilla Grande	1320	N/A	N/A	N/A	N/A
Crunchy Onion Rings	1230	N/A	N/A	N/A	N/A
Mini Bacon Cheeseburgers	1470	N/A	N/A	N/A	N/A
• Mozzarella Sticks	930	N/A	N/A	N/A	N/A
Nachos Nuevos	2070	N/A	N/A	N/A	N/A
Veggie Patch Pizza	940	N/A	N/A	N/A	N/A

RESTAURANTS & FAST-FOOD CHAINS

Applebee's (cont.)	Cal	Fat	Cbs	Fbr	Prtn
Burgers, Sandwiches & Rollups					
• Blacken Tilapia Sandwiches	710	N/A	N/A	N/A	N/A
• Brewtus Steak Burger	1390	N/A	N/A	N/A	N/A
Chicken Fajita Rollup	1080	N/A	N/A	N/A	N/A
Oriental Chicken Rollup	1170	N/A	N/A	N/A	N/A
Roasted Turkey and Bacon Ciabatta	1370	N/A	N/A	N/A	N/A
Zesty Ranch Chicken Sandwich	1170	N/A	N/A	N/A	N/A
Chicken					
Chicken Fingers Basket	1050	N/A	N/A	N/A	N/A
Chicken Fingers Platter	1300	N/A	N/A	N/A	N/A
Chicken Fried Chicken	1280	N/A	N/A	N/A	N/A
Chicken Parmesan	1430	N/A	N/A	N/A	N/A
Fiesta Lime Chicken	1290	N/A	N/A	N/A	N/A
Riblet and Chicken Fingers Basket	1360	N/A	N/A	N/A	N/A
• Riblet and Chicken Fingers Platter	1950	N/A	N/A	N/A	N/A
• Roasted Garlic & Asiago Chicken	770	N/A	N/A	N/A	N/A
Fresh-Made Sides					
• Baked Potato	380	N/A	N/A	N/A	N/A
Caesar Salad	220	N/A	N/A	N/A	N/A
Garden Salad	310	N/A	N/A	N/A	N/A
Garlic Mashed Potatoes	110	N/A	N/A	N/A	N/A
• Seasonal Vegetables	50	N/A	N/A	N/A	N/A
Pasta					
• Cheddar-Jack Mac & Cheese with Chicken	1110	N/A	N/A	N/A	N/A
Chicken Broccoli Pasta Alfredo Bowl	1220	N/A	N/A	N/A	N/A
• Crispy Orange Chicken Bowl	1910	N/A	N/A	N/A	N/A
Grilled Shrimp Pesto Alfredo Fettuccine	1790	N/A	N/A	N/A	N/A
Three-Cheese Chicken Penne	1210	N/A	N/A	N/A	N/A
Ribs & Fajitas					
• Applebee's Riblets	1740	N/A	N/A	N/A	N/A
• Applebee's Riblets Basket	1120	N/A	N/A	N/A	N/A
Honey BBQ Baby Backs	1430	N/A	N/A	N/A	N/A
Sizzling Fajitas	1440	N/A	N/A	N/A	N/A
Salads					
Blue Cheese Dressing, Full	460	N/A	N/A	N/A	N/A
Blue Cheese Dressing, Half	230	N/A	N/A	N/A	N/A
Buffalo Chicken Salad, Full	830	N/A	N/A	N/A	N/A
Buffalo Chicken Salad, Half	590	N/A	N/A	N/A	N/A
California Shrimp Salad, Full	370	N/A	N/A	N/A	N/A
California Shrimp Salad, Half	310	N/A	N/A	N/A	N/A
Creamy Avocado Dressing, Full	350	N/A	N/A	N/A	N/A
Creamy Avocado Dressing, Half	180	N/A	N/A	N/A	N/A
Garlic Caesar Dressing, Full	420	N/A	N/A	N/A	N/A
Garlic Caesar Dressing, Half	190	N/A	N/A	N/A	N/A
Grilled Chicken Caesar Salad, Full	380	N/A	N/A	N/A	N/A
• Grilled Chicken Caesar Salad, Half	210	N/A	N/A	N/A	N/A
Grilled Shrimp 'N Spinach Salad, Full	850	N/A	N/A	N/A	N/A
Grilled Shrimp 'N Spinach Salad, Half	580	N/A	N/A	N/A	N/A
Hot Bacon Vinaigrette Dressing, Full	310	N/A	N/A	N/A	N/A
Hot Bacon Vinaigrette Dressing, Half	150	N/A	N/A	N/A	N/A
Mexi-Ranch Dressing, Full	380	N/A	N/A	N/A	N/A
Mexi-Ranch Dressing, Half	190	N/A	N/A	N/A	N/A
Oriental Chicken Salad, Full	840	N/A	N/A	N/A	N/A
Oriental Chicken Salad, Half	450	N/A	N/A	N/A	N/A

(• = most healthy • = least healthy)

RESTAURANTS & FAST-FOOD CHAINS

Applebee's (cont.)

Applebee's (cont.)	Cal	Fat	Cbs	Fbr	Prtn
Salads (cont.)					
Oriental Grilled Chicken Salad, Full	630	N/A	N/A	N/A	N/A
Oriental Grilled Chicken Salad, Half	350	N/A	N/A	N/A	N/A
Oriental Vinaigrette Dressing, Full	590	N/A	N/A	N/A	N/A
Oriental Vinaigrette Dressing, Half	290	N/A	N/A	N/A	N/A
• Santa Fe Chicken Salad, Full	900	N/A	N/A	N/A	N/A
Santa Fe Chicken Salad, Half	800	N/A	N/A	N/A	N/A
Seafood					
• Double Crunch Shrimp	1330	N/A	N/A	N/A	N/A
• Garlic Herb Salmon	700	N/A	N/A	N/A	N/A
Parmesan Tilapia	880	N/A	N/A	N/A	N/A
Steak Toppings					
• Grilled Onions	90	N/A	N/A	N/A	N/A
Sauteed Garlic & Mushrooms	130	N/A	N/A	N/A	N/A
• Shrimp 'N Parmesan	350	N/A	N/A	N/A	N/A
Steaks					
Bourbon Street, 10 oz.	1570	N/A	N/A	N/A	N/A
• Chop Steak, 10 oz.	1820	N/A	N/A	N/A	N/A
• House Sirloin, 9 oz.	410	N/A	N/A	N/A	N/A
New York Strip, 12 oz.	590	N/A	N/A	N/A	N/A
Ribeye, 12 oz.	590	N/A	N/A	N/A	N/A
Shrimp 'N Parmesan Sirloin, 9 oz.	1420	N/A	N/A	N/A	N/A
Steak & Friend Shrimp, 7 oz.	1390	N/A	N/A	N/A	N/A
Steak & Grilled Shrimp, 7 oz.	530	N/A	N/A	N/A	N/A
Steak & Honey BBQ Chicken, 7 oz.	1280	N/A	N/A	N/A	N/A
Steak & Riblets, 7 oz.	1710	N/A	N/A	N/A	N/A
Ultimate Trios					
• Boneless Buffalo Wings	840	N/A	N/A	N/A	N/A
Dynamite Shrimp	730	N/A	N/A	N/A	N/A
Mini Bacon Cheese Burgers	750	N/A	N/A	N/A	N/A
Mini Chicken Ranchers	770	N/A	N/A	N/A	N/A
• Mozzarella Sticks	420	N/A	N/A	N/A	N/A
Spinach & Artichoke Dip	580	N/A	N/A	N/A	N/A
Steak Quesadilla Towers	690	N/A	N/A	N/A	N/A
Traditional Buffalo Wings	680	N/A	N/A	N/A	N/A

Arby's

Arby's	Cal	Fat	Cbs	Fbr	Prtn
Arby's Chicken Naturals®					
BBQ Dipping Sauce, 28 g	44	0	11	0	0
Buffalo Dipping Sauce, 28 g	10	1	2	0	0
Chicken Bacon & Swiss - Crispy, 214 g	624	29	52	2	36
Chicken Bacon & Swiss - Grilled, 209 g	462	17	38	2	38
Chicken Fillet Sandwich - Crispy, 249 g	577	30	50	3	30
Chicken Fillet Sandwich - Grilled, 244 g	414	17	36	3	32
Chicken Tenders - 3 piece, 131 g	379	18	28	2	25
Chicken Tenders - 5 piece, 218 g	630	31	47	3	42
• Chkn Cordon Bleu Sand - Crispy, 250 g	657	32	49	2	41
Chkn Cordon Bleu Sand - Grilled, 245 g	495	19	35	2	43
Honey Mustard Dipping, 28 g	129	12	6	0	0
Popcorn Chicken - Large, 184 g	531	26	39	3	35
• Popcorn Chicken - Regular, 126 g	365	18	27	2	24
Popcorn Chicken Shakers™, 240 g	585	27	51	3	36
Arby's® Roast Beef Sandwiches & Melts					
Arby's Melt, 146 g	302	12	36	2	16

Arby's (cont.)

	Cal	Fat	Cbs	Fbr	Prtn
Arby's® Roast Beef Sandwiches & Melts (cont.)					
Arby's Sauce, 14 g	15	0	4	0	0
Bacon Beef 'n Cheddar Sandwich, 212 g	521	27	45	2	27
BBQ Bacon 'n Jack 2 for, 169 g	360	16	42	2	19
Beef 'n Cheddar Sandwich, 195 g	445	21	44	2	22
French Dip & Swiss Sandwich, 224 g	473	18	38	3	32
• Ham & Swiss Melt Sandwich, 131 g	268	5	35	1	17
Kids Meal - Jr. Roast Beef Sand, 125 g	272	10	34	2	16
• Large Roast Beef Sandwich, 281 g	547	28	41	3	42
Medium Roast Beef Sandwich, 210 g	415	21	34	2	31
Regular Roast Beef, 154 g	320	14	34	2	21
Sourdough Ham Melt, 165 g	380	13	39	2	19
Sourdough Roast Beef Melt, 166 g	355	14	40	2	18
Super Roast Beef, 198 g	398	19	40	2	21
Swiss Melt, 146 g	303	12	37	2	16
Arby's® Toasted Subs					
Chicken Parmesan Toasted Sub, 317 g	843	38	80	3	47
Classic Italian Toasted Sub, 379 g	828	46	69	3	37
French Dip & Swiss Toasted Sub, 337 g	622	20	68	3	37
• Meatball Toasted Sub, 325 g	1000	62	71	5	43
Philly Beef Toasted Sub, 281 g	739	37	64	3	32
• Turkey Bacon Club Toasted Sub, 341 g	619	18	65	3	42
Breakfast					
Bacon & Egg Croissant, 120 g	337	22	23	1	11
Bacon Biscuit, 95 g	340	21	29	1	9
Bacon, Egg & Cheese Biscuit, 158 g	461	28	30	1	17
Bacon, Egg & Cheese Croissant, 133 g	378	22	23	1	14
Bacon, Egg & Cheese Sourdough, 173 g	437	16	40	2	20
Bacon, Egg, & Cheese Wrap, 193 g	515	29	50	2	16
Biscuit - Plain, 82 g	273	15	28	1	5
Blueberry Muffin, 85 g	320	12	49	1	4
Breakfast Syrup, 28 g	78	0	20	0	0
Chicken Biscuit, 132 g	417	23	39	1	15
Croissant, 57 g	190	10	21	1	3
Egg & Cheese Sourdough, 164 g	392	12	40	2	17
French Toastix, 124 g	312	13	44	1	6
Ham & Cheese Croissant, 113 g	274	12	22	1	13
Ham Biscuit, 132 g	323	17	29	1	14
Ham, Egg & Cheese Biscuit, 195 g	444	24	31	1	21
Ham, Egg & Cheese Croissant, 220 g	441	24	25	1	23
Ham, Egg & Cheese Sourdough, 214 g	442	14	41	2	26
Ham, Egg, & Cheese Wrap, 249 g	575	31	51	2	25
Sausage & Egg Croissant, 147 g	433	32	23	1	12
Sausage Biscuit, 122 g	436	31	28	1	10
• Sausage Gravy Biscuit, 238 g	961	68	107	1	7
• Sausage Patty, 51 g	210	20	0	0	6
Sausage, Egg & Cheese Biscuit, 185 g	557	38	30	1	18
Sausage, Egg & Cheese Croissant, 160 g	475	32	23	1	15
Sausage, Egg & Cheese Sourdough, 204 g	556	28	40	2	22
Sausage, Egg & Cheese Wrap, 239 g	689	45	50	2	21
Kids Menu					
Fruit Cup, 57 g	35	0	9	1	0
Junior Roast Beef Sandwich, 125 g	272	10	34	2	16
Market Fresh™ Mini Tkey & Chz Sandwich, 119 g	244	5	28	2	19

RESTAURANTS & FAST-FOOD CHAINS

Arby's (cont.)

	Cal	Fat	Cbs	Fbr	Prtn
Kids Menu (cont.)					
Market Fresh™ Mini Ham & Chz Sandwich, 119 g	235	5	28	2	15
Popcorn Chicken, 95 g	274	13	20	1	18
Market Fresh™ Salads					
Buttermilk Ranch Dressing, 64 g	325	34	4	0	1
Chicken Club Salad, 345 g	426	23	26	4	28
Garlic & Cheese Croutons, 14 g	77	5	7	0	2
Light Buttermilk Ranch Dressing, 64 g	112	6	13	1	1
Martha's Vineyard Salad™, 330 g	277	8	24	4	26
Raspberry Vinaigrette, 64 g	194	14	18	0	0
Santa Fe Ranch Dressing, 64 g	296	31	4	0	1
Santa Fe Salad™ w/ Grilled Chkn, 350 g	283	9	21	6	29
Santa Fe Salad™, 344 g	416	18	37	6	25
Seasoned Tortilla Strips, 14 g	71	3	9	1	1
Sliced Almonds, 14 g	81	8	2	1	4
Market Fresh™ Sandwiches & Wraps					
Corned Beef Reuben Sandwich, 295 g	590	32	55	3	32
Corned Beef Reuben Wrap, 266 g	560	29	42	1	36
Fish Sandwich, 210 g	535	25	59	2	21
Pecan Chicken Salad Sandwich, 322 g	769	39	79	9	30
Pecan Chicken Salad Wrap, 277 g	638	38	48	8	30
Roast Beef & Swiss Sandwich, 339 g	777	41	73	5	37
Roast Ham & Swiss Sandwich, 345 g	691	31	75	5	33
Roast Tkey Ranch & Bacon Sand, 367 g	818	38	75	5	46
Roast Turkey & Swiss Sandwich, 345 g	708	30	74	5	41
Roast Turkey Ranch & Bacon Wrap, 302 g	683	37	44	4	45
Roast Turkey Reuben Sandwich, 295 g	594	30	56	3	40
Roast Turkey Reuben Wrap, 266 g	564	27	43	1	44
Southwest Chicken Wrap, 254 g	567	29	42	4	36
Spicy Cajun Fish Sandwich, 217 g	595	32	59	3	21
Ultimate BLT Sandwich, 294 g	779	45	75	6	23
Ultimate BLT Wrap, 249 g	648	44	45	5	23
Shakes & Desserts					
Apple Turnover, 128 g	377	16	65	2	4
Cheesecake Poppers, 69 g	270	15	30	1	4
Cherry Turnover, 128 g	377	15	65	2	4
Chocolate Chip Cookie, 45 g	202	10	26	1	2
Chocolate Shake - Regular, 397 g	507	13	83	0	13
Jamocha Shake - Regular, 397 g	498	13	81	0	13
Raspberry Dipping Sauce, 28 g	60	0	14	0	0
Strawberry Banana Swirl Shake, 482 g	567	16	87	0	15
Strawberry Shake - Regular, 397 g	498	13	81	0	13
Vanilla Shake - Regular, 369 g	437	13	66	0	13
Sides & Sidekickers®					
Bronco Berry Dipping Sauce®, 57 g	122	0	30	0	0
Cheddar Cheese Sauce - side, 21 g	30	2	2	0	0
Cheddar Fries - Medium, 170 g	465	28	51	5	6
Chile Lime Ranch Dipping Sauce, 43 g	190	19	2	0	0
Cool Ranch Sour Crm Dipping Sauce, 43 g	158	16	2	0	1
Curly Fries - Medium, 125 g	397	24	46	4	5
Homestyle Fries - Medium, 142 g	377	25	55	4	4
Jalapeño Bites® - Regular (5), 110 g	305	21	29	2	5
Ketchup Packet, 14 g	13	0	3	0	0

Arby's (cont.)

Sides & Sidekickers® (cont.)	Cal	Fat	Cbs	Fbr	Prtn
Loaded Potato Bites® Regular (5), 112 g	353	22	27	2	11
Marinara Sauce, 43 g	30	2	4	1	1
Mozzarella Sticks - Regular (4), 137 g	426	28	38	2	18
Onion Petals - Regular, 113 g	331	23	35	2	4
Potato Cakes (2), 100 g	246	18	26	2	2
SW Egg rolls - Small (4 pieces), 90 g	225	7	29	3	11
Tangy Southwest Sauce®, 57 g	333	35	5	0	1
T.J. Cinnamons®					
• Chocolate Twist, 71 g	250	12	34	2	4
Cinnamon Twist, 71 g	260	14	33	1	3
Original Gourmet Cinnamon Roll®, 149 g	507	10	73	4	10
Pecan Sticky Bun 4 Pack, 738 g	2751	90	363	21	47
• Pecan Sticky Bun, 184 g	688	22	91	5	12
T.J. Cinnamons Mocha Chill®, 354 g	306	7	48	1	11
T.J. Icing, 28 g	117	5	18	0	1

Atlanta Bread Company

Baked Goods: Bagels	Cal	Fat	Cbs	Fbr	Prtn
Apple Spice, 4 oz.	360	3	73	3	11
• Asiago Cheese, 4 oz.	380	10	53	2	18
Blueberry, 4 oz.	270	1	55	2	10
Cinnamon Crisp, 4 oz.	330	3	68	4	11
Cinnamon Raisin, 4 oz.	270	1	56	3	10
Everything, 9 oz.	320	4	60	4	12
• Lower Carb Cranberry Walnut, 2 oz.	110	4	16	6	9
Onion, 4 oz.	290	1	59	3	11
Plain, 3 oz.	270	1	55	2	10
Poppy Seed, 4 oz.	320	5	57	3	12
Sesame, 4 oz.	360	9	57	4	14
Wheat, 4 oz.	270	2	54	4	10
Baked Goods: Breads					
ABC Roll, 4 oz.	260	1	54	3	10
Asiago Loaf, 2 oz.	160	2	29	1	7
Asiago Strip, 2 oz.	160	2	28	1	6
Challah, 2 oz.	160	3	29	0	6
Cinnamon Raisin Loaf, 2 oz.	150	2	28	1	5
Cracked Wheat, 2 oz.	160	2	30	2	6
Foccacia Round, Asiago, 2 oz.	180	5	26	1	7
Foccacia Round, Basil Pesto, 2 oz.	190	8	26	1	5
Foccacia Round, Tomato Onion, 2 oz.	150	3	27	1	5
Foccacia, Rosemary Tomato, 3 oz.	350	12	50	4	11
French Baguette, 2 oz.	140	1	30	1	5
French Loaf, 2 oz.	140	1	28	1	5
French Roll, 2 oz.	160	1	33	2	6
Honey Wheat, 2 oz.	150	2	28	2	5
Lower Carb Multigrain Bread, 2 oz.	100	2	16	6	11
Nine Grain, 2 oz.	160	3	28	2	6
Pumpernickel, 2 oz.	140	2	26	2	6
Rye, 2 oz.	150	2	28	3	6
• Sourdough Baguette, 2 oz.	140	0	29	1	5
• Sourdough Bread Bowl, 7 oz.	550	2	113	5	20
Sourdough Loaf, 2 oz.	140	0	29	1	5
Sourdough Roll, 2 oz.	160	0	34	1	6

RESTAURANTS & FAST-FOOD CHAINS

Atlanta Bread Company (cont.)

	Cal	Fat	Cbs	Fbr	Prtn
Baked Goods: Cream Cheese Spreads					
Garden Vegetable Cream Cheese, 2 oz.	170	17	4	0	4
Onion & Chive Cream Cheese, 2 oz.	190	17	4	0	4
• Plain Cream Cheese, 2 oz.	190	19	1	0	4
• Plain Cream Cheese, Light, 2 oz.	120	10	6	0	4
Strawberry Cream Cheese, 2 oz.	190	15	12	0	4
Beverages: Cold					
• Caramel Latte Caffechillo, 19 oz.	250	10	32	1	8
• Frozen Spiced Chai Tea, 16 oz.	260	6	43	1	8
Kona Mocha Caffechillo, 19 oz.	250	10	32	1	8
Vanilla Caffechillo, 19 oz.	250	10	32	1	8
Beverages: Hot					
Café Latte, tall, 16 oz.	170	6	18	0	10
Café Mocha, tall, 16 oz.	340	8	57	0	8
• Cappuccino, tall, 16 oz.	130	5	14	0	8
Caramel Macchiato, tall, 16 oz.	390	8	69	0	8
Espresso, single shot, 2 oz.	5	0	1	0	0
• Hot Chocolate, tall, 16 oz.	450	10	78	0	11
Hot Spiced Chai Tea, 15 oz.	260	6	43	1	8
House Latte, tall, 16 oz.	380	10	65	1	10
Beverages: Smoothies					
• Pineapple Mango Banana, 16 oz.	290	0	72	4	1
Strawberry Banana, 16 oz.	290	0	71	5	2
• Strawberry Blueberry Banana, 16 oz.	280	0	69	5	1
Breakfast: Gourmet Breakfast					
Belgian Waffle w/ syrup, 7 oz.	480	13	82	1	7
Belgian Waffle w/o syrup, 5 oz.	320	13	41	1	7
• French Toast w/ syrup, 9 oz.	560	9	103	3	16
French Toast w/o syrup, 7 oz.	400	9	61	3	16
• Scrambled eggs, 5 oz.	220	16	2	0	16
Breakfast: Hot Sandwiches					
Bacon, Egg & Cheese on Croissant, 5 oz.	530	34	39	1	16
• Egg & Cheese on Croissant, 5 oz.	480	30	39	1	14
Ham, Egg & Cheese on Croissant, 7 oz.	540	31	41	1	24
Sausage, Egg & Cheese on Croissant, 7 oz.	690	48	39	1	25
Breakfast: Omelets					
Florentine, 8 oz.	350	24	6	1	26
• Greek, 8 oz.	290	20	5	0	21
• Ham and Swiss, 8 oz.	390	26	4	0	33
Spanish, 8 oz.	350	24	6	1	25
Tomato Bacon, 8 oz.	370	27	4	1	27
Breakfast: Side Orders					
Bacon (3 slices), 1 oz.	80	7	0	0	4
Breakfast Potatoes, 4 oz.	170	9	20	4	3
• Ham, 2 oz.	60	2	2	0	9
• Sausage (2 patties), 3 oz.	310	27	1	0	17
Pastas					
Asiago Cream, 14 oz.	860	51	63	3	28
• Basil Pesto, 14 oz.	940	53	69	4	46
Chicken Parmesan, 15 oz.	780	27	75	3	57
• Kid's Pasta, 9 oz.	410	12	56	2	18
Pasta Puttanesca, 14 oz.	590	21	63	4	36
Penne Pomodoro Pasta, 18 oz.	920	44	66	4	50

Atlanta Bread Company (cont.)	Cal	Fat	Cbs	Fbr	Prtn
Pastries & Sweets: Cheesecakes					
• Carrot Cake Cheesecake, 1 slice	680	49	53	2	10
Chocolate Truffle Cheesecake, 1 slice	640	40	63	1	9
Oreo Cheesecake, 1 slice	630	39	60	1	10
Pecan Turtle Cheesecake, 1 slice	640	42	56	2	9
Plain Cheesecake, 1 slice	570	36	42	1	10
• Pumpkin Praline Cheesecake, 1 slice	510	31	50	2	8
Snickers Cheesecake, 1 slice	620	40	54	2	12
Pastries & Sweets: Cookies					
Chocolate Chunk, 3 oz.	400	19	51	2	3
• Chocolate Dipped Peanut, 4 oz.	530	30	52	2	10
Chocolate Dipped Shortbread, 4 oz.	440	23	55	2	4
• Oatmeal Raisin, 3 oz.	360	15	50	3	5
Peanut Butter, 3 oz.	430	24	42	1	9
Shortbread, 3 oz.	370	18	47	1	3
Toffee Chocolate Chunk, 3 oz.	400	21	49	2	4
White Macadamia, 3 oz.	410	22	49	1	5
Pastries & Sweets: Croissants					
• Almond Croissant, 6 oz.	660	38	67	4	13
Apple Croissant, 5 oz.	430	17	65	2	6
Cheese Croissant, 6 oz.	510	29	56	1	8
Chocolate Croissant, 4 oz.	520	27	61	3	8
• Plain Croissant, 3 oz.	360	20	39	1	7
Raspberry Cheese Croissant, 5 oz.	440	19	63	1	6
Pastries & Sweets: Danish					
Apple, 4 oz.	450	18	66	2	6
Cheese, 4 oz.	480	22	65	1	7
• Gooey Butter, 4 oz.	550	25	73	2	8
• Raspberry, 4 oz.	430	18	62	1	6
Pastries & Sweets: Muffins and Tops					
Banana Nut Muffin Top, 3 oz.	420	26	39	2	8
Banana Nut Muffin, 5 oz.	560	33	57	2	10
• Blueberry Muffin Top, 2 oz.	250	12	31	1	4
Blueberry Muffin, 4 oz.	430	21	54	1	7
Bran Raisin Muffin, 4 oz.	410	18	55	5	6
Chocolate Chip Muffin Top, 3 oz.	400	19	52	2	6
Chocolate Chip Muffin, 5 oz.	560	27	73	3	8
Cranberry Apple Muffin, 5 oz.	490	23	64	2	8
• Cranberry Orange Muffin, 5 oz.	560	34	55	3	10
Low Fat Apple Muffin, 4 oz.	340	5	66	2	6
Low Fat Pumpkin Muffin, 4 oz.	320	5	65	2	6
Mocha Muffin Top, 3 oz.	410	20	53	3	6
Mocha Muffin, 5 oz.	560	27	73	3	9
Pumpkin Muffin Top, 3 oz.	350	13	54	2	5
Pumpkin Muffin, 5 oz.	470	18	73	2	7
Pastries & Sweets: Scones					
Cinnamon Scone, 4 oz.	350	11	57	2	6
Raspberry Scone, 4 oz.	360	13	56	2	6
Pastries & Sweets: Other					
Austrian Pretzel, 4 oz.	550	34	55	2	7
Banana Nut Bread, 2 oz.	230	14	24	1	4
Bear Claw, 6 oz.	540	24	73	3	9
• Boston Cream Pound Cake, 2 oz.	200	12	21	0	3
Cinnamon Roll, 5 oz.	630	26	91	2	9

(•= most healthy •= least healthy)

RESTAURANTS & FAST-FOOD CHAINS

Atlanta Bread Company (cont.)

	Cal	Fat	Cbs	Fbr	Prtn
Pastries & Sweets: Other (cont.)					
Cranberry Orange Bread, 2 oz.	240	14	24	1	4
Key Lime Pie, 3 oz.	450	13	52	0	6
Lower Carb Chocolate Cake, 2 oz.	200	15	17	5	3
Marble Pound Cake, 2 oz.	230	15	22	1	4
• Pecan Roll, 6 oz.	860	60	72	4	11
Pumpkin Bread, 2 oz.	210	8	33	1	3
Sticky Bun, 5 oz.	560	30	66	2	6
Walnut Brownies, 4 oz.	490	24	63	3	7
Pizzas					
BBQ Chicken, 1/2 pizza	320	5	53	2	17
• Cheese (Kid's), 1/2 pizza	300	7	44	3	14
• Four Cheese, 1/2 pizza	530	23	46	3	35
Pepperoni, 1/2 pizza	340	10	44	3	18
White Pizza, 1/2 pizza	460	22	47	3	20
Salad Dressings					
• Balsamic Vinaigrette Dressing, 2 tbsp.	150	16	1	0	0
Bleu Cheese Dressing, 2 tbsp.	120	12	2	0	1
Caesar Dressing, 2 tbsp.	150	15	3	0	1
• Fat-Free Raspberry Vinaigrette, 2 tbsp.	35	0	8	0	0
Greek Dressing, 2 tbsp.	100	10	1	0	1
Honey Mustard Dressing, 2 tbsp.	130	12	6	0	0
Ranch Dressing, 2 tbsp.	130	13	2	0	1
Sesame Ginger Dressing, 2 tbsp.	130	11	8	0	0
Thousand Island Dressing, 2 tbsp.	120	11	5	0	0
Salads (w/o dressing)					
Add Grilled Chicken, 3 oz.	70	2	2	0	12
Balsamic Bleu Salad, 10 oz.	330	18	35	5	10
Caesar Salad, 8 oz.	190	10	11	2	14
Chicken Salad on Lettuce, 4 oz.	280	21	2	0	25
Chopstix Chicken Salad, 13 oz.	280	13	24	5	19
Extra Croutons, 1 oz.	50	2	6	0	1
Fruit Salad, 10 oz.	130	0	34	3	2
Greek Salad, 12 oz.	200	13	13	3	9
• House, 10 oz.	50	0	11	3	3
• Tuna Salad on Lettuce, 4 oz.	360	32	4	0	16
Sandwiches					
• Chicken Salad (Scoop), 4 oz.	280	21	2	0	25
Chicken Salad on Sourdough, 10 oz.	540	19	62	3	32
Grilled Cheese on French Bread, 5 oz.	390	11	57	3	17
Honey Maple Ham on Honey Wheat, 10 oz.	410	5	63	5	27
w/ Cheese and Mayo, 11 oz.	620	26	64	5	34
w/ Mayo, 10 oz.	520	17	64	5	27
w/ Cheddar Cheese, 11 oz.	520	15	63	5	34
Peanut Butter & Jelly on Fren Bread, 7 oz.	600	14	99	6	17
Roasted Turkey Breast on 9 Grain, 10 oz.	430	7	61	5	32
• w/ Cheese and Mayo, 11 oz.	630	26	62	5	38
w/ Cheese, 11 oz.	530	15	61	5	38
w/ Mayo, 10 oz.	530	18	62	5	32
Tuna Salad (Scoop), 4 oz.	360	32	4	0	16
Tuna Salad on French Bread, 10 oz.	610	29	62	4	27
Veggie Sandwich on Nine Grain, 9 oz.	340	5	63	6	13
w/ Cheese and Dill Sauce, 11 oz.	500	19	63	6	20
w/ Dill Sauce, 10 oz.	401	11	63	6	14

Atlanta Bread Company (cont.)

	Cal	Fat	Cbs	Fbr	Prtn
Sandwiches: Paninis (Full)					
• Chicken Pesto, 12 oz.	800	35	83	5	38
Cordon Bleu, 10 oz.	660	18	82	4	40
Cuban Pork Loin, 10 oz.	660	19	81	4	40
• Italian Vegetarian, 12 oz.	640	16	93	5	26
Turkey Club, 12 oz.	750	27	83	4	42
Soups					
Black Bean and Ham, 10 oz.	250	9	40	20	19
Chicken Tortilla, 10 oz.	190	9	20	0	8
Chunky Baked Potato, 10 oz.	290	16	30	1	5
Classic Chicken Noodle, 10 oz.	140	3	21	1	7
Cream of Broccoli, 10 oz.	200	11	19	0	6
Creamy Tomato, 10 oz.	130	9	10	1	3
French Onion with Toppings, 10 oz.	200	10	16	0	9
• French Onion, 10 oz.	80	3	10	0	3
Garden Vegetable, 10 oz.	100	2	19	4	3
• Homestyle Chicken and Dumpling, 10 oz.	290	18	25	0	8
New England Clam Chowder, 10 oz.	280	16	24	0	8
Pasta Fagioli, 10 oz.	170	6	24	1	6
Spicy Chicken Gumbo, 10 oz.	120	3	16	2	8
Wisconsin Cheese, 10 oz.	240	14	21	0	9
Soups: Chili					
Frontier Chicken Chili, 10 oz.	270	10	26	2	20
Hearty Beef Chili, 10 oz.	350	15	33	3	21
Specialty Sandwiches					
ABC Special on French Roll, 12 oz.	420	5	61	4	35
w/ Cheese and Mayo, 14 oz.	680	28	62	4	45
w/ Cheese, 14 oz.	570	16	61	4	45
w/ Mayo, 13 oz.	530	16	62	4	35
Bella Basil on Tom & Rosemary Focaccia, 10 oz.	660	35	58	5	29
w/ Cheese, 11 oz.	760	44	58	5	35
California Avocado on Tom Onion Focaccia, 12 oz.	690	40	71	14	14
w/ Cheese, 14 oz.	790	48	71	13	21
Hot Pastrami, 8 oz.	460	10	59	6	31
w/ Swiss Cheese, 9 oz.	570	18	59	6	39
• Tangy Roast Beef, 10 oz.	390	4	56	3	32
w/ Horseradish Cheddar & Mayo, 12 oz.	790	39	60	3	50
w/ Horseradish Cheddar, 12 oz.	690	28	59	3	50

Au Bon Pain

	Cal	Fat	Cbs	Fbr	Prtn
Bakery: Bagels					
Asiago Cheese Bagel, 4 oz.	340	6	55	0	15
• Cinnamon Crisp Bagel, 4 oz.	410	7	76	2	10
Cinnamon Raisin Bagel, 4 oz.	310	1	66	1	11
Everything Bagel, 4 oz.	340	5	62	1	13
Honey 9 Grain Bagel, 5 oz.	360	4	71	4	13
Jalapeño Double Cheddar Bagel, 5 oz.	340	10	52	0	17
Onion Dill Bagel, 4 oz.	290	1	58	1	11
• Plain Bagel, 4 oz.	280	1	57	0	11
Poppy Bagel, 4 oz.	320	4	58	1	12
Sesame Seed Bagel, 4 oz.	320	4	58	1	12
Bakery: Cookies & Desserts					
Banana Nut Pound Cake, 5 oz.	520	28	60	1	7
Blondie, 4 oz.	330	19	61	3	7

(•= most healthy •= least healthy)

RESTAURANTS & FAST-FOOD CHAINS

Au Bon Pain (cont.)

	Cal	Fat	Cbs	Fbr	Prtn
Bakery: Cookies & Desserts (cont.)					
Blueberry Tulip, 3 oz.	370	20	44	1	4
Cappuccino Poundcake, 5 oz.	530	26	68	1	3
Chocolate Bundt Cake, 4 oz.	440	21	61	1	3
Chocolate Cheesecake Brownie, 4 oz.	370	14	58	1	5
Chocolate Chip Brownie, 4 oz.	380	17	62	1	5
Chocolate Chip Cookie, 2 oz.	260	12	37	1	2
Choco Dipped Cranberry Almond Macaroon, 3 oz.	320	16	42	3	4
Chocolate Dipped Shortbread, 3 oz.	350	20	38	1	3
Chocolate Pound Cake, 134 g	500	29	58	3	7
Chocolate Raspberry Tulip, 4 oz.	430	21	55	1	5
Confetti Cookie With M&M's, 2 oz.	310	14	42	1	3
Crème De Fleur, 5 oz.	490	25	57	2	11
Crumb Cake, 4 oz.	470	25	56	1	5
English Toffee Cookie, 2 oz.	210	11	26	1	2
Gingerbread Cookie, 3 oz.	300	9	50	1	4
• Hazelnut Creme Pastry, 5 oz.	540	34	50	3	10
Hazelnut Dream Cookie, 3 oz.	390	24	41	2	4
Hazelnut Fudge Cookie, 2 oz.	290	16	34	3	4
Hazelnut Mocha Brownie, 4 oz.	430	21	58	3	6
Hazelnut Monkey Bread, 4 oz.	510	28	57	2	8
Holiday Tree Cookie, 2 oz.	170	5	31	0	2
Iced Cinnamon Roll, 4 oz.	400	15	60	2	8
Key Lime Sugar Cookie, 2 oz.	250	9	39	1	3
Key Lime Tulip, 4 oz.	440	22	55	1	5
Lemon Pound Cake, 139 g	520	27	64	0	5
Marble Pound Cake, 134 g	490	27	59	1	6
Mini Chocolate Chip Cookie, 1 oz.	70	3	9	0	1
• Mini Oatmeal Raisin Cookie, 1 oz.	60	2	9	1	1
Mint Chocolate Pound Cake, 5 oz.	530	28	65	3	7
Oatmeal Raisin Cookie, 2 oz.	230	8	36	2	3
Palmier, 4 oz.	440	23	53	1	1
Pecan Roll, 6 oz.	630	32	80	3	10
Rocky Road Brownie, 4 oz.	410	17	62	2	6
Shortbread Cookie, 4 oz.	310	18	34	1	3
Wh Choc Chunk Macadamia Nut Cookie, 2 oz.	280	15	34	1	3
Bakery: Croissants					
• Almond Croissant, 5 oz.	600	38	55	4	13
• Apple Croissant, 4 oz.	270	11	44	3	5
Chocolate Croissant, 4 oz.	430	22	58	3	7
Ham And Cheese Croissant, 4 oz.	400	20	38	2	16
Plain Croissant, 3 oz.	300	17	31	1	6
Raspberry Cheese Croissant, 4 oz.	320	15	41	2	7
Spinach And Cheese Croissant, 4 oz.	290	16	28	2	10
Sweet Cheese Croissant, 4 oz.	380	19	48	2	9
Bakery: Danish					
Cherry Danish, 4 oz.	420	20	54	2	7
Lemon Danish, 4 oz.	440	20	57	2	7
Bakery: Kids					
All Natural Grilled Chicken Sandwich, 7 oz.	490	14	59	2	24
• Chicken Nuggets, 3 oz.	180	7	14	0	14
• Grilled Cheese, 7 oz.	670	41	55	2	20
Kid's Buttered Penne Pasta, 4 oz.	260	12	31	1	6
Macaroni And Cheese, 6 oz.	220	14	15	0	9

Au Bon Pain (cont.)	Cal	Fat	Cbs	Fbr	Prtn
Bakery: Kids (cont.)					
Smoked Turkey Sandwich, 7 oz.	450	13	59	2	21
Bakery: Muffins					
Blueberry Muffin, 6 oz.	510	19	76	5	9
Carrot Walnut Muffin, 6 oz.	520	25	66	4	8
Corn Muffin, 6 oz.	460	16	69	2	9
Cranberry Walnut Muffin, 6 oz.	500	24	61	5	10
• Double Chocolate Chunk Muffin, 5 oz.	590	20	83	5	10
• Low-fat Triple Berry Muffin, 4 oz.	290	2	61	2	5
Mushroom, Gorgonzola & Rd Pepper Muffin, 5 oz.	490	28	50	1	8
Pumpkin Muffin, 6 oz.	490	17	75	2	9
Raisin Bran Muffin, 6 oz.	410	9	74	9	10
Southwest Jalapeño Muffin, 5 oz.	560	30	64	1	8
Bakery: Scones					
Cinnamon Scone, 4 oz.	530	27	60	2	9
Orange Scone, 4 oz.	470	23	57	1	10
Bakery: Strudel					
Apple Strudel, 4 oz.	430	24	48	1	5
Cherry Strudel, 5 oz.	460	26	49	2	5
Beverages: Blasts & Smoothies					
Banana Wildberry Smoothie Lg., 24 fl.oz.	530	8	119	11	3
Banana Wildberry Smoothie Medium, 16 fl.oz.	340	7	72	6	1
Caramel Blast Large, 24 fl.oz.	760	21	151	0	8
Caramel Blast Medium, 16 fl.oz.	540	17	104	0	6
Coffee Blast Large, 24 fl.oz.	690	29	119	0	11
Coffee Blast Medium, 16 fl.oz.	440	21	71	0	8
Mocha Blast Large, 24 fl.oz.	690	22	137	3	10
Mocha Blast Medium, 16 fl.oz.	440	17	80	2	7
Peach Smoothie Large, 24 fl.oz.	470	1	104	7	7
Peach Smoothie Medium, 16 fl.oz.	310	1	69	4	4
Strawberry Smoothie Large, 24 fl.oz.	470	1	100	4	7
• Strawberry Smoothie Medium, 16 fl.oz.	310	1	66	3	4
• Vanilla Blast Large, 24 fl.oz.	760	21	152	0	8
Vanilla Blast Medium, 16 fl.oz.	540	17	104	0	6
Wildberry Smoothie Large, 24 fl.oz.	530	8	104	4	7
Wildberry Smoothie Medium, 16 fl.oz.	380	7	71	3	4
Beverages: Coffee & Espresso					
• Caffe Americano Medium, 16 fl.oz.	10	0	2	0	0
Caffe Latte Medium, 16 fl.oz.	260	14	21	0	14
Cappuccino Medium, 16 fl.oz.	150	8	13	0	8
• Caramel Macchiato Medium, 16 fl.oz.	430	12	68	0	12
Chai Latte Medium, 16 fl.oz.	380	14	51	0	14
Iced Caffe Latte Medium, 16 fl.oz.	150	8	13	0	8
Iced Caramel Macchiato Med, 16 fl.oz.	390	10	65	0	10
Iced Chai Latte Medium, 16 fl.oz.	260	7	42	0	7
Iced Decaf French Roast Coffee Medium, 22 fl.oz.	10	0	2	0	0
Iced French Roast Coffee Med, 22 fl.oz.	10	0	2	0	0
Iced French Vanilla Coffee Med, 22 fl.oz.	10	0	2	0	1
Iced Mocha Latte Medium, 16 fl.oz.	300	15	40	2	9
Iced Vanilla Latte Medium, 16 fl.oz.	330	7	59	0	7
Iced White Chocolate Latte Medium, 16 fl.oz.	330	13	51	0	6
Mocha Latte Medium, 16 fl.oz.	390	20	48	2	13
Vanilla Latte Medium, 16 fl.oz.	410	12	66	0	12
White Chocolate Latte Medium, 16 fl.oz.	410	17	58	0	11

RESTAURANTS & FAST-FOOD CHAINS

▶ Au Bon Pain (cont.)

	Cal	Fat	Cbs	Fbr	Prtn
Breads					
Artisan Baguette Salad Size, 3 oz.	240	2	47	2	8
Artisan Baguette Sandwich Size, 4 oz.	310	2	62	3	10
Artisan Hny Multigrain Baguette Salad Size, 4 oz.	250	3	49	5	8
Artisan Hny Multigrain Baguette Sand Size, 5 oz.	340	4	66	6	11
Artisan Multigrain Bread, 4 oz.	280	3	53	5	10
Artisan Sundried Tomato Bread, 4 oz.	270	1	55	3	9
Asiago Breadstick, 2 oz.	180	4	28	0	8
Bacon And Cheese Mini Loaf, 5 oz.	570	33	52	1	15
Basil Pesto Cheese Toasts, 55 g	140	2	26	1	5
• Bread Bowl, 9 oz.	620	3	121	6	26
• Cheddar Jalapeño Breadstick, 2 oz.	130	2	25	0	6
Cheese Bread, 5 oz.	300	8	57	3	15
Ciabatta Small, 3 oz.	180	1	37	2	6
Cinnamon Raisin Breadstick, 2 oz.	180	0	40	1	6
Country White Bread, 4 oz.	270	1	56	2	9
Everything Breadstick, 2 oz.	170	3	31	0	7
Farm House Rolls, 5 oz.	320	6	57	3	10
Focaccia, 5 oz.	350	7	61	1	12
Lahvash, 4 oz.	280	4	56	4	9
Rosemary Garlic Bread Stick, 2 oz.	180	5	30	1	6
Sesame Breadstick, 2 oz.	180	4	30	1	7
Soft Roll, 5 oz.	410	11	65	2	12
Breakfast Sandwiches					
• Bacon And Bagel, 4 oz.	340	6	57	0	16
Bacon And Egg Melt On Ciabatta, 8 oz.	500	26	40	2	26
Breakfast Quesadilla Sandwich, 8 oz.	550	24	56	5	27
Egg On A Bagel With Bacon And Cheese, 8 oz.	500	15	59	0	30
Egg On A Bagel With Bacon, 7 oz.	420	8	60	0	25
Egg On A Bagel With Cheese, 8 oz.	430	10	58	0	25
Egg On A Bagel, 7 oz.	360	4	59	0	21
Mediterranean Spinach Breakfast Sandwich, 8 oz.	520	15	19	7	20
Portobello, Egg And Cheddar, 8 oz.	490	26	41	3	22
Prosciutto & Egg On Asiago Bagel, 9 oz.	530	17	59	1	34
• Sausage, Egg & Cheddar On Asiago Bagel, 10 oz.	810	47	58	1	38
Smoked Salmon & Wasabi On Onion Dill Bgl, 7 oz.	430	11	64	1	23
Breakfast: Café Sandwiches					
Arizona Chicken Sandwich, 12 oz.	750	29	61	4	49
Baja Turkey Sandwich, 13 oz.	640	24	63	4	43
Caprese Sandwich, 12 oz.	700	35	65	4	28
Chicken Pesto Sandwich, 13 oz.	720	26	62	2	44
Chicken Tarragon Sandwich, 11 oz.	740	31	61	1	39
• Chilean Chicken Sandwich, 14 oz.	790	29	64	6	51
Ham & Cheddar Sandwich (On Ciabatta), 12 oz.	650	20	80	4	40
Mozzarella Chicken Sandwich, 14 oz.	750	25	67	2	50
Portobello And Goat Cheese Sandwich, 10 oz.	560	26	61	6	18
Prosciutto Mozzarella Sandwich, 12 oz.	770	41	64	4	39
Roast Beef Caesar Sandwich, 10 oz.	680	27	65	3	40
Smoked Turkey Club Sandwich, 12 oz.	780	43	56	2	43
• Spicy Tuna Sandwich, 10 oz.	500	18	59	6	30
The Montana, 13 oz.	560	23	62	4	40
Turkey And Cranberry Chutney Sandwich, 11 oz.	530	10	77	4	30
Turkey And Swiss Sandwich (On Baguette), 12 oz.	650	24	66	3	41

Au Bon Pain (cont.)

	Cal	Fat	Cbs	Fbr	Prtn
Breakfast: Hot Sandwiches and Melts					
• BBQ Chicken On Farmhouse Roll, 14 oz.	860	31	78	4	50
Cajun Shrimp Hot Wrap, 15 oz.	660	20	95	5	20
Eggplant & Mozzarella Sandwich, 12 oz.	670	31	70	6	26
• Mayan Chicken Hot Wrap, 14 oz.	590	15	92	6	24
Steak Teriyaki Hot Wrap, 14 oz.	620	15	96	5	26
Steakhouse On Ciabatta, 13 oz.	720	31	71	4	43
Tuna Melt, 13 oz.	670	30	62	5	40
Turkey Melt, 12 oz.	780	34	73	3	45
Breakfast: Wraps					
Cajun Shrimp Hot Wrap, 15 oz.	660	20	95	5	20
Chicken Caesar Asiago Wrap, 11 oz.	660	28	62	5	36
Chopped Turkey Cobb Wrap, 12 oz.	620	31	63	6	29
Fields And Feta Wrap, 13 oz.	500	21	67	6	17
Mayan Chicken Hot Wrap, 14 oz.	590	15	92	6	24
• Mediterranean Wrap, 13 oz.	360	31	73	8	18
• Southwest Tuna Wrap, 14 oz.	760	42	65	7	40
Steak Teriyaki Hot Wrap, 14 oz.	620	15	96	5	26
Thai Peanut Chicken Wrap, 13 oz.	620	22	76	6	32
Turkey Spinach Sonoma Wrap, 12 oz.	530	13	83	7	26
Dressings					
Balsamic Vinaigrette Dressing, 2 oz.	190	16	11	0	0
Blue Cheese Dressing, 2 oz.	230	24	2	0	2
Caesar Dressing, 2 oz.	280	28	4	0	2
• Fat Free Raspberry Vinaigrette (Low Fat), 2 oz.	70	0	17	0	0
• Hazelnut Vinaigrette Dressing, 2 oz.	330	31	10	1	2
Light Olive Oil Vinaigrette, 2 oz.	130	10	9	0	0
Light Ranch Dressing, 2 oz.	150	13	3	0	2
Lite Honey Mustard Dressing, 2 oz.	180	11	21	1	1
Sesame Ginger Dressing, 2 oz.	280	25	13	0	1
Thai Peanut Dressing, 2 oz.	230	13	24	1	5
Harvest Rice Bowls					
Cajun Shrimp, 20 oz.	520	17	69	2	16
Cajun Shrimp w/ Brwn Rice, 20 oz.	560	20	73	5	14
• Mayan Chicken, 19 oz.	490	14	67	4	25
Mayan Chicken w/ Brown Rice, 19 oz.	540	16	71	7	23
Steak Teriyaki, 19 oz.	540	15	76	2	29
• Steak Teriyaki w/ Brown Rice, 19 oz.	590	18	80	5	27
Hot Entrées					
Beef Stroganoff, 1 oz.	35	3	2	0	2
Brown Rice, 1 oz.	35	1	6	0	0
Cheese Tortellini Primavera, 13 oz.	580	30	54	4	23
Chicken In Burgundy Wine Sauce, 1 oz.	30	1	2	0	2
Chicken Marsala, 1 oz.	30	2	2	0	2
• Chicken Penne Broccoli Alfredo, 17 oz.	700	31	47	5	47
Meat Lasagna, 11 oz.	480	28	29	2	28
Mediterranean Spinach & Chickpea Ragout, 1 oz.	20	0	4	1	1
Penne Marinara w/ Chicken And Vegetables, 1 oz.	30	1	3	1	2
Penne Marinara With Vegetables, 13 oz.	350	11	52	7	15
Penne w/ Chkn & Fire-Rsted Pepper Sauce, 17 oz.	620	19	58	7	42
Quinoa, 1 oz.	25	0	4	1	1
Roasted Carrots, 1 oz.	15	0	3	1	0
Roasted Green Beans With Almonds, 1 oz.	20	1	2	1	1
• Roasted Vegetable Provencal, 1 oz.	15	1	2	1	1

(• = most healthy • = least healthy) **RESTAURANTS & FAST-FOOD • 55**

RESTAURANTS & FAST-FOOD CHAINS

Au Bon Pain (cont.)

	Cal	Fat	Cbs	Fbr	Prtn
Hot Entrées (cont.)					
Salmon Provencal, 1 oz.	20	1	2	0	2
Spinach And Artichoke Lasagna, 12 oz.	410	16	43	5	24
White Bean Cacciatore, 1 oz.	20	1	3	1	1
Oatmeal					
• Oatmeal Large, 16 oz.	270	5	50	7	10
Oatmeal Medium, 12 oz.	210	4	38	5	8
• Oatmeal Small, 9 oz.	150	3	28	4	6
Pizzettas					
• Spinach And Artichoke Pizzetta, 7 oz.	520	27	56	6	13
• Three Cheese Pizzetta, 9 oz.	700	41	55	5	26
Tomato, Mozzarella, Basil Pizzetta, 8 oz.	650	41	53	5	15
Portions					
Apples, Blue Cheese & Cranberries, 5 oz.	200	10	27	3	4
• Asparagus And Almonds, 3 oz.	70	6	5	2	3
BBQ Chicken, 5 oz.	170	2	13	1	17
Brie, Fruit And Crackers, 4 oz.	190	10	17	1	6
Cheddar, Fruit And Crackers, 4 oz.	190	11	17	1	6
Chickpea And Tomato Salad, 6 oz.	100	1	19	6	5
Herb Cheese, Fruit And Crackers, 4 oz.	180	11	19	1	4
Honey Mustard Chicken, 4 oz.	170	2	12	1	17
Hummus And Cucumber, 4 oz.	130	8	10	3	4
Mediterranean Tuna Salad, 4 oz.	120	8	4	1	10
• Mozzarella And Tomato, 5 oz.	200	15	5	1	9
Mozzarella, Olives, Roasted Peppers & Tom., 4 oz.	180	14	4	1	9
Smkd Tkey, Asprgs, Cran Chutney & Grgnzla, 5 oz.	140	5	10	1	15
Thai Peanut Chicken And Snow Peas, 5 oz.	200	7	7	1	19
Salads					
Caesar Asiago Salad (Side), 3 oz.	120	6	11	2	6
Caesar Asiago Salad, 6 oz.	210	12	18	3	11
Chef's Salad, 9 oz.	250	15	8	3	23
Chickpea & Tom Cucumber Salad, 11 oz.	230	12	23	7	11
Garden Salad, 7 oz.	70	2	12	3	4
Green Bean And Beet Salad, 12 oz.	210	8	27	5	8
Grilled Chicken Caesar Asiago, 9 oz.	340	13	19	3	29
• Mandarin Sesame Chicken Salad, 10 oz.	350	18	30	3	21
Mediterranean Chicken Salad, 10 oz.	330	16	12	3	24
Riviera Salad, 10 oz.	260	7	46	5	7
• Side Garden Salad, 4 oz.	50	2	8	2	2
Thai Peanut Chicken Salad, 11 oz.	240	8	19	4	22
Tuna Garden Salad, 11 oz.	250	13	14	4	21
Turkey Medallion Cobb Salad, 11 oz.	340	19	15	4	27
Turkey Spinach Sonoma Salad, 9 oz.	230	11	16	5	19
Snacks					
Assorted Nuts, 4 oz.	730	64	24	10	21
Chocolate Covered Almonds, 2 oz.	220	14	24	2	3
Chocolate Covered Pretzels, 30 g	140	6	20	0	2
• Chocolate Covered Strawberry, 1 oz.	30	2	4	0	0
Chocolate Nonpareils, 1 oz.	190	12	25	3	2
Dark Chocolate Cranberries, 1 oz.	170	9	27	3	1
Fruit Cup Small, 6 oz.	70	0	16	1	1
Fruit Sours, 4 oz.	400	0	105	0	0
Kookaburra Red Licorice, 1 oz.	140	1	30	0	1
Majuka Fruit Trail Mix, 1 oz.	140	7	17	2	2

Au Bon Pain (cont.)	Cal	Fat	Cbs	Fbr	Prtn
Snacks (cont.)					
Maple Roasted Cashews, 4 oz.	650	49	45	4	16
Muesli, 8 oz.	390	8	76	7	11
New Trail Mix, 1 oz.	120	5	20	2	2
Peach Gummies, 1 oz.	150	0	36	0	2
Summit Blend, 4 oz.	500	27	63	7	10
Tamari Almonds, 1 oz.	180	14	5	3	9
• Tamari Roast, 4 oz.	770	61	41	20	28
The 19th Hole Snack Mix, 1 oz.	160	9	15	1	4
Turkish Apricots, 1 oz.	120	0	29	4	1
Walnuts, 4 oz.	740	74	16	8	17
Soups - Medium					
• Baked Stuffed Potato, 12 oz.	350	21	30	2	9
Broccoli Cheddar Soup, 12 oz.	310	21	20	2	11
Carrot Ginger Soup, 12 oz.	130	5	21	3	7
Chicken And Dumpling Soup, 12 oz.	210	7	28	2	11
Chicken Florentine Soup, 12 oz.	240	13	25	1	8
Chicken Gumbo Soup, 12 oz.	200	9	24	2	7
Chicken Noodle Soup (Low Fat), 12 oz.	130	3	20	2	9
Clam Chowder, 12 oz.	320	18	27	1	9
Corn And Green Chili Bisque, 12 oz.	250	14	29	3	5
Corn Chowder Medium, 12 oz.	350	18	40	3	9
Cream Of Chicken & Wild Rice Soup, 12 oz.	260	15	24	1	7
Curried Rice & Lentil Soup (Low Fat), 12 oz.	150	2	30	8	9
French Moroccan Tomato Lentil Soup, 12 oz.	180	2	32	8	10
French Onion Soup, 12 oz.	130	5	19	2	4
• Garden Vegetable Soup (Low Fat), 12 oz.	80	2	14	3	3
Gazpacho, 12 oz.	90	5	12	3	2
Harvest Pumpkin Soup, 12 oz.	190	10	26	2	8
Hearty Cabbage Soup, 12 oz.	110	5	14	3	4
Italian Wedding Soup, 12 oz.	170	7	19	2	8
Jamaican Black Bean Soup, 12 oz.	180	1	45	15	16
Mediterranean Pepper Soup, 12 oz.	100	3	18	5	5
Old Fashioned Tomato Rice, 12 oz.	120	1	24	3	4
Pasta E Fagioli Soup, 12 oz.	240	8	36	9	11
Portuguese Kale Soup, 12 oz.	120	5	15	3	5
Potato Cheese Soup, 12 oz.	250	14	25	2	7
Potato Leek Soup, 12 oz.	300	20	28	2	5
Rd Beans, Italian Sausage & Rice Soup, 12 oz.	200	5	38	16	15
Southern Black-eyed Pea Soup (Low Fat), 12 oz.	180	2	31	12	12
Southwest Tortilla Soup, 12 oz.	200	11	24	4	4
Southwest Vegetable Soup, 12 oz.	100	3	17	3	4
Split Pea With Ham Soup (Low Fat), 12 oz.	210	2	42	15	18
Thai Coconut Curry Soup, 12 oz.	150	7	20	2	3
Tomato Basil Bisque (Reduced Sodium), 12 oz.	210	8	29	5	6
Tomato Cheddar Soup, 12 oz.	240	15	17	2	12
Tomato Florentine Soup (Low Fat), 12 oz.	120	3	19	2	5
Tuscan Vegetable Soup, 12 oz.	170	5	24	3	7
Vegetable Beef Barley Soup (Low Fat), 12 oz.	140	3	21	4	9
Vegetarian Chili (Low Fat, Gluten Free), 12 oz.	230	3	40	11	12
Vegetarian Lentil Soup, 12 oz.	140	2	32	11	10
Vegetarian Minestrone Soup (Low Fat), 12 oz.	120	2	21	4	5
Wild Mushroom Bisque, 12 oz.	190	9	23	2	5

RESTAURANTS & FAST-FOOD CHAINS

Au Bon Pain (cont.)

	Cal	Fat	Cbs	Fbr	Prtn
Stews					
Beef Stew Medium, 12 oz.	300	16	25	3	18
• Chicken Vegetable Stew Medium, 12 oz.	290	17	26	3	11
• Macaroni And Cheese Medium, 12 oz.	440	26	31	2	19
Toppings					
All Natural Chicken Breast, 4 oz.	150	2	2	0	30
Bacon, 1 oz.	80	7	0	0	4
Bagged Croutons, 2 oz.	180	5	29	2	5
Brie Cheese, 2 oz.	150	14	0	0	8
Cheddar Cheese, 2 oz.	160	13	1	0	10
Goat Cheese, 1 oz.	110	9	1	0	6
Gorgonzola Cheese, 2 oz.	210	18	1	0	12
Granola Topping, 2 oz.	220	6	37	3	5
Guacomole, 30 g	60	6	2	2	1
Ham, 4 oz.	100	4	0	0	9
Mozzarella Cheese, 2 oz.	160	9	3	0	16
Prosciutto, 2 oz.	105	6	2	0	13
Provolone Cheese, 2 oz.	140	10	1	0	10
Roast Beef, 4 oz.	150	6	0	0	23
Roasted Red Pepper Hummus, 2 oz.	80	5	6	2	2
• Roasted Red Peppers, 2 oz.	45	4	4	1	1
Sausage Patty, 2 oz.	210	20	0	0	8
Swiss Cheese, 2 oz.	150	12	0	0	11
• Tarragon Mayonnaise Sauce, 2 oz.	420	45	2	0	0
Tuna Salad Mix, 4 oz.	180	12	2	1	18
Turkey Breast, 4 oz.	120	2	4	0	22
Toppings: Dressings					
Balsamic Vinaigrette Dressing, 2 oz.	190	16	11	0	0
Blue Cheese Dressing, 2 oz.	230	24	2	0	2
Caesar Dressing, 2 oz.	280	28	4	0	2
• Fat Free Raspberry Vinaigrette, 2 oz.	70	0	17	0	0
• Hazelnut Vinaigrette Dressing, 2 oz.	330	31	10	1	2
Light Ranch Dressing, 2 oz.	150	15	3	0	2
Lite Honey Mustard Dressing, 2 oz.	180	11	21	1	1
Sesame Ginger Dressing, 2 oz.	280	25	13	0	1
Thai Peanut Dressing, 2 oz.	230	11	24	1	5
Toppings: Spreads					
Artichoke Aioli, 1 oz.	70	7	2	0	1
Basil Pesto, 1 oz.	140	15	1	0	2
Chili Dijon, 1 oz.	120	12	3	1	1
Herb Bagel Spread, 56 oz.	130	11	5	0	4
• Herb Mayonnaise, 1 oz.	210	23	1	0	0
Honey Mustard, 3 oz.	210	13	23	1	1
Honey Pecan Cream Cheese, 2 oz.	120	10	5	0	4
Jalapeño Mayonnaise, 1 oz.	60	6	1	0	2
Lite Cream Cheese Spread, 2 oz.	120	9	5	0	4
Mayonnaise, 1 oz.	90	8	1	0	0
• Mustard, 6 g	0	0	0	0	0
Plain Cream Cheese, 2 oz.	170	16	4	0	3
Strawberry Cream Cheese, 2 oz.	180	15	9	0	3
Sundried Tomato Cream Cheese, 2 oz.	120	10	5	0	4
Sun-dried Tomato Spread, 1 oz.	70	6	4	0	1
Vegetable Cream Cheese, 2 oz.	170	16	3	0	3

Au Bon Pain (cont.)

	Cal	Fat	Cbs	Fbr	Prtn
Yogurt - Small					
• Blueberry Yogurt w/ Granola & Fruit, 9 oz.	310	6	56	2	10
Blueberry Yogurt With Fruit (Low Fat), 8 oz.	220	2	44	0	6
Strawberry Yogurt w/ Granola & Blueberries, 9 oz.	310	6	56	2	10
Strawberry Yogurt w/ Blueberries (Low Fat), 8 oz.	220	2	44	0	6
Vanilla Yogurt w/ Granola & Blueberries, 9 oz.	310	6	56	2	10
• Vanilla Yogurt w/ Blueberries (Low Fat), 8 oz.	190	2	32	0	10

Auntie Anne's

	Cal	Fat	Cbs	Fbr	Prtn
Beverages					
Auntie Anne's Lemonade, 22 fl.oz.	180	0	43	0	0
Auntie Anne's Strawberry Lemonade, 22 fl.oz.	190	0	48	0	0
• Blue raspberry Dutch Ice®, 14 fl.oz.	165	0	38	0	0
Blue raspberry Dutch Smoothie, 14 fl.oz.	230	8	34	0	3
Caramel Dutch latté™, 14 fl.oz.	350	15	49	0	4
Chocolate Dutch Shake, 14 fl.oz.	580	27	75	0	10
Coffee Dutch latté™, 14 fl.oz.	290	14	38	0	4
Coffee Dutch Shake, 14 fl.oz.	590	27	77	0	10
Grape Dutch Ice®, 14 fl.oz.	180	0	43	0	0
Grape Dutch Smoothie, 14 fl.oz.	230	8	36	0	3
Kiwi-Banana Dutch Ice®, 14 fl.oz.	190	0	44	0	0
Kiwi-Banana Dutch Smoothie, 14 fl.oz.	240	8	38	0	3
Lemonade Dutch Ice®, 14 fl.oz.	315	0	77	0	0
Lemonade Dutch Smoothie, 14 fl.oz.	300	8	53	0	3
Mocha Dutch Ice®, 14 fl.oz.	400	10	74	0	0
Mocha Dutch latté™, 14 fl.oz.	360	17	47	0	5
Mocha Dutch Smoothie, 14 fl.oz.	330	13	50	0	3
Orange Creme Dutch Ice®, 14 fl.oz.	280	0	64	0	0
Orange Creme Dutch Smoothie, 14 fl.oz.	280	8	46	0	3
Piña Colada Dutch Ice®, 14 fl.oz.	220	0	53	0	0
Piña Colada Dutch Smoothie, 14 fl.oz.	260	8	44	0	3
Strawberry Dutch Ice®, 14 fl.oz.	220	0	50	0	0
• Strawberry Dutch Shake, 14 fl.oz.	610	27	78	0	10
Strawberry Dutch Smoothie, 14 fl.oz.	250	8	40	0	3
Strawberry Lemonade Dutch Ice, 14 fl.oz.	330	0	81	0	0
Vanilla Dutch Shake, 14 fl.oz.	510	27	58	0	10
Watermelon Dutch Ice®, 14 fl.oz.	200	0	50	0	0
Wild Cherry Dutch Ice®, 14 fl.oz.	210	0	48	0	0
Wild Cherry Dutch Smoothie, 14 fl.oz.	250	8	41	0	3
Dip Flavors					
• Caramel Dip, 2 oz.	135	3	27	0	1
Cheese Sauce Dip, 1 oz.	100	8	4	0	3
Hot Salsa Cheese Dip, 1 oz.	100	8	4	0	2
Light Cream Cheese Dip, 1 oz.	70	6	1	0	3
• Marinara Sauce Dip, 1 oz.	10	0	4	0	0
Sweet Mustard Dip, 1 oz.	60	2	8	0	1
Sweet Pretzel Dip, 1 oz.	40	0	10	0	0
Pretzels & More					
Almond Pretzel, 1 oz.	400	8	72	2	9
Almond Pretzel, no Butter, 1 oz.	350	2	72	2	9
Cinnamon Sugar Pretzel, 1 oz.	450	9	83	3	8
Cinnamon Sugar Pretzel, no Butter, 1 oz.	350	2	74	2	9
Garlic Pretzel, 1 oz.	350	5	68	2	9
Garlic Pretzel, no Butter, 1 oz.	320	1	66	2	9

(• = most healthy • = least healthy) **RESTAURANTS & FAST-FOOD • 59**

RESTAURANTS & FAST-FOOD CHAINS

Auntie Anne's (cont.)

Pretzels & More (cont.)	Cal	Fat	Cbs	Fbr	Prtn
• Glazin' Raisin®	510	4	107	4	11
Glazin' Raisin®, no Butter	470	1	104	3	11
Jalapeño	310	5	59	2	8
• Jalapeño, no Butter	270	1	58	2	8
Original	370	4	72	3	10
Original, no Butter	340	1	72	3	10
Pretzel Dog	290	16	25	1	10
Sesame	410	12	64	7	12
Sesame, no Butter	350	6	63	3	11
Sour Cream & Onion	340	5	66	2	9
Sour Cream & Onion, no butter	310	1	66	2	9
Stix, 6 sticks	370	4	72	3	10
Stix, no Butter, 6 sticks	340	1	72	3	10
Whole Wheat	370	5	72	7	11
Whole Wheat, no Butter	350	2	72	7	11

Baja Fresh

	Cal	Fat	Cbs	Fbr	Prtn
Americano Soft Taco					
Breaded Fish, 129 g	240	11	23	2	10
Carnitas, 142 g	250	12	21	2	13
• Chicken, 142 g	230	10	20	2	16
Mahi Mahi, 150 g	240	10	20	2	17
Shrimp, 150 g	230	10	21	2	15
• Steak, 142 g	260	13	21	2	15
Baja Burrito					
Breaded Fish, 426 g	850	44	78	7	40
Carnitas, 440 g	830	45	67	8	45
Chicken, 440 g	790	38	65	8	52
Mahi Mahi, 451 g	780	38	66	7	51
• Shrimp, 454 g	760	37	66	7	47
• Steak, 437 g	850	46	67	7	49
Baja Ensalada®					
Charbroiled Chicken, 473 g	310	7	18	7	46
• Charbroiled Shrimp, 445 g	230	6	18	6	28
• Charbroiled Steak, 473 g	450	18	18	6	54
Savory Pork Carnitas, 473 g	370	18	20	7	35
Baja Fish Taco - Fried					
• Breaded Fish, 134 g	250	13	27	2	8
Complimentary Chips, 43 g	210	9	29	3	3
• Mahi Mahi Taco - Grilled, 177 g	230	9	26	4	12
Bean and Cheese Burritos					
Breaded Fish, 477 g	1030	41	108	20	54
Carnitas, 491 g	1010	42	98	21	59
Chicken, 491 g	970	35	96	21	67
Mahi Mahi, 502 g	960	35	96	20	65
• No Meat, 392 g	840	33	96	20	39
Shrimp, 505 g	950	34	96	20	61
• Steak, 488 g	1030	43	97	20	64
Burrito Mexicano					
Breaded Fish, 499 g	850	19	129	18	37
Carnitas, 514 g	830	20	119	19	42
Chicken, 514 g	790	13	117	20	50
Mahi Mahi, 525 g	791	13	117	18	49

Baja Fresh (cont.)	Cal	Fat	Cbs	Fbr	Prtn
Burrito Mexicano (cont.)					
• Shrimp, 528 g	770	13	117	18	44
• Steak, 511 g	860	21	118	18	47
Burrito Ultimo					
Breaded Fish, 465 g	940	42	96	8	41
Carnitas, 480 g	920	44	86	9	46
Chicken, 481 g	880	36	84	9	54
Mahi Mahi, 491 g	880	36	84	8	52
• Shrimp, 494 g	860	36	85	8	48
• Steak, 477 g	950	44	85	8	50
Chicken Tortilla Soup					
With Charbroiled Chicken, 388 g	320	14	29	4	17
Without Charbroiled Chicken, 354 g	270	14	29	4	8
"Enchilado" Style					
To Burrito add, 420 g	630	40	45	7	23
To "Burrito Dos Manos"® add, 839 g	1260	80	91	15	46
Fajitas					
Breaded Fish w/ Corn Tortillas, 817 g	1060	37	130	22	51
• Breaded Fish w/ Flour Tortillas, 876 g	1340	46	172	25	59
Breaded Fish w/ Mix Tortillas, 869 g	1260	43	162	24	57
Carnitas w/ Corn Tortillas, 788 g	920	34	108	23	50
Carnitas w/ Flour Tortillas, 847 g	1190	43	150	26	58
Carnitas w/ Mix Tortillas, 840 g	1120	40	140	26	55
Chicken w/ Corn Tortillas, 788 g	860	24	105	24	61
Chicken w/ Flour Tortillas, 847 g	1140	33	147	27	69
Chicken w/ Mix Tortillas, 840 g	1070	30	137	26	67
• Mahi Mahi w/ Corn Tortillas, 794 g	840	23	105	22	57
Mahi Mahi w/ Flour Tortillas, 853 g	1120	32	147	25	64
Mahi Mahi w/ Mix Tortillas, 846 g	1050	29	138	24	62
Shrimp w/ Corn Tortillas, 817 g	840	23	106	22	55
Shrimp w/ Flour Tortillas, 876 g	1120	32	148	25	62
Shrimp w/ Mix Tortillas, 869 g	1040	29	138	24	60
Steak w/ Corn Tortillas, 788 g	960	36	107	22	58
Steak w/ Flour Tortillas, 847 g	1240	45	149	25	65
Steak w/ Mix Tortillas, 840 g	1170	42	139	24	63
Grilled Veggie					
Grilled Veggie, 506 g	800	33	94	16	32
Kids' Faves					
Chicken Taquitos, 304 g	630	33	60	4	18
Mini Bean & Cheese Burrito w/ Chicken, 382 g	590	15	84	12	28
• Mini Bean & Cheese Burrito, 348 g	540	14	84	11	18
• Mini Cheese Quesadilla w/ Chicken, 317 g	650	27	72	5	28
Mini Cheese Quesadilla, 283 g	610	26	72	5	19
Nachos					
Breaded Fish, 867 g	2090	116	176	31	78
Charbroiled Chicken, 882 g	2020	110	164	32	91
Charbroiled Mahi Mahi, 893 g	2020	110	164	31	90
Charbroiled Shrimp, 893 g	2000	110	164	31	85
• Charbroiled Steak, 879 g	2120	118	163	31	96
• Cheese, 782 g	1890	108	163	31	63
Savory Pork Carnitas, 882 g	2060	117	166	32	83
Original Baja Taco					
Carnitas, 116 g	220	7	29	2	10
Chicken, 116 g	210	5	28	2	12

(•= most healthy •= least healthy)

RESTAURANTS & FAST-FOOD CHAINS

Baja Fresh (cont.)

	Cal	Fat	Cbs	Fbr	Prtn
Original Baja Taco (cont.)					
• Shrimp, 125 g	200	5	28	2	11
• Steak, 113 g	230	8	28	2	11
Quesadilla					
Breaded Fish, 539 g	1400	86	96	8	62
Charbroiled Chicken, 553 g	1330	80	84	9	75
Charbroiled Mahi Mahi, 565 g	1330	79	84	8	73
Charbroiled Shrimp, 567 g	1310	79	84	8	69
• Charbroiled Steak, 550 g	1430	87	84	8	80
• Cheese, 454 g	1200	78	84	8	47
Savory Pork Carnitas, 553 g	1370	87	86	9	67
Veggie, 565 g	1260	78	96	11	48
Salad Dressing					
• Fat Free Salsa Verde, 71 g	15	0	3	1	0
• Olive Oil Vinaigrette, 71 g	290	31	2	0	0
Ranch Dressing, 71 g	260	26	4	0	2
Sides					
Black Beans, 327 g	360	3	61	26	23
Corn Tortilla Chips, 43 g	210	9	29	3	3
Pinto Beans, 300 g	320	1	56	21	19
• Pronto Guacamole, 170 g	560	34	60	8	9
Rice and Beans Plate, 325 g	420	5	72	18	18
Rice, 181 g	280	4	55	4	5
• Side Salad, 186 g	130	6	16	4	5
Tostada Salad					
Breaded Fish, 744 g	1200	61	111	25	47
Charbroiled Chicken, 758 g	1140	55	98	27	60
Charbroiled Fish, 769 g	1130	55	99	25	59
Charbroiled Shrimp, 772 g	1120	55	99	25	55
• Charbroiled Steak, 755 g	1230	63	98	25	65
• No Meat, 659 g	1010	53	94	25	32
Savory Pork Carnitas, 758 g	1180	62	100	26	52

Baker's Drive-Thru

	Cal	Fat	Cbs	Fbr	Prtn
American Menu: Chicken Specialties					
• Caribbean Chicken Sandwich	398	18	41	1	19
• Grilled Chicken Sandwich w/o Dressing	273	8	31	3	19
• Grilled Chicken Sandwich	380	18	35	3	19
Teriyaki Chicken Sandwich	386	18	36	3	19
American Menu: French Fries					
1/2 Pound Fries	759	40	96	8	10
• Budget Meal French Fries	223	12	28	2	3
• Chili Cheese Fries	988	59	102	9	25
Regular French Fries	357	19	45	4	5
American Menu: Hamburgers					
Boca Burger w/Cheese & Dressing	391	19	39	6	19
• Boca Burger w/o Cheese & Dressing	211	2	35	6	15
Budget Meal Hamburger	294	12	28	0	18
Chicken Sandwich w/o Dressing	273	8	31	3	19
• Double Baker	696	43	34	1	42
Grilled Boca Burger w/o Cheese or Dressing	211	2	35	6	15
Grilled Boca Burger	391	19	39	6	18
Grilled Cheese Sandwich	363	22	28	2	13
Grilled Cheese	363	22	28	2	13

RESTAURANTS & FAST-FOOD CHAINS

Baker's Drive-Thru (cont.)

	Cal	Fat	Cbs	Fbr	Prtn
American Menu: Hamburgers (cont.)					
Old Fashioned Cheeseburger	462	26	33	1	23
Old Fashioned Hamburger	382	20	33	1	19
American Menu: Platters					
Chicken Burrito Platter	1013	47	108	11	29
Chicken Mexican Salad	678	38	50	11	40
Chicken Soft Taco Platter	726	34	71	10	35
• Combination Burrito Platter	1089	47	123	18	48
Ground Beef Mexican Salad	762	47	49	12	42
Ground Beef Taco Platter	753	38	69	11	35
Shredded Beef Burrito Platter	1035	44	107	10	56
Shredded Beef Mexican Salad	695	38	50	11	42
Shredded Beef Soft Taco Platter	672	26	72	9	38
• Vegetarian Mexican Salad - (all beans)	642	33	64	17	29
Breakfast					
Add Potato to any Breakfast Burrito	247	13	32	2	4
Chili & Egg Burrito	534	23	55	5	26
Chorizo & Egg Burrito	657	34	55	5	32
• Egg Burrito w/Beans & Meat	744	31	75	12	42
Egg Burrito	535	24	56	5	26
Egg Sandwich	467	31	33	1	15
• Egg Taco	177	11	11	2	9
Hash Browns	433	23	56	4	6
Machaca Burrito	623	26	57	5	40
Sausage & Egg Burrito	639	32	56	5	32
Sausage & Egg Sandwich	579	40	34	1	21
Mexican: Burritos					
• All Chicken Burrito w/o Cheese	438	14	56	3	23
All Chicken Burrito	524	21	57	3	10
Bean & Cheese Burrito	442	10	70	9	17
Cheese Burrito	650	35	54	3	29
Combination Burrito	601	22	72	10	30
Green Burrito	621	17	90	18	27
Ground Beef Burrito	675	32	55	4	42
Make it Big!	73	6	4	1	2
Mexican Rice & Bean Burrito	442	13	74	5	11
Red Burrito	621	17	90	16	28
Shredded Beef Burrito	546	18	57	3	37
• Veggie Wrap	736	27	108	14	21
Mexican: Extras					
Bean Cup w/o cheese	229	3	37	13	14
Bean Cup	315	10	37	13	19
Cheese Quesadilla	588	39	45	5	18
• Chili & Bean Cup	222	9	26	8	14
Guacamole & Chips	426	28	44	4	7
Mexican Rice Cup	284	6	52	1	5
• Nachos	1407	81	120	24	61
Taco Burger	270	10	30	1	16
Tostada	285	10	38	10	11
Mexican: Tacos					
Bean Taco	150	6	18	4	6
Chicken Soft Taco	169	9	12	2	11
• Soft Taco w/Shredded Beef	141	5	12	1	13
• Taco	182	11	11	2	11

(•= most healthy •= least healthy)   **RESTAURANTS & FAST-FOOD • 63**

RESTAURANTS & FAST-FOOD CHAINS

Baker's Drive-Thru (cont.)

	Cal	Fat	Cbs	Fbr	Prtn
Milkshake					
Butterfinger® Milkshake	715	36	88	1	15
• Chocolate Milkshake	624	29	84	1	13
Oreo® Milkshake	718	35	90	2	14
• Snickers® Milkshake	722	38	85	1	16
Strawberry Milkshake	637	28	88	0	12
Vanilla Milkshake	634	28	86	0	12
Vegetarian					
• Boca Burger w/o Cheese or Dressing	211	2	35	6	15
Cheese Burrito	650	35	54	3	29
Green Burrito	621	17	90	18	27
Grilled Boca Burger	391	19	39	6	19
Grilled Cheese Sandwich	363	22	28	2	13
Red Burrito	621	17	90	18	27
Tostada Salad - Vegetarian Style	700	36	61	11	42
Vegetarian Combination w/o cheese	478	8	76	10	24
Vegetarian Combination	563	15	77	10	30
Vegetarian Sandwich	240	5	35	3	16
Vegetarian Soft Taco	145	3	19	3	10
Vegetarian Taco	170	6	19	4	11
• Veggie Wrap	736	27	108	14	21

Baker's Square

	Cal	Fat	Cbs	Fbr	Prtn
Breakfast					
Rise & Shine Breakfast	510	19	66	5	20
Sunrise Omelette	650	25	70	6	37
Entrees					
Chicken and Vegetable Stir-Fry	465	14	61	2	20
• Grilled Catch of the Day	390	19	32	3	23
Lemon Chicken	440	20	33	2	31
• Small Sirloin Steak	500	25	32	2	35
Pitas & Wraps					
Fajita Pita	610	22	65	4	38
Stir-Fry Pita	660	23	74	5	40
Salads					
Chicken Caesar Salad	315	15	14	5	32
Stir-Fry Salad	555	22	53	7	34

Baskin Robbins

	Cal	Fat	Cbs	Fbr	Prtn
Cappuccino Blasts®					
Caramel Medium, 24 fl.oz.	720	24	121	0	10
• Low Fat Small, 16 fl.oz.	220	2	45	0	6
Mocha Medium, 24 fl.oz.	240	18	87	0	8
Mocha w/ Whipped Cream Medium, 24 fl.oz.	620	21	100	0	9
Nonfat Medium, 24 fl.oz.	340	0	78	0	11
• Oreo® N' Cookies Medium, 24 fl.oz.	800	31	118	2	13
Original Medium, 24 fl.oz.	460	19	66	0	9
Turtle - Medium, 24 fl.oz.	710	23	121	0	10
Whipped Cream Medium, 24 fl.oz.	480	21	67	0	9
Fruit Blast - Medium					
• Berry Pomegranate Fruit Blast, 24 fl.oz.	210	0	128	1	1
• Strawberry Citrus Fruit Blast, 24 fl.oz.	480	1	122	4	2
Wild Mango Fruit Blast, 24 fl.oz.	470	2	116	2	1

Baskin Robbins (cont.)	Cal	Fat	Cbs	Fbr	Prtn
Fruit Blast Smoothie - Medium					
Berry Pomegranate Banana, 24 fl.oz.	710	1	172	3	7
• Mango Fruit Blast Smoothie, 24 fl.oz.	620	2	148	3	7
Strawberry Banana, 24 fl.oz.	730	2	178	7	9
Holiday & Special Occasion Ice Cream Cakes					
• Choco Chip Ice Cream/Devil's Food Heart, 125 g	330	18	40	1	5
• Vanilla Ice Crm/Devil's Food Heart, 125 g	340	19	39	1	5
Ice Cream: Classic Flavors					
Cherries Jubilee, 4 oz.	240	12	30	1	4
Choco Chip Cookie Dough Ice Crm, 4 oz.	290	15	36	1	5
Chocolate Chip Ice Cream, 4 oz.	270	16	28	1	5
Chocolate Fudge Ice Cream, 4 oz.	270	15	35	0	4
Chocolate Ice Cream, 4 oz.	260	14	33	0	5
French Vanilla Ice Cream, 4 oz.	280	18	26	0	4
Gold Medal Ribbon® Ice Cream, 4 oz.	260	13	34	0	5
Heath® Bar Crunch Ice Cream, 4 oz.	300	15	38	0	5
Jamoca® Almond Fudge Ice Cream, 4 oz.	270	15	31	1	6
Jamoca® Ice Cream, 4 oz.	240	13	26	0	5
Mint Chocolate Chip Ice Cream, 4 oz.	270	16	28	1	5
Nutty Coconut Ice Cream, 4 oz.	300	20	28	1	6
Old Fashioned Butter Pecan Ice Crm, 4 oz.	280	18	24	1	5
Oreo® Cookies 'n Cream Ice Crm, 4 oz.	280	15	32	1	5
• Peanut Butter 'n Chocolate Ice Crm, 4 oz.	320	20	31	1	7
Pistachio Almond Ice Cream, 4 oz.	290	19	25	1	7
Pralines 'n Cream Ice Cream, 4 oz.	270	14	34	0	5
Reese's® PB Cup Ice Cream, 4 oz.	300	18	31	0	6
Rocky Road Ice Cream, 4 oz.	290	15	36	1	5
Strawberry Cheesecake Ice Cream, 4 oz.	270	14	32	0	5
Vanilla Ice Cream, 4 oz.	260	16	26	0	4
• Very Berry Strawberry Ice Cream, 4 oz.	220	11	28	0	4
World Class® Chocolate Ice Cream, 4 oz.	280	16	31	0	5
Ice Cream: Seasonal Flavors					
Baseball Nut™ Ice Cream, 4 oz.	270	14	32	0	5
Black Walnut Ice Cream, 4 oz.	280	19	25	1	6
Chocolate Almond Ice Cream, 4 oz.	300	18	32	1	7
• Choco Mousse Royale® Ice Cream, 4 oz.	310	18	35	1	5
Chocolate Oreo® Ice Cream, 4 oz.	300	16	38	2	5
Creole Cream Cheese Ice Cream, 4 oz.	190	7	28	0	28
Egg Nog Ice Cream, 4 oz.	200	7	30	0	5
German Chocolate Cake Ice Cream, 4 oz.	300	16	37	1	5
Icing on the Cake Ice Cream, 4 oz.	290	15	35	0	5
Jamoca® Oreo® Ice Cream, 4 oz.	270	12	36	1	4
Lemon Custard Ice Cream, 4 oz.	260	13	30	0	4
Mississippi Mud Ice Cream, 4 oz.	270	13	38	1	4
New York Cheesecake Ice Cream, 4 oz.	230	10	30	0	4
Peppermint Ice Cream, 4 oz.	270	14	32	0	4
Pink Bubblegum Ice Cream, 4 oz.	260	12	36	0	4
• Pumpkin Pie Ice Cream, 4 oz.	180	6	29	0	4
Quarterback Crunch Ice Cream, 4 oz.	250	12	33	0	5
Rum Raisin Ice Cream, 4 oz.	250	11	34	0	4
Winter White Chocolate Ice Cream, 4 oz.	220	9	30	1	4
Lighter Side: Ice					
Lime Daiquiri Ice, 4 oz.	130	0	33	0	0

RESTAURANTS & FAST-FOOD CHAINS

Baskin Robbins (cont.)

	Cal	Fat	Cbs	Fbr	Prtn
Lighter Side: Low Fat Ice Cream - No Sugar Added					
• Berries 'n Banana, 4 oz.	110	2	25	1	5
• Chocolate Chocolate Chip, 4 oz.	150	5	31	1	6
Pineapple Coconut, 4 oz.	120	2	27	0	5
Lighter Side: Low Fat Yogurt					
Raspberry Cheese Louise Frozen Yogurt, 4 oz.	190	4	35	1	5
Lighter Side: Nonfat Soft Serve Yogurt - No Sugar Added					
• Truly Free® Cafe Mocha, 88 g	90	0	18	1	4
• Truly Free® Chocolate, 1/2 cup, 88 g	80	0	15	0	4
Truly Free® Vanilla, 1/2 cup, 88 g	90	0	17	1	4
Lighter Side: Nonfat Yogurt					
Vanilla Nonfat Yogurt, 4 oz.	150	0	32	0	6
Lighter Side: Sherbet					
Orange Sherbet, 4 oz.	160	2	34	0	1
Rainbow Sherbet, 4 oz.	160	2	34	0	1
• Rock 'n Pop Swirl Sherbet, 4 oz.	190	4	37	0	1
• Wild 'N Reckless Sherbet, 4 oz.	160	2	33	0	1
Roll Ice Cream Cakes					
• Chocolate Chip Ice Cream/Chocolate, 117 g	290	15	41	2	4
Mint Chocolate Chip Ice Cream/Chocolate, 117 g	290	14	36	2	5
• Vanilla Ice Cream/Chocolate, 117 g	270	14	39	2	4
Round Ice Cream Cakes					
• Choco Chp Cookie Dgh Ice Crm/Dvl's Fd 6, 161 g	460	23	59	1	7
Choco Chip Ice Cream/Devil's Food 9, 161 g	410	23	51	2	6
• Oreo® Cookies 'n Crm Ice Crm/Dvl's Fd 6, 161 g	440	23	56	1	7
Oreo® Cookies 'n Crm Ice Crm/Dvl's Food 9, 161 g	430	23	55	1	7
Pralines 'n Cream Ice Crm/White Sponge 9, 161 g	430	20	65	1	6
• Vanilla & Choco Ice Cream/Fudge Crunch 9, 123 g	340	18	41	1	5
Shakes - Medium					
• Choco Oreo® Shake, 633 g	1350	69	172	6	23
Choco Shake with Choco Ice Cream, 24 fl.oz.	990	40	149	1	20
Choco Shake with Vanilla Ice Cream, 24 fl.oz.	1000	45	133	0	19
Heath® Bar Crunch Shake, 24 fl.oz.	1340	66	167	1	22
Jamoca® Oreo® Shake, 625 g	1170	44	177	2	21
Mint Chocolate Chip Shake, 24 fl.oz.	970	47	116	2	21
Peppermint Shake, 612 g	930	32	145	0	20
Reese's® Peanut Butter Cup Shake, 24 fl.oz.	1340	92	105	7	37
• Strawberry w/ Very Brry Strwbrry Ice Crm, 24 fl.oz.	650	19	104	1	18
Vanilla Shake, 24 fl.oz.	980	45	125	0	19
Sheet Ice Cream Cakes					
Chocolate Chip Ice Cream/Devil's Food, 126 g	330	18	41	1	5
Mint Chocolate Chip Ice Cream/Devil's Food, 126 g	330	18	41	1	5
Oreo® Cookies 'n Crm Ice Crm/Wh Spnge, 126 g	350	16	47	1	5
• Pralines 'n Cream Ice Cream/White Sponge, 126 g	360	16	49	1	5
Vanilla & Choco Ice Cream/Fudge Crunch, 126 g	330	18	40	1	5
Vanilla Ice Cream/Devil's Food, 126 g	340	19	39	1	5
• Very Brry Strawberry Ice Crm/White Spnge, 126 g	310	13	44	1	4
Sundaes					
• 2 Scoop Hot Fudge Sundae, 203 g	530	29	62	0	8
3 Scoop Hot Fudge Sundae, 288 g	750	41	86	0	11
Banana Royale Sundae, 316 g	630	27	91	5	9
Banana Split Sundae, 570 g	1030	39	168	7	12
Brownie Sundae, 303 g	890	42	123	1	10
Candy Rush Sundae, 258 g	850	40	115	2	8

Baskin Robbins (cont.)

Sundaes (cont.)	Cal	Fat	Cbs	Fbr	Prtn
Heath® Bar Crunch Sundae, 370 g	1210	59	160	2	13
Oreo® Sundae, 347 g	1030	47	147	3	11
• Peppermint Brownie Sundae, 512 g	1580	75	221	2	18
Reese's® Peanut Butter Cup Sundae, 372 g	1400	90	124	7	29

BD's Mongolian Barbecue

Meats	Cal	Fat	Cbs	Fbr	Prtn
Chicken, 3 oz.	102	3	0	0	18
Lamb, 3 oz.	126	7	0	0	17
• NY Strip, 3 oz.	79	1	1	0	16
Pork, 3 oz.	123	5	0	0	18
Ribeye, 3 oz.	123	4	0	0	18
• Sausage, 3 oz.	273	26	2	0	9
Turkey, 3 oz.	102	3	0	0	19
Noodles					
• Lo Mein, 2 oz.	161	1	33	2	6
• Pasta, 2 oz.	210	1	42	2	7
Rice					
Rice, 3/4 cup	160	0	35	0	3
Salad Dressings					
Balsamic Vinaigrette, 1 oz.	60	5	4	0	0
• Blue Cheese, 1 oz.	160	17	2	0	1
Caesar, 1 oz.	150	16	29	0	1
• FAT FREE French, 1 oz.	30	0	8	1	0
Greek Feta, 1 oz.	70	5	1	1	5
Honey Mustard, 1 oz.	160	16	5	0	0
Raspberry Vinaigrette, 1 oz.	35	0	8	0	0
Sauces					
Barbecue, 1 oz.	41	0	9	0	0
Black Bean, 1 oz.	34	1	3	0	1
Chili Garlic, 1 oz.	40	3	3	1	0
Fajita, 1 oz.	27	2	2	0	0
Kung Pao, 1 oz.	34	1	7	0	1
Lemon, 1 oz.	23	0	6	0	0
• Lite Soy, 1 oz.	10	0	1	0	1
Mongo Marinara, 1 oz.	17	0	3	0	1
Mongolian Ginger, 1 oz.	42	1	7	0	1
• Peanut, 1 oz.	96	8	4	0	2
Sesame Oil, 0.5 oz.	60	7	0	0	0
Shiitake Mushroom, 1 oz.	27	0	5	0	1
Spicy Buffalo, 1 oz.	40	5	0	0	0
Sweet & Sour, 1 oz.	35	0	8	0	0
Teriyaki, 1 oz.	27	0	7	0	0
Seafood					
Calamari, 3 oz.	78	1	3	0	15
Cod, 3 oz.	69	1	0	0	15
Crawfish, 3 oz.	80	2	0	0	15
Krab (Surimi), 3 oz.	85	1	9	0	10
• Salmon, 3 oz.	156	10	0	0	17
Scallops, 3 oz.	84	1	3	0	16
• Shrimp, 3 oz.	65	0	0	0	14
Tuna, 3 oz.	112	4	0	0	20

RESTAURANTS & FAST-FOOD CHAINS

BD's Mongolian Barbecue (cont.)

	Cal	Fat	Cbs	Fbr	Prtn
Soups					
• Chicken Noodle, 8 oz.	70	2	10	1	4
Clam Chowder, 8 oz.	200	9	18	1	11
Country Potato, 8 oz.	220	10	21	1	10
Hearty Vegetable, 8 oz.	60	5	12	2	3
Hot and Sour, 8 oz.	90	4	10	1	4
Mangia Mangia Mushroom, 8 oz.	220	15	18	2	5
Mushroom Bisque, 8 oz.	180	9	16	1	7
• Tomato Bisque, 8 oz.	310	26	17	2	3
Vegetarian Chili, 8 oz.	140	2	26	6	7
Tortillas					
Tortillas, 1 oz.	100	3	15	1	2
Vegetables					
Artichoke, 1 oz.	8	0	2	1	1
Bean Sprouts, 1 oz.	29	0	2	0	1
Beets, 1 oz.	10	0	2	1	1
Black Olives, 1 oz.	53	5	2	0	0
Bok Choy, 1 oz.	2	1	0	0	0
Broccoli, 1 oz.	8	1	2	0	1
Cabbage (Green), 1 oz.	7	1	2	1	1
Cabbage (Red), 1 oz.	6	1	1	1	1
Carrots, 1 oz.	12	1	3	1	1
Celery, 1 oz.	5	0	1	0	1
• Cheddar Cheese, 1 oz.	120	10	1	0	7
• Cilantro, 1 tsp	0	0	0	1	0
Corn (Baby), 1 oz.	6	0	1	0	0
Crouton, 7 pieces	35	2	4	0	1
Cucumbers, 1 oz.	4	1	1	1	1
Head Lettuce, 1 leaf	1	0	0	0	0
Lemons, 1 wedge	2	0	1	0	0
Limes, 1 lime	20	1	7	2	0
Mushrooms, 1 oz.	7	1	1	0	1
Onions (Yellow), 1 oz.	11	1	2	1	1
Pea Pods, 1 oz.	11	1	3	1	1
Peppers (Green), 1 oz.	8	0	2	1	1
Peppers (Red), 1 oz.	9	1	2	1	1
Pineapple, 1 oz.	14	0	3	1	1
Romaine Lettuce, 1 oz.	1	0	0	0	0
Water Chestnuts, 1 oz.	9	0	2	1	1

Ben & Jerry's

	Cal	Fat	Cbs	Fbr	Prtn
Scoop Shop					
Banana Split, 85 g	210	12	22	1	3
Bananas On The Run, 90 g	210	10	27	0	3
• Berry Berry Extraordinary Sorbet, 92 g	100	0	27	1	0
Black Raspberry Frozen Yogurt, 93 g	140	2	28	1	3
Butter Pecan, 86 g	260	25	17	0	4
Cake Batter, 92 g	243	15	25	0	3
Cherry Garcia, 92 g	200	11	23	0	3
Chocolate Chip Cookie Dough, 87 g	220	12	26	0	4
Chocolate Fudge Brownie Frozen Yogurt, 94 g	160	3	32	1	4
Chocolate Fudge Brownie, 87 g	220	11	27	1	3
Chocolate Peanut Butter Swirl, 89 g	250	17	22	2	6
Chocolate Therapy, 86 g	210	12	25	2	4

RESTAURANTS & FAST-FOOD CHAINS

Ben & Jerry's (cont.)

	Cal	Fat	Cbs	Fbr	Prtn
Scoop Shop (cont.)					
Chocolate, 88 g	200	12	21	1	3
Chunky Monkey, 87 g	240	14	24	1	4
Cinnamon Buns, 88 g	240	12	30	0	3
Coconut Almond Fudge Chip, 88 g	230	17	21	1	5
• Coconut Seven Layer Bar, 92 g	277	18	26	1	3
Coffee, 88 g	190	11	18	0	3
Coffee, Coffee BuzzBuzzBuzz!, 88 g	230	14	23	1	4
Half Baked Frozen Yogurt, 85 g	160	3	31	1	4
Imagine Whirled Peace, 1/2 cup	252	15	27	0	3
Jamaican Me Crazy Sorbet, 144 g	140	0	37	1	0
Lemonade Sorbet, 88 g	100	0	26	1	0
Mango Mango Sorbet, 91 g	100	0	27	1	0
Mint Chocolate Chunk, 88 g	230	14	23	1	3
New York Super Fudge Chunk, 1/2 cup	250	17	24	2	4
One Cheesecake Brownie, 92 g	235	14	24	0	3
Phish Food, 88 g	230	11	33	1	3
Pumpkin Cheesecake, 88 g	230	12	26	0	3
Strawberry Cheesecake, 87 g	210	11	24	0	3
Strawberry Kiwi Sorbet, 92 g	100	0	27	1	0
Strawberry, 87 g	170	9	20	1	3
Sweet Cream & Cookies, 88 g	220	13	24	0	4
Triple Cream Chunk, 88 g	230	12	28	0	3
Vanilla Frozen Yogurt, 94 g	130	2	25	0	4
Vanilla Fudge Chip, 80 g	180	13	20	3	3
Vanilla Heath Bar Crunch, 82 g	240	14	24	0	3
Vanilla, 88 g	190	12	18	0	3

Big Apple Bagels

	Cal	Fat	Cbs	Fbr	Prtn
BAB's Choice Bagels					
Blueberry Cobbler, 70 g	196	4	35	1	5
• Cheddar Nacho, 70 g	176	3	30	2	7
Cinnamon Apple Pie, 70 g	193	4	34	1	5
• Cinnamon Bun, 70 g	200	4	35	1	5
Cinnamon Danish, 70 g	198	4	36	2	5
French Toast, 70 g	186	2	37	1	6
Quiche Lorraine, 70 g	177	4	27	1	8
Strawberry White Chocolate, 70 g	182	2	36	2	6
Swiss Melt, 70 g	184	4	29	1	9
White Chocolate Swirl, 70 g	198	4	35	1	5
Big Apple Bagels® Regular Bagels					
Apple Cinnamon, 70 g	166	1	35	2	6
Banana Nut, 70 g	170	1	34	2	6
Blueberry, 70 g	165	1	34	2	6
Cheddar Herb, 70 g	176	3	30	1	7
Chocolate Chip, 70 g	174	1	34	2	6
Cinnamon Raisin, 70 g	168	1	35	2	6
Cinnamon Sugar, 70 g	175	1	37	1	6
Cranberry Walnut, 70 g	176	1	36	2	6
Egg, 70 g	164	1	33	1	6
Everything, 70 g	168	1	34	2	6
Garlic, 70 g	165	1	34	2	6
Honey Oat, 70 g	160	1	34	1	6
Jalapeño, 70 g	175	1	30	1	6

RESTAURANTS & FAST-FOOD CHAINS

Big Apple Bagels (cont.)

	Cal	Fat	Cbs	Fbr	Prtn
Big Apple Bagels® Regular Bagels (cont.)					
Onion, 70 g	168	1	35	2	6
Plain, 70 g	167	1	34	2	6
Poppy, 70 g	172	1	34	2	6
Pumpernickel, 70 g	166	1	34	2	6
Salt, 70 g	162	1	33	1	6
• Sesame, 70 g	179	2	33	2	7
Spinach, 70 g	178	1	36	2	7
Strawberry, 70 g	171	1	36	2	6
Tomato Basil, 70 g	161	1	33	2	6
• Vegetable, 70 g	159	1	33	2	6
Wheat, 70 g	165	1	34	2	6
Breakfast Sandwiches					
• Breakfast B.L.T., 9 oz.	704	31	83	4	22
Lox & Cream Cheese, 11 oz.	602	21	78	4	29
• Morning Classic, 8 oz.	486	11	73	3	23
Northern Omelette, 10 oz.	699	31	73	3	31
So. Tradition (w/bacon), 8 oz.	566	18	73	3	27
So. Tradition (w/ham), 8 oz.	547	15	73	3	29
So. Tradition (w/sausage), 10 oz.	696	31	73	3	31
Build Your Own Sandwiches					
Ham, 10 oz.	490	9	77	4	27
Roast Beef, 10 oz.	480	6	77	4	29
• Tuna, 10 oz.	547	14	77	4	27
• Turkey, 10 oz.	465	3	77	4	32
Classic Recipe Cream Cheese					
Cheddar Jalapeño, 30 g	90	8	2	0	1
• Garden Vegetable, 30 g	90	9	2	0	1
Onion Chive, 30 g	80	8	2	0	1
• Plain Lite, 30 g	60	5	3	0	2
Plain, 30 g	90	9	2	0	1
Strawberry, 30 g	90	7	5	0	1
Gourmet Salads					
Calypso Chicken Salad, 14 oz.	637	49	34	3	20
Chicken Caesar Salad, 12 oz.	524	41	15	3	23
Classic Caesar Cafe Salad, 4 oz.	225	19	9	2	5
Classic Caesar Salad, 8 oz.	414	36	12	3	9
• Garden Mix Cafe Salad (w/o egg), 7 oz.	63	2	9	2	2
Garden Mix Cafe Salad, 7 oz.	100	5	9	2	5
Garden Mix Salad (w/o egg), 12 oz.	123	4	18	4	3
Garden Mix Salad, 12 oz.	197	9	18	4	9
Grilled Chicken Club Salad, 18 oz.	820	69	16	3	35
• Mediterranean Bread Salad, 19 oz.	973	73	52	5	30
Gourmet Sandwiches					
Classic Turkey, 10 oz.	552	14	74	4	32
• Holey Guacamole, 11 oz.	476	5	76	4	33
• Kick-N Roast Beef, 11 oz.	579	15	79	4	29
Mediterranean Veg-Out, 11 oz.	506	9	90	8	20
Icepresso Drinks					
Caramel Decadence Icepresso, 16 oz.	300	12	42	2	6
Classic Icepresso, 16 oz.	300	5	52	0	8
• Java Chip Icepresso, 16 oz.	360	18	48	2	6
Latte Icepresso, 16 oz.	300	12	42	2	6
Mocha Icepresso, 16 oz.	301	12	42	2	6

Big Apple Bagels (cont.)	Cal	Fat	Cbs	Fbr	Prtn
Icepresso Drinks (cont.)					
Strawberry Icepresso, 16 oz.	340	12	56	0	2
Low Carb Entrees					
Chicken Caesar Salad, 11 oz.	482	39	9	2	22
Deli Meat & Cheese Plate, 8 oz.	533	37	3	0	45
Garden Mix Salad, 15 oz.	564	51	12	4	14
Ham & Cheese Omelette, 13 oz.	679	49	6	1	52
Kick-n Chicken Plate, 9 oz.	382	22	10	0	35
• Three Cheese Omelette, 13 oz.	860	61	8	1	66
• Tuna Salad Plate, 9 oz.	356	25	3	1	28
Muffins					
• Fat Free Blueberry, 55 g	108	0	26	1	2
Fat Free Cherry Pie, 55 g	109	0	26	0	2
Fat Free Chocolate Marble, 55 g	125	0	29	1	2
• Fat Free Cinnamon Bun, 55 g	168	0	42	0	1
Fat Free Raspberry Amaretto, 55 g	127	0	31	1	2
My Favorite Muffin® Bagels					
• Blueberry, 113 g	320	2	66	2	11
Cinnamon Raisin, 113 g	310	1	66	3	11
Honey Grain, 113 g	310	3	61	4	11
Plain, 113 g	310	1	64	2	11
Russian Black Bread, 113 g	320	1	67	4	11
• Sour Dough, 113 g	310	1	64	2	11
Whole Wheat, 113 g	310	2	66	5	12
Other Specialty Drinks					
• Americano, 16 oz.	12	0	2	0	0
Black Forest Coffee, 16 oz.	198	5	37	1	1
• Cafe Caramello, 16 oz.	212	8	31	0	2
Overstuffed Sandwiches					
Classic Reuben, 14 oz.	962	43	57	4	60
Corned Beef, 11 oz.	661	19	77	3	43
Ham and Cheese, 14 oz.	889	36	79	4	60
• Manhattan Club, 16 oz.	1122	40	120	6	69
• Pastrami, 11 oz.	661	19	77	3	43
TD California Club, 16 oz.	759	12	113	8	49
TD Classic Club, 19 oz.	1119	43	122	5	61
TD The Clubhouse, 15 oz.	1079	37	117	5	69
Pizzaah! Sandwiches (per piece)					
• Bruschetta Pizzaah, 13 oz.	162	12	7	3	7
Cheese Pizzaah, 11 oz.	189	7	23	3	10
Grilled Chicken Bruschetta Pizzaah, 14 oz.	343	21	24	3	17
• Pepperoni Pizzaah, 14 oz.	398	26	23	3	19
Sausage Pizzaah, 14 oz.	211	17	6	2	11
Veggie Pizzaah, 12 oz.	238	10	32	7	12
Regular Muffins					
Pumpkin Spice, 55 g	181	8	26	0	2
Lemon Poppyseed, 55 g	201	10	25	0	3
Golden Corn Bread, 55 g	197	9	26	1	3
Double Chocolate, 55 g	201	9	28	1	2
Deep Dish Apple Pie, 55 g	177	8	25	0	2
• Cinnamon Swirl Cheesecake, 55 g	214	11	28	0	2
Cinnamon Crumb Cake, 55 g	212	13	21	0	3
Chocolate Chip, 55 g	211	11	27	1	3
Chocolate Cheesecake, 55 g	202	12	22	0	2

(• = most healthy • = least healthy)   **RESTAURANTS & FAST-FOOD • 71**

RESTAURANTS & FAST-FOOD CHAINS

Big Apple Bagels (cont.)	Cal	Fat	Cbs	Fbr	Prtn
Regular Muffins (cont.)					
Cherry Cheesecake, 55 g	170	10	19	0	2
Boston Cream Pie, 55 g	176	7	26	0	2
• Blueberry, 55 g	168	8	22	0	2
Blueberry Cheesecake, 55 g	199	12	20	0	3
Banana Nut, 55 g	195	11	21	1	4
Salads: Prepared with Lite Italian Dressing					
Calypso Chicken Salad, 14 oz.	317	17	22	3	20
Chicken Caesar Salad, 12 oz.	268	12	17	3	20
• Classic Caesar Salad, 8 oz.	158	8	14	3	6
Grilled Chicken Club Salad, 18 oz.	500	31	18	3	35
• Mediterranean Bread Salad, 19 oz.	626	32	55	5	30
Snacks					
• Enchilada Bagellata, 8 oz.	522	11	84	4	22
• Pizza Bagel, 8 oz.	481	6	85	5	22
Soups					
Beef Barley Mushroom, 8 oz.	100	3	12	N/A	6
Beef Pot Roast, 8 oz.	110	4	12	N/A	6
Boston Clam Chowder, 8 oz.	210	13	20	N/A	2
California Medley, 8 oz.	170	9	16	N/A	7
• Cheese & Bacon, 8 oz.	310	21	18	N/A	11
Chicken & Dumplings, 8 oz.	250	14	20	N/A	9
Chicken & Wild Rice, 8 oz.	190	9	22	N/A	5
Chicken Gumbo, 8 oz.	130	3	19	N/A	8
Chicken Noodle, 8 oz.	110	4	12	N/A	7
Country Bean, 8 oz.	140	2	24	N/A	6
Cream of Broccoli (w/Cheese), 8 oz.	170	11	15	N/A	5
Cream of Broccoli (w/o Cheese), 8 oz.	230	17	17	N/A	3
Cream of Potato, 8 oz.	240	14	24	N/A	4
• French Onion, 8 oz.	60	2	9	N/A	2
Garden Vegetable, 8 oz.	110	1	22	N/A	3
Hearty Vegetable Beef, 8 oz.	100	1	16	N/A	5
Minestrone, 8 oz.	150	3	26	N/A	5
Navy Bean w/Ham, 8 oz.	110	2	23	N/A	6
New England Clam Chowder, 8 oz.	220	13	21	N/A	6
Potato Chowder, 8 oz.	210	13	20	N/A	4
Sirloin Beef w/Pasta, 8 oz.	190	7	22	N/A	8
Split Pea w/Ham, 8 oz.	90	2	15	N/A	5
Turkey & Sausage Gumbo, 8 oz.	190	10	14	N/A	10
Vegetable Beef, 8 oz.	110	3	16	N/A	5
Wisconsin Cheese, 8 oz.	210	11	20	N/A	8
Specialty Drinks (prepared with 2% milk)					
Cappuccino, 16 oz.	195	7	20	0	13
Cinnamon Toast Latte, 16 oz.	299	7	45	0	13
Creme Caramel Latte, 16 oz.	303	7	47	0	13
Italiano, 16 oz.	131	5	13	0	9
Jittery Monkey, 16 oz.	482	11	82	1	13
Latte, 16 oz.	212	7	22	0	14
Mocha w/whipped cream, 16 oz.	454	12	71	2	15
Oregon Chai® Tea Latte, 16 oz.	274	5	48	0	9
Raspberry Cheesecake Latte, 16 oz.	319	7	51	0	13
• Turtle Mocha, 16 oz.	577	17	91	1	14
Vanilla Creme Latte, 16 oz.	275	7	39	0	13

RESTAURANTS & FAST-FOOD CHAINS

Big Apple Bagels (cont.)	Cal	Fat	Cbs	Fbr	Prtn
Specialty Drinks (prepared with fat free milk)					
Cappuccino, 16 oz.	133	1	18	0	12
Cinnamon Toast Latte, 16 oz.	240	1	44	0	11
Creme Caramel Latte, 16 oz.	244	1	45	0	11
• Italiano, 16 oz.	89	1	12	0	8
Jittery Monkey, 16 oz.	429	6	80	1	12
Latte, 16 oz.	145	1	20	0	13
Mocha w/whipped cream, 16 oz.	392	6	70	2	14
Oregon Chai® Tea Latte, 16 oz.	231	1	47	0	8
Raspberry Cheesecake Latte, 16 oz.	259	1	50	0	11
Turtle Mocha, 16 oz.	522	12	90	1	12
Vanilla Creme Latte, 16 oz.	132	1	18	0	12
Specialty Sandwiches					
All-American Duo, 13 oz.	752	28	78	4	46
• Big Apple Club, 11 oz.	797	37	75	4	41
Chicken Caesar, 11 oz.	611	19	78	4	31
• Grilled Chicken, 10 oz.	571	17	77	4	28
Roma Italian, 13 oz.	764	34	76	4	40
Turkey Club, 11 oz.	782	34	75	4	43
Toasted Sandwiches					
• Cafe Chicken Melt, 14 oz.	815	32	80	4	51
Deli-Style Turkey, 12 oz.	732	25	76	4	48
• Roast Beef Parmesan Grinder, 11 oz.	583	15	76	4	36
Spicy Italian Sub, 14 oz.	770	34	77	4	40
Tuna Melt, 10 oz.	641	23	75	4	32
Whipped Cream Cheese					
Brown Sugar Cinnamon, 20 g	70	5	5	0	1
• Classic Plain, 20 g	70	7	1	0	1
• Reduced Fat Spring Veggie, 20 g	60	5	2	0	1

Big Boy	Cal	Fat	Cbs	Fbr	Prtn
Beverages					
Chocolate Float w/Pepsi	195	5	38	0	1
Chocolate Malt	290	16	31	1	7
Chocolate Milk Shake, Plain	276	15	30	1	6
w/ Chocolate Syrup	382	16	57	1	7
w/ Fudge Topping	377	18	48	1	8
French Vanilla Malt	300	17	29	1	10
French Vanilla Milk Float w/Pepsi	200	6	37	0	3
French Vanilla Milk Shake, Plain	286	16	28	1	9
Strawberry Waffle Topping Add	386	16	53	1	9
w/ Caramel Topping	387	19	46	1	11
• w/ Chocolate Syrup	392	17	55	2	10
w/ Fudge Topping	387	19	46	1	11
French Vanilla Root Beer Float	202	6	36	0	3
• Frozen Yogurt Shake	158	0	33	0	7
Fruit Works Large, 16 fl.oz.	168	0	43	0	0
Sierra Mist Float	200	6	36	0	3
Strawberry Float w/Pepsi	190	5	37	0	1
Strawberry Malt	280	16	31	1	7
Strawberry Milk Shake, Plain	266	15	29	1	6
w/ Strawberry Topping	366	15	54	1	6
Breakfast					
Belgian Waffle w/Powdered Sugar, 1 waffle	526	25	65	2	14

RESTAURANTS & FAST-FOOD CHAINS

▶ Big Boy (cont.)

	Cal	Fat	Cbs	Fbr	Prtn
Breakfast (cont.)					
w/ Apple Topping, 1 waffle	746	26	122	5	14
w/ Strawberry Topping, 1 waffle	836	26	145	5	14
Big Boy Fave No Meat No Grain Product , 2 eggs	440	32	25	2	14
Biscuits Buttered, 2 Biscuits	460	24	54	2	8
Biscuits Plain, 2 Biscuits	424	20	54	2	8
Canadian Bacon, 2 sl.	146	7	2	0	19
Cinnamon French Toast, 2 sl.	472	8	88	6	14
Cinnamon Roll, 2 oz.	218	8	34	1	4
Country Biscuits& Sausage Gravy	924	54	93	4	21
Country Gravy w/ Sausage, 2 oz.	96	8	4	0	3
Danish, Pieces, 1 oz.	100	4	15	6	1
Deli Rye Bread Toasted Buttered, 2 sl.	284	7	45	6	9
Deli Rye Bread Toasted Plain, 2 sl.	248	3	45	6	9
Egg (Texas Toast) Bread Plain, 2 sl.	284	4	52	3	9
Egg (Texas Toast) Buttered, 2 sl.	320	8	52	3	9
Eggs Benedict	947	61	60	4	40
English Muffin Plain, 1 muffin	140	2	27	2	5
English Muffin w/ Butter, 1 muffin	176	6	27	2	5
French Toast, 2 sl.	365	7	363	3	12
H.S Egg Beaters Chz Omelet w/2 Sl. Dry Toast	322	8	39	2	20
H.S Egg Beaters Plain Omelet w/2 Sl. Dry Toast	283	6	38	2	18
H.S Egg Beaters Scrambled Eggs w/2 Sl. Dry Toast	283	6	38	2	18
H.S Egg Beaters Veggie Omelet w/2 Sl. Dry Toast	317	6	45	3	19
Hash Brown Potatoes, 4 oz.	254	18	23	2	0
Hot Cakes w/ Apple Top, no syrup, 3 hot cakes	1330	26	243	9	36
Hot Cakes w/ Blueberries, no syrup, 3 hot cakes	1115	26	187	6	36
● Hot Cakes w/ Strwbrry Top, no syrup, 3 hot cakes	1420	26	266	9	36
Hot Cakes, No syrup, 3 hot cakes	1110	25	186	6	36
Multi-Grain Hot cakes Plain, 1 order	698	25	105	14	25
Omelet Cheese w/ Toast	866	53	61	4	30
w/ 2-2 oz. Hotcakes, No Syrup	1002	54	87	4	36
w/ Biscuits	1092	70	79	4	32
Omelet Farmer's w/ Toast	899	51	69	5	33
w/ 2-2 oz. Hotcakes, No Syrup	1035	53	95	5	39
w/ Biscuits	1125	68	87	5	35
Omelet Ham &Cheese w/ Toast	902	53	61	4	39
w/ 2-2 oz. Hotcakes, No Syrup	1038	54	87	4	45
w/ Biscuits	1128	70	79	4	41
Omelet Mexican Fiesta w/ Toast	896	52	67	4	34
w/ 2-2 oz. Hotcakes, No Syrup	1032	53	93	4	40
w/ Biscuits	1112	69	85	4	36
Omelet Plain w/ Toast	749	44	59	4	24
w/ 2 Hotcakes, No Syrup	885	45	85	4	30
w/ Biscuits	975	61	77	4	26
Omelet Southern Country w/ Toast	1102	70	72	5	39
w/ 2-2 oz. Hotcakes, No Syrup	1234	71	98	5	45
w/ Biscuits	1328	87	90	5	41
Omelet Vegetarian w/ Toast	782	44	66	6	26
w/ 2-2 oz. Hotcakes, No Syrup	918	46	92	6	32
w/ Biscuits	1008	61	84	6	28
Pecan Roll Plain, 1 Roll	419	30	35	4	7
Pork Sausage Links, 2 links	133	11	1	0	7
Pork Sausage Patties, 1 patty	134	11	3	0	8

Big Boy (cont.)

	Cal	Fat	Cbs	Fbr	Prtn
Breakfast (cont.)					
Potato Pancakes Plain, 1 order	404	14	68	4	12
Seasoned Brawny Lad Patty, 1 patty	246	17	0	0	22
• Sliced Bacon, 2 sl.	75	1	0	0	5
Sliced Breakfast Ham, 1/2 sl.	311	21	1	0	27
White Bread Toasted Buttered, 2 sl.	234	7	36	2	6
White Bread Toasted Plain, 2 sl.	198	3	36	2	6
Whole Wheat Bread Toasted Buttered, 2 sl.	228	7	36	3	6
Whole Wheat Bread Toasted Plain, 2 sl.	192	3	36	3	6
Desserts					
Apple and Ice Cream Puff	579	30	73	2	6
Banana Cream Pie, 1 slice	368	22	39	1	4
• Banana Split	709	26	114	4	9
Butter Pecan Ice Cream, 2 scoops	200	12	20	1	2
Butter Pecan Super Sunday	221	13	23	1	2
w/ Caramel Topping	433	19	62	1	3
w/ Chocolate Syrup	433	14	76	2	3
w/ Fudge Topping	422	19	59	2	5
Chocolate Ice Cream, 2 scoops	190	10	22	1	2
Chocolate Super Sundae, Plain	211	11	25	1	2
w/ Caramel Topping	421	17	64	1	3
w/ Chocolate Syrup	423	12	78	2	3
w/ Fudge Topping	412	17	61	2	5
Coconut Cream Pie, 1 slice	402	29	34	2	3
Crumb Cherry Pie, 1 slice	466	10	60	2	4
French Silk Cream Pie, 1 slice	524	35	48	2	6
French Vanilla Ice Cream	200	11	20	1	5
French Vanilla Sundae, Plain	121	7	13	25	5
French Vanilla Super Sundae, Plain	221	12	23	1	5
w/ Caramel Topping	431	18	62	1	3
w/ Chocolate Syrup	433	13	76	2	3
w/ Fudge Topping	422	18	59	2	8
w/ Strawberry Topping	421	12	73	1	5
• Frozen Yogurt, 2 scoops	118	0	27	1	3
Hot Fudge Cake, 1 slice	662	27	100	3	11
No Sugar Added (NSA) Apple Pie, 1 slice	329	14	47	3	4
Oreo Mud Pie, 1 slice	495	24	66	2	6
Peanut Butter Ice cream Pie, 1 slice	607	42	47	4	21
Plain Cheese Cake, 1 slice	360	26	27	1	6
Pumpkin Pie Plain, 1 slice	366	16	48	4	6
Strawberry Cheese Cake, 1 slice	475	26	55	2	6
Strawberry Ice Cream, 2 scoops	180	10	21	1	2
Strawberry Pie, 1 slice	404	12	70	4	3
Strawberry Super Sundae, Plain	201	11	24	1	2
w/ Strawberry Topping	401	11	74	1	2
Dinner					
Baked Spaghetti Dinner	1056	47	108	7	54
Broiled Chicken Crumb Cod No Potato	671	51	14	0	37
Broiled Lemn Cod w/ Plain Bkd Potato	446	4	66	5	39
Cajun Chicken w/ Plain Baked Potato	396	5	57	5	31
Chicken & Veggie Stir Fry w/ Plain Baked Potato	717	8	128	11	35
Chicken Breast Mozz w/ Plain Baked Potato	436	8	58	5	34
Chicken Breast Tenders Only, 2 tenders	280	11	24	0	24
Chicken Parmesan Dinner	904	44	95	7	45

(• = most healthy • = least healthy) **RESTAURANTS & FAST-FOOD • 75**

RESTAURANTS & FAST-FOOD CHAINS

Big Boy (cont.)

	Cal	Fat	Cbs	Fbr	Prtn
Dinner (cont.)					
Chicken Pasta Primavera Dinner	919	28	117	10	54
Chicken Wisconsin Dinner No Potato	307	17	3	0	34
Country Fried Steak Dinner	990	66	68	5	41
• Fish & Chips	1252	84	87	6	34
Fried Lake Perch No Potato	504	55	25	1	26
Meatloaf (no Vegetable)	479	22	32	4	39
N.Y. Strip Steak No Potato	845	45	37	1	69
• Pot Roast Dinner, No Veg, No Potato	251	7	8	1	37
Sauteed Lake Perch No Potato	645	49	25	1	26
Shrimp (7 Pieces) No Potato	512	20	55	3	29
Spaghetti Dinner	612	13	105	8	22
Spaghetti Marinara Dinner	364	4	71	1	12
Turkey Dinner	642	18	83	5	39
Veal Parmesan	833	31	92	8	
Vegetable Stir Fry w/ Plain Baked Potato	567	3	128	11	10
Kiddie Menu					
Cinnamon French Toast, 1 slice	236	4	44	3	7
Combination Plate	685	31	69	3	35
Fish& Chips	796	60	44	3	20
• French Toast, 1 slice	183	4	32	2	6
Hot Cakes w/ App Waffle Top, No Syrup, 2 ht cks	894	18	162	6	24
Hot Cakes w/ Blueberries, No Syrup, 2 hot cakes	743	17	125	4	24
• Hot Cakes w/ Strawberry Top, No Syrup, 2 ht cks	957	17	177	6	24
Hot Cakes, No Syrup, 2 hot cakes	740	17	124	4	24
Macaroni & Cheese	330	12	45	2	11
Salads					
3 -Cheese Grilled Chicken Montreal Salad	749	58	10	2	46
Blackened Chicken & Melon Salad	599	8	102	9	28
Buffalo Chicken Tenders Salad	1196	93	55	3	44
Caesar Salad, Side	66	4	7	1	2
Chicken Breast Caesar Salad	278	12	13	2	28
Chicken Fajita Salad w/Salsa Ranch Dressing	800	55	29	5	41
Chipotle Krab Salad	1106	100	39	6	13
Cole Slaw	120	10	9	2	1
• Dinner Salad, No Dressing	44	0	6	1	1
• Grilled Chicken Chipotle Salad	1697	152	32	1	40
Grilled Ham Steak w/ Grilled Melons & Pineapple	702	29	66	5	37
Lo Carb Cheddar Burger Salad	1081	87	10	2	54
Trop Garden Chicken w/ Roll & Promise Margarine	577	16	74	8	33
Turkey Club Super Salad	421	24	7	2	44
Sandwiches					
Bacon Lettuce & Tomato Sandwich	535	33	39	3	21
BBQ Pot Roast Sandwich Only	895	26	122	2	43
Big Cheese& Bacon Chicken w/ am Cheese (only)	847	50	40	2	59
w/ Mozz. Cheese (only)	849	50	40	2	61
w/ Swiss Cheese (only)	876	52	40	2	63
Big Ringer Burger (only)	958	59	50	2	60
Big Ringer Chicken (only)	615	30	50	2	40
Big Shrooms & Onion's (only)	801	44	45	3	57
Brawny Lad (only)	471	25	36	3	27
Breast of Chicken Fillet (only)	621	41	54	4	22
Chkn Brst & Mozz. Pita (only) w/ Greek Pita Bread	463	13	48	3	36
Chkn Brst & Mozz. Pita (only) w/ Med Pita Bread	494	11	57	2	38

Big Boy (cont.)

	Cal	Fat	Cbs	Fbr	Prtn
Sandwiches (cont.)					
Chkn Club Ciabatta Wrap	1103	66	76	4	50
Chkn Santa Fe Ciabatta Wrap	926	40	90	7	53
Club Sandwich Only	778	39	58	4	45
• Corned Beef Reuben Sandwich Only	1132	78	57	6	52
Grilled Cheese Sandwich Only	531	22	58	3	20
Hot Meat Loaf	677	25	68	4	45
Hot Turkey w/ Gravy	477	11	59	4	37
• Kiddie Grilled Cheese Only	312	13	37	2	10
Patty Melt	900	54	36	5	63
Philly Steak & Cheese Sandwich Only	620	28	38	2	53
Plain Big Topping Burger (only)	694	38	38	2	51
Plain Chicken Burger Sandwich (only)	351	9	39	2	30
Roast Beef Ciabatta Wrap	1052	59	80	5	64
Sandwich Only	635	40	35	2	35
Slim Jim (only)	548	27	51	2	26
Super Big Boy (only)	853	55	35	2	54
Super Slim Jim Sandwich	858	44	77	4	40
Swiss Miss (only)	604	37	33	2	36
Tuna Melt Sandwich Only	791	48	51	6	41
Tuna salad Pita (only) w/ Greek Pita Bread	546	29	47	3	27
Tuna Salad Pita (only) w/ Med Pita Bread	577	27	56	2	29
Tuna Salad Sandwich Only	524	29	40	3	26
Turkey & Swiss Ciabatta Wrap	1040	58	78	4	49
Turkey Pita (only) w/ Greek Pita Bread	394	6	48	3	33
Turkey Pita (only) w/ Med Pita Bread	425	5	57	2	35
Sides					
6 Mozzarella Cheese Sticks- Plain	480	21	87	0	24
Beef Gravy, 2 oz.	31	1	3	0	2
Big Boy Sauce, 2 oz.	250	25	8	0	1
Big Boy Special Chili, 7 oz.	212	7	18	4	18
Broccoli Plain, 4 oz.	32	0	6	3	4
• Buffalo Style Chkn Tenders w/ Hot Sauce	658	30	52	1	48
Caesar Salad, Dressing, 2 oz.	338	32	12	0	1
Café Crackers, 1 pkg	25	1	3	0	0
• Cauliflower Plain, 4 oz.	21	0	4	3	2
Chicken Gravy, 2 oz.	57	3	7	0	1
Corn Plain, 4 oz.	104	1	25	1	5
Dinner Roll Plain, 1 Roll	123	3	20	1	3
Flavoured Sauce - Chipotle, 2 fl.oz.	424	44	4	0	2
Flavoured Sauce - Horseradish, 2 fl.oz.	324	33	6	1	2
French Fries (Combo & Side), 5 oz.	490	26	57	5	6
French Fries, (Kiddie Portion) 2 1/2 oz.	245	13	29	3	3
Garlic & Oil Dressing, 2 oz.	250	27	2	0	0
Green Beans Plain, 4 oz.	32	0	8	3	2
Grilled Grecian Roll (Garlic), 1 Roll	203	7	32	2	5
Grilled Texas Toast (Garlic), 1 slice	178	6	26	1	4
Mashed Potatoes Plain, 1 #8 Scoop	112	5	18	2	2
Ohio Big Boy Sauce, 2 oz.	354	38	2	0	1
Onion Rings, 8 Rings	304	16	36	0	4
Oyster Crackers, 1 pkg	60	3	9	1	1
Peas Plain, 4 oz.	91	7	16	5	7
Plain Bagel Plain, 1 Bagel	363	2	71	3	13
Plain Baked Potato, 8 oz.	246	0	57	6	4

RESTAURANTS & FAST-FOOD CHAINS

Big Boy (cont.)

	Cal	Fat	Cbs	Fbr	Prtn
Sides (cont.)					
Salsa Ranch Dressing, 2 fl.oz.	123	11	6	1	1
Shrimp Sauce, 2 oz.	54	0	15	1	0
Sour Cream, 1 oz.	60	6	2	0	2
Stir Fry Sauce, 2 oz.	222	1	55	1	1
Stir Fry Vegetables Plain, 6 oz.	53	0	11	4	3
Sweet Baby Rays Barbecue Sauce, 2 oz.	160	0	40	0	0
Tarter Sauce, 2 oz.	340	36	0	0	4
Tomato & Spice Dressing, 2 oz.	290	30	7	0	0
Turkey Gravy, 2 oz.	32	1	3	0	2
Vegetable Rice Pilaf, 5 oz.	206	4	38	1	3
Soups & Chili					
Bean w/ Bacon Soup, 6 oz.	170	13	8	2	6
• Cabbage Soup, 6 oz.	42	0	8	2	2
• Canadian Cheese Soup, 6 oz.	270	17	18	1	11
Chicken Noodle Soup, 6 oz.	110	2	17	1	7
Chicken w/ Rice Soup, 6 oz.	60	2	6	0	4
Chili Original, 6 oz.	230	11	20	5	15
Clam Chowder Soup, 6 oz.	109	6	10	1	5
Cream of Broccoli w/ Ham Soup, 6 oz.	110	9	8	1	6
Cream of Potato Soup, 6 oz.	180	10	17	1	5
Minestrone Soup, 6 oz.	70	2	12	2	4
Split Pea w/ Ham Soup, 6 oz.	80	3	9	1	6
Vegetable Beef Barley Soup, 6 oz.	80	3	10	2	4
Vegetarian Vegetable Soup, 6 oz.	45	1	9	1	2

Blackjack Pizza

	Cal	Fat	Cbs	Fbr	Prtn
Pizza					
Blackjack Pizza 14" Lg Cheese Pepperoni, 108 g	250	9	28	2	13
Blackjack Pizza 14" Lg Cheese Sausage, 109 g	240	8	28	2	13
Blackjack Pizza 14 Large Cheese, 98 g	200	5	28	2	12
• Cheesebread, 163 g	410	15	52	3	16
• Cinnabread, 2 oz.	190	5	31	1	5
Mediterranean Chicken, 78 g	190	11	15	1	8
Santa Fe, 98 g	210	11	17	1	10

Blimpie

	Cal	Fat	Cbs	Fbr	Prtn
Breads/Wraps					
Cheddar Jalapeño, 6", 3 oz.	213	4	36	1	8
Ciabatta, 4 oz.	230	3	43	2	8
Honey Oat 6", 4 oz.	259	8	41	5	10
Marble Rye 6", 4 oz.	242	2	46	2	9
• Wheat, 6", 3 oz.	190	4	34	4	9
White, 6", 3 oz.	213	3	40	1	7
Wrap, Spinach Herb 12", 4 oz.	310	8	52	3	9
• Wrap, Traditional 12", 4 oz.	310	8	52	5	9
Zesty Parmesan, 6", 3 oz.	236	4	39	2	9
Breakfast Items					
Biscuit, Bacon Egg & Cheese, 5 oz.	387	21	33	1	16
Biscuit, Egg & Cheese, 4 oz.	339	18	33	1	13
Biscuit, Golden Buttermilk, 2 oz.	224	9	31	1	5
Biscuit, Ham Egg & Cheese, 5 oz.	375	19	34	1	18
Biscuit, Sausage Egg & Cheese, 6 oz.	489	32	33	1	19
Bluffin, Bacon Egg & Cheese, 5 oz.	293	14	27	2	16

Blimpie (cont.)	Cal	Fat	Cbs	Fbr	Prtn
Breakfast Items (cont.)					
Bluffin, Egg & Cheese, 4 oz.	245	10	27	2	13
Bluffin, Ham Egg & Cheese, 5 oz.	280	11	29	2	18
• Bluffin, Plain, 2 oz.	129	1	25	2	5
Bluffin, Sausage Egg & Cheese, 6 oz.	395	24	27	2	19
Burrito, Bacon Egg & Cheese, 10 oz.	553	24	56	5	31
Burrito, Egg & Cheese, 10 oz.	506	20	56	5	28
Burrito, Ham Egg & Cheese, 12 oz.	559	21	58	5	36
Burrito, Sausage Egg & Cheese, 12 oz.	656	34	56	5	34
Croissant, Bacon Egg & Cheese, 5 oz.	393	24	29	1	16
Croissant, Egg & Cheese, 4 oz.	345	21	29	1	12
Croissant, Ham Egg & Cheese, 5 oz.	381	21	30	1	17
Croissant, Plain, 2 oz.	232	12	27	1	5
Croissant, Sausage Egg & Cheese, 6 oz.	495	35	29	1	18
Donut, Long John Cream Filled, 4 oz.	370	15	51	1	7
Donut, Yeast, 4 oz.	404	25	52	2	10
Gourmet Cinnamon Roll, 6 oz.	566	233	9	3	10
Muffin, Banana Walnut, 4 oz.	420	19	56	2	6
Muffin, Blueberry, 4 oz.	440	23	54	1	5
Panini Breakfast, 4", 8 oz.	494	14	67	2	26
• Panini Breakfast, 6", 13 oz.	773	24	96	3	43
Cheese					
American Y&W, 1 oz.	104	9	1	N/A	6
• Cheddar, serving, 1 oz.	75	6	1	N/A	4
Four Blend, serving, 0.5 oz.	52	4	1	0	4
• Mild Cheddar Shredded, serving, 1 oz.	114	9	0	0	7
Pepper Jack, serving, 1 oz.	77	7	0	0	6
Provolone, serving, 1 oz.	76	6	0	N/A	5
Swiss, serving, 1 oz.	79	6	0	0	6
Desserts					
• Brownie, Chocolate Chip, 4 oz.	430	18	63	2	4
Cookie, Chocolate Chunk, 2 oz.	191	9	25	1	2
• Cookie, Oatmeal Raisin Walnut, 2 oz.	191	8	28	1	3
Cookie, Peanut Butter, 2 oz.	220	12	23	1	4
Cookie, Sugar, 3 oz.	327	17	41	1	3
Cookie, White Chocolate Macadamia Nut, 2 oz.	206	10	26	0	2
Strudel Stick, Apple, 3 oz.	264	16	27	1	3
Strudel Stick, Cherry, 3 oz.	289	16	33	1	3
Strudel Stick, Raspberry, 3 oz.	290	18	29	1	3
Strudel Stick, Strawberry Cream Cheese, 3 oz.	289	182	27	0	3
Turnover, Apple, 4 oz.	357	23	35	1	3
Turnover, Cherry, 4 oz.	358	23	35	1	4
Dressings/Sauces					
• Dressing, Blue Cheese, 2 oz.	230	24	2	N/A	2
Dressing, Buttermilk Ranch, 2 oz.	230	24	2	N/A	1
Dressing, Creamy Caesar, 2 oz.	210	21	2	N/A	1
Dressing, Creamy Italian, 2 oz.	180	18	4	0	0
Dressing, Dijon Honey Mustard, 2 oz.	180	17	8	N/A	1
Dressing, Fat-Free Italian, 2 oz.	25	0	5	0	0
Dressing, Honey French, 2 oz.	210	18	14	N/A	0
Dressing, Light Buttermilk Ranch, 2 oz.	70	4	8	N/A	1
Dressing, Light Italian, 2 oz.	20	1	2	N/A	0
Dressing, Special, 1 oz.	70	7	0	N/A	0
Dressing, Thousand Island, 2 oz.	210	20	6	0	0

(•= most healthy •= least healthy)

RESTAURANTS & FAST-FOOD CHAINS

▶ Blimpie (cont.)

	Cal	Fat	Cbs	Fbr	Prtn
Dressings/Sauces (cont.)					
Mayonnaise, 1 oz.	202	22	0	0	0
Mayonnaise, Chipotle, 1 oz.	100	10	4	0	0
Mayonnaise, Horseradish, 1 oz.	100	10	4	0	0
Mustard, Deli Style, 0.5 oz.	5	0	0	0	0
Mustard, Honey, 1 oz.	43	1	7	1	1
• Mustard, Spicy Brown, 0.5 oz.	5	0	0	N/A	0
Oil, Blend, 0.5 oz.	130	14	0	0	0
Red Hot Original Sauce, 1 oz.	10	0	2	0	0
Red Wine Vinegar, 0.5 oz.	5	0	1	0	0
Kids Meals					
3" Ham & American Cheese, 6 oz.	262	9	32	2	15
• 3" Tuna, 6 oz.	277	11	30	2	14
• 3" Turkey, 5 oz.	187	2	31	2	10
Meats/Protein					
Bacon, 1 oz.	105	8	0	0	7
Cappacola, 1 oz.	18	1	0	N/A	3
Chicken Strips, 3 oz.	93	3	0	0	16
Corned Beef, 3 oz.	106	2	2	0	18
Egg, 2 oz.	45	3	2	0	4
Ham, 1 oz.	35	1	2	N/A	5
Meatballs, 5 oz.	220	15	10	3	11
Pastrami, 3 oz.	114	6	1	0	14
Pepperoni, 0.5 oz.	66	6	1	N/A	3
• Prosciuttini, 0.5 oz.	13	0	1	0	2
Roast Beef, 2 oz.	46	1	0	0	8
Salami, serving, 0.5 oz.	36	3	0	0	2
Seafood Salad, 3 oz.	92	4	10	1	4
Steak & Onion, 4 oz.	210	15	5	N/A	13
• Tuna, 3 oz.	241	18	0	0	16
Turkey, 1 oz.	30	0	1	N/A	5
Salads					
Chef Regular, 9 oz.	176	7	10	2	18
Chef Stacked, 10 oz.	209	8	12	2	23
Chicken Caesar Regular, 9 oz.	124	3	7	2	18
Chicken Caesar Stacked, 10 oz.	170	5	7	2	26
Chicken, 4 oz.	260	20	9	1	11
Cole Slaw, 4 oz.	160	9	20	2	1
• Garden Vegetable, 7 oz.	55	2	8	3	3
Macaroni, 5 oz.	330	22	28	2	5
Northwest Potato, 5 oz.	260	17	22	3	3
Potato, 5 oz.	230	12	28	3	3
Seafood, Regular, 9 oz.	122	4	17	3	6
Seafood, Stacked, 10 oz.	168	6	22	3	8
Sicilian Regular, 10 oz.	351	25	11	2	19
• Sicilian Stacked, 12 oz.	404	28	13	2	25
Tuna, Regular, 9 oz.	272	18	7	2	18
Tuna, Stacked, 10 oz.	393	28	7	2	26
Sandwiches/Wraps					
Blimpie Best, 6" Regular, 10 oz.	420	14	49	3	25
Blimpie Best, 6" Stacked, 12 oz.	478	16	51	3	32
BLT, 6" Regular, 8 oz.	346	11	46	3	15
BLT, 6" Stacked, 8 oz.	399	15	46	3	19
Buffalo Chicken, 6" Regular, 11 oz.	521	23	46	2	31

Blimpie (cont.)

	Cal	Fat	Cbs	Fbr	Prtn
Sandwiches/Wraps (cont.)					
Buffalo Chicken, 6" Stacked, 13 oz.	591	25	47	2	42
Chicken Teriyaki (LTO), 8 oz.	428	9	50	1	35
Ciabatta, Buffalo Chicken (LTO), 12 oz.	583	27	50	3	32
Ciabatta, Grilled Chicken Caesar, 11 oz.	617	24	63	3	34
Ciabatta, The Mediterranean, 10 oz.	447	8	65	3	26
Ciabatta, The Sicilian, 11 oz.	637	25	68	3	33
Ciabatta, The Tuscan, 10 oz.	600	23	65	3	29
Ciabatta, Turkey Italiano, 10 oz.	502	11	64	3	30
Club, 6" Regular, 10 oz.	386	10	49	3	25
Club, 6" Stacked, 11 oz.	419	10	51	3	29
Cuban, 6" Regular, 8 oz.	413	11	43	1	29
Cuban, 6" Stacked, 20 oz.	515	12	55	1	37
Garden Burger, White 6", 10 oz.	382	8	64	6	14
Grilled Chicken, 6" Regular, 10 oz.	334	6	46	3	29
Grilled Chicken, 6" Stacked, 11 oz.	380	7	46	3	32
Ham & Swiss, 6" Regular, 10 oz.	391	10	50	3	25
Ham & Swiss, 6" Stacked, 11 oz.	427	11	51	3	30
Ham, Salami & Cheese, 6" Regular, 10 oz.	443	16	49	3	25
Ham, Salami & Cheese, 6" Stacked, 11 oz.	498	20	50	3	29
Meatball 6" Regular, 9 oz.	509	24	50	4	24
Meatball 6" Stacked, 14 oz.	706	40	54	10	36
Pastrami Special, 6" Regular, 11 oz.	463	14	47	3	32
Pastrami Special, 6" Stacked, 12 oz.	524	16	47	3	40
Pastrami, 6" Regular, 11 oz.	454	17	48	3	30
Pastrami, 6" Stacked, 13 oz.	522	20	49	3	39
Reuben, 6" Regular, 10 oz.	571	24	54	3	34
Reuben, 6" Stacked, 11 oz.	624	25	54	3	43
Roast Beef & Cheese, 6" Regular, 11 oz.	408	11	47	3	31
Roast Beef & Cheese, 6" Stacked, 13 oz.	454	12	47	3	39
Roast Beef, Turkey & Cheese, 6" Regular, 11 oz.	571	30	48	3	27
Roast Beef, Turkey & Cheese, 6" Stacked, 12 oz.	609	31	48	3	34
• Seafood, 6" Regular, 10 oz.	333	7	56	4	13
Seafood, 6" Stacked, 12 oz.	379	9	61	4	15
Steak & Onion, 6" Regular, 7 oz.	499	24	45	1	26
Steak & Onion, 6" Stacked, 11 oz.	709	39	50	1	39
Tuna, 6" Regular, 10 oz.	483	21	46	3	25
Tuna, 6" Stacked, 12 oz.	603	30	46	3	33
Turkey & Cheese, 6" Regular, 11 oz.	393	10	49	3	26
Turkey & Cheese, 6" Stacked, 13 oz.	431	10	51	3	32
Turkey Italian 6" Regular, 11 oz.	459	17	47	3	26
Ultimate Club, 6" Regular, 6 oz.	395	13	43	1	26
Ultimate Club, 6" Stacked, 8 oz.	443	14	44	1	32
Veggie Supreme, 6", 10 oz.	553	28	48	3	29
Wrap, Chicken Caesar, Regular, 10 oz.	607	29	56	4	30
Wrap, Chicken Caesar, Stacked, 11 oz.	653	30	56	4	38
Wrap, Roast Beef & Cheddar, Regular, 12 oz.	684	36	59	6	32
Wrap, Roast Beef & Cheddar, Stacked, 14 oz.	729	37	59	6	41
Wrap, Southwestern Regular, 10 oz.	530	22	61	4	23
Wrap, Southwestern Stacked, 11 oz.	575	23	63	4	29
Wrap, Steak & Onion, Regular, 11 oz.	774	47	62	6	28
• Wrap, Steak & Onion, Stacked, 15 oz.	984	62	67	6	41
Wrap, Ultimate BLT, Regular, 12 oz.	703	39	60	6	29
Wrap, Ultimate BLT, Stacked, 13 oz.	755	42	61	6	36

RESTAURANTS & FAST-FOOD CHAINS

Blimpie (cont.)

	Cal	Fat	Cbs	Fbr	Prtn
Sandwiches/Wraps (cont.)					
Wrap, Zesty, Regular, 10 oz.	569	26	59	6	28
Wrap, Zesty, Stacked, 11 oz.	655	31	61	6	34
Soups					
Bean w/ Ham, 9 oz.	140	1	23	11	8
Beef Steak & Noodle, 9 oz.	120	3	14	0	8
Beef Stew, 9 oz.	170	4	18	2	17
Captain's Corn Chowder, 9 oz.	210	7	29	4	6
Cheddar Cauliflower, 9 oz.	130	6	15	5	4
Chicken & Dumpling, 9 oz.	170	5	19	3	11
Chicken Gumbo, 9 oz.	90	2	13	2	6
Chicken Noodle, 9 oz.	130	4	18	2	7
• Chicken w/ White & Wild Rice, 9 oz.	250	10	15	4	14
Cream of Broccoli w/ Cheese, 9 oz.	190	8	15	3	6
Cream of Potato, 9 oz.	190	9	24	3	5
French Onion, 9 oz.	80	4	11	1	2
Grande Chili w/ Bean & Beef, 9 oz.	250	9	30	18	18
Harvest Vegetable, 9 oz.	100	1	19	3	4
Italian Style Wedding, 9 oz.	130	4	17	0	7
Minestrone, 9 oz.	90	3	14	4	4
New England Clam Chowder, 9 oz.	170	3	28	2	7
Pasta Fagioli w/ Sausage, 9 oz.	150	5	22	4	7
Pilgrim Turkey Vegetables w/ Rice, 9 oz.	110	2	19	2	4
Seafood Gumbo, 9 oz.	100	2	16	2	4
Split Pea w/ Ham, 9 oz.	130	2	21	6	8
Tomato Basil w/ Raviolini, 9 oz.	110	1	22	0	4
• Yankee Pot Roast, 9 oz.	80	2	12	2	5
Toppings					
• Guacamole, 1 oz.	45	4	2	1	0
Lettuce, serving, 2 oz.	6	0	1	0	0
Olives, serving, 0.5 oz.	16	2	1	0	0
Onion, serving, 3 oz.	11	0	3	0	0
• Peppers, Hot Ring, 12 pcs., 1 oz.	0	0	1	0	0
Peppers, Jalapeño, 18 pcs., 1 oz.	10	0	2	0	0
Peppers, Red Roasted, serving, 2 oz.	11	0	2	0	0
Peppers, Sweet Strips, 6 pcs., 1 oz.	20	0	5	0	0
Tomato, serving, 2 oz.	7	0	2	0	0

Bob Evans Restaurants

	Cal	Fat	Cbs	Fbr	Prtn
Breakfast					
Bacon & Cheese Omelet, 10 oz.	825	66	6	1	49
Bacon & Cheese Omelet, egg beaters, 10 oz.	615	47	7	1	57
Blueberry Hotcake, 6 oz.	328	9	55	2	6
• Bob Evans Sausage Country Benedict, 14 oz.	936	66	40	0	44
Border Scramble Burrito, 21 oz.	110	64	80	12	51
Border Scramble Omelet, 15 oz.	756	58	15	3	42
Border Scramble Omelet, egg beaters, 15 oz.	517	37	16	3	48
Buttermilk Hotcake, 6 oz.	318	9	53	2	6
Cinnamon Hotcake, 6 oz.	417	15	66	2	6
Country Biscuit Breakfast, 10 oz.	659	45	40	1	24
Egg Beaters, 3 eggs, 7 oz.	173	12	3	0	28
Egg Beaters, omelet shell, 7 oz.	173	12	3	0	28
Farmer's Market Omelet, 15 oz.	778	60	13	2	42

Bob Evans Restaurants (cont.)	Cal	Fat	Cbs	Fbr	Prtn
Breakfast (cont.)					
Farmer's Market Omelet, egg beaters, 15 oz.	569	41	14	2	49
French toast, 2 oz.	131	2	13	1	3
Fruit & Yogurt Plate, 21 oz.	403	2	93	9	9
Garden Harvest Omelet, 14 oz.	654	50	13	2	33
Garden Harvest Omelet, egg beaters, 14 oz.	444	31	14	2	40
Grits, 7 oz.	178	7	28	2	3
Ham & Cheddar Omelet, 11 oz.	634	48	3	1	44
Ham & Cheddar Omelet, egg beaters, 11 oz.	426	29	5	1	51
Ham & Cheese Benedict, 15 oz.	826	52	44	0	44
• Hard Cooked Eggs, 2 oz.	60	4	1	0	6
Multigrain Hotcake, 6 oz.	322	10	52	3	7
Mush, 2 oz.	79	3	11	2	1
Oatmeal, 11 oz.	172	3	32	4	6
Omelet Shell, 7 oz.	383	31	2	0	20
Over Easy Egg, 2 oz.	101	8	1	0	7
Plain Crepe, 5 oz.	459	36	27	1	6
Pot Roast Hash, 13 oz.	652	39	34	4	38
Raspberry Crepes, 13 oz.	102	72	81	6	12
Roasted Apple Crepes, 13 oz.	102	73	76	4	11
Sausage & Cheddar Omelet, 10 oz.	741	61	3	1	42
Sausage & Cheddar Omelet, egg beaters, 10 oz.	502	40	4	1	48
Sausage & Egg Sandwich, breakfast, 7 oz.	577	37	32	1	27
Sausage Gravy, bowl, 10 oz.	268	17	21	0	7
Sausage Gravy, cup, 5 oz.	134	9	10	0	4
Sausage Link, 1 oz.	125	11	0	0	5
Sausage Patty, 2 oz.	141	11	0	0	8
Scrambled Eggs, 6 oz.	255	17	2	0	20
Smoked Ham, 4 oz.	87	2	2	0	14
Spinach, Bacon & Tom Country Benedict, 12 oz.	729	48	42	1	30
Stacked & Stuffed Crml Apple Crm Htcks, 24 oz.	128	50	192	5	26
Stacked & Stuffed Crml Banaca Pcn Htcks, 23 oz.	154	77	198	8	21
Stacked & Stuffed Cinnamon Crm Htcks, 16 oz.	103	49	136	4	14
Strawberry Yogurt, 5 oz.	145	1	28	1	6
Stuffed French Toast, plain, 10 oz.	599	20	53	3	11
Sunshine Skillet, 17 oz.	842	60	36	4	37
Sweet Cream Waffles, 10 oz.	598	12	100	3	15
Three Cheese Omelet, 9 oz.	645	52	4	1	35
Three Cheese Omelet, egg beaters, 9 oz.	435	34	5	1	43
Turkey Florentine Omelet, 14 oz.	736	54	6	1	49
Turkey Florentine Omelet, egg beaters, 14 oz.	496	33	7	2	55
Turkey Sausage (1 link), 11 oz.	329	13	35	3	30
Turkey Sausage, (1 link), 2 oz.	72	4	1	0	9
Western Omelet, 13 oz.	654	48	8	2	44
Western Omelet, egg beaters, 14 oz.	447	30	10	2	52
Breakfast Condiments					
Apple Butter, 1 oz.	33	0	8	0	0
Apple Jelly, 1 oz.	35	0	9	0	0
Butter Cups (1), 0.5 oz.	37	4	0	0	0
Captain Wafers Crackers, 1 oz.	65	2	8	0	1
• Diet Blackberry Jam, 0.5 oz.	5	0	2	0	0
Grape Jelly, 1 oz.	36	0	9	0	0
Half and Half Cups, 1 oz.	40	3	1	0	1
Honey, 1 oz.	43	0	12	0	0

(• = most healthy • = least healthy)   **RESTAURANTS & FAST-FOOD • 83**

RESTAURANTS & FAST-FOOD CHAINS

Bob Evans Restaurants (cont.)

	Cal	Fat	Cbs	Fbr	Prtn
Breakfast Condiments (cont.)					
• Margarine Buttery Taste Sprd Cp, 0.5 oz.	102	3	0	0	0
Condiments					
• Mayonnaise, 1 oz.	90	10	0	0	0
• Non-Dairy Creamer Cups, 1 oz.	19	1	1	0	0
Non-Dairy Creamer, 2 oz.	44	3	4	0	0
Orange Marmalade, 1 oz.	35	0	9	0	0
Saltine Crackers, 1 oz.	52	2	8	0	1
Sour Cream, 1 oz.	57	5	2	0	1
Desserts					
Apple Dumpling Pie a la mode, 13 oz.	769	37	105	4	7
Apple Dumpling Pie, 9 oz.	589	28	83	4	4
Coconut Cream Pie, 7 oz.	534	27	65	2	8
French Silk Pie, 6 oz.	693	47	62	2	6
NSA Apple Pie, 11 oz.	650	38	74	4	7
NSA Apple Pie, 7 oz.	491	30	55	4	4
• Pecan Pie, 8 oz.	909	46	127	2	9
Pumpkin Pie, 8 oz.	575	30	71	1	7
• Vanilla Ice Cream, 3 oz.	116	6	14	0	2
Dinner					
Bacon, 1 oz.	36	4	0	0	1
Chicken Parmesan, 23 oz.	611	29	45	4	40
Chicken Salad Plate, 21 oz.	763	46	72	11	22
Chicken Stir-Fry, 27 oz.	636	20	77	6	38
Chicken-N-Noodles Deep-Dish, 21 oz.	845	43	67	2	32
Country Fried Steak with Gravy, 8 oz.	553	38	37	0	19
Country Fried Steak, no gravy, 5 oz.	496	33	31	0	18
Fried Chicken Breast (1), 5 oz.	285	13	13	1	29
Fried Chicken Strips (1), 2 oz.	137	8	10	0	7
Fried Haddock, 7 oz.	363	18	27	0	24
Fruit Dish, 5 oz.	71	0	18	1	1
Garden Vegetable Alfredo, 27 oz.	713	45	59	11	22
Garden Vegetable Alfredo, chicken, 27 oz.	764	44	45	6	47
Garden Vegetable Alfredo, salmon, 30 oz.	888	52	46	6	59
Garden Vegetable Alfredo, shrimp, 28 oz.	814	52	45	6	41
Green Pepper and Onion Pasta, 22 oz.	372	19	43	6	9
Grilled Chkn Breast, garlic butter, 5 oz.	271	16	3	0	30
Grilled Chkn Breast, plain, 4 oz.	232	13	0	0	29
Grilled Chkn Breast, Wildfire Sauce, 6 oz.	325	13	22	2	29
• Grilled Chkn Tenders (1), 2 oz.	93	6	0	0	10
Italian Sausage and Pepper Pasta, 22 oz.	636	40	37	4	27
Meatloaf, 5 oz.	282	19	9	1	33
Open-Faced Roast Beef Dinner, 10 oz.	510	25	24	1	33
Pot Roast Beef Stew Deep-Dish, 20 oz.	763	39	65	2	26
Potato-Crusted Flounder, 5 oz.	254	17	8	0	17
Salmon Stir-Fry, 29 oz.	750	27	77	6	50
Salmon, garlic butter, 9 oz.	326	16	2	0	40
Salmon, plain, 8 oz.	287	13	0	0	40
Salmon, Wildfire Sauce, 9 oz.	380	13	22	2	40
Sausage Sandwich Patty, 3 oz.	222	17	0	0	13
Shrimp Stir-Fry, 29 oz.	686	28	77	6	32
Sirloin Steak, 5 oz.	403	27	3	0	33
Slow-Roasted Chicken-N-Noodles, 11 oz.	296	16	23	1	13
Slow-Roasted Pork Loin, 2 pieces, 12 oz.	519	30	30	0	57

Bob Evans Restaurants (cont.)

	Cal	Fat	Cbs	Fbr	Prtn
Dinner (cont.)					
Slow-Roasted Pork Loin, 7 oz.	324	20	18	0	29
• Slow-Roasted Pot Pie, 19 oz.	908	60	64	5	33
Slow-Roasted Turkey, 3 oz.	114	4	1	0	16
Steak Tips and Noodles, 28 oz.	822	43	44	3	66
Steak Tips Stir-Fry, 30 oz.	102	47	84	6	69
Steak Tips, 4 oz.	279	16	3	0	29
Turkey and Dressing Dinner, 14 oz.	551	28	33	1	37
Vegetable Stir-Fry, 27 oz.	505	15	86	9	13
Kids Menu					
Fruit & Yogurt Dippers, 13 oz.	275	2	61	5	7
Fudge Blast Sundae, 4 oz.	244	11	33	0	3
Grilled Cheese Sandwich, 3 oz.	290	16	26	1	9
Hotcakes, 9 oz.	501	17	79	2	9
Macaroni and Cheese, kids, 7 oz.	320	11	45	2	11
• Pasta, 8 oz.	113	5	15	1	3
Reese I'm Smiling Sundae, 5 oz.	330	17	41	1	5
• Smiley Face Potatoes, 6 oz.	524	31	57	3	5
Salads					
Avocado Ranch Dressing, dinner, 3 oz.	411	43	3	0	1
Bleu Cheese Dressing, dinner, 3 oz.	440	47	6	0	3
Buttermilk Ranch Dressing, dinner, 3 oz.	312	31	3	0	3
Chili and Cheese Taco Salad, 17 oz.	715	46	62	11	23
• Chili and Cheese Taco Salad, 24 oz.	928	62	73	16	30
Cobb Salad, 13 oz.	469	30	10	3	41
Cobb Salad, 20 oz.	698	46	14	5	60
Colonial Dressing, dinner, 3 oz.	464	41	23	0	0
Colonial Dressing, side, 2 oz.	232	21	12	0	0
Cranberry Pecan Chicken Salad, 14 oz.	801	47	49	5	31
• Cranberry Pecan Chicken Salad, 22 oz.	114	64	63	7	46
French Dressing, dinner, 3 oz.	439	41	19	0	0
French Dressing, side, 2 oz.	219	21	10	0	0
Garden Salad, 5 oz.	137	4	22	3	4
Heritage Chef Salad, 11 oz.	259	15	9	3	23
Heritage Chef Salad, 17 oz.	456	26	14	5	41
Honey Mustard Dressing, dinner, 3 oz.	384	36	16	0	0
Honey Mustard Dressing, side, 2 oz.	192	18	8	0	0
Hot Bacon Dressing, dinner, 3 oz.	213	6	35	0	0
Hot Bacon Dressing, side, 2 oz.	106	3	18	0	0
Lite Ranch Dressing, dinner, 3 oz.	206	20	5	1	2
Lite Ranch Dressing, side, 2 oz.	103	10	2	0	1
Specialty Side Salad, 6 oz.	171	9	14	2	9
Spinach Salad, 10 oz.	504	35	11	4	40
Spinach Salad, 13 oz.	608	40	13	5	52
Sweet Italian Dressing, dinner, 3 oz.	346	21	16	0	0
Sweet Italian Dressing, side, 2 oz.	173	10	8	0	0
Swiss Bacon Dressing, dinner, 3 oz.	454	51	3	0	3
Swiss Bacon Dressing, side, 2 oz.	227	26	1	0	1
Thousand Island Dressing, dinner, 3 oz.	425	40	14	0	0
Thousand Island Dressing, side, 2 oz.	213	20	7	0	0
Vinegar & Oil Dressing, dinner, 3 oz.	54	6	0	0	0
Vinegar & Oil Dressing, side, 2 oz.	27	3	0	0	0
Wildfire Chicken Salad, fried, 14 oz.	631	30	68	8	26
Wildfire Chicken Salad, fried, 19 oz.	789	38	81	10	34

(• = most healthy • = least healthy)   **RESTAURANTS & FAST-FOOD • 85**

RESTAURANTS & FAST-FOOD CHAINS

Bob Evans Restaurants (cont.)	Cal	Fat	Cbs	Fbr	Prtn
Salads (cont.)					
Wildfire Chicken Salad, grilled, 14 oz.	541	26	49	7	31
Wildfire Chicken Salad, grilled, 20 oz.	654	32	53	9	43
Wildfire Ranch Dressing, dinner, 3 oz.	241	19	18	0	1
Wildfire Ranch Dressing, side, 2 oz.	121	9	9	0	1
Sandwiches					
Bacon Cheeseburger, 8 oz.	716	48	32	3	38
Bob's BLT & E, 9 oz.	645	38	27	2	19
Cheeseburger, 8 oz.	645	41	32	3	37
Chicken Salad Sandwich, 7 oz.	649	38	53	6	22
Chicken Salad Sandwich, half, 5 oz.	331	19	28	3	12
Double Sausage Sandwich, 9 oz.	716	46	31	1	34
Fried Chicken Club Sandwich, 9 oz.	660	35	44	3	40
Fried Chicken Sandwich, plain, 7 oz.	503	21	43	2	34
Fried Haddock Sandwich, 11 oz.	786	34	78	2	40
Grilled Cheese Sandwich, 5 oz.	396	16	25	2	9
Grilled Chicken Club Sandwich, 9 oz.	606	35	31	2	41
Grilled Chicken Sandwich, plain, 6 oz.	399	15	30	1	35
Hamburger Patty, 5 oz.	321	24	1	1	26
Hamburger, plain, 7 oz.	539	32	31	3	31
Homemade Meat Loaf Knife & Fork Sand, 16 oz.	716	38	41	3	28
Knife & Fork Meatloaf Sandwich, 16 oz.	716	38	41	3	28
Knife & Fork Pork Loin Sandwich, 17 oz.	844	48	58	3	36
Knife & Fork Turkey Sandwich, 15 oz.	696	36	46	2	24
Mini Cheeseburgers, 3 oz.	306	19	21	1	12
Pot Roast Sandwich, 9 oz.	610	28	58	3	31
Pot Roast Sandwich, half, 6 oz.	390	19	31	2	23
• Ranch Steak Burger, 11 oz.	937	68	35	3	42
Sausage Sandwich Patty, 6 oz.	494	29	31	1	21
Slow Roasted Pork Loin Knife & Fork Sand, 17 oz.	844	48	58	3	36
Turkey Bacon Melt, 9 oz.	617	29	53	3	33
• Turkey Bacon Melt, half, 4 oz.	306	14	26	1	16
Sauces & Toppings					
American Cheese, 1 oz.	53	4	1	0	3
Apple Butter, 1 oz.	33	0	8	0	0
Apple Jelly, 1 oz.	35	0	9	0	0
Beef Gravy, 2 oz.	22	1	3	0	1
Bleu Cheese, 1 oz.	97	8	0	0	6
Brown Sugar, 1 oz.	79	0	20	0	0
Butter Cups, 0.5 oz.	37	4	0	0	0
Chicken-Roasted Gravy, 2 oz.	53	4	3	0	1
Citrus Stir-Fry Sauce, 2 oz.	51	0	12	0	1
Country Gravy, 3 oz.	56	4	6	0	0
Cranberries, 1 oz.	68	0	17	1	0
Diet Blackberry Jam, 0.5 oz.	5	0	2	0	0
Garlic Butter, 1 oz.	40	3	2	0	0
Grape Jelly, 1 oz.	36	0	9	0	0
Hollandaise, 2 oz.	50	3	5	0	1
Honey Roasted Pecans, 1 oz.	142	14	6	2	2
Honey, 1 oz.	43	0	12	0	0
• Lettuce & Tomato, 1 oz.	4	0	1	0	0
Lettuce, Tomato and Pickle, 1 oz.	6	0	1	0	0
Margarine Buttery Taste Sprd Cup, 0.5 oz.	102	3	0	0	0
Marinara, 3 oz.	35	1	5	1	1

Bob Evans Restaurants (cont.)	Cal	Fat	Cbs	Fbr	Prtn
Sauces & Toppings (cont.)					
Mayonnaise, 1 oz.	90	10	0	0	0
Milk, 2 oz.	28	1	3	0	2
Monterey Jack Cheese, 1 oz.	76	6	0	0	4
Non-Dairy Creamer Cups (1), 1 oz.	19	1	1	0	0
Non-Dairy Creamer, 2 oz.	44	3	4	0	0
Orange Marmalade, 1 oz.	35	0	9	0	0
• Pancake Syrup, 3 oz.	213	0	55	0	0
Pork-Roasted Gravy, 2 oz.	63	5	3	0	1
Raisins, 1 oz.	70	0	17	1	1
Ranchero Picante, 1 oz.	38	0	0	0	7
Raspberry, 3 oz.	108	0	27	4	1
Roasted-Apple Topping, 3 oz.	102	1	24	1	0
Saltine Crackers, 1 oz.	52	2	8	0	1
Sour Cream, 1 oz.	57	5	2	0	1
Strawberry Jam, 1 oz.	36	0	9	0	0
Sugar Free Pancake Syrup, 3 oz.	39	0	10	0	0
Tarter Sauce, 1 oz.	166	18	1	0	0
Whipped Topping, 1 oz.	92	7	7	0	0
Wildfire Sauce, 2 oz.	94	0	22	2	0
Seniors					
Chicken Parmesan, 17 oz.	522	26	33	3	38
Chicken Stir-Fry, 16 oz.	368	13	44	5	21
Garden Vegetable Alfredo, 14 oz.	363	23	29	5	11
Garden Vegetable Alfredo, chicken, 16 oz.	452	26	29	5	26
Garden Vegetable Alfredo, shrimp, 17 oz.	537	37	29	5	22
Green Pepper and Onion Pasta, 14 oz.	259	14	28	4	6
Italian Sausage and Pepper Pasta, 14 oz.	523	36	21	3	24
Shrimp Stir-Fry, 17 oz.	456	24	44	5	18
• Steak Tip Stir-Fry, 18 oz.	560	26	48	5	37
Steak Tips and Noodles, 15 oz.	422	22	23	2	33
Turkey and Dressing Dinner, 11 oz.	438	23	33	1	21
• Vegetable Stir-Fry, 14 oz.	281	10	44	5	7
Sides					
Applesauce, 4 oz.	83	0	21	2	0
Baked Potato, 11 oz.	207	0	54	6	8
Bread and Celery Dressing, 6 oz.	272	15	29	1	5
Broccoli Florets, 4 oz.	32	0	6	3	3
Caramelized Onions, 2 oz.	38	2	6	1	1
Coleslaw, 4 oz.	209	14	19	2	1
Corn, 5 oz.	169	8	25	3	4
Cottage Cheese, 4 oz.	115	5	4	0	14
Cranberry Relish, 1 oz.	57	0	13	1	0
• Dill Pickle Slices, 1 oz.	1	0	0	0	0
French Fries, 5 oz.	354	15	51	1	5
Fruit Cup, 5 oz.	150	1	38	4	2
Garden Vegetables, 6 oz.	121	7	14	5	3
Glazed Carrots, 4 oz.	83	3	14	4	1
Green Beans, 6 oz.	79	3	9	3	5
Grilled Mushrooms, 8 oz.	152	12	10	5	4
Home Fries, 5 oz.	186	7	27	3	3
• Loaded Baked Potato, 12 oz.	373	13	56	7	19
Mashed Potatoes, 6 oz.	205	7	17	1	3
Rice Pilaf, 6 oz.	129	4	20	1	2

(•= most healthy •= least healthy) **RESTAURANTS & FAST-FOOD • 87**

RESTAURANTS & FAST-FOOD CHAINS

Bob Evans Restaurants (cont.)	Cal	Fat	Cbs	Fbr	Prtn
Sides (cont.)					
Tomato Slice, 1 oz.	4	0	1	0	0
Soups					
Bean Soup, bowl, 10 oz.	205	5	27	7	14
Bean Soup, cup, 7 oz.	144	3	19	5	10
Cheddar Baked Potato Soup, bowl, 14 oz.	371	25	24	2	13
Cheddar Baked Potato Soup, cup, 11 oz.	294	20	19	1	10
• Sausage Chili, bowl, 11 oz.	376	24	26	10	22
Sausage Chili, cup, 8 oz.	268	17	18	7	16
Vegetable Beef Soup, bowl, 10 oz.	193	7	25	4	9
• Vegetable Beef Soup, cup, 7 oz.	135	5	17	3	6

Bojangles	Cal	Fat	Cbs	Fbr	Prtn
Biscuit Sandwiches					
Bacon	290	17	26	1	8
Bacon, Egg & Cheese	550	42	27	1	17
• Biscuit (plain)	243	12	29	2	4
Cajun Filet	454	21	46	1	20
Country Ham	270	15	26	1	9
Egg	400	30	26	1	8
Sausage	350	23	26	1	9
Smoked Sausage	380	26	27	1	10
• Steak	649	49	37	1	14
Cajun Spiced Chicken					
Breast	278	17	12	1	18
• Leg	264	16	11	1	19
Thigh	310	23	11	1	15
• Wing	355	25	11	1	21
Individual Fixin'					
Botato Rounds	235	11	31	3	3
Cajun Pintos	110	0	18	6	6
Corn on the Cob	140	2	34	2	5
Dirty Rice	166	6	24	1	5
• Green Beans	25	0	5	2	0
Macaroni & Cheese	198	14	12	1	7
Marinated Cole Slaw	136	3	26	3	1
Potatoes w/o gravy	80	1	16	1	2
• Seasoned Fries	344	19	39	4	5
Sandwiches					
Cajun Filet	337	11	41	3	22
• Cajun Filet w/mayo	437	22	41	3	22
• Grilled Filet	235	5	25	2	23
Grilled Filet w/mayo	335	16	25	2	23
Snacks					
Buffalo Bites	180	5	5	0	27
Chicken Supremes	337	16	26	1	21
Southern Style Chicken					
Breast	261	16	12	1	16
• Leg	254	15	11	1	19
Thigh	308	21	14	1	16
• Wing	337	21	19	1	17
Sweet Biscuits					
Bo Berry™	220	10	29	1	3
Cinnamon	320	18	37	1	4

RESTAURANTS & FAST-FOOD CHAINS

Boston Market	Cal	Fat	Cbs	Fbr	Prtn
Desserts					
Apple Pie (slice), 6 oz.	420	20	56	2	3
• Chocolate Cake, 5 oz.	600	32	75	2	5
Chocolate Chip Fudge Brownie, 5 oz.	580	23	81	3	9
• Cornbread, 2 oz.	180	5	31	0	4
Nestle Toll House Chocolate Chip Cookie, 3 oz.	370	19	49	2	4
Family Meals					
Award Winning Sirloin, 5 oz.	290	15	0	0	39
• Boneless Holiday Turkey Breast, 5 oz.	180	3	0	0	38
• Meatloaf, 8 oz.	480	33	23	2	29
Roasted Turkey, 5 oz.	180	3	0	0	38
Rotisserie Chicken, 6 oz.	290	14	4	0	39
Spiral Sliced Holiday Ham, 8 oz.	450	26	13	0	40
Whole Holiday Turkey, 8 oz.	310	18	0	0	40
Individual Meals					
1 Thigh & 1 Drumstick, 6 oz.	300	17	6	0	32
1/4 White Rotisserie Chicken, 6 oz.	290	11	4	0	45
1/4 White Rotisserie Chicken, No Skin, 6 oz.	210	2	6	0	42
3 Piece Dark (2 thighs & 1 drumstick), 9 oz.	510	30	8	0	52
3 Piece Dark Individual Meal, 7 oz.	380	19	7	0	45
3 Piece Dark Skinless (2 thighs & drumstick), 7 oz.	310	13	6	0	42
3 Piece Dark Skinless (thigh & 2 drumsticks), 6 oz.	240	8	7	0	37
Award Winning Roasted Sirloin, 5 oz.	290	15	0	0	39
Half Rotisserie Chicken, 348 g	590	27	10	0	77
Meatloaf, 8 oz.	480	33	23	2	29
• Pastry Top Chicken Pot Pie, 15 oz.	780	47	60	4	29
• Roasted Turkey, 5 oz.	180	3	0	0	38
Salads					
• Caesar Salad Entree, 7 oz.	500	45	12	3	13
Dressing, 3 oz.	360	38	4	1	2
Lite Ranch Dressing, 2 oz.	70	4	8	0	1
Roasted Sirloin, 3 oz.	160	6	0	0	26
Roasted Turkey, 3 oz.	140	6	1	0	19
Rotisserie Chicken, 5 oz.	160	1	3	0	35
w/o dressing, 7 oz.	140	8	8	2	11
• Market Chopped Salad, 18 oz.	580	48	30	9	10
Dressing, 3 oz.	360	39	2	0	0
Lite Ranch Dressing, 2 oz.	70	4	8	0	1
Roasted Sirloin, 3 oz.	160	6	0	0	26
Roasted Turkey, 3 oz.	140	6	1	0	19
Rotisserie Chicken, 5 oz.	160	1	3	0	35
w/o dressing, 17 oz.	210	9	28	9	10
Sandwiches					
Beef Au jus, 4 oz.	20	0	4	0	1
Boston Chicken Carver, 11 oz.	700	29	68	3	44
Boston Meatloaf Carver, 15 oz.	940	45	96	6	49
• Boston Sirloin Dip Carver, 13 oz.	1000	51	70	3	67
Boston Turkey Carver, 14 oz.	770	27	68	3	66
Boston Turkey Dip Carver, 16 oz.	770	27	67	3	66
• Half Boston Chicken Carver, 7 oz.	340	15	29	1	24
Half Boston Sirloin Dip Carver, 7 oz.	500	25	35	1	33
Half Boston Turkey Carver, 7 oz.	390	14	34	2	33
Half Turkey Dip Carver, 7 oz.	380	14	33	1	33
Poultry Au Jus, 4 oz.	15	1	4	0	1

(•= most healthy •= least healthy)   **RESTAURANTS & FAST-FOOD • 89**

RESTAURANTS & FAST-FOOD CHAINS

Boston Market (cont.)

	Cal	Fat	Cbs	Fbr	Prtn
Soups & Sides					
Beef Gravy, 3 oz.	35	2	4	0	1
Broccoli with Garlic Butter, 4 oz.	80	6	6	3	3
Butternut Squash R, 5 oz.	140	5	25	2	2
Caesar Salad Dressing, 3 oz.	360	38	4	1	2
• Caesar Side Salad w/o Dressing, 3 oz.	40	2	3	1	3
Caesar Side Salad, 5 oz.	400	40	7	2	5
Chicken Noodle Soup, 6 oz.	170	5	17	1	13
Chicken Tortilla Soup with toppings, 6 oz.	340	22	24	1	12
Chicken Tortilla Soup w/o toppings, 6 oz.	90	5	7	1	5
Cinnamon Apples, 5 oz.	210	3	47	3	0
Cranberry Walnut Relish LF, 3 oz.	140	2	30	2	1
Creamed Spinach, 7 oz.	280	23	12	4	9
Fresh Steamed Vegetables LF, 5 oz.	60	2	8	3	2
Fresh Vegetable Stuffing, 5 oz.	190	8	25	2	3
Garden Fresh Coleslaw, 4 oz.	170	9	21	2	2
Garlic Dill New Potatoes LF, 5 oz.	140	3	24	3	3
Green Bean Casserole, 6 oz.	60	2	9	2	2
Green Beans, 3 oz.	60	4	7	3	2
Macaroni and Cheese, 8 oz.	330	12	39	1	14
Market Chopped Salad Dressing, 3 oz.	360	39	2	0	0
Market Chopped Side Salad w/o Dressing, 5 oz.	80	4	10	3	3
Market Chopped Side Salad, 7 oz.	440	43	12	3	4
Mashed Potatoes, 8 oz.	270	11	36	4	5
Poultry Gravy, 4 oz.	15	1	4	0	1
Seasonal Fresh Fruit Salad LF, 5 oz.	60	0	15	1	1
Spinach Artichoke Dip, 2 oz.	100	8	3	1	3
Spinach with Garlic Butter Sauce, 6 oz.	130	9	9	5	5
Squash Casserole, 8 oz.	320	24	21	3	9
Sweet Corn, 6 oz.	170	4	37	2	6
• Sweet Potato Casserole, 7 oz.	460	17	77	3	4

Brown's Chicken & Pasta

	Cal	Fat	Cbs	Fbr	Prtn
Main Chicken Items					
• Chicken breast	284	15	12	N/A	26
Chicken legs	287	16	9	N/A	26
Chicken thigh	355	24	13	N/A	21
• Chicken wing	385	25	17	N/A	23
Miscellaneous Items					
• Chicken Gizzards	387	N/A	26	N/A	24
Chicken Livers	341	N/A	20	N/A	23
• Mushrooms	289	N/A	30	N/A	6
Pasta Items					
• Mostaccioli (in Marinara)	792	10	146	N/A	24
• Spaghetti (in Marinara)	792	10	146	N/A	24
Premium Side Items					
• Cheezy Potatoes, 12 oz.	188	11	16	N/A	7
• Mostaccioli (in Marinara)	792	10	146	N/A	24
Spaghetti (in Marinara)	792	10	146	N/A	24
Regular Side Items					
Cole slaw	131	10	9	N/A	2
• Corn fritters	415	25	42	N/A	5
• Potato salad	95	4	13	N/A	2

Bruegger's	Cal	Fat	Cbs	Fbr	Prtn
Alternative Breads					
• Bruegger's Bagel Bowl, Per Container	720	9	133	8	30
• Single Ciabatta, 113 g	250	3	48	2	9
Wheat Wrap, 4 oz.	310	8	53	4	10
Bagels					
Asiago Parmesan, 123 g	330	4	62	4	14
Baked Apple Bagel, 113 g	310	2	65	4	10
Blueberry, 120 g	330	2	67	4	11
Chocolate Chip, 121 g	350	5	64	4	12
Cinnamon Raisin, 123 g	330	2	69	4	11
Cinnamon Sugar, 129 g	350	2	73	6	12
Cranberry Orange, 121 g	330	2	68	4	11
Everything, 123 g	320	2	64	4	12
Fortified, 130 g	350	4	68	6	12
Garlic, 122 g	320	2	65	4	12
Honey Grain, 124 g	330	3	65	5	13
Jalapeño, 121 g	320	2	64	4	12
Onion, 122 g	320	2	64	4	12
Plain, 121 g	320	2	64	4	12
Poppy, 122 g	320	3	64	4	12
Pretzel Bagel, 123 g	320	2	64	4	12
Pumpernickel, 124 g	330	3	67	5	12
• Pumpkin Bagel, 120 g	310	2	63	4	11
Rosemary Olive Oil, 123 g	350	7	64	4	12
Salt, 123 g	320	2	64	4	12
Sesame, 130 g	360	3	68	4	13
Sourdough, 134 g	340	2	68	4	13
Sun Dried Tomato, 121 g	320	2	64	4	12
• Whole Wheat, 136 g	390	6	73	9	16
Breakfast Sandwich					
Classic Wrap with Bacon, 269 g	520	45	52	4	36
Classic Wrap with Ham, 312 g	510	41	54	4	40
Classic Wrap with Sausage, 312 g	660	60	52	4	38
Denver, 272 g	460	18	74	5	30
• Egg & cheese, 208 g	420	18	71	4	23
Egg, cheese & bacon, 210 g	460	23	65	4	28
Egg, cheese & ham, 244 g	460	18	73	4	31
Egg, cheese & sausage, 265 g	640	38	72	5	32
Rio Grande Wrap with Bacon, 284 g	560	49	55	4	34
Rio Grande Wrap with Ham, 298 g	630	34	55	4	31
Rio Grande Wrap with Sausage, 284 g	510	47	53	4	27
• Western Wheat Softwich, 308 g	820	58	76	8	30
Bruegger's Salmon					
Smoked Salmon, 2 oz.	90	3	1	0	15
Cream Cheese					
Bacon Scallion, 43 g	140	12	5	0	3
Cucumber Dill, 43 g	140	13	3	0	3
Garden Veggie Light, 43 g	90	6	3	0	6
Garden Veggie, 43 g	130	11	5	1	3
Herb & Garlic Light, 43 g	100	6	4	0	6
• Honey Walnut, 43 g	150	12	8	1	3
Jalapeño, 43 g	140	13	4	0	3
Olive Pimento, 43 g	140	13	3	0	3
Onion and Chive, 43 g	140	13	3	0	3

RESTAURANTS & FAST-FOOD CHAINS

Bruegger's (cont.)

	Cal	Fat	Cbs	Fbr	Prtn
Cream Cheese (cont.)					
Plain Light, 43 g	100	6	4	1	3
Plain, 43 g	130	11	6	1	3
Pumpkin, 43 g	120	11	4	0	3
• Smoked Salmon, 2 oz.	90	3	1	0	15
Strawberry, 43 g	140	13	4	0	3
Wildberry, 43 g	140	12	5	0	3
Deli Sandwiches					
BLT with Mayo, 213 g	570	23	72	5	20
Chicken Breast, 318 g	660	11	87	5	47
Chicken Salad, 268 g	630	26	73	5	25
Ham, 275 g	460	7	76	5	27
• Hummus, 54 g	110	6	10	0	5
• Roast Beef w/ Mayo, Lettuce & Tomato, 289 g	730	39	71	5	30
Tuna Salad, 247 g	620	27	73	5	23
Turkey, 261 g	510	14	70	5	26
Deli Softwiches					
BLT with Mayo, 218 g	600	25	73	5	22
Chicken Breast, 325 g	630	11	81	5	47
Chicken Salad, 316 g	670	27	76	5	32
• Ham, 302 g	510	6	85	5	29
Hummus, 288 g	540	13	85	11	20
• Roast Beef w/ Mayo, Lettuce & Tomato, 325 g	750	40	72	5	33
Roasted Tkey w/ Chz, Let, Tom & Mayo, 302 g	550	15	74	5	32
Tuna Salad, 288 g	720	34	76	5	26
Desserts					
Chocolate Chunk Brownies, 73 g	330	18	40	2	4
Chocolate Chunk Cookie, 113 g	500	22	71	3	5
Lemon Pound Cake, 94 g	320	13	48	1	5
Luscious Lemon Bars, 78 g	300	16	36	0	3
• Marshmallow Chew, 69 g	250	6	55	0	2
Oatmeal Raisin Cookie, 113 g	460	19	71	3	5
Oreo® Dream Bar, 107 g	470	28	49	2	5
Peanut Butter Cookie, 113 g	480	23	63	2	8
Pecan Chocolate Chunks, 34 g	310	19	32	1	3
Raspberry Sammies, 73 g	340	16	44	1	3
• Seven Layer Bar, 133 g	650	43	58	5	10
Toffee Almond Bars, 89 g	400	19	53	1	4
Triple Chocolate Chunk Cookie, 121 g	560	28	71	3	6
White Choco Macadamia Cookie, 121 g	580	31	70	1	6
Iced Coffee					
Raspberries and Cream, 20 fl.oz.	210	10	27	0	3
Muffins					
• Blueberry Muffin, 43 g	450	19	64	3	8
• Chocolate Muffin, 128 g	460	24	57	3	6
Salad Wraps					
• Tossed Chicken Caesar, 354 g	660	28	73	5	36
Tossed Mandarin Medley, 328 g	630	25	87	7	17
• Tossed Sesame Chicken, 338 g	77	36	80	5	31
Softwiches (Square Bagels)					
Asiago, 130 g	360	5	66	4	15
BLT, 218 g	600	25	73	5	22
Chicken Breast, 325 g	630	11	81	5	47
• Everything, 123 g	320	2	64	4	12

RESTAURANTS & FAST-FOOD CHAINS

Bruegger's (cont.)

	Cal	Fat	Cbs	Fbr	Prtn
Softwiches (Square Bagels) (cont.)					
Garden Veggie, 285 g	380	3	76	6	15
Ham, 285 g	380	3	76	6	15
Hummus, 285 g	380	3	76	6	15
Plain, 5 oz.	350	2	70	4	13
Roast Beef, 285 g	380	3	76	6	15
Sesame, 5 oz.	360	3	68	4	13
• Tuna Salad, 288 g	720	34	76	5	26
Whole Wheat, 130 g	350	4	70	7	13
Soups					
Beef Chili, 8 oz.	190	8	18	6	10
Butternut Squash, 285 g	380	3	76	6	15
Chicken Spaetzle Soup, 8 oz.	200	12	15	1	8
Chicken Tortilla Soup, 8 oz.	140	8	11	1	6
Chicken Wild Rice Soup, 285 g	380	3	76	6	15
Fire Roasted Tomato Soup, 285 g	380	3	76	6	15
• Four Cheese & Broccoli Soup, 285 g	380	3	76	6	15
New England Clam Chowder, 8 oz.	230	14	16	1	12
• Steak and Onion Soup, 8 oz.	90	4	11	1	4
Speciality Bagel Sandwiches					
Chicken Fajita, 311 g	530	11	81	6	30
Cranberry Gobbler, 274 g	620	21	78	5	32
Cuban Chicken, 319 g	680	25	74	4	44
• Garden Veggie, 285 g	380	3	76	6	15
Herby Turkey, 259 g	560	14	78	5	30
Leonardo Da Veggie, 244 g	480	12	74	5	21
Radishy Roast Beef, 269 g	560	18	73	5	35
• Roadhouse Chicken, 315 g	710	19	84	4	50
Santa Fe Turkey, 294 g	490	9	75	5	30
Smoked Salmon, 253 g	490	10	74	5	28
Supreme Club, 250 g	470	9	72	5	28
Specialty Softwiches					
Chicken Fajita, 311 g	570	10	81	6	39
Cranberry Gobbler, 312 g	730	28	80	5	40
• Cuban Chicken, 376 g	810	32	77	4	56
Garden Veggie, 285 g	380	3	76	6	15
Herby Turkey, 276 g	580	14	80	5	3
Leonardo Da Veggie, 329 g	550	15	79	6	25
Mediterranean Softwich, 303 g	790	33	90	11	30
Radishy Roast Beef, 310 g	670	26	75	5	43
Roadhouse Chicken, 296 g	670	19	74	4	50
Santa Fe Turkey, 328 g	520	10	78	5	33
Smoked Salmon, 282 g	520	11	76	5	30
• Supreme Club, 219 g	270	8	21	11	31
Thai Peanut Chicken Softwich, 332 g	590	12	82	5	36
Tossed Salads					
• Caesar, 234 g	270	17	22	2	9
Chicken Caesar, 319 g	370	20	23	2	27
Mandarin Medley, 286 g	340	17	36	4	8
• Sesame Chicken, 298 g	480	28	30	2	22

Buca di Beppo

	Cal	Fat	Cbs	Fbr	Prtn
Entrees					
• Chicken Marsala, 1/6 of large serving	380	24	11	1	21

(• = most healthy • = least healthy)   **RESTAURANTS & FAST-FOOD • 93**

RESTAURANTS & FAST-FOOD CHAINS

Buca di Beppo (cont.)

	Cal	Fat	Cbs	Fbr	Prtn
Entrees (cont.)					
• Fresh Salmon, 1/2 of small serving	465	26	26	4	31
Green Beans, 1/6 of large serving	70	5	7	3	1
Pasta					
Linguini Frutti Di Mare, 1/4 of sm serving	360	22	18	1	25
• Penne Campofiore, 1/4 of sm serving	380	19	41	5	14
• Spaghetti with Marinara Sauce, 1/4 of sm serving	260	2	50	4	9
Pizza					
Pizza Margherita, Small 2 slices	325	12	26	7	28
Salad					
Apple Gorgonzola Salad, 1/4 of sm serving	210	14	17	4	7
Warm Tomato and Spinach Salad, 1/4 of sm serving	90	6	7	2	3

Buck's Pizza

	Cal	Fat	Cbs	Fbr	Prtn
14 Canadian Bacon Pizza, 1 sl.	313	9	47	3	13
• 14 Cheese Pizza, 1 sl.	296	8	47	3	10
14 Pepperoni Pizza, 1 sl.	361	14	47	3	13
14 Sausage Pizza, 1 sl.	362	14	47	3	14
16 Cheese Pizza, 1 sl.	309	8	48	3	10
16 Pepperoni Pizza, 1 sl.	374	14	48	3	13
• 16 Sausage Pizza, 1 sl.	377	15	49	3	14

Burger King

	Cal	Fat	Cbs	Fbr	Prtn
Breakfast					
Bacon, Egg & Cheese Biscuit, 146 g	410	25	31	1	16
Breakfast Syrup, 28 g	80	0	21	0	15
Cini-minis, 108 g	390	18	51	2	7
Croissan'wich® Bcn, Egg & Chz, 122 g	340	20	26	1	15
Egg & Cheese, 115 g	300	17	26	1	12
Ham, Egg & Cheese, 149 g	340	18	26	1	18
Sausage & Cheese, 106 g	370	25	23	1	14
Sausage, Egg & Cheese, 159 g	470	32	26	1	19
Double Croissan'wich™ w/Bcn, Egg, & Chz, 142 g	430	27	27	1	21
w/ Ham, Bcn, Egg, & Chz, 169 g	420	24	27	1	24
w/ Ham, Egg, & Cheese, 196 g	420	23	27	1	27
w/ Ham, Sausage, Egg, & Chz, 206 g	550	37	27	1	28
w/ Sausage, Bacon, Egg, & Chz, 179 g	550	39	27	1	25
w/ Sausage, Egg, & Cheese, 215 g	680	51	26	1	29
• Enormous Omelet Sandwich, 266 g	730	45	44	2	37
French Toast Kid's Meal (With Syrup), 494 g	680	24	100	3	0
• French Toast Sticks (3 Piece), 65 g	240	13	26	1	4
French Toast Sticks (5 Piece), 109 g	390	22	43	2	7
Grape Jam, 12 g	30	0	7	0	0
Ham Omelet Sandwich, 139 g	330	14	35	1	16
Ham, Egg, & Cheese Biscuit, 156 g	390	22	31	1	16
Hash Browns - Large, 202 g	620	40	60	6	5
Hash Browns - Medium, 140 g	430	28	42	4	4
Hash Browns - Small, 84 g	260	17	25	2	2
Sausage Biscuit, 118 g	390	26	28	1	12
Sausage, Egg, & Cheese Biscuit, 183 g	530	37	31	1	20
Strawberry Jam, 12 g	30	0	7	0	0
Vanilla Icing (For Cini-minis), 28 g	110	3	21	0	0
Desserts					
• Dutch Apple Pie, 108 g	300	13	45	1	2

RESTAURANTS & FAST-FOOD CHAINS

Burger King (cont.)

	Cal	Fat	Cbs	Fbr	Prtn
Desserts (cont.)					
• Hershey®'s Sundae Pie, 79 g	310	19	32	1	3
Fire-grilled Burgers					
Bk™ Double Stacker, 190 g	610	39	32	1	34
• Bk™ Quad Stacker, 311 g	1000	68	34	1	62
• Bk™ Triple Stacker, 250 g	800	54	33	1	48
Cheeseburger, 133 g	330	16	31	1	17
Double Cheeseburger, 189 g	500	29	31	1	30
Double Hamburger, 164 g	410	21	30	1	25
• Hamburger, 121 g	290	12	30	1	15
The Angus Steak Burger, 273 g	640	33	55	3	33
Salad Dressings & Toppings & Condiments					
Garlic Parmesan Croutons, 14 g	60	2	9	0	1
Ken's® Creamy Caesar Dressing, 2 oz.	210	21	4	0	3
Ken's® Fat Free Ranch Dressing, 2 oz.	60	0	15	2	0
• Ken's® Honey Mustard Dressing, 2 oz.	270	23	15	0	1
Ken's® Light Italian Dressing, 2 oz.	120	11	5	0	0
Ken's® Ranch Dressing, 2 oz.	190	20	2	0	1
• Ketchup (Packet), 10 g	10	0	3	0	0
Mayonnaise (Packet), 12 g	80	9	1	0	0
Salads					
Garden Salad (No Chicken), 184 g	90	5	7	3	5
• Side Garden Salad, 98 g	15	0	3	1	1
• Tendercrisp™ Chkn Garden Salad, 306 g	410	22	26	5	29
Tendergrill™ Chkn Garden Salad, 292 g	240	9	8	4	33
Shakes, Milk, & Iced Coffee					
• Chocolate Milk Shake - Medium, 447 g	690	20	114	2	11
• Mocha Bk Joe® Iced Coffee, 452 g	380	10	66	1	6
Oreo® Sundae Shake - Chocolate - Med, 369 g	680	24	105	2	9
Oreo® Sundae Shake - Strawberry - Med, 367 g	660	23	103	1	9
Oreo® Sundae Shake - Vanilla - Med, 351 g	610	24	87	1	9
Strawberry Milk Shake - Med, 444 g	660	19	111	0	10
Vanilla Milk Shake - Medium, 412 g	560	21	79	0	11
Sides					
Cheesy Tots™ Potatoes - Medium (9 pcs.), 115 g	320	18	30	2	10
French Fries - Medium (Salt Not Added), 116 g	360	20	41	4	4
• French Fries - Medium (Salted), 116 g	360	20	41	4	4
• Mott's® Strawberry Flavored Apple Sauce, 113 g	90	0	23	1	0
Onion Rings - Medium, 91 g	310	15	37	3	4
Zesty Onion Ring Dipping Sauce (1 oz), 28 g	150	15	3	1	0
Whopper® Sandwiches					
Bacon (1 Strip), 3 g	15	1	0	0	1
Barbecue Dipping Sauce, 1 oz.	40	0	11	0	0
Bk Big Fish® Sandwich w/o Tartar Sauce, 220 g	470	13	65	3	23
Bk Big Fish® Sandwich, 249 g	640	32	67	3	24
Bk Veggie® Burger w/ Cheese, 228 g	470	20	47	7	25
Bk Veggie® Burger w/o Mayo, 205 g	340	8	46	7	23
Bk Veggie® Burger, 215 g	420	16	46	7	23
Bk™ Chicken Fries 12 pcs., 170 g	520	31	35	4	25
Bk™ Chicken Fries 6 pcs., 85 g	260	15	18	2	12
Bk™ Chicken Fries 9 pcs., 128 g	390	23	26	3	18
Buffalo Dipping Sauce (1 oz), 28 g	80	8	2	0	0
Chicken Tenders® 5 pcs., 77 g	210	12	13	0	12
Chicken Tenders® 8 pcs., 123 g	340	20	21	1	19

(• = most healthy • = least healthy) **RESTAURANTS & FAST-FOOD • 95**

RESTAURANTS & FAST-FOOD CHAINS

Burger King (cont.)

Whopper® Sandwiches (cont.)	Cal	Fat	Cbs	Fbr	Prtn
Chicken Tenders® Big Kid's Meal 6 pcs, 92 g	250	15	16	0	14
• Chicken Tenders® Kid's Meal 4 pcs., 62 g	170	10	11	0	9
Double Whopper® Sandwich, 373 g	900	57	51	3	47
w/o Mayo, 352 g	740	39	51	3	47
with Cheese w/o Mayo, 376 g	830	47	52	3	52
with Cheese, 398 g	990	64	52	3	52
Honey Mustard Dipping Sauce, 1 oz.	90	6	8	0	0
Original Chicken Sandwich w/o Mayo, 190 g	450	17	52	4	23
Original Chicken Sandwich, 219 g	660	40	52	4	24
Ranch Dipping Sauce, 1 oz.	140	15	1	0	1
Spicy Chick'n Crisp™ Sandwich w/o Mayo, 122 g	320	13	36	1	15
Spicy Chick'n Crisp™ Sandwich, 144 g	480	31	36	1	15
Sweet and Sour Dipping Sauce, 1 oz.	45	0	11	0	0
Tendercrisp® Chicken Sandwich, 284 g	790	44	68	5	33
w/ Mayo, 258 g	510	19	49	4	37
w/o Mayo, 244 g	400	7	49	4	36
Triple Whopper® Sandwich, 456 g	1130	74	51	3	67
w/o Mayo, 434 g	980	57	51	3	66
with Cheese w/o Mayo, 459 g	1070	65	52	3	71
• with Cheese, 480 g	1230	82	52	3	71
Whopper Jr.® Sandwich, 158 g	370	21	31	2	15
w/o Mayo, 147 g	290	12	31	2	15
with Cheese w/o Mayo, 149 g	330	16	31	2	17
with Cheese, 170 g	410	24	32	2	18
Whopper® Sandwich, 290 g	670	39	51	3	28
w/o Mayo, 269 g	510	22	51	3	28
with Cheese w/o Mayo, 294 g	600	30	52	3	32
with Cheese, 315 g	760	47	52	3	33

Burgerville, USA

Breakfast	Cal	Fat	Cbs	Fbr	Prtn
2 Eggs, Any Style	200	14	2	0	14
American Cheese, 2 slices	90	7	0	0	5
Bagel, Bacon, Egg	450	11	64	2	23
Bagel, Ham, Egg	450	8	65	2	28
• Bagel, Sausage, Egg	600	26	64	2	27
Biscuit, Bacon, Egg	400	23	32	1	16
Biscuit, Ham, Egg	400	20	33	1	21
Biscuit, Sausage, Egg	470	29	32	1	20
Cheese Bagel	290	6	53	2	12
• Ham, 2 oz.	55	2	1	0	9
Hash Browns	220	13	23	0	3
Plain Bagel	310	1	63	2	12
Sausage Patty, 2 oz.	210	20	0	0	8
Tillamook Cheese, 1 slices	120	10	1	0	7
Condiments/Dressings					
BBQ Sauce Dip	60	1	13	0	1
Blue Cheese Dressing	240	24	3	0	1
Honey Mustard Dressing	210	20	6	0	0
Italian Dressing	140	15	1	0	0
Ranch Dressing	250	27	1	0	0
• Raspberry Vinaigrette	45	2	6	0	0
• Spread Cups, 2 oz.	280	30	4	0	0

RESTAURANTS & FAST-FOOD CHAINS

Burgerville, USA (cont.)	Cal	Fat	Cbs	Fbr	Prtn
Condiments/Dressings (cont.)					
Tartar Cups, 2 oz.	260	28	2	0	0
Cones					
Ice Cream Cone	250	11	32	0	5
Yogurt Cone	190	0	39	0	4
Cookies					
Chocolate Chunk	320	14	48	0	4
• Heath Toffee	340	14	46	0	4
• Oatmeal Raisin	290	8	50	1	4
White Chocolate Macadamia	340	16	46	0	4
Entrees					
Cheeseburger	350	19	29	2	14
Chicken Strips, 5 pcs.	550	30	36	0	33
Colossal	520	30	30	5	30
Crispy Chicken	450	18	55	3	20
Deluxe Crispy Chicken	610	30	56	3	30
Double Beef Cheeseburger	430	25	29	2	22
Gardenburger	460	19	53	8	18
Grilled Chicken	350	3	45	3	37
• Half Pound Colossal	730	45	31	5	48
Halibut Fillet Sandwich	480	27	42	2	20
Halibut Fish, 3 pcs.	330	16	25	0	20
Halibut Fish, 4 pcs.	410	20	32	0	25
• Hamburger	300	15	29	2	12
Pepper Bacon Cheeseburger	680	45	28	5	38
Protein Platter	530	40	6	3	38
Spicy Black Bean Gardenburger	550	32	45	10	24
Tillamook Cheeseburger	630	40	32	5	34
Turkey Burger	540	29	33	5	36
Turkey Club Sandwich	540	32	38	3	27
French Fries					
• Kid's	220	12	24	2	3
• Large	510	29	57	6	7
Regular	390	22	44	5	5
Kids Meal					
• Apple Slices	29	0	9	2	0
• Cheeseburger	370	20	29	2	17
Chicken Strips, 3 pcs.	200	8	15	0	14
Hamburger	320	16	29	2	15
Kid's French Fries	220	12	24	2	3
Kids Caramel Sundae	210	7	35	0	2
Kids Chocolate Sundae	180	6	31	0	3
Kids Hot Fudge Sundae	210	10	30	0	3
Milkshakes					
Black Forest	820	32	130	3	13
• Chocolate Hazelnut	900	44	117	0	15
Fresh Strawberry	770	31	116	2	12
Mocha Perk	830	39	112	3	17
NW Blackberry	870	36	129	3	14
NW Huckleberry	790	36	105	0	14
NW Raspberry	870	36	126	3	14
Pumpkin Spice	770	35	105	1	14
Regular Chocolate	520	23	73	0	9
Regular Strawberry	500	20	74	0	8

(• = most healthy • = least healthy)   **RESTAURANTS & FAST-FOOD • 97**

RESTAURANTS & FAST-FOOD CHAINS

Burgerville, USA (cont.)

	Cal	Fat	Cbs	Fbr	Prtn
Milkshakes (cont.)					
Regular Vanilla	500	20	74	0	8
Salads					
• Chicken Strip Salad	750	51	39	7	38
Grilled Chicken Salad	520	35	18	7	36
NW Smoked Salmon Salad	540	34	20	7	34
NW Smoked Turkey Salad	500	36	25	7	34
• Side Salad	70	4	5	3	5
Seasonal					
Blackberry Shortcake	340	7	70	5	4
• Onion Rings, 5 pcs.	810	48	83	3	12
• Raspberry Shortcake	330	7	63	4	4
Strawberry Shortcake	290	5	62	N/A	3
Sweet Potato Fries	530	29	60	3	4
Walla Walla Onion Cheeseburger	679	44	39	4	31
Smoothies					
• Chocolate Hazelnut	460	4	93	1	11
Chocolate Monkey	450	3	100	4	10
Fresh Strawberry	410	0	90	1	8
NW Blackberry	420	0	92	2	9
NW Huckleberry	390	0	82	0	9
NW Raspberry	420	0	91	2	9
Pumpkin Spice	390	2	79	1	10
• Strawberry Splash	310	1	68	2	6
Triple Berry Blast	350	0	75	0	7
Sundaes					
Caramel	380	15	56	0	6
Chocolate	360	15	52	0	6
• Hot Fudge	380	18	51	0	7
• Raspberry	360	14	53	1	6

Captain D's Seafood

	Cal	Fat	Cbs	Fbr	Prtn
Appetizers					
Cheese Sticks w/o sauce, 133 g	440	24	32	0	N/A
• Cheese Sticks with sauce, 154 g	560	36	35	0	N/A
Fried Pickles w/ Ranch Dressing, 143 g	360	30	17	1	N/A
• Gumbo Soup with Rice, 227 g	210	8	26	2	N/A
Jalapeño Cheese Bites, 136 g	350	19	36	4	N/A
D's Classics					
2 Piece Fish & Chicken Dinner, 502 g	1460	93	121	7	N/A
2 Piece Fish Dinner, 443 g	1290	83	110	7	N/A
3 Piece Fish Dinner, 508 g	1450	93	120	7	N/A
Batter Dipped Fish, 65 g	160	10	10	0	N/A
Bite Size Shrimp Platter, 432 g	1140	62	121	8	N/A
• Butterfly Shrimp, 15 g	45	3	3	0	N/A
Catfish Dinner, 404 g	1040	63	87	7	N/A
• Catfish Feast, 737 g	1990	141	128	11	N/A
Chicken Dinner, 438 g	1200	72	102	7	N/A
Chicken Strip, 58 g	170	10	11	0	N/A
Clam Platter, 490 g	1440	87	134	13	N/A
Country Style Fish Dinner, 440 g	1180	69	99	7	N/A
Crab & Fish Dinner, 492 g	1320	83	118	7	N/A
Crab & Shrimp Dinner, 450 g	1080	63	104	7	N/A

RESTAURANTS & FAST-FOOD CHAINS

Captain D's Seafood (cont.)	Cal	Fat	Cbs	Fbr	Prtn
D's Classics (cont.)					
Crab Dinner, 490 g	1050	60	106	7	N/A
Deluxe Seafood Platter, 630 g	1700	106	144	7	N/A
Fish & Fries, 330 g	1120	71	97	5	N/A
Fish & Shrimp Dinner, 516 g	1510	96	126	7	N/A
Fish, Shrimp & Chicken Platter, 568 g	1700	107	138	7	N/A
Flounder Dinner, 584 g	1530	94	116	8	N/A
Jumbo Fish Platter, 573 g	1610	102	130	7	N/A
Oyster Dinner, 416 g	1000	58	100	7	N/A
Shrimp Dinner, 409 g	1110	67	102	8	N/A
Stuffed Crab, 57 g	100	5	9	0	N/A
Super Shrimp Platter, 496 g	1380	83	122	9	N/A
Desserts					
Carrot Cake, 99 g	390	19	50	1	N/A
• Cheesecake w/ Strawberry Topping, 142 g	430	26	45	1	N/A
• Chocolate Cake, 85 g	300	11	49	2	N/A
Pecan Pie, 113 g	470	26	56	2	N/A
Pineapple Cream Cheese Pie, 106 g	320	14	43	2	N/A
Dressing Packets					
Blue Cheese Dressing, 2 oz.	230	24	2	0	N/A
• Fat Free Italian Dressing, 2 oz.	15	0	3	0	N/A
Fat Free Raspberry Vinaigrette, 2 oz.	50	0	13	0	N/A
• Honey Mustard Dressing, 2 oz.	250	25	8	0	N/A
Ranch Dressing, 2 oz.	180	18	2	0	N/A
Thousand Island Dressing, 2 oz.	180	17	8	0	N/A
Family Packs					
• 10 Piece Chicken Only, 146 g	440	26	27	0	N/A
10 Piece Chicken Pack, 406 g	1110	66	96	7	N/A
10 Piece Fish Only, 213 g	690	47	45	0	N/A
• 10 Piece Fish Value Pack, 473 g	1360	87	114	7	N/A
Seafood Feast, 456 g	1350	85	115	6	N/A
Slaw, Fries, Hush Puppies, 260 g	670	40	69	7	N/A
Kids Meal					
• Kid's Chicken, 535 g	680	32	85	4	N/A
• Kid's Fish, 593 g	960	55	105	4	N/A
Kid's Shrimp, 562 g	740	33	100	5	N/A
Kitchen Selections					
Chicken Breast Combo, 288 g	470	15	54	2	N/A
• Coastal Flounder Dinner, 302 g	360	10	31	1	N/A
Mahi-Mahi, 315 g	490	15	52	2	N/A
Parmesan Chicken Scampi, 352 g	610	27	59	2	N/A
Premium Shrimp Dinner, 186 g	470	15	18	2	N/A
• Seafood Lover's Mixed Grill, 605 g	910	25	80	2	N/A
Seafood Scampi Platter, 409 g	530	20	36	2	N/A
Shrimp Skewers Combo, 315 g	510	10	53	2	N/A
Tilapia Combo, 316 g	490	14	52	2	N/A
Wild Alaskan Salmon, 330 g	590	22	56	2	N/A
Pasta					
Chicken Broccoli Alfredo, 540 g	900	37	98	4	N/A
• Chicken Broccoli Alfredo, 554 g	970	44	98	4	N/A
Classic Chicken Parmesan, 519 g	850	30	105	5	N/A
Savory Shrimp Scampi, 473 g	800	33	92	4	N/A
Shrimp Broccoli Alfredo, 517 g	870	36	97	5	N/A

RESTAURANTS & FAST-FOOD CHAINS

Captain D's Seafood (cont.)

	Cal	Fat	Cbs	Fbr	Prtn
Pasta (cont.)					
• Shrimp Marinara, 502 g	670	15	94	5	N/A
Salads					
Blackened Chicken Salad, 325 g	250	9	10	3	N/A
Breadstick, 43 g	150	5	21	1	N/A
Crispy Chicken Caesar Salad, 440 g	920	70	52	4	N/A
Fried Chicken Salad, 335 g	500	29	31	3	N/A
Fried Shrimp Salad, 388 g	610	29	60	4	N/A
• Garden Salad, 218 g	150	8	9	3	N/A
• Grilled Chicken Caesar Salad, 510 g	910	68	44	4	N/A
Grilled Seasoned Shrimp, 400 g	420	12	41	4	N/A
Grilled Wild Alaskan Salmon, 466 g	570	25	44	4	N/A
Southern Style Fried Chicken Salad, 354 g	460	20	51	4	N/A
Sandwiches					
Deluxe Classic Fish Sandwich, 306 g	890	59	62	2	N/A
• Double Bacon Ranch Crispy Chkn Sand, 331 g	1000	67	67	2	N/A
Double Bacon Ranch Grilled Chkn Sand, 310 g	870	60	45	2	N/A
Grilled Alaskan Salmon Sandwich, 328 g	790	49	46	2	N/A
• Seasoned Tilapia Sandwich, 314 g	690	42	42	2	N/A
Sauces					
• Cocktail Sauce, 3/4 oz.	25	0	6	0	N/A
Ginger Teriyaki Sauce, 2 fl.oz.	60	0	13	0	N/A
• Honey Mustard Sauce, 3/4 oz.	120	12	3	0	N/A
Scampi Sauce, 2 fl.oz.	120	10	5	0	N/A
Sweet & Sour Sauce, 3/4 oz.	45	0	10	0	N/A
Sweet Chili Sauce, 2 fl.oz.	100	0	25	1	N/A
Tartar Sauce, 3/4 oz.	100	10	1	0	N/A
Sides					
Baked Potato plain, 255 g	240	0	54	6	N/A
Breadstick, 85 g	300	11	42	2	N/A
Broccoli, 100 g	40	1	5	2	N/A
Cole Slaw, 109 g	170	12	13	2	N/A
Corn on the Cob, 163 g	190	3	37	4	N/A
French Fries, 3 oz.	310	15	38	4	N/A
Fried Okra, 113 g	230	14	23	4	N/A
Fried Pickles w/ Ranch Dressing, 143 g	360	30	17	1	N/A
Garlic Mashed Potatoes, 113 g	100	3	16	1	N/A
Green Beans, 113 g	60	2	10	3	N/A
• Hush Puppies, 99 g	400	26	36	3	N/A
Lemon Herb Rice, 113 g	150	1	31	1	N/A
Macaroni & Cheese, 113 g	160	7	17	1	N/A
Roasted Red Potatoes, 124 g	170	7	25	3	N/A
• Sliced Tomatoes, 60 g	10	0	2	1	N/A
Vegetable Medley, 144 g	140	11	9	3	N/A

Caribou Coffee

	Cal	Fat	Cbs	Fbr	Prtn
Amy's Blend Pink Ribbon Bagel, 113 g	310	4	61	3	9
Blackberry & White Choco Scone, 128 g	490	22	70	2	6
Blueberry Muffin, 135 g	410	18	55	1	7
Caprese Salad, 287 g	378	32	8	2	19
Caribou Coffee Snack Bars, 35 g	140	4	26	1	2
Cheddar Cheese Bagel, 113 g	290	4	53	3	11
Chocolate Chocolate Chip Muffin, 135 g	480	24	62	3	6
Chocolate Chunk Cookie, 94 g	441	25	58	2	5

RESTAURANTS & FAST-FOOD CHAINS

Caribou Coffee (cont.)	Cal	Fat	Cbs	Fbr	Prtn
Cinnamon Chip Scone, 120 g	500	22	68	2	7
Cinnamon Hoof Mints, 1 g	0	0	1	0	0
Cinnamon Raisin Bagel, 113 g	300	2	63	3	10
Cinnamon Roll Popover, 159 g	580	30	70	3	8
Cinnamon Streusel Muff w/ Wh Choco Chp, 135 g	530	25	71	2	6
Dark Chocolate Graham, 28 g	140	8	18	1	2
Double Chocolate Biscotti, 57 g	250	10	36	2	4
• Fruit Salad, 250 g	105	0	27	2	2
Italian Beef Sandwich, 272 g	626	30	56	1	32
Lemon Poppy Seed Loaf Cake, 128 g	470	26	56	1	6
Milk Chocolate Graham, 28 g	140	8	18	1	2
Multi Grain Bagel, 113 g	360	7	63	6	13
Orange Walnut White Chocolate Biscotti, 57 g	250	11	34	1	4
Original Almond Biscotti, 57 g	230	8	34	1	5
Peanut Butter Cookie, 94 g	450	23	55	2	9
Peppermint Hoof Mints, 1 g	0	0	1	0	0
Pumpkin Bread, 124 g	430	22	54	2	6
Reduced Fat Banana Bread, 129 g	380	11	72	2	5
Reduced Fat Cranberry Orange Scone, 128 g	450	14	78	3	6
Reduced Fat Mountain Brry Muffin, 135 g	300	6	54	1	6
Roasted Chicken Sandwich, 238 g	540	19	53	3	29
Roasted Vegetable Sandwich, 296 g	622	36	61	10	14
Rosemary Romano Chicken Salad Sandwich, 258 g	637	65	49	4	29
Smoked Turkey Sandwich, 245 g	590	29	53	1	31
Tomato Gorgonzola Pasta Salad, 258 g	397	19	45	3	10
• Tortellini Salad, 278 g	820	48	72	4	22
Turkey and Pesto Sandwich, 239 g	431	16	42	2	28
Turkey Cherry Pasta Salad, 247 g	571	33	44	3	23
White Chocolate Macadamia Nut Cookie, 94 g	420	20	55	1	5
White Chocolate Pretzel, 24 g	110	5	17	0	2
Wintergreen Hoof Mints, 1 g	0	0	1	0	0
Beverages					
Small Açaí Smoothie, 16 fl.oz.	290	3	65	2	1
• Small Americano, 12 fl.oz.	5	0	1	0	0
Small Blended Chai w/ 2% Milk, 16 fl.oz.	180	4	31	0	6
Small Blended Chai w/ Skim Milk, 16 fl.oz.	150	0	31	0	6
Small Breve, 12 fl.oz.	310	26	11	0	7
• Small Campfire Mocha, 12 fl.oz.	460	16	71	0	9
Small Cappuccino, 12 fl.oz.	140	5	14	0	9
Small Caramel Cooler, 16 fl.oz.	340	12	56	0	3

Carl's Jr.	Cal	Fat	Cbs	Fbr	Prtn
Breakfast					
Bacon & Egg Burrito, 208 g	570	33	37	1	30
• Breakfast Burger™, 309 g	830	47	65	3	37
• French Toast Dips® - No Syrup (5 pieces), 129 g	430	18	58	1	9
Hash Brown Nuggets, 108 g	330	21	32	3	3
Loaded Breakfast Burrito, 328 g	820	51	52	2	38
Sourdough Breakfast Sandwich, 193 g	460	21	39	2	28
Steak & Egg Burrito, 322 g	660	36	44	2	40
Sunrise Croissant™ Sandwich, 172 g	560	41	27	1	20
Charbroiled Burgers					
Big Hamburger, 209 g	470	17	54	3	24
Double Western Bacon Cheeseburger™, 323 g	970	52	71	3	52

RESTAURANTS & FAST-FOOD CHAINS

Carl's Jr. (cont.)

	Cal	Fat	Cbs	Fbr	Prtn
Charbroiled Burgers (cont.)					
Famous Star™ with Cheese, 278 g	660	39	53	3	27
Jalapeño Burger™, 286 g	720	45	50	3	27
• Kid's Hamburger, 195 g	460	17	53	2	24
Philly Cheesesteak Burger, 297 g	830	55	52	3	40
Super Star® with Cheese, 385 g	930	59	54	3	47
The Bacon Cheese Six Dollar Burger™, 409 g	1070	76	50	3	46
• The Double Six Dollar Burger™, 602 g	1520	111	60	3	69
The Guacamole Bacon Six Dollar Burger™, 447 g	1140	85	54	6	43
The Low Carb Six Dollar Burger™, 267 g	490	37	6	2	33
The Original Six Dollar Burger™, 430 g	1010	68	60	3	40
The Western Bacon Six Dollar Burger®, 382 g	1130	66	83	4	47
Western Bacon Cheeseburger®, 241 g	710	33	70	3	32
Chicken & Other Choices					
• Bacon Swiss Crispy Chicken™ Sandwich, 318 g	720	35	64	3	35
Carl's Catch™ Fish Sandwich, 291 g	660	31	75	3	22
• Charbroiled BBQ Chicken™ Sandwich, 239 g	360	5	48	4	34
Charbroiled Chicken Club™ Sandwich, 264 g	550	25	43	4	40
Charbroiled Santa Fe Chicken™ Sandwich, 264 g	610	32	43	4	37
Chicken Breast Strips (3 pieces), 129 g	420	25	28	1	23
Chicken Breast Strips (5 pieces), 215 g	710	41	46	2	38
Spicy Chicken Sandwich, 213 g	560	30	59	2	15
Desserts					
Chocolate Cake, 85 g	300	12	48	1	3
• Chocolate Chip Cookie, 71 g	350	18	46	1	3
• Strawberry Swirl Cheesecake, 99 g	290	17	30	0	6
Hand-Scooped Ice Cream Shakes & Malts™					
Chocolate Malt, 414 g	780	35	98	1	17
Chocolate Shake, 397 g	710	33	85	1	14
• OREO® Cookie Malt, 414 g	790	39	91	1	18
OREO® Cookie Shake, 397 g	720	37	79	1	16
Strawberry Malt, 414 g	770	35	97	0	17
• Strawberry Shake, 397 g	700	33	84	0	14
Vanilla Malt, 414 g	780	35	99	0	17
Vanilla Shake, 397 g	710	33	86	0	14
Salad Dressings					
• Blue Cheese Dressing, 2 oz.	320	34	1	0	2
House Dressing, 2 oz.	220	22	2	0	1
• Low Fat Balsamic Dressing, 2 oz.	35	2	5	0	0
Thousand Island Dressing, 2 oz.	250	2	7	0	0
Salads - Without Dressings					
Charbroiled Chicken Salad, 417 g	260	7	16	5	34
Side Salad, 139 g	50	3	5	2	3
Sides					
• Chicken Stars™ (6 pieces), 85 g	260	16	14	1	13
CrissCut® Fries, 139 g	410	24	43	4	5
• Fish & Chips, 258 g	630	28	68	3	26
French Fries (Medium), 147 g	460	22	59	5	7
Fried Zucchini, 139 g	320	19	31	0	6
Onion Rings, 128 g	430	21	53	2	6

Carvel Ice Cream

	Cal	Fat	Cbs	Fbr	Prtn
Classic Sundaes (Regular)					
• Bittersweet Fudge	690	38	77	1	8

RESTAURANTS & FAST-FOOD CHAINS

Carvel Ice Cream (cont.)	Cal	Fat	Cbs	Fbr	Prtn
Classic Sundaes (Regular) (cont.)					
Caramel	670	34	81	0	8
Hot Fudge	670	38	73	1	8
No Fat Classic Sundae (Fudge)	380	0	81	0	8
• No Fat Classic Sundae (Strawberry)	320	0	69	1	8
Strawberry	580	33	63	1	7
Cones - Regular					
• Cake Cone with Chocolate	440	21	51	2	10
Cake Cone with Vanilla	470	26	50	0	6
Sugar Cone with Chocolate	460	21	59	2	11
Sugar Cone with Vanilla	500	26	58	0	7
Waffle Cone with Chocolate	500	22	66	3	11
• Waffle Cone with Vanilla	530	26	65	1	8
Fountain Regular					
Brown Bonnet®, 16 fl.oz.	370	21	40	0	3
Chipsters, 16 fl.oz.	330	16	44	4	4
Deluxe Flying Saucer™, 16 fl.oz.	330	15	47	1	4
Flying Saucer™ (Chocolate), 16 fl.oz.	230	10	33	1	4
Flying Saucer™ (Vanilla), 16 fl.oz.	240	11	33	1	4
• Mini Sundae (Chocolate Syrup), 16 fl.oz.	200	9	27	0	2
No Fat Carvelanche® (Strwbrry), 16 fl.oz.	430	0	91	1	12
No Fat Chocolate Shake, 16 fl.oz.	440	0	104	0	5
No Fat Mocha Shake, 16 fl.oz.	440	0	97	0	10
No Fat Vanilla Shake, 16 fl.oz.	300	0	62	0	9
Olde Fashion Sundae, 16 fl.oz.	340	15	47	0	4
• Sinful Love Bar, 16 fl.oz.	460	29	47	5	4
Sprinkle Cup, 16 fl.oz.	230	15	28	0	2
Ice Cream Regular Cup					
Chocolate, 7 oz.	410	21	48	2	10
No Fat Chocolate, 7 oz.	270	0	62	0	4
• No Fat Vanilla, 7 oz.	270	0	55	0	9
No Sugar Added Vanilla, 7 oz.	300	7	57	0	11
Sherbet, 7 oz.	300	3	66	0	2
• Vanilla, 7 oz.	450	26	47	0	6
Novelties					
• 98% Fat Free Flying Saucer™ (chocolate)	180	3	34	1	5
98% Fat Free Flying Saucer™ (vanilla)	180	3	35	1	5
No Fat Miniature Sundae	190	0	45	0	4
No Fat Olde Fashioned Sundae	300	0	67	0	6
No Fat Parfait	190	0	42	0	4
No Sugar Added Miniature Sundae	200	3	42	0	5
• No Sugar Added Olde Fashioned Sundae	360	5	76	0	8
No Sugar Added Parfait	200	3	42	0	5

Charley's Grilled Subs	Cal	Fat	Cbs	Fbr	Prtn
Chicken Tenders					
5 piece	334	20	17	2	22
Kid's	200	12	10	1	13
Fries					
Cheddar & Bacon	1089	87	55	2	16
Cheddar Cheese	1054	84	55	2	14
• Cheddar, Ranch & Bacon	1249	103	57	2	16
Ranch & Bacon	1149	95	51	2	15
• Regular	611	46	42	2	5

(• = most healthy • = least healthy)   **RESTAURANTS & FAST-FOOD • 103**

RESTAURANTS & FAST-FOOD CHAINS

Charley's Grilled Subs (cont.)

	Cal	Fat	Cbs	Fbr	Prtn
Grilled Salads					
• Buffalo Chicken	296	13	17	6	32
Chicken Teriyaki	292	13	16	5	32
• Fresh Garden	141	8	13	5	7
Grilled Chicken	281	13	14	5	31
Grilled Steak	291	16	14	5	26
Lemonade					
Kiwi or Strawberry, 16 oz.	202	0	50	0	2
Original, 16 oz.	162	0	40	0	2
Sandwiches					
• Bacon 3 cheese Steak	645	30	55	2	43
Bacon 3 cheese Steak Low Fat	490	18	53	2	32
BBQ Cheddar Steak	586	20	70	3	36
BBQ Cheddar Steak Low Fat	476	11	69	3	29
Chicken Bacon Club	580	23	54	2	45
Chicken Bacon Club Low Fat	480	15	53	2	37
Chicken Buffalo	531	16	61	4	42
Chicken Buffalo Low Fat	431	8	60	4	35
Chicken Cordon Bleu	595	22	58	2	46
Chicken Cordon Bleu Low Fat	495	14	57	2	38
Chicken Teriyaki	527	16	60	3	43
Chicken Teriyaki Low Fat	427	8	59	3	35
Italian Deli	427	12	55	2	28
Italian Deli Low Fat	327	4	54	2	21
Philly Cheesesteak	526	19	58	3	36
Philly Cheesesteak Low Fat	426	11	57	3	29
Philly Chicken	519	16	59	3	41
Philly Chicken Low Fat	419	8	58	3	34
Philly Ham & Swiss	439	13	59	3	26
Philly Ham & Swiss Low Fat	339	5	58	3	19
Philly Steak Deluxe	529	19	59	3	36
Philly Steak Deluxe Low Fat	429	11	58	3	29
Philly Veggie	452	15	63	3	22
• Philly Veggie Low Fat	297	3	61	3	11
Steak Sicilian	570	24	54	2	37
Steak Sicilian Low Fat	520	20	54	2	34
Turkey Cheddar Melt	444	12	55	2	31
Turkey Cheddar Melt Low Fat	334	3	54	2	24
Ultimate Club	517	20	55	2	32
Ultimate Club Low Fat	407	11	54	2	25

Chevy's Fresh Mex

	Cal	Fat	Cbs	Fbr	Prtn
Grande Salads					
Santa Fe Chopped Salad	682	41	25	10	53
No cheese	480	25	25	10	41
• No cheese, bacon or avocado	258	6	21	7	31
No cheese or bacon	338	13	25	10	32
• Tostada Salad with Chicken	1228	77	63	18	78
No tortilla strips	1088	71	44	17	76
No tortilla strips, cheese or sour cream	542	23	40	17	48
No tortilla strips, cheese, sour cream, or guac	463	16	35	14	47
No tortilla strips or cheese	663	35	42	17	50
Grilled Tacos					
Grilled Chicken Tacos	911	41	86	6	49

Chevy's Fresh Mex (cont.)	Cal	Fat	Cbs	Fbr	Prtn
Grilled Tacos (cont.)					
No tamalito	827	37	73	5	48
No tamalito or rice	651	32	44	4	45
No tamalito, rice, cheese or Chipotle Aioli	504	17	43	4	42
No tamalito, rice or cheese	595	27	44	4	42
• Grilled Fish Tacos (Salmon)	1092	64	70	10	62
No tamalito	1008	60	57	9	61
No tamalito or rice	832	55	28	8	58
No tamalito, rice or sour cream	711	43	26	8	56
No tamalito, rice, sour cream or guacamole	632	36	21	5	55
Grilled Fish Tacos (Sea Bass)	845	39	88	7	36
No tamalito	761	35	75	6	35
No tamalito or rice	585	30	46	5	32
No tamalito, rice or cheese	529	25	46	5	29
• No tamalito, rice, cheese or Chipotle Aioli	438	15	45	5	29
Grilled Steak Tacos	972	51	87	6	44
No tamalito	888	47	74	5	43
No tamalito or rice	712	42	45	4	40
No tamalito, rice or cheese	656	37	45	4	37
Homemade Beans					
Beans a la Charra	230	5	33	11	14
No cheese	202	3	33	11	12
No cheese or pico de gallo	198	3	32	11	12
Black Beans	207	3	33	11	13
No cheese	179	1	33	11	11
• No cheese or pico de gallo	175	1	32	11	11
• Refried Beans	298	15	29	9	12
No cheese	270	13	29	9	10
No cheese or pico de gallo	266	13	28	9	10
Sizzling Fajitas					
• Juicy Shrimp Fajitas, no tortillas	1212	85	70	10	47
No tortillas, tamalito	1128	81	57	9	46
No tortillas, tamalito or rice	952	76	28	8	43
No tortillas, tamalito, rice or sour cream	831	64	26	8	41
No tortillas, tamalito, rice, sour crm or guac	752	57	21	5	40
Mix & Match (Chicken & Steak) Fajitas, no tortillas	959	52	67	9	58
No tortillas, tamalito	875	48	54	8	57
No tortillas, tamalito or rice	699	43	25	7	54
No tortillas, tamalito, rice or sour cream	578	31	23	7	52
No tortillas, tamalito, rice, sour cream or guac	499	24	18	4	51
Original Famous Chicken Fajitas, no tortillas	913	45	67	9	63
No tortillas or tamalito	829	41	54	8	62
No tortillas, tamalito or rice	653	36	25	7	59
No tortillas, tamalito, rice or sour cream	532	24	23	7	57
No tortillas, tamalito, rice, sour cream or guac	453	17	18	4	56
Portobello Mushroom & Asprgs Fajitas, no tortillas	878	57	69	14	15
No tortillas, tamalito	794	53	73	13	14
No tortillas, tamalito or rice	618	48	44	12	11
No tortillas, tamalito, rice or sour cream	497	36	42	12	9
• No tortillas, tamalito, rice, sour cream or guac	418	29	37	9	8
Sizzling Steak Fajitas, no tortillas	1066	59	67	9	54
No tortillas or tamalito	922	55	54	8	53
No tortillas, tamalito or rice	746	50	25	7	50
No tortillas, tamalito, rice or sour cream	625	38	23	7	48

RESTAURANTS & FAST-FOOD CHAINS

Chevy's Fresh Mex (cont.)	Cal	Fat	Cbs	Fbr	Prtn
Sizzling Fajitas (cont.)					
No tortillas, tamalito, rice, sour cream or guac	546	31	18	4	47

Chick-Fil-A	Cal	Fat	Cbs	Fbr	Prtn
Breakfast					
Bacon Egg & Cheese Biscuit, 6 oz.	470	26	39	1	18
Biscuit with Gravy, 7 oz.	330	15	43	1	5
Chicken, Egg & Chz on Sunflower Mltgrn Bagel, 8 oz.	500	20	49	3	31
Chick-Fil-A Chicken Burrito, 7 oz.	410	16	42	4	22
Chick-Fil-A Chicken, 5 oz.	420	19	44	2	18
Chick-Fil-A Chick-N-Minis (3 Count), 3 oz.	280	11	29	2	14
Chick-Fil-A Chick-N-Minis (4 Count), 4 oz.	370	15	38	3	19
Chick-Fil-A Sausage Burrito, 7 oz.	450	23	39	3	20
Cinnamon Cluster, 1 oz.	400	15	61	3	8
• Fruit Cup (medium), 4 oz.	70	0	16	2	1
Hashbrowns, 3 oz.	260	17	25	3	2
Hot Buttered Biscuit, 3 oz.	270	12	38	1	4
• Sausage & Egg Biscuit, 7 oz.	570	37	39	2	19
Sunflower Multigrain Bagel, 3 oz.	220	3	41	2	7
Chick-Fil-A Coolwrap					
Chargrilled Chicken Coolwrap, 9 oz.	410	12	46	8	34
• Chicken Caesar Coolwrap, 8 oz.	480	16	44	7	41
• Spicy Chicken Coolwrap, 8 oz.	410	12	44	8	35
Croutons/Kernels					
• Garlic & Butter Croutons, 0.5 oz.	70	3	9	0	1
• Honey Roasted sunflower Kernels, 0.5 oz.	80	7	3	1	3
Tortilla Strips, 0.5 oz.	70	4	9	1	2
Desserts					
Cheesecake (1 slice), 3 oz.	340	21	30	2	6
Fudge Nut Brownie (1 Brownie), 3 oz.	330	15	45	2	4
Hand-Spun Milk Shake (Chocolate), 20 oz.	760	28	113	1	16
• Hand-Spun Milk Shake (Cookies & Cream), 20 oz.	790	33	111	1	17
Hand-Spun Milk Shake (Strawberry), 20 oz.	730	28	109	1	16
Hand-Spun Milk Shake (Vanilla), 20 oz.	660	27	90	0	16
• Icedream (Small Cone), 5 oz.	160	4	28	0	4
Icedream (Small Cup), 8 oz.	240	6	41	0	6
Lemon Pie (1 slice), 4 oz.	350	11	59	1	6
Dipping Sauces					
Barbecue Sauce, 1 oz.	45	0	11	0	0
• Buttermilk Ranch Sauce, 1 oz.	110	12	1	0	0
• Chick-Fil-A Buffalo Sauce, 1 oz.	15	2	1	0	0
Honey Mustard Sauce, 1 oz.	45	0	10	0	0
Honey Roasted BBQ Sauce, 0.5 oz.	60	6	2	0	0
Polynesian Sauce, 1 oz.	110	6	13	0	0
Dressings					
Blue Cheese, 29 g	150	16	1	0	1
Buttermilk Ranch, 30 g	160	16	1	0	0
• Caesar, 29 g	160	17	1	0	1
Fat Free Honey Mustard, 35 g	60	0	14	0	0
• Light Italian, 32 g	15	5	2	0	0
Reduced Fat Raspberry Vinaigrette, 37 g	80	2	15	0	0
Spicy, 29 g	140	14	2	0	0
Thousand Salad, 30 g	150	14	5	0	0

RESTAURANTS & FAST-FOOD CHAINS

Chick-Fil-A (cont.)	Cal	Fat	Cbs	Fbr	Prtn
Salads					
• Chick-Fil-A Chargrilled Chicken Green Salad, 10 oz.	180	6	9	3	22
Chick-Fil-A Chick-N-Strips Salad, 11 oz.	400	20	21	4	34
Chick-Fil-A Southwest Chargrilled Salad, 11 oz.	240	8	17	5	25
Sandwiches: Classics					
• Chargrilled Chicken Club Sandwich, 8 oz.	221	11	33	3	35
Chick-Fil-A Chargrilled Chicken Sandwich, 7 oz.	270	4	33	3	28
Chick-Fil-A Chicken Salad Sandwich, 5 oz.	350	15	32	5	20
Chick-Fil-A Chicken Sandwich, 6 oz.	410	16	38	1	28
Chick-Fil-A Chick-N-Strips, 5 oz.	310	15	15	1	28
Chick-Fil-A Nuggets, 4 oz.	260	13	10	2	27
Sides					
Carrot & Basin Salad (small), 4 oz.	170	6	28	2	1
• Chick-Fil-A Waffle Potato Fries (sm), 3 oz.	270	13	34	4	3
Cole Slaw, 5 oz.	260	21	17	2	2
Fruit Cup (small), 4 oz.	70	0	17	2	1
Hearty Breast of Chicken Soup, 9 oz.	140	4	18	1	8
• Side Salad, 4 oz.	60	3	4	2	3

Chili's Restaurant	Cal	Fat	Cbs	Fbr	Prtn
Baby Back Ribs					
• Blazin' Habanero Ribs w/ Habanero BBQ Sauce	1220	66	94	5	58
Brown Sugar Chile Ribs w/ Sauce	1000	70	37	3	55
Honey BBQ Ribs w/ Honey BBQ Sauce	1060	65	82	3	55
Honey Chipotle Ribs w/ Sauce	1160	65	82	3	56
Memphis Dry Rub Ribs w/ Dijon BBQ Sauce	1000	70	37	3	55
• Original BBQ Ribs w/ Classic BBQ Sauce	970	66	33	3	56
Big Mouth Burgers®					
Bacon Burger	1080	71	54	3	55
• BBQ Ranch Burger	1110	71	60	3	56
Big Mouth Bun only (with butter)	460	20	55	2	12
• Burger Patty only (without bun or toppings)	360	25	0	0	31
Chipotle Bleu Cheese Bacon Burger	1090	71	57	3	51
Ground Peppercorn Burger	1050	68	61	3	44
Mushroom-Swiss Burger	1100	71	60	4	53
Oldtimer Burger®	800	44	54	3	43
Oldtimer Burger® w/ Cheese	880	51	54	3	48
Chicken					
Cajun Chicken Pasta w/ Garlic Toast	1500	78	123	8	67
Chicken Club Tacos	1140	45	126	10	53
Chicken Crispers®	1880	130	133	8	67
Chicken Tacos	1200	41	137	12	57
Country Fried Chicken Crispers (no dressing)	1660	101	141	9	68
Crispy Honey Chipotle Crispers (no dressing)	1890	99	203	9	70
• Margarita Grilled Chicken	690	18	81	9	48
Monterey Chicken®	1130	67	67	11	73
Create Your Own Combo					
Sizzle & Spice Classic Sirloin	540	42	1	0	36
Sizzle & Spice Firecracker Tilapia	270	7	16	1	30
• Sizzle & Spice Garlic & Lime Grilled Shrimp	260	13	6	0	24
Sizzle & Spice Half Rack Baby Back Ribs	490	33	16	1	28
Sizzle & Spice Honey BBQ Sirloin	730	57	17	1	48
Sizzle & Spice Margarita Grilled Chicken	320	13	13	1	36
Sizzle & Spice Monterey Chicken®	460	27	14	1	44

▶ Chili's Restaurant (cont.)	Cal	Fat	Cbs	Fbr	Prtn
Desserts					
Cheesecake	720	44	68	1	11
• Chocolate Chip Paradise Pie® w/ Vanilla Ice Cream	1600	78	215	6	19
Frosty Chocolate Shake w/ Chocolate Sprinkles	850	36	123	1	13
Molten Chocolate Cake w/ Vanilla Ice Cream	1270	62	172	6	14
Sweet Shot – Dutch Apple Caramel	230	6	41	1	2
Sweet Shot – Seven Layers of Chocolate	310	16	40	1	2
• Sweet Shot – Strawberry Vanilla Cheesecake	220	11	26	5	2
Dressings & Sauces					
Asian Sesame Ginger Dressing, 2 fl.oz.	260	26	6	0	0
Avocado Ranch Dressing, 2 fl.oz.	150	15	3	1	3
• Awesome Blossom Sauce, 2 fl.oz.	350	36	5	0	0
Balsamic Ranch Dressing, 2 fl.oz.	270	27	4	0	3
Balsamic Vinaigrette Dressing, 2 fl.oz.	270	27	4	0	3
Balsamic Vinaigrette Dressing, low fat, 2 fl.oz.	50	0	9	0	0
BBQ Sauce, 2 fl.oz.	80	0	18	1	0
Bleu Cheese Dressing, 2 fl.oz.	320	35	1	0	2
Caesar Dressing, 2 fl.oz.	350	37	3	0	2
Carolina BBQ Sauce, 2 fl.oz.	130	0	31	5	0
Chimichurri Sauce, 2 fl.oz.	250	29	3	1	1
Chipotle Ranch Dressing, 2 fl.oz.	170	18	2	0	3
Citrus Balsamic Vinaigrette Dressing, 2 fl.oz.	340	33	7	0	0
Creamy Cilantro Dressing, 2 fl.oz.	300	32	2	0	1
Dijon BBQ Sauce, 2 fl.oz.	145	0	35	0	0
Habanero BBQ Sauce, 2 fl.oz.	170	0	39	1	0
Honey Chipotle Sauce, 2 fl.oz.	200	0	49	0	0
Honey Lime Dressing, 2 fl.oz.	270	22	17	0	1
Honey Mustard Dressing, 2 fl.oz.	260	28	2	0	1
Honey Mustard Dressing, no fat, 2 fl.oz.	90	1	14	1	0
Jalapeño Ranch Sauce, 2 fl.oz.	200	20	3	0	3
Mango Sauce, 2 fl.oz.	170	15	9	0	2
Peanut Dipping Sauce (Lettuce Wraps), 2 fl.oz.	190	13	15	1	4
Ranch Dressing, 2 fl.oz.	240	25	3	0	4
Ranch Dressing, low fat, 2 fl.oz.	110	6	12	0	1
• Salsa Picante Sauce, 2 fl.oz.	40	0	4	1	2
Sesame-Ginger Dipping Sauce (Lett Wrps), 2 fl.oz.	70	0	11	1	2
Thousand Island Dressing, 2 fl.oz.	270	26	9	0	1
Wasabi-Ranch Dressing, 2 fl.oz.	180	18	3	0	3
Fire-Grilled Steaks					
Cajun Ribeye	870	76	3	1	40
• Classic Sirloin	540	42	1	0	36
• Country-Fried Steak w/ Sides	1890	107	148	7	99
Flame-Grilled Ribeye	960	87	1	0	40
Honey BBQ Sirloin	800	56	19	1	48
NY Strip	790	64	1	0	48
Guiltless Grill®					
Big Mouth Bun, unbuttered	330	6	55	2	12
• Black Bean Brgr Patty only (w/o bun or toppings)	200	2	25	20	21
• Guiltless Black Bean Burger	650	12	96	26	38
Guiltless Chicken Platter	580	9	85	5	39
Guiltless Chicken Sandwich	490	8	63	11	39
Guiltless Salmon	480	14	31	10	54
Small Whole Wheat Bun, unbuttered	80	2	16	1	3

Chili's Restaurant (cont.)	Cal	Fat	Cbs	Fbr	Prtn
Pepper Pals®					
Cheese Pizza, 1 Pizza	570	24	67	3	23
Corn Dog	250	17	18	1	5
Country-Fried Chipotle Crispers, 3 each	610	41	26	1	37
• Crispy Honey Chipotle Crispers, 3 each	770	41	65	1	37
Grilled Cheese Sandwich	420	27	26	1	16
• Grilled Chicken Platter	140	3	3	1	26
Grilled Chicken Sandwich	170	3	16	1	20
Kraft® Macaroni & Cheese	510	18	69	3	16
Little Chicken Crispers	590	42	19	0	34
Little Mouth Burger	280	15	14	1	20
Little Mouth Cheeseburger	350	21	14	1	24
Pepper Pals® Pasta w/ Alfredo Sauce	410	17	47	2	15
Pepper Pals® Pasta w/ Marinara Sauce	290	5	52	2	7
Ribs Basket, 1 basket	370	24	16	1	20
Pepper Pals Sides & Desserts					
Black Beans	115	0	19	5	6
Cinnamon Apples	210	8	35	5	0
• Frosty Choc-A-Lot Shake w/ Chocolate Sprinkles	640	27	92	1	9
Homestyle Fries	260	16	27	3	2
Mashed Potatoes	190	11	19	3	4
Rice	160	1	33	1	3
• Steamed Broccoli	80	6	6	3	3
Sweet Corn on the Cob	230	7	55	3	6
Vanilla Ice Cream, 1 Scoop	400	22	44	0	4
Salads					
Boneless Buffalo Chicken Salad	910	58	51	6	44
• Caesar Salad w/ Chicken & Dressing	1010	76	39	7	38
Caesar Salad w/ Lime Grlld Shrimp & Dressing	980	77	39	6	30
Dinner Salad – Caesar w/ Dressing	520	43	27	5	6
• Dinner Salad – House	140	7	12	2	6
Grilled Caribbean Salad	440	10	51	6	33
Lettuce Wraps w/ Dipping Sauces	580	35	55	8	14
Mesquite Chicken Salad	800	43	53	10	53
Quesadilla Explosion Salad w/ Ranch Drizzle	980	48	81	11	58
Southwestern Cobb Salad	970	60	56	7	53
Sandwiches & Pitas					
Cajun Chicken Sandwich	820	43	66	4	45
• Chicken Ranch Sandwich	1150	70	82	3	45
Chili's Cheesesteak Sandwich	1010	55	72	4	61
Grilled Chicken Sandwich	840	47	57	2	48
Pita – Chicken Caesar	650	41	31	4	36
• Pita – Chicken Fajita	450	17	35	3	43
Pita – Steak Fajita	580	33	32	3	36
Smoked Turkey Sandwich	930	57	65	4	43
Smoked Turkey Sandwich w/ Bacon	1030	64	66	4	49
Seafood					
• Add On Garlic & Lime Grilled Shrimp, 4 each	160	10	3	0	12
Firecracker Tilapia	540	14	63	6	37
Grilled Salmon w/ Garlic & Herbs	700	33	53	5	48
• Grilled Shrimp Alfredo Pasta w/ Garlic Toast	1540	84	123	6	77
Southwest Cedar Plank Tilapia	680	34	53	6	40
Sides & Extras					
Black Beans w/ Pico de Gallo	115	0	19	5	6

(• = most healthy • = least healthy)   **RESTAURANTS & FAST-FOOD • 109**

RESTAURANTS & FAST-FOOD CHAINS

Chili's Restaurant (cont.)

	Cal	Fat	Cbs	Fbr	Prtn
Sides & Extras (cont.)					
Cinnamon Apples	210	8	35	5	0
Garlic Toast, 1 Piece	200	12	18	1	3
Homestyle Fries Basket	520	31	53	5	5
Homestyle Fries w/ Entrée	430	26	43	4	4
• Mashed Potatoes – Loaded	500	32	37	6	15
Mashed Potatoes w/ Black Pepper Gravy	450	28	44	3	7
Rice	210	2	45	1	4
Sautéed Mushrooms, Onions & Bell Peppers	120	10	6	2	3
Steamed Broccoli	80	6	6	3	3
Steamed Seasonal Veggies w/ Parmesan Cheese	80	5	8	3	3
• Steamed Seasonal Veggies w/ Parmesan Cheese	50	1	8	3	4
Sweet Corn on the Cob, unbuttered	180	2	55	3	6
Sizzling Fajitas & Quesadillas					
Add On Cadillac Style (rice & black beans only)	350	3	68	8	12
Add On Guacamole	60	5	3	3	0
Buffalo Chicken Fajitas	1090	76	56	6	51
Citrus Fire Chicken & Shrimp Fajitas	720	42	34	4	51
• Classic Chicken Fajitas	330	11	23	3	40
Classic Combo Chicken & Steak Fajitas	560	30	21	3	52
Classic Steak Fajitas	790	49	20	4	63
Fajita Chicken Quesadillas	1830	95	151	12	86
Fajita Combo Chicken & Steak Quesadillas	1690	87	133	12	89
• Fajita Steak Quesadillas	1830	95	151	12	86
Fajita Trio - Garlic Lime Shrmp, Grlld Stk & Chkn	870	51	28	5	71
Flour Tortillas, 4 each	400	12	79	2	9
Guac, Sour Crm, Cheese & Pico de Gallo, 1 boat	240	19	8	3	8
Mushroom Jack Fajitas	750	45	31	5	59
Rice, Black Beans, Sour Cream & Pico de Gallo	480	10	79	8	14
Steak & Portobello Fajitas	1130	84	26	5	65
Soups					
Baked Potato Soup, 1 cup	220	16	12	1	8
Broccoli Cheese Soup, 1 cup	160	9	12	2	7
Chicken Enchilada Soup, 1 cup	220	14	11	2	13
• Chicken Noodle Soup, 1 cup	50	1	7	1	2
Chicken Tortilla Soup, 1 cup	140	7	10	2	8
Chili - Terlingua w/ Toppings, 1 cup	180	8	15	3	12
• New England Clam Chowder Soup, 1 cup	470	33	27	3	17
Southwestern Vegetable Soup, 1 cup	110	5	13	2	5
Starters					
• Awesome Blossom® w/ Seasoned Sauce	2710	203	194	15	24
Blazin' Boneless Bfflo Wng w/ Mango Sau, 9 ea.	1050	67	60	4	52
Boneless Bfflo Wings w/ Bleu Cheese, 9 ea.	1170	85	50	4	51
Boneless Shanghai Wngs w/ Wasabi-Ranch, 9 ea.	1140	62	91	4	53
Bottomless Tostada Chips w/ Ht Sauce, 1 basket	480	36	26	4	6
• Bottomless Tostada Chips, 1 basket	400	36	18	3	3
Classic Nachos w/ Fajita Beef	1740	127	55	10	89
Classic Nachos w/ Fajita Chicken	1630	112	55	12	99
Classic Nachos w/ Pico de Gallo & Sour Cream	1450	108	53	10	65
Fried Cheese w/ Marinara Sauce, 9 ea.	1210	89	82	3	42
Hot Spinach & Artichoke Dip	510	17	39	18	24
w/ Tostada Chips	905	36	74	21	30
Skillet Queso	670	53	12	3	35
w/ Tostada Chips	1071	89	30	5	38

RESTAURANTS & FAST-FOOD CHAINS

Chili's Restaurant (cont.)

Starters (cont.)	Cal	Fat	Cbs	Fbr	Prtn
SW Egg rolls w/ Avocado-Ranch Dressing, 3 each	810	51	59	10	29
Texas Cheese Fries w/ Jalapeño-Ranch, 1 skillet	2070	160	73	8	85
Triple Dipper - Blazin' BBQ Wngs w/Mngo Sau, 5	620	41	35	2	28
Boneless Bfflo Wngs w/Trtll Strips & Bleu Chz, 5	760	57	0	3	28
Chicken Crispers w/ Honey Mustard, 3	780	63	21	0	34
Country Fried Chicken Crispers, 3	610	41	26	1	35
Fried Cheese Option w/ Marinara, 5	680	50	34	1	22
Honey Fried Chicken Crispers w/ Honey-Chipotle, 3	960	41	115	2	37
Hot Spinach & Artichoke Dip w/Tostada Chips	630	53	27	4	11
Shanghai Wings w/ Wasabi-Ranch, 5	780	45	63	3	30
SW Egg rolls w/ Avocado-Ranch Dressing, 2	550	35	39	6	20
Wings Over Buffalo® w/ Bleu Cheese, 5	740	67	3	0	33
Celery & Carrot Sticks Garnish	20	0	5	3	1
Wings Over Buffalo® w/ Bleu Cheese, 10	1340	117	4	0	68

Chipotle

	Cal	Fat	Cbs	Fbr	Prtn
Barbacoa, 4 oz.	170	7	2	0	24
Black Beans, 4 oz.	130	1	22	12	9
Burrito Size Flour Tortilla, 1 ea	290	9	44	2	7
Carnitas, 4 oz.	210	11	2	0	26
Cheese, 1 oz.	110	9	0	0	7
Chicken, 4 oz.	200	7	2	0	33
• Chips, 4 oz.	570	27	73	8	8
Corn Salsa, 4 oz.	100	1	22	3	3
Crispy Taco Shells, 3 ea	180	7	26	2	3
Fajita Vegetables, 3 oz.	100	8	6	1	1
Green Tomatillo, 2 oz.	15	1	3	1	1
Guacamole, 4 oz.	140	10	10	10	2
• Lettuce, 1 oz.	5	0	0	1	1
Pinto Beans, 4 oz.	138	1	23	10	9
Red Tomatillo, 2 oz.	28	1	4	1	1
Rice, 4 oz.	160	4	30	1	3
Sour Cream, 2 oz.	120	10	2	0	2
Steak, 4 oz.	190	7	2	0	29
Taco Size Flour Tortilla, 3 ea	255	8	38	2	6
Tomato Salsa, 4 oz.	20	0	3	0	2
Vinaigrette, 2 oz.	330	31	12	0	0

Chuck E. Cheese

	Cal	Fat	Cbs	Fbr	Prtn
Appetizers					
• Buffalo Wings, 12 ea	660	45	3	0	60
Italian Bread Sticks, 1 stick	193	8	27	1	4
• Mozzarella Sticks, 1 stick	105	6	7	0	3
Birthday Cakes					
8" Chocolate/white, 1 slice	310	13	45	1	3
8" White/white, 1 slice	310	13	44	1	3
Desserts					
Apple Pie Pizza, 1 slice	194	2	40	1	3
Cinnamon Sticks, 1 stick	197	5	33	1	4
French Fries					
French fries, 5 oz.	241	9	37	3	4
French fries, ala carte, 10 oz.	482	17	74	6	9

RESTAURANTS & FAST-FOOD CHAINS

Chuck E. Cheese (cont.)

	Cal	Fat	Cbs	Fbr	Prtn
Pizzas					
• Individual w/ cheese, 1 slice	155	5	22	1	6
Pepperoni, 1 slice	172	6	22	1	6
Large w/ cheese, 1 slice	262	8	36	2	10
• All Meat Combo, 1 slice	332	14	37	2	14
BBQ Chicken, 1 slice	296	8	47	2	12
Canadian Bacon & Pineapple, 1 slice	272	8	38	2	11
Pepperoni & Sausage, 1 slice	313	13	37	2	12
Pepperoni, 1 slice	289	10	36	2	11
Super Combo, 1 slice	305	12	39	2	12
Vegetarian, 1 slice	264	8	40	2	10
Medium w/ cheese, 1 slice	237	7	33	2	9
All Meat Combo, 1 slice	292	12	33	2	12
BBQ Chicken, 1 slice	269	8	43	2	11
Canadian Bacon & Pineapple, 1 slice	245	7	34	2	10
Pepperoni & Sausage, 1 slice	281	11	33	2	11
Pepperoni, 1 slice	263	10	33	2	10
Super Combo, 1 slice	270	10	35	2	10
Vegetarian, 1 slice	237	7	36	2	9
Small w/ cheese, 1 slice	192	6	27	1	7
All Meat Combo, 1 slice	227	9	27	1	9
BBQ Chicken, 1 slice	214	6	34	2	9
Canadian Bacon & Pineapple, 1 slice	199	6	28	1	8
Pepperoni & Sausage, 1 slice	230	9	27	1	8
Pepperoni, 1 slice	216	8	27	1	8
Super Combo, 1 slice	220	8	29	1	8
Vegetarian, 1 slice	194	6	30	2	7
Salad Dressings					
• Blue Cheese, 29 g	150	16	1	0	1
• French, 33 g	35	0	8	0	0
Lite Ranch, 30 g	80	8	1	0	1
Olive Oil & Vinegar, 31 g	100	11	1	0	0
Thousand Island, 30 g	150	15	5	0	0
Sandwiches					
Grilled Chicken Sub	652	31	70	5	36
Ham & Cheese	622	28	70	5	33
• Hot Dog	170	17	27	1	12
Hot Dog w/Cheese	335	30	28	1	22
• Italian Sub	729	40	69	5	33

Church's Chicken

	Cal	Fat	Cbs	Fbr	Prtn
Condiments					
BBQ Sauce, 21 g	30	0	7	0	0
Creamy Jalapeño Sauce, 21 g	100	11	1	0	0
Honey Mustard Sauce, 21 g	110	11	4	0	0
Honey, 9 g	27	0	7	0	0
• Hot Sauce, 7 g	18	0	0	0	0
Ketchup, 17 g	18	0	5	0	0
Purple Pepper Sauce, 21 g	45	0	12	0	0
• Ranch Sauce, 30 g	130	13	1	0	0
Sweet & Sour Sauce, 21 g	30	0	8	0	0
Desserts					
• Edward's Double Lemon Pie, 85 g	300	14	39	0	5
Edward's Strawberry Cream Cheese, 78 g	280	15	32	2	4

RESTAURANTS & FAST-FOOD CHAINS

Church's Chicken (cont.)

	Cal	Fat	Cbs	Fbr	Prtn
Desserts (cont.)					
• Pie Apple Pie, 88 g	260	11	39	1	2
Main Course					
Bigger Better Chicken Sandwich w/ Cheese, 182 g	510	27	46	4	20
Chkn. Fried Steak w/ White Gravy, 164 g	470	28	36	1	21
• Chkn. Fried Steak, w/ White Gravy, 213 g	610	43	31	2	24
Chicken Fried Steak Sandwich, 142 g	490	32	38	2	13
Crunchy Tenders, 54 g	120	6	6	0	12
Original Breast, 1 piece	200	11	3	1	22
• Original Leg, 1 piece	110	6	3	0	10
Original Thigh, 1 piece	330	23	8	1	21
Original Wing, 1 piece	300	19	7	3	27
Spicy Breast, 1 piece	320	20	12	2	21
Spicy Crunchy Tenders, 54 g	135	7	7	4	11
Spicy Fish Fillet, 65 g	160	9	13	1	7
Spicy Fish Sandwich, 108 g	320	20	25	2	10
Spicy Leg, 1 piece	180	11	8	1	12
Spicy Thigh, 1 piece	480	35	20	2	22
Spicy Wing, 1 piece	430	27	17	2	29
Sides					
Cajun Rice, 88 g	130	7	16	1	1
Cole Slaw, 118 g	150	10	15	2	1
Collard Greens, 100 g	25	0	5	2	2
Corn on the Cob, 1 ear	140	3	24	9	4
French Fries, 100 g	290	14	38	4	3
Honey Butter Biscuits, 60 g	240	12	28	1	3
Jalapeño Bombers®, 113 g	240	10	29	3	8
Macaroni & Cheese, 150 g	210	11	23	1	8
Mashed Potatoes & Gravy, 104 g	70	2	12	1	2
Okra, 113 g	350	22	36	5	3
• Sweet Corn Nuggets, 210 g	600	29	72	5	7
• Whole Jalapeño Peppers, 36 g	10	0	2	1	0

Cici's Pizza

	Cal	Fat	Cbs	Fbr	Prtn
Extras & Desserts					
• Apple Pizza, 1 slice	149	4	26	1	3
Brownies, 1 slice	143	6	22	1	1
Cinnamon Rolls, 1 slice	139	6	20	1	2
Garlic Bread, 1 slice	99	5	10	0	4
Pizza: 15" To-Go Pizzas					
Alfredo, 1 slice	216	2	27	2	8
Bacon Cheddar, 1 slice	257	8	36	4	10
BBQ, 1 slice	289	10	36	2	13
Beef, 1 slice	260	10	28	3	14
Cheese, 1 slice	223	8	28	3	11
Ham & Pineapple, 1 slice	225	8	27	24	11
• Ole, 1 slice	169	4	26	3	7
Pepperoni & Jalapeño, 1 slice	221	9	25	3	10
Pepperoni, 1 slice	240	10	27	3	11
• Sausage, 1 slice	290	10	28	3	12
Spinach Alfredo, 1 slice	243	8	32	3	11
Zesty Ham & Cheddar, 1 slice	229	11	24	2	11
Zesty Pepperoni, 1 slice	246	12	26	2	10
Zesty Tomato Alfredo, 1 slice	217	8	27	2	8

RESTAURANTS & FAST-FOOD CHAINS

Cici's Pizza (cont.)

	Cal	Fat	Cbs	Fbr	Prtn
Pizza: 15" To-Go Pizzas (cont.)					
Zesty Veggie, 1 slice	213	9	25	2	9
Pizza: Buffet Pizza					
12" Alfredo, 1 slice	139	5	18	1	6
12" Bacon Cheddar, 1 slice	145	5	18	3	6
12" BBQ, 1 slice	172	6	21	2	8
12" Beef, 1 slice	170	7	18	1	9
12" Cheese, 1 slice	152	5	20	1	7
12" Ham & Pineapple, 1 slice	141	4	19	1	7
• 12" Ole, 1 slice	108	4	13	2	5
12" Pepperoni & Jalapeño, 1 slice	163	6	20	2	8
12" Pepperoni, 1 slice	175	7	21	2	8
• 12" Sausage, 1 slice	197	7	19	1	8
12" Spinach Alfredo, 1 slice	151	5	20	2	7
12" Zesty Ham & Cheddar, 1 slice	153	6	18	1	6
12" Zesty Pepperoni, 1 slice	157	7	18	1	6
12" Zesty Tomato Alfredo, 1 slice	136	5	18	2	6
12" Zesty Veggie, 1 slice	124	4	17	1	5

Cinnabon

	Cal	Fat	Cbs	Fbr	Prtn
Classic Cinnabon	813	32	117	4	15
• The Caramel Pecanbon	1100	56	141	8	16
• The Minibon	339	13	49	2	6

Cold Stone Creamery

	Cal	Fat	Cbs	Fbr	Prtn
6" Cakes - per slice					
A Cheesecake Named Desire™, 145 g	420	19	56	1	5
Butterfinger® Bonanza, 140 g	450	21	59	1	6
• Cake Batter Confetti™, 130 g	350	17	46	1	5
Caramel Nut Nirvana™, 144 g	510	29	57	3	7
Chocolate Chipper™, 133 g	450	26	49	3	6
• Coffeehouse Crunch™, 146 g	530	31	59	3	6
Cookie Dough Delirium™, 136 g	420	21	53	1	5
Cookies & Creamery™, 129 g	390	20	49	1	6
Midnight Delight™, 151 g	510	28	60	4	5
MMMMMM Chip™, 127 g	380	19	46	2	5
Peanut Butter Playground™, 139 g	490	29	54	3	7
Raspberry Truffle Temptation™, 145 g	470	25	55	3	6
Strawberry Passion™, 141 g	390	19	50	1	5
Zebra Stripes Dark, 146 g	480	29	53	3	6
Zebra Stripes, 137 g	400	22	46	1	5
Grab and Go Ice Cream					
Chocolate Devotion™, 74 g	200	11	26	1	3
Coffee Lovers Only®, 74 g	210	13	22	1	3
Crème De La Berry™, 74 g	180	9	23	0	3
Founder's Favorite®, 74 g	210	12	24	1	3
Peanut Butter Cup Perfection™, 74 g	220	13	24	1	4
• Rocky Off Road™, 74 g	230	14	25	2	4
Shock-A-Cone™, 74 g	220	13	26	0	2
• Zenilla™, 74 g	170	11	17	0	3
Ice Cream (Love It)					
Amaretto Ice Cream, 227 g	530	31	53	0	8
Banana Ice Cream, 227 g	500	29	53	0	8
Black Cherry Ice Cream, 227 g	530	30	58	0	8

RESTAURANTS & FAST-FOOD CHAINS

Cold Stone Creamery (cont.)	Cal	Fat	Cbs	Fbr	Prtn
Ice Cream (Love It) (cont.)					
Bubble Gum Ice Cream, 227 g	520	27	64	0	7
Butter Pecan Ice Cream, 227 g	520	31	53	0	8
Cake Batter Ice Cream™, 227 g	550	30	66	0	8
Candy Cane Ice Cream, 227 g	560	32	64	0	7
Cheesecake Ice Cream, 227 g	520	29	59	0	8
Chocolate Ice Cream, 227 g	520	32	53	2	9
• Cinnamon Bun Ice Cream, 227 g	600	33	68	0	7
Cinnamon Ice Cream, 227 g	530	32	55	1	8
Coconut Ice Cream, 227 g	520	31	52	0	8
Coffee Ice Cream, 227 g	530	31	54	0	8
Cookie Batter Ice Cream, 227 g	600	32	71	0	7
Cotton Candy Ice Cream, 227 g	530	31	55	0	8
Dark Chocolate Ice Cream, 227 g	540	32	51	5	11
Dark Chocolate Peppermint Ice Cream, 227 g	540	32	54	5	11
French Toast Ice Cream, 227 g	530	31	56	0	8
French Vanilla Ice Cream, 227 g	540	30	60	0	8
Irish Cream Ice Cream, 227 g	530	32	54	0	8
Macadamia Nut Ice Cream, 227 g	530	31	540	0	8
Mango Ice Cream, 227 g	490	29	53	0	7
Mint Ice Cream, 227 g	530	30	57	0	8
Mocha Ice Cream, 227 g	520	31	53	2	9
Oatmeal Cookie Batter Ice Cream, 227 g	540	31	58	1	9
Orange Dreamsicle Ice Cream, 227 g	510	30	55	0	8
Peach Ice Cream, 227 g	500	27	58	1	7
Peanut Butter Ice Cream, 227 g	590	39	53	1	12
Pecan Praline Ice Cream, 227 g	530	30	58	0	8
Pistachio Ice Cream, 227 g	520	31	54	0	8
Pumpkin Ice Cream, 227 g	460	24	53	2	7
Raspberry Ice Cream, 227 g	520	30	57	0	8
• Sinless Sans Fat™Sweet Cream, 227 g	220	0	55	1	10
Strawberry Ice Cream, 227 g	510	30	55	0	8
Sweet Cream Ice Cream, 227 g	530	32	53	0	8
Vanilla Bean Ice Cream, 227 g	530	31	52	0	8
White Chocolate Ice Cream, 227 g	520	31	53	0	8
Light Ice Cream (Love It)					
• Cake Batter Light Ice Cream, 227 g	390	10	68	0	11
Chocolate Light Ice Cream, 227 g	350	10	57	1	12
Coffee Light Ice Cream, 227 g	350	9	56	0	11
• Vanilla Light Ice Cream, 227 g	350	9	56	0	11
Mix-Ins: Candy					
Almond Joy® Candy, 35 g	170	9	21	2	1
Butterfinger® Candy, 30 g	140	6	22	1	2
Chocolate Chips, 1 oz.	130	7	16	1	1
Chocolate Shavings, 0.5 oz.	90	5	9	2	1
Gumballs, 1 oz.	90	0	23	1	0
Gummi Bears, 1 oz.	120	0	30	0	0
Heath® Candy Bar, 20 g	110	7	12	0	1
Kit Kat® Candy Bar, 20 g	110	5	13	0	1
• Kool-Aid® Infusions, 05 oz.	80	3	14	0	0
M&M's® Candy, 1 oz.	170	7	25	1	2
Nestle® Crunch Bar, 25 g	130	7	16	1	2
Peanut M&M's®, 1 oz.	150	8	18	1	3
• Reese's® Peanut Butter Cup, 35 g	190	11	19	1	4

RESTAURANTS & FAST-FOOD CHAINS

Cold Stone Creamery (cont.)	Cal	Fat	Cbs	Fbr	Prtn
Mix-Ins: Candy (cont.)					
Reese's® Pieces, 1 oz.	180	9	21	1	4
Snickers® Candy, 35 g	170	9	21	1	3
Twix® Candy, 30 g	150	7	20	0	1
White Chocolate Chips, 1 oz.	160	9	18	0	2
Whoppers® Candy, 1 oz.	120	4	19	0	1
York® Peppermint Patties, 1 oz.	120	2	24	1	1
Mix-Ins: Fruit					
Apple Pie Filling, 3/4 oz.	60	0	16	1	0
Bananas, 60 g	50	0	14	2	1
• Black Cherries, 3/4 oz.	80	0	18	0	0
Blackberries, 3/4 oz.	10	0	2	1	0
Blueberries, 3/4 oz.	10	0	2	0	0
Cherry Pie Filling, 3/4 oz.	50	0	13	0	0
• Maraschino Cherries, 1 g	5	0	1	0	0
Peach Pie Filling, 1 oz.	60	0	16	1	0
Pineapple Chunks, 3/4 oz.	15	0	4	0	0
Raisins, 1 oz.	70	0	20	1	0
Raspberries, 3/4 oz.	25	0	5	1	0
Strawberries, 3/4 oz.	20	0	7	1	0
Nuts					
Cashews, 1 oz.	170	14	9	1	5
Macadamia Nuts, 1 oz.	180	19	3	2	2
Peanuts, 1 oz.	210	18	5	3	10
• Pecan Pralines, 1 oz.	210	21	5	2	2
Pecans, 1 oz.	140	15	3	2	2
Pistachio Nuts, 1 oz.	200	16	10	4	7
Roasted Almonds, 1 oz.	150	14	4	3	5
Sliced Almonds, 1 oz.	210	20	6	4	7
• Walnuts, 1 oz.	130	13	3	1	3
Other Mix-Ins					
Brownies, 40 g	170	4	32	1	2
Coconut, 0.5 oz.	80	5	7	1	0
• Cookie Dough, 40 g	180	8	26	0	1
Graham Cracker Pie Crust, 1 oz.	130	6	17	1	1
Granola, 1 oz.	120	2	23	2	2
Marshmallows, 1 oz.	100	0	24	0	1
• Nilla Wafers, 15 g	70	3	11	0	1
OREO® Cookies, 25 g	120	5	18	1	1
OREO® Pie Crust, 1 oz.	180	8	19	0	0
Peanut Butter, 3/4 oz.	150	13	5	1	6
Toasted Coconut, 0.5 oz.	90	7	7	1	1
Yellow Cake, 25 g	80	3	13	0	2
Shakes (Love It)					
Cake 'n Shake™, 629 g	1480	76	186	1	24
Cherry Cheeseshake™, 636 g	1290	66	157	1	19
Cream de Menthe™, 571 g	1280	74	138	2	20
Lotta Caramel Latte™, 660 g	1530	72	200	0	20
Milk and Cookies™, 598 g	1400	80	154	1	22
Oh Fudge!™, 773 g	1660	91	191	4	27
• PB&C™, 687 g	1690	111	149	8	39
• Savory Strawberry™, 636 g	1200	67	138	2	19
Very Vanilla™, 607 g	1390	69	173	0	20

RESTAURANTS & FAST-FOOD CHAINS

Cold Stone Creamery (cont.)	Cal	Fat	Cbs	Fbr	Prtn
Smoothies (Like It)					
2 to Mango™, 437 g	330	0	86	1	0
Berry Lemony™, 470 g	370	0	97	2	1
Berry Trinity™ (Soy), 437 g	270	3	57	4	7
• Berry Trinity™ (Yogurt), 417 g	260	0	60	2	8
Citrus Sunsation™, 549 g	420	0	107	2	1
• Dew Iced™, 390 g	570	0	151	1	0
Man-Go Bananas™ (Soy), 457 g	360	3	80	4	7
Man-Go Bananas™ (Yogurt), 437 g	360	0	83	2	8
On the YoGo™ (Soy), 445 g	370	3	82	3	7
On the YoGo™ (Yogurt), 425 g	360	0	85	1	7
Strawberry Bananza™, 516 g	350	0	91	4	2
Sorbet (Love It)					
Green Apple Gummy Bear, 227 g	250	0	65	1	0
• Lemon Sorbet™, 227 g	250	0	64	0	0
• Raspberry Sorbet™, 227 g	260	0	67	0	0
• Watermelon Sorbet™, 227 g	260	0	66	0	0
Toppings					
Butterscotch Fat Free, 1 oz.	80	0	0	0	1
Caramel Fat Free, 1 oz.	80	0	0	0	1
Chocolate Sprinkles, 1 oz.	25	0	0	0	0
• Cinnamon, 1 oz.	0	0	0	0	0
Fudge Fat Free, 1 oz.	80	0	0	0	1
Honey, 1 oz.	90	0	0	0	0
Marshmallow Crème, 1 oz.	100	0	0	0	0
Rainbow Sprinkles, 1 oz.	25	0	0	0	0
Reddi Whip® Original, 20 g	45	3	0	0	1
Smuckers Caramel, 1 oz.	100	0	0	0	0
• Smuckers Fudge, 1 oz.	100	3	0	0	1
Waffle Products					
• Dipped Waffle, 68 g	310	15	46	2	3
• Sugar Cone, 13 g	50	0	11	0	1
Waffle Cone or Bowl, 38 g	160	4	29	0	2

Corner Bakery Café	Cal	Fat	Cbs	Fbr	Prtn
Breakfast					
All American Scrambler no potatoes or bread	310	22	3	0	23
Anaheim Scrambler no potatoes or bread	490	36	10	4	30
Baked French Toast	570	15	86	1	13
Buckhead Cheese Grits	350	22	19	2	11
Crunchy Honey Banana Oatmeal	380	3	78	5	12
Farmer's Scrambler, no potatoes or bread	430	31	6	1	31
Fresh Berry Parfait	330	4	67	5	9
Ham & Cheddar Panini	720	34	57	2	42
Oatmeal	280	7	41	3	12
• Seasonal Fruit Medley	90	0	24	2	1
Smoked Bacon & Cheddar Panini	680	34	56	2	33
Swiss Oatmeal	330	1	79	6	4
• The Commuter Croissant	720	46	44	2	29
Entree Salads					
• Caesar Salad	520	44	19	5	11
with Roasted Chicken	640	49	19	5	29
with Roasted Chicken, no croutons	540	44	8	5	27
Chopped Salad, no bread	810	61	27	10	40

RESTAURANTS & FAST-FOOD CHAINS

Corner Bakery Café (cont.)

	Cal	Fat	Cbs	Fbr	Prtn
Entree Salads (cont.)					
Harvest Salad	860	68	53	10	19
• with Roasted Chicken	980	72	53	10	37
Santa Fe Ranch	680	44	56	10	19
with Roasted Chicken	800	49	56	10	37
Panini					
• California Grille Panini	700	41	59	8	29
Chicken Pomodori Panini	890	45	74	5	47
Club Panini	900	48	72	4	50
• Corned Beef Reuben Panini	930	48	76	2	44
Grilled Ham & Swiss Panini	880	44	75	4	45
Pasta					
Chicken Carbonara	740	28	70	4	51
Half Moon Cheese Ravioli	550	21	63	4	28
• Penne with Marinara	550	11	92	14	20
• Pesto Cavatappi	930	40	93	13	52
Salad Dressings					
Balsamic Vinaigrette	300	31	4	0	0
• Caesar	310	32	2	0	1
House Dressing	280	27	8	0	0
Ranch	160	16	2	0	2
Sandwiches					
Bavarian with Ham	720	25	78	4	40
Bavarian with Turkey	690	22	78	4	39
• Chicken Pesto	840	41	75	5	41
D.C. Chicken Salad	750	37	81	4	27
Southwest Roast Beef	840	37	78	5	44
Tomato Mozzarella	670	26	73	5	28
• Tuna Salad on Olive Bread	450	16	42	3	29
Turkey Derby	650	29	60	5	39
Turkey Harvest	560	7	91	7	29
Uptown Turkey	660	29	61	9	39
Side Salads					
Cucumber Tomato Salad, 6 oz.	140	9	13	1	1
D.C. Chicken Salad, 6 oz.	560	46	18	4	20
• Egg Salad, 6 oz.	570	53	2	0	16
Roasted Potato Bacon Salad, 6 oz.	370	23	29	3	8
• Seasonal Fruit Medley, 6 oz.	90	0	22	2	1
Tomato Mozzarella Pasta Salad, 6 oz.	205	8	24	4	7
Tuna Salad, 6 oz.	310	16	3	1	34
Soup					
Big Al's Chili with cheddar cheese, 10 oz.	380	17	29	8	23
• Butternut Bisque, 10 oz.	166	6	27	3	3
Cheddar Broccoli, 10 oz.	310	23	16	2	9
Chicken Wild Mushroom Brie Stew, 10 oz.	260	14	20	2	11
Chicken Wild Mushroom Brie Stew, bread bowl	420	30	21	2	12
Chkn. Wild Mushroom Brie Stew, Cup w/ Caesar	510	35	28	5	17
Chkn. Wild Mushroom Brie Stew, Cup w/ Greens	480	31	35	6	14
Loaded Baked Potato, 10 oz.	420	29	29	2	13
Mom's Chicken Noodle lower fat, 10 oz.	170	4	23	1	8
Old Fashioned Beef Stew, 10 oz.	260	13	20	2	7
Old Fashioned Beef Stew, bread bowl	420	29	21	2	8
• Old Fashioned Beef Stew, Cup w/ Caesar Salad	510	34	28	5	12
Old Fashioned Beef Stew, Cup w/ Mixed Greens	480	29	34	6	9

RESTAURANTS & FAST-FOOD CHAINS

Corner Bakery Café (cont.)	Cal	Fat	Cbs	Fbr	Prtn
Soup (cont.)					
Roasted Tomato Basil, 10 oz.	170	5	27	4	3
Zesty Chicken Tortilla w/ tortilla strips, 10 oz.	230	11	26	5	8

Cosi	Cal	Fat	Cbs	Fbr	Prtn
Arctics					
Arctic Latte - Grande, 16 oz.	527	16	94	0	6
Arctic Mocha - Grande, 16 oz.	539	14	101	1	6
• Arctic Raspberry Chai - Grande, 16 oz.	404	11	75	0	3
• Double Oh! Arctic - Grande, 16 oz.	758	29	123	2	9
Smores Latte - Grande, 16 oz.	509	23	61	1	14
Bagels					
Asiago Cheese, 6 oz.	327	1	68	2	9
• Cinnamon Raisin, 6 oz.	438	1	90	5	10
Cranberry Orange, 6 oz.	372	1	80	2	9
Etruscan Whole Grain, 5 oz.	331	3	66	4	10
Everything, 6 oz.	353	3	71	3	10
• Plain, 6 oz.	326	1	68	2	9
Poppy Seed, 6 oz.	346	3	69	3	10
Sesame, 6 oz.	347	3	69	3	10
Baked Omelette Sandwiches					
• Bacon & Cheddar, 5 oz.	326	16	1	0	24
Ham & Swiss, 5 oz.	225	15	1	0	20
• Plain, 4 oz.	131	9	1	0	10
Spinach & Tomato, 5 oz.	142	9	3	1	11
Beverage Favorites					
Chai Tea Latte - Grande, 12 oz.	163	3	23	0	6
• Hot Chocolate - Grande, 16 oz.	502	31	49	1	12
Iced Tea - Grande, 12 oz.	22	0	6	0	0
Lemonade, 15 oz.	112	0	26	0	0
• Mint Hot Chocolate, 10 oz.	10	10	10	10	10
Mocha Latte - Grande, 13 oz.	358	18	40	1	9
Steamer, 10 oz.	10	10	10	10	10
Beverages: Coffee & Espresso					
• Café Americano, 10 oz.	10	10	10	10	10
Café Au Lait, 10 oz.	10	10	10	10	10
Cappuccino, 10 oz.	10	10	10	10	10
Caramel Mocha - Grande, 12 oz.	420	22	50	1	7
• Egg Nog Latte - Grande, 14 oz.	527	26	65	0	12
Espresso, 10 oz.	10	10	10	10	10
House Coffee, 10 oz.	10	10	10	10	10
Latté, 10 oz.	10	10	10	10	10
Mint Mocha, 10 oz.	10	10	10	10	10
Breakfast Favorites					
Apple Crumb Cake, 6 oz.	540	30	62	1	7
• Bagel Club Sandwich, 8 oz.	719	31	70	2	39
Biscotti Amaretto, 3 oz.	240	8	34	0	5
Biscotti Chocolate, 3 oz.	280	13	38	3	5
Cosi Break Bar, 1 oz.	463	24	54	4	11
Croissant - Almond, 3 oz.	340	16	42	2	7
Croissant - Butter, 3 oz.	330	17	38	1	7
Croissant - Chocolate, 3 oz.	370	18	45	2	8
Dried Fruits & Yogurt Parfait, 12 oz.	586	6	112	11	15
Fruit Salad, 8 oz.	216	1	54	5	4

(• = most healthy • = least healthy) **RESTAURANTS & FAST-FOOD • 119**

RESTAURANTS & FAST-FOOD CHAINS

Cosi (cont.)

	Cal	Fat	Cbs	Fbr	Prtn
Breakfast Favorites (cont.)					
Granola Cereal, 9 oz.	564	12	107	8	14
Granola Peach Parfait, 12 oz.	389	6	74	3	13
Granola Strawberry Parfait, 12 oz.	426	6	84	4	13
Plain Crumb Cake, 6 oz.	600	36	61	1	8
Cream Cheese					
Fruit Trio, 2 oz.	159	14	7	0	2
Low Fat Plain, 2 oz.	121	12	2	0	6
• Low Fat Veggie, 2 oz.	113	9	2	0	4
• Plain, 2 oz.	182	18	2	0	4
Desserts					
Apple Tart, 6 oz.	396	6	83	4	5
Blondie Brownie, 4 oz.	570	36	57	2	6
Cheesecake Brownie, 4 oz.	470	26	55	1	5
Cheesecake, 6 oz.	567	33	62	0	7
Chocolate Chunk Cookie, 4 oz.	480	20	72	0	8
Cinnamon Apple Pie, 14 oz.	960	40	147	4	10
Creme Brulee Cheesecake, 3 oz.	307	21	25	0	5
• Double Scoop Ice Cream, 6 oz.	225	14	22	0	4
• Double Trouble Brownie Sundae, 18 oz.	1586	77	198	4	18
Extra chocolate Bar, 2 oz.	230	13	24	1	3
Large Sundae, 11 oz.	520	31	55	1	6
Medium Sundae, 8 oz.	408	24	43	1	6
Mississippi Mud Pie, 9 oz.	850	49	109	9	9
Oatmeal Raisin Cookie, 4 oz.	440	14	76	3	8
Plain Cheesecake, 3 oz.	307	21	25	0	5
Rocky Road Brownie, 6 oz.	550	33	49	2	13
S'mmm...Oreos ™ (For 4), 14 oz.	1535	45	271	7	21
S'mmm...Oreos ™ (For 2), 7 oz.	827	24	147	4	12
S'mores (For 4), 14 oz.	1382	39	244	6	19
S'mores (For 2), 7 oz.	751	21	133	3	10
Triple Scoop Ice Cream, 9 oz.	338	20	34	0	7
White Chocolate Mac Cookie, 4 oz.	520	24	72	0	8
Dinner Flatbread Pizza					
Margherita Pizza, 25 oz.	1656	71	228	16	72
• Meat Trio, 28 oz.	1986	97	227	16	93
Pan Asian Chicken, 33 oz.	1668	67	267	22	42
Pepperoni Pizza, 25 oz.	1829	86	226	16	77
• Traditional Cheese, 23 oz.	1539	62	225	16	64
Every Day Soups					
Pollo E Pasta (Reg/Cup), 10 oz.	122	3	12	1	10
Tomato Basil Aurora (Reg/Cup), 10 oz.	374	34	18	2	5
Fruit Smoothies					
Blueberry Pomegranate - Grande, 16 oz.	725	1	179	1	0
• Citrus Passion Fruit - Grande, 16 oz.	753	0	186	1	1
• Mango Mania - Grande, 16 oz.	715	0	177	1	0
Strawberry - Banana - Grande, 16 oz.	720	0	179	3	1
Hearth-Baked Dinners					
• Alpine Chicken, 13 oz.	973	63	28	2	77
Grilled Wild Alaskan Salmon, 11 oz.	623	13	35	23	93
• Turkey & Stuffing, 18 oz.	458	21	41	1	32
Individual Flatbread Pizza					
Margherita Pizza, 13 oz.	829	36	114	8	36
• Meat Trio, 14 oz.	994	49	113	8	46

Cosi (cont.)	Cal	Fat	Cbs	Fbr	Prtn
Individual Flatbread Pizza (cont.)					
Pan Asian Chicken, 16 oz.	833	33	133	11	21
Pepperoni Pizza, 13 oz.	911	43	112	8	38
• Traditional Cheese, 12 oz.	769	31	112	8	32
Kid's Pizza					
Cheese Pizza, 23 oz.	1257	34	187	8	53
Pepperoni Pizza, 28 oz.	1901	93	190	8	76
Kids Menu					
• Gooey Grilled Cheese, 4 oz.	357	21	26	2	21
Tuna Sandwich, 5 oz.	333	13	27	2	25
• Turkey Sandwich, 5 oz.	289	7	48	1	8
Melts					
Bacon Turkey Cheddar, 12 oz.	682	25	74	4	45
Chicken TBM Melt, 15 oz.	926	47	68	8	64
Grilled Chicken Parmesan, 12 oz.	701	27	64	8	50
Pesto Chicken, 12 oz.	809	39	64	7	54
• Tomato, Basil & Mozzarella Melt, 10 oz.	666	34	67	7	31
• Tuna Melt, 13 oz.	1012	60	56	4	64
Muffins					
Banana Nut Muffin, 5 oz.	480	22	63	3	9
Blueberry Muffin, 5 oz.	440	19	60	2	8
Carrot Muffin, 5 oz.	470	22	62	3	8
• Chocolate Chocolate Chip Muffin, 5 oz.	506	27	67	2	8
Corn Muffin, 5 oz.	450	25	50	3	7
• Low Fat Bran Muffin, 5 oz.	351	6	70	8	8
Salads					
• Bombay Chicken, 13 oz.	176	3	13	4	27
Caesar Dressing, 2 oz.	301	32	2	0	2
Caesar w/ Grilled Chicken, 10 oz.	340	16	21	3	33
Caesar, 7 oz.	182	8	20	2	8
Cosi Cobb, 11 oz.	419	28	8	4	43
Cosi Vinaigrette, 2 oz.	357	39	2	0	0
Fat Free Balsamic Vinaigrette, 2 oz.	45	0	11	0	0
Greek Salad, 12 oz.	236	17	9	4	11
Italian Dressing, 2 oz.	279	30	2	0	2
Low Fat Ginger Soy Dressing, 2 oz.	74	2	13	1	1
Pepperanch Dressing, 2 oz.	262	28	2	0	2
Reduced Fat Roasted Shallot Sherry, 2 oz.	85	5	3	0	0
Roasted Shallot Sherry Vinaigrette, 2 oz.	308	31	8	0	0
• Salad Bruschetta, 18 oz.	474	13	67	26	60
Shanghai Chicken, 9 oz.	221	9	16	5	26
Signature Salad, 10 oz.	375	21	40	7	15
Wild Alaskan Salmon Salad, 15 oz.	339	15	20	7	34
Sandwiches					
Buffalo Blue, 10 oz.	649	30	57	5	44
Classic Turkey & Stuffing, 13 oz.	440	10	65	2	26
Così Club, 10 oz.	702	35	59	4	37
Green Market, 12 oz.	555	17	74	7	23
Grilled Chicken T.B.M., 10 oz.	791	43	60	6	48
• Hummus & Fresh Veggies, 12 oz.	432	8	77	8	13
Italiano, 10 oz.	834	47	58	4	43
Meatball Aurora, 11 oz.	796	40	63	8	39
Roasted Turkey & Brie, 11 oz.	772	36	71	3	41

RESTAURANTS & FAST-FOOD CHAINS

Cosi (cont.)

Sandwiches (cont.)	Cal	Fat	Cbs	Fbr	Prtn
Sesame Ginger Chicken, 11 oz.	508	11	70	6	38
Smoked Ham & Brie, 10 oz.	639	25	69	3	33
T.B.M., 11 oz.	729	42	61	6	26
Tandoori Chicken, 10 oz.	633	26	58	4	40
• Tuna Cheddar, 12 oz.	956	55	55	4	60
Turkey Light, 10 oz.	476	9	73	4	30
Turkey Rustica, 12 oz.	619	27	60	4	37
Tuscan Pesto Chicken, 10 oz.	571	22	58	6	43
Vegi Muffaletta, 12 oz.	824	51	24	4	24
Wasabi Roast Beef, 11 oz.	626	28	64	5	31
Scones					
Blueberry Scones, 4 oz.	410	17	60	2	8
Cranberry Scones, 4 oz.	400	15	61	3	7
Shareables					
• Brie & Fruit, 6 oz.	277	15	26	2	9
• Fresh Guacamole, 10 oz.	10	10	10	10	10
Hummus Dip, 4 oz.	121	4	18	3	3
Spinach Artichoke, 3 oz.	182	15	9	3	6
Weekly Soups					
• Autumn Vegetable & Mushroom, 10 oz.	93	3	14	1	2
Beef with Winter Garden Vegetable, 10 oz.	136	7	12	1	8
Moroccan Lentil, 10 oz.	199	3	32	7	13
• New England Clam Chowder, 10 oz.	440	29	24	1	22
Sausage, Chicken & Orzo, 10 oz.	238	10	10	1	12

Country Buffet

Bread and Other Items	Cal	Fat	Cbs	Fbr	Prtn
• Biscuits, 51 g	180	7	24	1	3
Breadsticks, 47 g	140	5	21	1	4
Buns, Hot Dog, 43 g	120	2	22	1	4
• Cinnamon Bread, 50 g	45	1	10	0	1
Cinnamon Sugared Donut Holes, 11 g	50	3	5	0	1
Dinner Rolls, Wheat, 36 g	110	3	18	1	4
Dinner Rolls, White, 36 g	120	4	20	1	3
English Muffin, 26 g	60	1	13	1	2
Flour Tortilla, 38 g	120	3	20	1	4
French Toast, 74 g	170	8	24	1	5
Glazed Donuts, 34 g	130	7	16	0	2
Pancakes, 49 g	120	4	19	1	2
Taco Shells, 11 g	50	3	7	0	1
Waffles, 41 g	120	3	19	1	3
Condiments					
Bacon Bits, 7 g	25	2	0	0	3
Black Olives, sliced, 15 g	15	2	1	1	0
• Blueberry Syrup, 2 fl.oz.	250	0	63	0	0
Brown Sugar, 9 g	35	0	9	0	0
Butter, packet, 5 g	35	4	0	0	0
Cheese, Grated Parmesan, 7 g	30	2	0	0	3
Cheese, Shredded Cheddar, 10 g	40	4	0	0	3
Cherry Peppers, 11 g	4	0	1	0	0
Cocktail Sauce, 30 g	30	0	8	0	0
Coffee Creamers, packet, 11 g	15	1	0	0	0
Cranberry Sauce, 30 g	45	0	12	0	0

Country Buffet (cont.)	Cal	Fat	Cbs	Fbr	Prtn
Condiments (cont.)					
Crushed Red Pepper, 2 g	10	1	1	1	0
Diced Onions, 15 g	5	0	2	0	0
Hollandaise Sauce, 2 fl.oz.	130	13	3	0	1
Honey, packet, 14 g	45	0	11	0	0
Horseradish Sauce, 30 g	60	5	2	0	1
• Hot Sauce, 5 g	0	0	0	0	0
Jalapeño Peppers, 11 g	2	0	1	0	0
Jelly, packet, 14 g	35	0	9	0	0
Ketchup, 15 g	15	0	4	0	0
Lemons, 8 g	2	0	1	0	0
Lettuce, shredded, 14 g	0	0	0	0	0
Maple Syrup, 2 fl.oz.	180	0	47	0	0
Margarine, melted, 2 fl.oz.	410	45	1	0	1
Margarine, packet, 5 g	25	3	0	0	0
Mayonnaise, 14 g	100	11	0	0	0
Mustard, 15 g	10	1	1	1	1
Non-Dairy Creamers, packet, 11 g	10	1	1	0	0
Peanut Butter, 16 g	100	8	3	1	4
Pepperoncini Peppers, 11 g	2	0	1	0	0
Salsa, 30 g	10	0	2	0	0
Sautéed Green Peppers, 54 g	25	2	4	1	1
Sautéed Mushrooms, 51 g	30	3	2	1	2
Sautéed Onions, 51 g	30	1	5	1	1
Sliced Pickles, 11 g	2	0	1	0	0
Sliced/Diced Tomatoes, 15 g	2	0	1	0	0
Sour Cream, 12 g	25	3	1	0	0
Soy Sauce, 5 g	2	0	1	0	0
Sweet Pickle Relish, 15 g	25	0	6	0	0
Tabasco Sauce, 5 g	0	0	0	0	0
Desserts					
Apple Crisp, 94 g	150	4	31	2	1
Apple Pie, Reduced Sugar, 116 g	190	11	24	2	1
Bread Pudding, 96 g	190	8	27	1	3
Butterfinger Pieces, 15 g	70	3	11	0	1
Butterscotch Topping, 75 g	230	1	56	0	0
Cheesecake, Plain, 80 g	220	10	29	0	3
Chocolate Chips, 15 g	90	5	10	0	0
Chocolate Cream Pie-Reduced Sugar, 79 g	190	12	18	1	2
Chocolate Decadence Cake, 64 g	200	9	27	0	2
Chocolate Syrup, 37 g	80	0	21	0	0
Cone, Ice Cream, 4 g	15	0	3	0	0
Cookie-Sugar Free Ranger, 20 g	100	5	11	1	2
FunE Chips, 15 g	80	3	12	0	0
Gummy Bears, 20 g	60	0	15	0	1
Honey Nut Topping, 28 g	150	12	7	2	6
Hot Fudge Sundae Cake, 86 g	160	4	32	1	1
Hot Fudge Topping, 41 g	120	3	23	0	1
Hydrox Cookies, Crushed, 8 g	35	2	6	0	0
Malted Milk Balls, Ground, 15 g	70	3	11	0	0
Nestle Crunch Pieces, 15 g	80	4	10	0	1
Pudding, Chocolate, 86 g	150	7	19	0	2
• Pudding, Chocolate, Reduced Sugar, 86 g	70	1	14	0	2

RESTAURANTS & FAST-FOOD CHAINS

Country Buffet (cont.)

	Cal	Fat	Cbs	Fbr	Prtn
Desserts (cont.)					
Pudding, Vanilla, 86 g	140	6	19	0	2
Pudding, Vanilla, Reduced Sugar, 86 g	70	1	14	0	2
• Pumpkin Pie, 119 g	270	9	31	2	5
Rainbow Sprinkles, 15 g	70	2	13	0	0
Reduced Sugar Pie-Cherry, 95 g	160	9	16	0	3
Reduced Sugar Pie-Lemon, 95 g	160	9	16	0	3
Reduced Sugar Pie-Lime, 95 g	160	9	16	0	3
Reduced Sugar Pie-Orange, 95 g	160	9	16	0	3
Reduced Sugar Pie-Raspberry, 95 g	160	9	16	0	3
Reduced Sugar Pie-Strawberry, 95 g	160	9	16	0	3
Soft Serve Froz Yog, Nonfat, Strawberry, 4 fl.oz.	100	0	23	0	3
Soft Serve Froz Yog, Nonfat, Vanilla, 4 fl.oz.	110	0	23	0	3
Soft Serve, Chocolate, 4 fl.oz.	140	5	24	1	4
Soft Serve, Vanilla, 4 fl.oz.	150	5	25	1	3
SS Froz Yog, Nonfat, Nutrasweet, Vanilla, 4 fl.oz.	80	0	17	0	4
Strawberry Topping, 47 g	100	0	23	0	1
Whipped Topping, Non-Dairy, 21 g	60	5	5	0	0
Dressings					
• Bleu Cheese, 30 g	170	18	1	0	1
Creamy Italian, 29 g	110	11	3	0	0
Fat Free French, 30 g	35	0	8	1	0
French, 33 g	150	12	12	0	0
Italian, 32 g	120	11	5	0	0
• Low Fat Italian, 30 g	25	2	2	0	0
Ranch, 30 g	110	11	1	0	1
Reduced Fat Ranch, 30 g	60	6	2	0	1
Entrees					
• BBQ Beef Ribs, 143 g	300	23	7	0	17
BBQ Smoked Sausage, 80 g	140	10	9	1	4
Beef Liver and Onion, 45 g	80	3	4	0	9
Carved Beef Brisket, 3 oz.	200	11	1	0	25
Carved Ham, 3 oz.	140	9	0	0	13
Carved Peppered Pork Loin, 3 oz.	160	8	0	0	23
Carved Roast Beef, 3 oz.	230	15	0	0	23
Carved Roast Turkey, 3 oz.	170	8	0	0	24
Carved Salmon Filet, 3 oz.	190	12	0	0	21
Chicken and Dumplings, 136 g	190	7	24	1	7
Chicken Cacciatore, 140 g	220	11	3	1	26
Chicken, Hand Breaded Fried-breast, 143 g	310	16	3	0	38
Chicken, Hand Breaded Fried-drumstick, 39 g	90	6	2	0	8
Chicken, Hand Breaded Fried-thigh, 89 g	210	14	4	0	18
Chicken, Traditional Baked-breast, 149 g	280	12	0	0	44
Chicken, Traditional Baked-drumstick, 40 g	90	6	0	0	10
Chicken, Traditional Baked-thigh, 91 g	160	11	0	0	16
Chinese Chicken Livers, 200 g	200	12	17	1	8
Country BBQ Chicken-breast, 143 g	300	12	5	0	44
Country BBQ Chicken-drumstick, 40 g	110	6	3	0	10
Country BBQ Chicken-thigh, 91 g	210	13	4	0	20
Country BBQ Chicken-wing, 37 g	70	3	3	0	8
Denver Scrambled Eggs, 77 g	140	11	2	0	8
Egg, Poached, 50 g	70	5	0	0	6
Eggs Benedict, 134 g	250	15	15	1	15
Fish Patties, 73 g	160	9	13	0	8

RESTAURANTS & FAST-FOOD CHAINS

Country Buffet (cont.)

	Cal	Fat	Cbs	Fbr	Prtn
Entrees (cont.)					
Fish, Fried, 37 g	80	4	9	0	4
Hamburger Patties, 74 g	220	19	0	0	13
Hot Dogs, Turkey, 56 g	130	11	2	0	6
Hot Wings-Drummies, 15 g	35	2	0	0	4
• Hot Wings-Wing, 10 g	25	2	0	0	2
Mini Corn Dogs, 19 g	50	2	6	0	2
Mostaciolli, Baked, 102 g	120	5	13	1	6
Orange Chicken, 99 g	240	11	24	0	10
Quiche, Breakfast, 106 g	220	15	12	0	10
Sauerkraut , 28 g	5	0	1	0	0
Scrambled Eggs, 62 g	130	11	1	0	7
Shrimp, fried, 54 g	110	5	11	0	4
Smoked Sausage, 56 g	190	17	2	0	7
Spanish Rice, 86 g	140	9	9	1	7
Taco Meat, Beef, 2 fl.oz.	100	5	3	0	11
Teriyaki Chicken Wings-Drummie, 26 g	50	3	2	0	5
Teriyaki Chicken Wings-Wing, 13 g	50	3	2	0	4
Fruits					
Cantaloupe, 85 g	25	0	6	1	1
• Grapes, 80 g	60	0	15	1	1
Honeydew, 88 g	30	0	8	1	1
Pineapple, 78 g	35	0	10	1	0
Strawberries, 72 g	25	0	6	1	1
• Watermelon, 76 g	25	0	6	0	1
Gravies and Sauces					
• Au Jus, 2 fl.oz.	0	0	0	0	0
Gravy, Beef, 2 fl.oz.	30	2	5	0	1
Gravy, Chicken, 2 fl.oz.	30	1	5	0	1
• Gravy, Country, 2 fl.oz.	120	8	12	0	0
Gravy, Roasted Pork, 2 fl.oz.	50	4	3	0	0
Gravy, Turkey, 2 fl.oz.	10	0	1	0	0
Meat Sauce, 2 fl.oz.	70	3	4	1	7
Salad Toppers					
Bacon Bits, Imitation, 7 g	30	1	2	1	3
Black Olives, sliced, 15 g	15	2	1	1	0
Carrots, julienne, 8 g	5	5	1	0	0
Cherry Tomatoes, 17 g	5	0	1	0	0
Chow Mein Noodles, 7 g	35	2	4	1	1
Croutons, 7 g	35	2	5	0	1
Cucumbers, sliced, 15 g	2	0	1	0	0
Eggs, hard cooked, diced, 15 g	20	2	0	0	2
Feta Cheese, 40 g	35	3	1	0	2
• Mushrooms, sliced, 10 g	2	0	1	0	0
Parmesan Cheese, grated, 7 g	30	2	0	0	3
Peas, 15 g	10	0	2	1	1
Pepperoncini, 11 g	2	0	1	0	0
Raisins, 12 g	40	0	10	1	0
Red Onions, sliced, 6 g	2	0	1	0	0
Shredded Cheese, Imitation, 10 g	25	2	2	0	1
Spinach Leaves, 32 g	5	0	1	1	1
• Sunflower Seeds, 11 g	70	6	2	1	2
Salads					
Ambrosia, 89 g	140	5	23	1	1

(•= most healthy •= least healthy)

RESTAURANTS & FAST-FOOD CHAINS

	Cal	Fat	Cbs	Fbr	Prtn
Salads (cont.)					
BLT Salad, 70 g	150	14	3	1	2
Broccoli Apple Salad, 100 g	160	11	13	2	3
Caesar Salad, 65 g	80	6	5	1	2
California Coleslaw, 100 g	90	1	22	1	1
Carrot and Raisin Salad, 100 g	140	8	18	2	1
Chicken Pasta Salad, 100 g	230	18	11	1	6
Creamy Pea Salad, 100 g	160	11	11	4	7
Cucumber Tomato Salad, 100 g	30	1	6	1	1
Dilled Potato Salad, 83 g	110	8	9	1	1
Flavored Gelatin, 70 g	40	0	10	0	1
Gelatin Whip, 68 g	80	3	14	0	1
Greek Salad, 75 g	120	8	11	1	3
Macaroni Vegetable Salad, 100 g	230	15	20	1	4
Marinated Vegetables, 100 g	60	4	6	1	1
Oriental Pasta, 100 g	110	6	11	2	6
Pickled Beets, 100 g	100	0	25	2	1
Potato Salad, 75 g	110	5	14	1	2
Prunes, Stewed, 71 g	100	0	28	2	1
Raisin Fluff, 80 g	140	4	25	1	2
• Seafood Salad, 117 g	310	26	16	1	4
Seven Layer Salad, 75 g	180	17	4	1	4
Sicilian Pasta Salad, 100 g	150	9	15	2	3
• Spring Mix, 45 g	5	0	1	1	1
Strawberry Whip, 76 g	200	14	17	0	2
Strawberry-Banana Salad, 85 g	70	1	16	1	1
Strawberry-Peach-Banana, 79 g	80	1	20	1	1
Tarragon Potato Salad, 82 g	120	7	13	1	1
Three Bean Salad, 100 g	90	5	12	3	2
Tossed Green Salad, 45 g	5	0	1	1	1
Waldorf Salad, 60 g	110	7	12	1	1
Whipped Pineapple/Banana, 114 g	180	2	33	0	8
Sides					
Bacon, 6 g	30	3	0	0	2
Baked Beans, 110 g	120	1	29	4	4
Bread Dressing, 100 g	130	4	21	1	4
Cabbage, German Boiled, 85 g	40	4	3	1	1
Cabbage, Green, 85 g	40	3	3	1	1
Carrots, steamed, 85 g	40	0	9	3	1
Chesapeake Corn, 85 g	80	3	13	2	2
Corn on the Cob, 72 g	100	3	16	1	3
Corn, steamed, 85 g	100	1	21	2	3
Creamy Cheese Sauce, 2 fl.oz.	50	2	9	0	1
French Fries, 51 g	190	9	24	2	2
Fried Rice w/Ham, 100 g	170	6	23	1	7
Green Bean Casserole, 110 g	60	3	9	2	2
Green Beans El Greco, 85 g	20	0	5	2	1
• Green Beans, 85 g	15	0	3	1	1
Grits, 4 fl.oz.	70	0	16	0	2
Joe's Cracked Pepper Green Beans, 85 g	70	6	5	2	2
Montreal Vegetable Medley, 85 g	40	4	3	1	1
Oatmeal, 4 fl.oz.	70	1	13	2	3
Pinto Beans w/ Ham, 85 g	90	1	21	7	7
Potatoes, Baked Sweet, 192 g	160	0	47	6	3

RESTAURANTS & FAST-FOOD CHAINS

Country Buffet (cont.)	Cal	Fat	Cbs	Fbr	Prtn
Sides (cont.)					
Potatoes, Baked, 180 g	160	0	39	3	4
Potatoes, Hash Brown Patties, 57 g	120	8	11	1	1
Potatoes, Hash Browns, 80 g	110	6	13	1	2
Potatoes, Jo Jo, 84 g	210	15	18	2	2
Potatoes, O'Brien, 110 g	120	6	16	2	2
Potatoes, Red, 113 g	100	3	18	2	2
Red Beans w/ Ham, 85 g	90	1	18	7	8
Sausage Links, 25 g	100	10	0	0	4
Spaghetti, 85 g	90	1	19	1	3
• Spinach Marie, 110 g	210	17	8	1	8
Squash, winter, 85 g	150	9	18	1	1
Turnip or Collard Greens w/ Bacon, 110 g	40	3	2	1	1
Vegetable Stir Fry, 85 g	25	1	6	2	1
White Rice, 100 g	90	0	22	1	2
Wild Rice Vegetable Pilaf, 100 g	90	1	17	1	3
Yams, Candied, 118 g	140	2	30	1	3
Zucchini, Sautéed, 85 g	50	4	3	1	1
Soups					
Chicken Noodle Soup, 4 fl.oz.	70	2	7	1	7
Chicken Rice Soup, 4 fl.oz.	70	2	8	1	6
Chili Bean Soup, 4 fl.oz.	100	4	9	1	9
Corn Chowder, 4 fl.oz.	140	8	15	1	2
Cream of Broccoli Soup, 4 fl.oz.	80	7	5	1	1
• Navy Bean Soup w/ Ham, 4 fl.oz.	50	1	10	4	5
• New England Clam Chowder, 4 fl.oz.	300	12	9	0	3
Potato Cheese Soup, 4 fl.oz.	130	9	11	1	3

Cousins Subs	Cal	Fat	Cbs	Fbr	Prtn
5" Mini Subs					
5" Mini BLT, 125 g	298	19	24	1	9
5" Mini Chicken Cheddar Deluxe, 169 g	329	19	26	1	16
5" Mini Club, 195 g	337	18	27	1	19
• 5" Mini Garden Veggie, 146 g	216	7	26	1	11
5" Mini Ham & Provolone, 174 g	316	18	26	1	15
5" Mini Hot Veggie, 144 g	254	10	28	1	13
• 5" Mini Italian Special, 178 g	403	25	25	1	16
5" Mini Meatball & Provolone, 140 g	361	19	27	1	20
5" Mini Pepperoni Melt, 169 g	348	21	26	1	15
5" Mini Pizza Sub, 157 g	336	18	28	1	15
5" Mini Seafood with Crab, 170 g	323	19	31	1	10
5" Mini Three Cheese, 156 g	363	23	25	1	15
5" Mini Tuna, 169 g	335	20	25	1	16
5" Mini Turkey Breast, 172 g	279	14	26	1	15
7 1/2" Subs					
7½" BLT, 225 g	591	38	47	1	19
7½" Cheese Steak, 290 g	503	19	49	1	31
7½" Chicken Breast, 314 g	569	27	50	1	35
7½" Chicken Cheddar Deluxe, 330 g	669	39	51	1	34
7½" Club, 361 g	657	35	51	1	38
7½" Double Cheese Steak, 393 g	747	36	49	1	52
• 7½" Garden Veggie, 253 g	390	12	51	1	20
7½" Gyro, 344 g	710	41	61	2	32
7½" Ham & Provolone, 308 g	612	34	50	1	28

RESTAURANTS & FAST-FOOD CHAINS

▶ Cousins Subs (cont.)

	Cal	Fat	Cbs	Fbr	Prtn
7 1/2" Subs (cont.)					
7½" Hot Veggie, 277 g	472	17	55	2	24
• 7½" Italian Special, 343 g	817	51	50	1	36
7½" Meatball & Provolone, 280 g	723	38	54	2	40
7½" Pepperoni Melt, 331 g	730	45	50	1	32
7½" Philly Cheese Steak, 326 g	531	19	55	2	32
7½" Pizza Sub, 324 g	709	39	55	2	33
7½" Roast Beef, 301 g	607	30	50	1	35
7½" Seafood with Crab, 314 g	642	38	60	1	20
7½" Spicy Chicken Sedona, 308 g	530	18	54	3	37
7½" Three Cheese, 276 g	685	44	50	1	26
7½" Tuna, 312 g	666	40	49	1	32
7½" Turkey Breast, 301 g	537	28	50	1	26
Better Bunch Salads					
Chef Salad (Better Bunch), 295 g	131	3	10	2	18
Garden Salad (Better Bunch), 201 g	40	0	8	2	2
• Garden Salad w/Chicken Brst (Better Bunch), 315 g	154	1	10	3	26
• Side Salad (Better Bunch), 96 g	19	0	4	1	1
Better Bunch Subs					
5" Mini Club (Better Bunch), 169 g	193	3	26	1	16
• 5" Mini Garden Veggie (Better Bunch), 123 g	136	1	26	1	6
5" Mini Ham (Better Bunch), 149 g	178	2	26	1	13
5" Mini Hot Veggie (Better Bunch), 112 g	144	1	27	1	6
5" Mini Turkey Breast (Better Bunch), 157 g	177	2	26	1	15
7½" Chicken Breast (Better Bunch), 286 g	366	2	50	1	35
7½" Club (Better Bunch), 312 g	381	5	51	1	32
7½" Garden Veggie (Better Bunch), 218 g	266	2	50	1	11
7½" Ham (Better Bunch), 258 g	336	4	50	1	23
7½" Hot Veggie (Better Bunch), 223 g	287	2	55	2	12
• 7½" Roast Beef (Better Bunch), 272 g	405	6	50	1	35
7½" Turkey Breast (Better Bunch), 272 g	335	3	50	1	26
Limited Time Specials					
• 5" Mini Chicken Salad, 170 g	280	11	32	1	12
7½" Black Forest Bliss, 330 g	545	17	69	4	31
7½" Chicken Italiana, 371 g	520	12	57	3	44
• 7½" Chicken Salad, 314 g	556	23	62	3	25
Salads					
Chef Salad, 345 g	332	14	26	2	29
Chicken Sedona Salad, 365 g	232	5	16	5	28
Garden Salad, 251 g	241	11	24	2	13
w/ Chicken Breast, 365 g	355	12	26	3	37
Italian Salad, 329 g	409	24	25	2	24
Seafood Salad, 336 g	320	11	35	2	22
• Side Salad, 124 g	135	6	14	1	7
• Tuna Salad, 379 g	629	46	24	2	36
Sides & Other					
Chocolate Chip Cookie, 43 g	210	11	26	0	2
Chocolate Chip with M&Ms, 43 g	190	9	26	0	2
Coconut Toffee Chip Cookie, 43 g	200	9	23	0	2
Double Chocolate Chip Cookie, 43 g	190	9	25	1	2
• French Fries (Medium), 113 g	367	19	43	3	5
Oatmeal Cranberry Walnut Cookie, 43 g	170	7	26	1	2
Oatmeal Raisin Cookie, 43 g	170	7	25	1	2
Peanut Butter w/ Reese's Pieces Cookie, 43 g	210	11	22	0	4

Cousins Subs (cont.)

	Cal	Fat	Cbs	Fbr	Prtn
Sides & Other (cont.)					
Snickerdoodle Cookie, 43 g	190	9	25	0	2
Sugar Cookie, 43 g	180	8	26	0	2
White Chunk Macadamia Nut Cookie, 43 g	200	11	24	0	2
Soups					
Beef Steak & Noodle (Regular), 198 g	105	3	12	0	7
Cheddar Cauliflower (Regular), 198 g	114	5	13	4	4
Cheddar Cheese (Regular), 198 g	201	11	18	1	7
Chicken & Dumplings (Regular), 198 g	149	4	17	3	10
Chicken Noodle (Regular), 198 g	114	4	16	2	6
Chicken with Wild Rice (Regular), 198 g	219	9	13	4	12
• Chili (Regular), 198 g	219	8	26	16	16
Cream of Broccoli w/ Cheese (Regular), 198 g	166	7	13	3	5
Cream of Mushroom (Regular), 198 g	193	11	13	0	4
Cream of Potato (Regular), 198 g	166	8	21	3	4
Eight Bean Soup with Ham (Regular), 198 g	105	1	18	5	7
Fiesta Tortilla Soup with Chicken (Regular), 198 g	114	5	11	2	6
New England Clam Chowder (Regular), 198 g	149	3	25	2	6
Tomato Basil w/ Raviolini (Regular), 198 g	96	1	19	0	4
• Vegetable Beef (Regular), 198 g	70	2	11	2	4

Culver's

	Cal	Fat	Cbs	Fbr	Prtn
ButterBurger Classics					
ButterBurger, Cheese, Double, 9 oz.	580	32	37	1	38
• ButterBurger, Cheese, Single, 6 oz.	398	20	36	1	22
ButterBurger, Cheese, Triple, 12 oz.	763	45	38	1	55
Bacon ButterBurger Deluxe, Double, 10 oz.	751	50	34	1	43
Bacon ButterBurger Deluxe, Single, 9 oz.	573	38	34	1	26
• Bacon ButterBurger Deluxe, Triple, 13 oz.	931	63	34	1	59
ButterBurger, Low Carb, 6 oz.	443	32	1	0	37
ButterBurger Original, Double, 8 oz.	480	23	36	1	33
ButterBurger Original, Single, 5 oz.	346	15	35	1	19
ButterBurger Original, Triple, 10 oz.	613	31	37	1	47
The Culver's ButterBurger Deluxe, Double, 10 oz.	671	43	34	1	39
The Culver's ButterBurger Deluxe, Single, 8 oz.	494	31	34	1	22
The Culver's ButterBurger Deluxe, Triple, 12 oz.	851	56	34	1	55
Classic Sundaes					
Banana Split, 2-Scoop, 18 oz.	1081	64	115	6	16
• Banana Split, 3-Scoop, 21 oz.	1345	75	152	6	20
• Bananas Foster Sundae, 1-Scoop, 8 oz.	420	20	53	2	6
Bananas Foster Sundae, 2-Scoop, 13 oz.	784	41	93	2	11
Bananas Foster Sundae, 3-Scoop, 18 oz.	1015	51	123	4	15
Caramel Cashew, 1- Scoop, 7 oz.	585	33	58	1	11
Caramel Cashew, 2-Scoop, 13 oz.	957	51	104	1	17
Caramel Cashew, 3-Scoop, 15 oz.	1133	62	121	1	21
Strawberry Shortcake Sundae, 1-Scoop, 9 oz.	577	28	73	1	9
Strawberry Shortcake Sundae, 2-Scoop, 15 oz.	939	48	115	1	14
Strawberry Shortcake Sundae, 3-Scoop, 18 oz.	1115	58	132	1	17
Turtle Sundae, 1-Scoop, 7 oz.	605	41	53	2	10
Turtle Sundae, 2-Scoop, 13 oz.	977	60	97	2	16
Turtle Sundae, 3-Scoop, 15 oz.	1153	71	114	2	19
Concrete Mixers					
Chocolate Concrete Mixer, Medium, 16 oz.	992	49	122	0	16
• Turtle Concrete Mixer, Medium, 15 oz.	1153	71	114	2	19

RESTAURANTS & FAST-FOOD CHAINS

Culver's (cont.)

	Cal	Fat	Cbs	Fbr	Prtn
Concrete Mixers (cont.)					
• Vanilla Concrete Mixer, Medium, 13 oz.	832	49	82	0	15
Condiments					
BBQ Sauce, 1 oz.	48	0	12	0	0
Dill Pickles, Sliced, 0 oz.	1	0	0	0	0
Honey Mustard, 2 oz.	130	6	20	0	0
Horseradish Sauce, 1 oz.	150	14	6	0	0
Ketchup, 1 oz.	15	0	4	0	0
Mayonnaise, 0.5 oz.	100	11	0	0	0
Mustard, Mild, 0.5 oz.	0	0	0	0	0
• Mustard, Spicy Brown, 0.5 oz.	0	0	0	0	0
Picante Sauce, Mild and Medium, 1 oz.	10	0	2	0	0
Shrimp Cocktail Sauce, 2 oz.	50	0	12	2	2
Steak Sauce, 0.5 oz.	10	0	2	0	0
Sweet & Sour Dipping Sauce, 2 oz.	90	0	23	0	0
• Tartar Sauce, 1 oz.	188	18	1	0	0
Cones & Custard					
• Baby Scoop Chocolate Cake Cone, 3 oz.	193	8	25	1	4
Baby Scoop Vanilla Cake Cone, 3 oz.	200	10	22	0	3
Chocolate Cake Cone, 1-Scoop, 5 oz.	319	14	40	1	6
Chocolate Cake Cone, 2-Scoop, 10 oz.	592	27	73	3	12
Chocolate Cake Cone, 3-Scoop, 12 oz.	739	34	90	3	15
Chocolate Dipped Waffle Cone w/Sprinkles, 2 oz.	306	13	47	2	3
Chocolate Dipped Waffle Cone, 1-Scoop, 7 oz.	533	24	72	3	9
Chocolate Dipped Waffle Cone, 2 oz.	239	10	37	2	3
Chocolate, Dish, 1-Scoop, 5 oz.	294	14	35	1	6
Chocolate, Dish, 2-Scoop, 10 oz.	567	27	68	3	12
Chocolate, Dish, 3-Scoop, 12 oz.	714	34	85	3	15
Chocolate, Waffle Cone, 1-Scoop, 6 oz.	384	15	55	2	8
Chocolate, Waffle Cone, 2-Scoop, 10 oz.	657	28	88	4	14
Chocolate, Waffle Cone, 3-Scoop, 13 oz.	804	35	105	4	17
No Sugar Added Caramel Fudge Swirl, 3 oz.	205	11	30	7	5
Plain Cake Cone, 0.5 oz.	25	0	5	0	0
Plain Waffle Cone, 1 oz.	90	1	20	1	2
Vanilla Cake Cone, 1-Scoop, 5 oz.	332	18	35	0	6
Vanilla Cake Cone, 2-Scoop, 10 oz.	616	35	63	0	11
Vanilla Cake Cone, 3-Scoop, 12 oz.	770	44	78	0	14
Vanilla, Choc. Dipped Waffle Cone, 1-Scoop, 7 oz.	546	28	67	2	9
Vanilla, Dish, 1-Scoop, 5 oz.	307	18	30	0	6
Vanilla, Dish, 2-Scoop, 10 oz.	591	35	58	0	11
Vanilla, Dish, 3-Scoop, 12 oz.	745	44	73	0	14
Vanilla, Waffle Cone, 1-Scoop, 6 oz.	397	19	50	1	8
Vanilla, Waffle Cone, 2-Scoop, 10 oz.	681	36	78	1	13
• Vanilla, Waffle Cone, 3-Scoop, 13 oz.	835	45	93	1	16
Dinner Plates					
• Beef Pot Roast Dinner, 21 oz.	635	24	74	5	33
Breaded Shrimp (about 8 pieces), 18 oz.	1250	61	148	9	28
Chicken, 2 pcs., 25 oz.	1755	94	140	6	87
• Chicken, 4 pcs., 32 oz.	2185	116	158	6	124
Chopped Steak Dinner, 22 oz.	683	29	67	6	40
Crispy Shrimp Basket, 8 pcs., 11 oz.	760	34	92	7	23
Fish n' Chips, 6 pcs., 16 oz.	1381	83	104	4	45
North Atlantic Cod Fillet, 2 pcs., 23 oz.	1831	116	135	8	54
North Atlantic Cod Fillet, 3 pcs., 28 oz.	2122	134	147	9	76

RESTAURANTS & FAST-FOOD CHAINS

Culver's (cont.)	Cal	Fat	Cbs	Fbr	Prtn
Favorites					
Angus Philly Steak Sandwich, 10 oz.	518	20	46	2	38
Beef Frank w/ Bun, 7 oz.	392	22	38	1	13
• Beef Pot Roast Sandwich, 6 oz.	363	16	33	1	24
Blackened Chicken Sandwich, 8 oz.	369	8	48	2	31
Cheese Dog w/ Bun, 6 oz.	461	31	27	1	20
Chicken Salad Wrap, 7 oz.	518	26	39	4	32
Chicken Tenders, Breaded, 4 pcs., 6 oz.	440	20	32	4	36
Chili Dog w/Bun, 6 oz.	379	24	28	1	15
Crispy Chicken Fillet Sandwich, 9 oz.	625	29	68	3	26
Grilled Chicken Breast, 8 oz.	374	8	47	2	32
Grilled Ham n' Swiss on Rye, 8 oz.	497	25	33	2	37
• North Atlantic Cod Fillet Sandwich, 10 oz.	740	42	58	3	33
Pork Tenderloin Sandwich, 9 oz.	593	29	62	2	26
Tuna Salad Wrap, 8 oz.	485	24	39	4	29
Turkey Sourdough BLT, 9 oz.	562	31	36	0	34
Turkey, Stacked, Sandwich, 8 oz.	450	19	47	2	26
Garden Fresh Salads					
Avocado Pecan Bleu w/ Blackened Chicken, 13 oz.	557	41	16	8	36
Chicken Cashew w /Grilled Chicken, 11 oz.	441	25	17	3	38
Classic Caesar w/ Grilled Chicken, 10 oz.	358	14	15	2	43
Cobb Salad, 13 oz.	531	31	19	6	44
• Crispy Chicken Salad, 11 oz.	616	42	34	6	32
Garden Fresco, 9 oz.	225	11	25	7	16
• Side Caesar, 3 oz.	82	4	5	1	7
Side Salad, 4 oz.	86	5	6	1	5
Kids Meals					
ButterBurger, 5 oz.	346	15	35	1	19
• ButterBurger, Cheese, 6 oz.	396	20	36	1	22
• Chicken Tenders, Breaded, 2 pcs., 3 oz.	220	10	16	2	18
Corn Dog, 3 oz.	260	14	26	0	6
French Fries, 4 oz.	275	12	38	3	4
Grilled Cheese on Sourdough, 4 oz.	290	14	33	0	11
Hot Dog w/Bun, 5 oz.	366	22	30	1	13
Malts & Shakes					
• Chocolate Malt, Medium, 16 oz.	968	45	122	0	18
Chocolate Shake, Medium, 16 oz.	912	44	114	0	16
• Old Fashioned Cherry Soda, 16 oz.	516	25	63	0	9
Vanilla Malt, Medium, 14 oz.	872	45	98	0	17
Vanilla Shake, Medium, 13 oz.	752	44	74	0	15
Salad Dressing					
• Bleu Cheese, Fancy, Chunky, 2 oz.	310	33	2	0	1
Caesar Dressing, 2 oz.	220	23	2	0	2
French, 2 oz.	190	13	19	0	0
French, Reduced Calorie, 2 oz.	140	9	16	0	0
Ranch, Buttermilk, Gourmet, 2 oz.	230	24	3	0	1
Ranch, Reduced Calorie, 2 oz.	130	12	5	0	1
• Raspberry Vinaigrette, 2 oz.	45	0	11	0	0
Sesame Ginger Dressing, 2 oz.	70	0	16	0	1
Thousand Island, Gourmet, 2 oz.	220	18	14	0	0
Sides					
Chili Cheddar Fries, 9 oz.	661	34	73	5	18
Cole Slaw, 5 oz.	350	21	37	2	1
Dinner Roll, 2 oz.	140	6	19	0	4

(• = most healthy • = least healthy) **RESTAURANTS & FAST-FOOD · 131**

RESTAURANTS & FAST-FOOD CHAINS

Culver's (cont.)

	Cal	Fat	Cbs	Fbr	Prtn
Sides (cont.)					
French Fries, Regular, 5 oz.	385	17	53	4	5
Green Beans, 7 oz.	203	18	12	3	2
Mashed Potatoes & Gravy, 7 oz.	140	2	26	2	3
• Mashed Potatoes, 6 oz.	120	1	24	2	2
Onion Rings, Breaded, 7 oz.	630	36	70	3	7
• Wisconsin Dairyland Cheese Curds, 7 oz.	670	38	54	3	28
Soups					
Baja Chicken Enchilada, 11 oz.	352	23	21	4	16
Bean with Ham, 11 oz.	190	3	33	9	9
Black Bean, 11 oz.	188	3	32	11	9
Boston Clam Chowder, 11 oz.	252	11	25	1	12
Bread Bowl, 9 oz.	665	3	135	0	25
Broccoli Cheese with Florets, 11 oz.	240	14	16	1	11
California Medley, 11 oz.	204	11	18	2	9
Cauliflower Cheese, 11 oz.	252	14	23	1	8
Cheesy Chicken Tortilla, 11 oz.	180	7	16	1	12
Chicken & Dumpling, 11 oz.	300	22	19	1	9
Chicken Gumbo, 11 oz.	120	6	13	1	5
Chicken Noodle, 11 oz.	112	2	14	1	9
Chicken Pot Pie, 11 oz.	260	16	22	1	8
Chicken Tortilla, 11 oz.	168	3	26	6	10
Corn Chowder, 11 oz.	276	13	35	4	7
Cream of Asparagus Spears, 11 oz.	250	11	26	1	11
Cream of Broccoli, 11 oz.	185	10	16	1	8
Cream of Potato, 11 oz.	288	13	26	1	7
Creamy Garden Vegetable, 11 oz.	188	11	19	4	4
Creamy Tomato Bisque, 11 oz.	180	9	20	2	6
Creamy Turkey Vegetable, 11 oz.	216	9	19	1	12
• Fire Roasted Vegetable, 11 oz.	72	2	12	2	2
French Onion, 11 oz.	155	8	12	0	10
• George's Chili Supreme, 11 oz.	456	30	27	5	23
George's Chili, 11 oz.	336	18	27	6	18
Harvest Grain w/ Portabello Mushrooms, 11 oz.	185	7	26	4	5
Italian Style Wedding, 11 oz.	275	6	44	2	11
Lumberjack Mixed Vegetable, 11 oz.	150	6	21	7	4
Minestrone, 11 oz.	100	1	19	4	4
Mushroom Medley, 11 oz.	252	16	20	1	6
Oven Roasted Turkey Noodle, 11 oz.	175	5	21	1	11
Pasta Fagioli, 11 oz.	172	3	28	5	8
Potato Au Gratin, 11 oz.	350	22	28	1	11
Potato with Bacon, 11 oz.	225	9	28	4	8
Seven Bean Medley, 11 oz.	150	2	25	6	8
Split Pea with Ham, 11 oz.	262	9	32	12	13
Stuffed Green Pepper with Beef, 11 oz.	150	3	25	1	6
Tomato Basil Ravioletti, 11 oz.	112	3	18	1	4
Tomato Florentine, 11 oz.	112	1	21	1	4
Vegetable Beef & Barley, 11 oz.	112	4	14	3	7
Wild and Brown Rice with Chicken, 11 oz.	452	22	27	1	37
Wisconsin Cheese, 11 oz.	375	24	29	1	11
Special Treats					
Cookies n' Cream Concrete Cake, 4 oz.	245	14	26	0	4
• Culver's Root Beer Float, 15 oz.	467	18	70	0	6
Lemon Ice Smoothie, 11 oz.	403	16	61	0	5

RESTAURANTS & FAST-FOOD CHAINS

Culver's (cont.)	Cal	Fat	Cbs	Fbr	Prtn
Special Treats (cont.)					
• Lemon Ice, 7 oz.	140	0	35	0	0
Turtle Concrete Cake, 4 oz.	280	17	30	1	4
Specialty Burgers & Sandwiches					
• Cheddar Burger with Bacon, 11 oz.	871	48	56	2	52
Cheddar Burger, Double, 8 oz.	641	37	31	1	43
Cheddar Burger, Single, 5 oz.	421	22	31	1	24
Cheddar Burger, Triple, 11 oz.	861	52	31	1	62
Grilled Reuben Melt, 11 oz.	588	31	41	2	39
Mushroom & Swiss Burger, Double, 9 oz.	633	35	35	1	45
Mushroom & Swiss Burger, Single, 6 oz.	417	21	33	1	25
Mushroom & Swiss Burger, Triple, 13 oz.	849	49	37	1	65
Sourdough Melt, Double, 9 oz.	636	35	33	0	44
Sourdough Melt, Single, 6 oz.	413	20	33	0	25
Sourdough Melt, Triple, 12 oz.	858	50	34	0	63
Wisconsin Swiss Melt, Double, 9 oz.	616	34	34	2	46
• Wisconsin Swiss Melt, Single, 6 oz.	403	20	33	2	26
Wisconsin Swiss Melt, Triple, 12 oz.	828	48	35	2	66
Toppings					
Almond, 0.5 oz.	84	8	3	2	3
Andes Creme De Menthe Thins, 1 oz.	151	10	16	1	2
Apple, 0.5 oz.	23	0	6	0	0
Black Cherry, 0.5 oz.	18	0	5	0	0
Blackberry, 0.5 oz.	14	0	4	0	0
Blueberry, 0.5 oz.	17	0	4	0	0
• Brownie Pieces, 3 oz.	361	16	52	2	3
Butterfinger®, 1 oz.	110	5	18	1	1
Butterscotch, 0.5 oz.	43	0	10	0	0
Cashew, 0.5 oz.	90	7	4	1	3
Cherry, 0.5 oz.	20	0	5	0	0
Chocolate Chip Cookie Dough, 1 oz.	120	5	17	0	1
Crème De Menthe, 0.5 oz.	45	1	10	0	0
Culver's Chocolate Syrup, 1 oz.	64	0	16	0	0
Heath® Toffee Chunks, 1 oz.	155	9	17	0	1
Hershey's Take Five, 1 oz.	141	7	17	1	3
M&M Minis, 1 oz.	140	7	18	2	2
Marshmallow Creme, 0.5 oz.	39	0	10	0	0
Milk Chocolate Flakes, 1 oz.	142	9	17	2	2
Nestle Crunch, 1 oz.	140	7	19	1	1
Novelty Coating, 0.5 oz.	87	7	6	1	0
Oreo® Cookie Crumbs, 0.5 oz.	62	2	9	1	1
Peach, 0.5 oz.	15	0	4	0	0
Peanut Butter, 1 oz.	179	15	6	1	6
Pecan Halves, 0.5 oz.	100	11	2	1	2
Pineapple, 0.5 oz.	20	0	5	0	0
Raspberry, 0.5 oz.	18	0	4	1	0
Reese's Pieces® Minis, 1 oz.	142	7	16	1	4
Reese's® Peanut Butter Cups, 1 oz.	150	9	16	1	3
Snickers® Candy Bar Pieces, 0.5 oz.	67	4	8	1	1
Spanish Peanuts, 1 oz.	160	14	5	2	8
Sprinkles, Blue and White, 1 oz.	140	7	21	0	0
Sprinkles, King Decorette, 1 oz.	134	6	20	0	0
• Strawberry, 0.5 oz.	13	0	3	0	0

RESTAURANTS & FAST-FOOD CHAINS

D'Angelo	Cal	Fat	Cbs	Fbr	Prtn
D'Lite Sandwiches					
ChixSFry D'Lite, 354 g	426	6	57	7	37
Classic Veggie, 345 g	362	7	63	8	15
Fresh Veggie, 267 g	348	7	62	7	13
Grilled Chicken Breast, 261 g	388	7	52	6	31
Roast Beef, 234 g	338	5	51	6	25
• Turkey Cranberry, 291 g	444	4	75	6	28
• Turkey, 234 g	347	4	51	6	28
D'Lite Wraps					
• Chicken Caesar Salad, 373 g	374	7	43	4	34
• Tuna, 288 g	725	59	20	10	33
Turkey & Bacon, 263 g	491	30	19	10	39
Wrap LC Steak & Provolone, 227 g	469	27	15	9	46
Dressing					
Bleu Cheese, 30 g	152	15	3	0	1
• Caesar, 85 g	397	43	6	0	6
Creamy Italian, 85 g	340	37	9	0	0
• Fat Free Caesar, 85 g	57	0	9	0	0
Greek w/ Feta Cheese, 85 g	227	26	6	0	0
Honey Mustard, 30 g	150	14	7	0	0
Lite Ranch, 85 g	240	19	6	1	2
Olive Oil Vinaigrette, 85 g	170	17	9	0	0
Kidz Meals					
Cheeseburger Sub, 123 g	294	13	28	3	15
• Cookie Chocolate Chip, 43 g	171	6	26	0	3
Ham & Cheese Sub, 103 g	227	5	32	1	14
• Kidz Tuna Sub, 128 g	438	29	30	1	15
Meatball Sub, 153 g	330	15	37	4	15
Turkey D'Lite, 113 g	217	3	30	3	19
Pokket® Sandwiches					
Big Papi, 340 g	469	11	53	3	39
BLT & Cheese, 255 g	397	17	38	3	22
Caesar Salad, 312 g	616	39	54	3	20
Capicola & Cheese, 230 g	362	13	35	2	26
Cheese, 230 g	519	27	41	2	29
Cheeseburger, 231 g	459	25	31	2	27
Chicken Caesar Salad, 390 g	674	39	47	3	40
Chicken Club, 296 g	526	28	36	2	34
Chicken Honey Dijon, 323 g	508	20	40	2	41
Chicken Salad, 238 g	623	42	34	2	27
Chicken Stir Fry, 277 g	380	9	39	2	35
Classic Vegetable Pokket, 341 g	368	13	46	4	19
Classic Vegetable, 341 g	368	13	46	4	19
Classic Veggie No Cheese, 312 g	212	1	44	4	9
• Greek, 450 g	790	61	49	4	16
Grilled Chicken, 261 g	303	5	35	2	29
Ham & Salami, 202 g	386	17	34	2	23
Ham & Cheese, 222 g	326	10	38	2	22
Ham, 177 g	229	3	35	2	17
Hamburger, 212 g	399	20	29	2	24
Italian, 232 g	525	30	36	2	28
Lobster, 255 g	530	31	34	2	29
Meatball, 346 g	574	31	52	4	26
Mortadella & Cheese, 205 g	410	21	35	2	21

RESTAURANTS & FAST-FOOD CHAINS

D'Angelo (cont.)	Cal	Fat	Cbs	Fbr	Prtn
Pokket® Sandwiches (cont.)					
Number 9, 258 g	407	18	31	2	31
Pastrami, 184 g	438	25	33	1	24
Pepperoni, 184 g	407	20	35	3	21
Roast Beef, 202 g	247	3	33	2	23
• Salad, 298 g	196	1	40	4	8
Salami & Cheese, 216 g	509	30	33	2	25
Seafood Salad, 234 g	449	22	50	3	14
Steak & Cheese, 186 g	377	17	26	1	29
Steak Bomb, 343 g	631	32	44	3	43
Steak Tip, 310 g	452	16	45	2	27
Steak, 164 g	305	12	24	1	25
Tuna, 238 g	664	49	33	2	24
Turkey Club, 284 g	332	7	32	2	34
Turkey, 202 g	256	2	33	2	26
Salads					
Antipasto, 389 g	284	18	17	6	16
Caesar, 326 g	474	39	25	4	15
Chicken Caesar, 404 g	533	38	19	4	35
Chicken Stir Fry, 366 g	168	3	11	4	25
Cobb, 333 g	292	17	11	4	27
Greek, 387 g	299	23	17	4	11
Lobster, 415 g	376	26	12	4	26
Roast Beef, 352 g	131	3	10	4	19
• Steak Tip Caesar, 383 g	661	50	21	3	32
• Tossed, 274 g	49	1	11	4	3
Turkey, 366 g	157	2	10	4	26
Soup (Small)					
Beef Stew, 227 g	220	8	23	2	12
Beef Stew, 227 g	220	8	23	2	12
Chicken Noodle, 227 g	110	3	14	1	6
Ex. Broc. & Cheddar Cheese, 227 g	270	21	11	2	9
• Hearty Vegetable, 227 g	40	0	7	2	2
Italian Wedding, 227 g	120	6	11	2	6
• Lobster Bisque, 227 g	360	29	16	1	8
NE Clam Chowder, 227 g	320	18	31	1	9
Portuguese Kale, 227 g	130	4	16	3	8
Subs: Small Subs					
Big Papi, 340 g	525	15	60	7	40
BLT & Cheese, 244 g	463	19	51	6	23
Capicola & Cheese, 225 g	408	13	48	5	25
Cheese, 244 g	589	28	55	5	30
Cheeseburger, 246 g	526	26	44	5	29
Chicken Club, 289 g	593	29	49	5	35
Chicken Honey Dijon, 316 g	575	22	53	5	42
Chicken Salad, 252 g	692	44	48	5	29
Chicken Stir Fry, 291 g	449	11	53	6	37
Classic Veggie, 364 g	462	15	64	8	21
Grilled Chicken, 254 g	369	7	48	5	30
Ham & Cheese, 236 g	395	11	52	2	24
Ham & Salami, 216 g	456	19	48	2	25
Ham, 208 g	302	5	49	2	18
Hamburger, 227 g	466	22	42	5	25
Italian, 253 g	614	31	54	3	30

(• = most healthy • = least healthy)   **RESTAURANTS & FAST-FOOD • 135**

RESTAURANTS & FAST-FOOD CHAINS

D'Angelo (cont.)	Cal	Fat	Cbs	Fbr	Prtn
Subs: Small Subs (cont.)					
Lobster, 255 g	598	33	48	5	30
Meatball, 360 g	644	33	66	7	28
Mortadella & Cheese, 219 g	479	23	49	5	23
Number 9, 263 g	450	19	41	4	31
Pastrami, 227 g	613	34	47	5	34
Peppercorn Steak, 230 g	508	39	7	1	33
Pepperoni, 226 g	603	33	49	7	28
Roast Beef, 234 g	320	5	48	5	25
• Salad, 397 g	281	3	57	8	10
Salami & Cheese, 230 g	579	32	47	5	27
Seafood Salad, 227 g	498	23	61	6	14
Steak & Cheese, 202 g	446	19	40	4	31
Steak Bomb, 343 g	670	33	52	6	43
Steak Tip, 333 g	545	18	63	3	29
Steak, 181 g	373	14	37	4	27
Toasted BBQ Steak, 273 g	623	25	62	5	35
Toasted Italian Bistro, 210 g	585	31	49	5	29
Toasted Pastrami Ruben, 298 g	750	47	55	7	30
Toasted Roast Beef & Cheddar, 234 g	564	26	51	5	35
• Toasted Spicy Meatball, 453 g	933	57	71	9	61
Toasted Tuna & Swiss, 283 g	796	54	49	5	32
Toasted Turkey & Ham, 255 g	532	24	49	5	33
Toasted Turkey Thanksgiving, 234 g	705	20	80	6	32
Tuna, 241 g	685	46	47	2	24
Turkey Club, 291 g	401	9	49	3	33
Turkey, 163 g	317	4	45	5	27
Toppings					
Bacon, 14 g	64	5	0	0	5
Buffalo Sauce, 1 oz.	10	0	2	0	0
Cheese Cheddar, 28 g	114	9	1	0	7
Cucumber, 3 slices, 28 g	4	0	1	0	0
Fat Free Mayonnaise, 1 packet, 12 g	10	0	2	0	0
• Hot Peppers, 1 oz.	0	0	1	0	0
Lettuce, 1 oz.	4	0	1	0	0
Mayonnaise (2 tbsp.), 30 g	225	25	1	0	0
Mushrooms, 1 oz.	7	0	1	1	1
Mustard, Honey Dijon, 2 tbsp, 36 g	60	0	18	0	0
Mustard Yellow, 2 tbsp., 30 g	20	1	2	1	1
• Olive Oil Blend, 2 tbsp., 27 g	239	27	0	0	0
Onions, 0.5 oz.	6	0	1	0	0
Pickles 8 slices, 14 g	0	0	1	0	0
Processed American Cheese, 1 oz.	95	7	3	0	5
Provolone Cheese, 1 oz.	100	8	1	0	7
Sweet Peppers, 1 oz.	8	0	2	0	0
Swiss Cheese, 1 oz.	106	8	1	0	8
Tomato 3 slices, 60 g	11	0	2	1	1
Turkey Gravy, 85 g	84	5	4	0	1
Vinegar, 2 tbsp., 30 g	1	0	0	0	0
Wraps					
Big Papi, 347 g	593	23	56	4	41
BLT & Cheese, 229 g	544	26	54	4	24
Buffalo Chicken Salad, 400 g	823	44	67	4	40
Caesar Salad, 329 g	711	44	65	5	20

D'Angelo (cont.)

	Cal	Fat	Cbs	Fbr	Prtn
Wraps (cont.)					
Capicola & Cheese, 242 g	494	20	53	4	25
Cheese, 261 g	675	35	59	4	30
Cheeseburger, 263 g	609	33	48	3	30
Chicken Caesar Salad, 421 g	830	47	65	5	42
• Chicken Cobb, 433 g	931	55	71	6	36
Chicken Filet & Bacon, 342 g	639	28	58	3	38
Chicken Honey Dijon, 396 g	672	29	60	5	43
Chicken Salad, 286 g	782	51	53	4	29
Chicken Stir, 308 g	535	17	57	4	37
ChixSFry D'Lite, 439 g	422	5	56	5	39
Classic Veggie, 389 g	486	13	68	5	24
Greek, 436 g	765	61	44	4	15
Grilled Chicken, 349 g	422	6	59	4	34
Ham & Cheese, 251 g	435	10	60	3	26
Ham & Salami, 260 g	513	18	57	3	30
Hamburger, 258 g	509	21	50	2	28
Italian, 277 g	631	29	59	3	32
Lobster, 315 g	749	43	57	3	33
Meatball, 392 g	687	31	75	5	31
Mortadella & Cheese, 251 g	522	21	58	3	25
Number 9, 276 g	517	24	44	3	32
Pastrami, 230 g	550	25	55	2	28
Peppercorn Steak, 315 g	702	40	45	3	41
Pepperoni, 230 g	519	21	57	4	25
Roast Beef, 249 g	448	13	58	4	26
• Salad, 429 g	324	2	66	6	13
Salami & Cheese, 258 g	605	29	56	3	29
Seafood Salad, 258 g	541	22	69	3	17
Steak & Cheese, 222 g	464	18	43	2	33
Steak Bomb, 343 g	670	33	52	6	43
Steak Tip, 298 g	432	16	41	2	26
Steak, 200 g	392	13	41	2	28
Tuna, 284 g	731	44	56	3	27
Turkey Club, 284 g	415	7	52	3	34
Turkey, 249 g	369	3	55	3	30

Dairy Queen

	Cal	Fat	Cbs	Fbr	Prtn
Blizzard Treats					
• Med. Banana Split Blizzard®, 382 g	580	17	97	1	12
• Med. Choc. Chip Cookie Dough Blizzard®, 446 g	1030	40	151	1	17
Med. Reese's® P. Butter Cup Blizzard®, 383 g	790	28	114	0	18
Med. Strawberry CheeseQuake™ Blizzard®, 376 g	730	29	105	1	13
Medium Oreo® Cookies Blizzard®, 334 g	690	26	103	1	13
Burgers					
Bacon Cheddar GrillBurger™, 229 g	650	37	41	2	36
Classic GrillBurger™ with Cheese, 231 g	560	30	42	2	29
Classic GrillBurger™, 212 g	470	23	42	2	24
• DQ Homestyle Burger, 142 g	350	14	33	1	17
DQ® Homestyle® Bacon Double, 245 g	730	41	35	1	41
DQ® Homestyle® Cheeseburger, 156 g	400	18	34	1	19
DQ® Homestyle® Double Cheeseburger, 226 g	640	34	34	1	34
DQ® Ultimate® Burger, 259 g	780	48	33	1	41
• FlameThrower® GrillBurger, 1/2 lb.	1030	73	41	2	53

RESTAURANTS & FAST-FOOD CHAINS

Dairy Queen (cont.)

	Cal	Fat	Cbs	Fbr	Prtn
Burgers (cont.)					
FlameThrower® GrillBurger, 1/4 lb.	780	54	41	2	33
GrillBurger™ with Cheese, 1/2 lb.	820	49	47	2	51
GrillBurger™, 1/2 lb.	670	37	42	2	42
Mushroom Swiss GrillBurger™, 210 g	630	40	39	2	29
Cones					
DQ® Chocolate Soft Serve, 1/2 Cup, 94 g	150	5	22	0	4
• DQ® Vanilla Soft Serve, 1/2 Cup, 94 g	150	5	22	0	3
Medium Chocolate Cone, 199 g	340	10	54	0	9
• Medium Dipped Cone, 220 g	490	23	61	1	8
Medium Vanilla Cone, 199 g	340	10	54	0	8
DQ® Blizzard® Cakes					
• Chocolate Xtreme Blizzard® Cake, 249 g	660	31	85	2	10
• Oreo® Cookies Blizzard® Cake, 220 g	490	20	67	1	8
Reese's® PB Cup Blizzard® Cake, 220 g	490	20	67	1	9
Fries/Onion Rings					
DQ® Medium French Fries, 196 g	510	23	70	7	6
DQ® Regular Onion Rings, 113 g	470	30	45	3	6
Hot Dogs					
All-Beef Chili Cheese Dog, 150 g	380	24	24	1	16
All-Beef Hot Dog, 115 g	300	15	30	1	11
Malts, Shakes and Arctic Rush					
• Medium Arctic Rush™ Slush, 595 g	310	0	63	0	0
• Medium Chocolate Malt, 567 g	900	21	157	0	19
Medium Chocolate Shake, 550 g	780	20	133	0	17
MooLatté® Frozen Blended Coffee					
• Cappuccino MooLatté®, 16 oz.	500	18	73	0	7
• Caramel MooLatté®, 16 oz.	630	19	103	0	7
French Vanilla MooLatté®, 16 oz.	570	18	90	0	7
Mocha MooLatté®, 16 oz.	590	23	84	0	8
Novelties					
• Buster Bar®, 148 g	480	31	45	2	11
Chocolate Dilly® Bar, 87 g	240	15	24	1	4
• DQ® Fudge Bar – no sugar added, 66 g	50	0	13	0	4
DQ® Sandwich, 85 g	190	5	32	1	4
DQ® Vanilla Orange Bar – no sugar added, 66 g	60	0	17	0	2
StarKiss®, 85 g	80	0	21	0	0
Royal Treats®					
• Banana Split, 374 g	530	14	98	3	8
• Brownie Earthquake™, 304 g	740	28	149	1	10
Peanut Buster® Parfait, 304 g	710	30	96	2	16
Salad Dressings					
DQ® Blue Cheese Dressing, 57 g	210	20	4	0	2
DQ® Honey Mustard Dressing, 57 g	260	21	18	0	1
• DQ® Ranch Dressing, 57 g	310	33	3	0	1
• Fat Free Italian Dressing, 43 g	10	0	3	0	0
Salads					
• Crispy Chicken Salad – no dressing, 424 g	420	22	90	6	28
Grilled Chicken Salad – no dressing, 424 g	270	11	92	4	32
• Side Salad - no dressing, 182 g	45	0	27	3	2
Sandwiches/Baskets					
Chicken Strip Basket™, 4 pcs., 446 g	1030	54	105	8	37
• Chicken Strip Basket™, 6 pcs., 531 g	1270	67	121	10	51
Crispy Chicken Sandwich, 198 g	540	29	47	1	23

RESTAURANTS & FAST-FOOD CHAINS

Dairy Queen (cont.)	Cal	Fat	Cbs	Fbr	Prtn
Sandwiches/Baskets (cont.)					
• Grilled Chicken Sandwich, 177 g	350	16	49	1	23
Sundaes					
Medium Chocolate Sundae, 234 g	410	10	72	0	7
Medium Strawberry Sundae, 248 g	370	10	63	1	7

Damon's Grill	Cal	Fat	Cbs	Fbr	Prtn
Aloha Chicken	515	12	45	8	57
Chimi Chicken	450	9	37	7	57
• Maui Salmon	535	21	40	7	50
• Grilled Chicken Breast Salad	340	10	18	4	45

Del Taco	Cal	Fat	Cbs	Fbr	Prtn
Breakfast					
5-Piece Hash Brown Sticks, 80 g	250	19	20	0	0
8-Piece Hash Brown Sticks, 128 g	410	30	32	0	0
Bacon & Egg Quesadilla, 175 g	450	23	40	2	21
Big Fat Breakfast Taco, 167 g	559	17	36	1	19
• Breakfast Burrito, 107 g	250	11	24	1	10
Egg & Cheese Burrito, 213 g	450	24	39	3	23
• Macho Bacon & Egg Burrito ™, 454 g	1030	60	82	6	40
Shredded Beef Breakfast Burrito, 297 g	785	33	41	3	38
Steak & Egg Burrito, 255 g	580	34	41	3	33
Burgers					
Bacon Double Del Cheeseburger™, 212 g	610	39	35	4	29
Bun Taco, 191 g	440	0	37	4	24
Cheeseburger, 131 g	330	13	37	3	16
Del Cheeseburger ™, 161 g	430	25	35	4	16
Double Del Cheeseburger ™, 202 g	560	35	35	4	26
• Hamburger, 118 g	280	21	37	3	13
Burritos					
Bean & Cheese Cup, 220 g	415	9	47	11	16
Bean & Cheese Green Burrito, 142 g	280	8	38	6	11
• Bean & Cheese Red Burrito, 142 g	270	8	38	6	11
Chicken Works Burrito, 312 g	520	23	57	4	26
Del Beef Burrito ™, 227 g	550	30	42	3	31
Del Classic Chicken Burrito ™, 227 g	560	36	41	3	24
Del Combo Burrito, 269 g	530	22	61	11	28
Deluxe Combo Burrito™, 340 g	570	25	64	12	29
Deluxe Del Beef Burrito™, 298 g	590	33	45	4	32
Half Pound Green Burrito, 241 g	430	12	59	13	20
Half Pound Red Burrito, 241 g	430	12	65	13	20
• Macho Beef Burrito ™, 539 g	1170	62	89	7	60
Macho Chicken Burrito ™, 524 g	930	33	111	16	47
Macho Combo Burrito ™, 553 g	1050	44	113	17	49
Shredded Beef Combo Burrito, 297 g	815	30	61	8	35
Spicy Chicken Burrito, 290 g	510	17	68	8	28
Steak Works Burrito, 312 g	590	31	58	5	27
Veggie Works Burrito, 319 g	490	18	69	9	18
Fries					
Chili Cheese Fries, 298 g	670	46	51	5	17
Deluxe Chili Cheese Fries ™, 340 g	710	49	53	6	17
• Medium Fries, 198 g	490	32	47	5	5

RESTAURANTS & FAST-FOOD CHAINS

Del Taco (cont.)

	Cal	Fat	Cbs	Fbr	Prtn
Nachos					
Macho Nachos ®, 468 g	1100	63	113	15	31
Nachos, 113 g	380	24	40	2	5
Quesadilla					
Cheddar Quesadilla, 151 g	500	27	39	2	23
• Chicken Cheddar Quesadilla, 194 g	580	31	41	2	33
Spicy Jack Chicken Quesadilla, 194 g	570	30	40	2	32
• Spicy Jack Quesadilla, 151 g	490	26	38	2	23
Salads					
Mexican Caesar Salad (Large) w/ Dressing, 306 g	557	47	16	3	9
w/o Dressing, 246 g	257	13	14	3	7
w/Dressing +Chicken, 418 g	677	51	24	3	25
w/o Dressing +Chicken, 358 g	377	17	32	3	23
Mexican Caesar Salad (Side) with Dressing, 155 g	415	40	9	1	5
• w/o Dressing, 95 g	115	6	7	1	3
Deluxe Chicken Salad, 526 g	740	34	77	15	33
• Deluxe Taco Salad ™, 541 g	780	40	76	14	33
Taco Salad, 177 g	350	30	10	2	10
Shakes					
• Chocolate Shake, 425 g	680	16	117	1	16
• Strawberry Shake, 425 g	540	8	100	1	14
Vanilla Shake, 425 g	550	10	97	0	16
Sides					
Beans 'n Cheese Cup, 220 g	415	9	47	11	16
• Large Chips and Salsa, 255 g	465	21	65	5	8
Medium Chips and Salsa, 170 g	310	14	43	3	5
Rice Cup, 113 g	140	2	27	1	3
• Side of Bacon (2 slices), 10 g	50	4	0	0	3
Small Chips and Salsa, 85 g	155	7	22	1	2
Tacos					
Big Fat Chicken Taco ™, 153 g	340	13	38	3	18
• Big Fat Steak Taco ™, 153 g	390	19	38	3	18
Big Fat Taco ™, 153 g	320	11	39	3	16
Carne Asada Taco, 142 g	237	8	22	2	9
Chicken Soft Taco, 106 g	293	11	18	1	10
Chicken Taco Del Carbon, 98 g	170	5	19	2	12
Crispy Fish Taco ™, 131 g	290	16	30	2	7
Macho Taco ®, 170 g	308	17	16	1	23
Shredded Beef Taco Del Carbon, 92 g	199	11	17	2	11
• Soft Taco, 80 g	160	8	16	1	8
Steak Taco Del Carbon, 98 g	220	11	19	2	12
Taco, 63 g	160	10	11	1	7

Denny's

	Cal	Fat	Cbs	Fbr	Prtn
Appetizers and Entrees					
Applesauce Musselman's®, 3 oz.	60	0	15	1	0
Baked Potato, plain w/skin, 7 oz.	220	0	51	5	5
Bread Stuffing, plain, 3 oz.	110	5	13	1	2
Buffalo Chicken Strips (5), 10 oz.	734	42	43	0	48
Buffalo Wings (9), 19 oz.	974	72	11	2	67
Chicken Strips (5), 10 oz.	720	33	56	0	47
Chicken Strips, 10 oz.	635	25	55	0	47
Corn, 4 oz.	110	2	23	3	3
Cottage Cheese, 3 oz.	73	3	2	0	9

RESTAURANTS & FAST-FOOD CHAINS

Denny's (cont.)	Cal	Fat	Cbs	Fbr	Prtn
Appetizers and Entrees (cont.)					
Country Fried Steak, 9 oz.	644	46	30	11	28
Fish & Chips, 17 oz.	958	54	83	6	34
Fried Shrimp Dinner, 5 oz.	260	12	18	2	21
Grilled Chicken Alfredo, 24 oz.	1290	67	111	4	58
Grilled Chicken Dinner, 10 oz.	280	5	4	0	55
Grilled Shrimp Skewers/Pilaf/garlic brd, 13 oz.	650	29	59	3	31
Grilled Tilapia Dinner, 11 oz.	530	18	33	1	53
Lemon Pepper Tilapia, 15 oz.	810	48	38	3	55
Mashed Potatoes, plain, 5 oz.	170	7	23	2	4
Meat Loaf Dinner, 11 oz.	930	60	51	2	42
• Mini Burgers (6) w/Onion Rings, 25 oz.	2180	133	173	9	78
Mozzarella Sticks (8), 8 oz.	710	41	49	6	36
Mushroom Swiss Chopped Steak, 13 oz.	930	76	13	1	46
Nacho, 23 oz.	1278	64	117	11	54
Roast Turkey & Stuffing (incl. gravy), 12 oz.	510	14	66	3	27
Sampler ™, 17 oz.	1405	80	124	4	47
• Sliced Tomatoes (3 slices), 2 oz.	13	0	3	1	1
Smothered Cheese Fries, 9 oz.	767	48	69	0	27
Steakhouse Strip Dinner, 8 oz.	390	14	0	0	59
T-bone Steak Dinner, 13 oz.	630	29	0	0	88
Vegetable Blend, 4 oz.	60	4	5	1	1
Vegetable Rice Pilaf, 5 oz.	173	3	33	1	4
Breakfast					
All American Slam ® w/ hashbrowns, 14 oz.	950	75	21	2	48
Belgian Waffle Platter, 8 oz.	619	45	28	0	22
Buttermilk Pancake, 9 oz.	420	5	82	3	9
Cntry Fried Steak & Eggs w/ hashbrwns, 19 oz.	740	46	49	2	32
Country Fried Potatoes, 5 oz.	394	20	23	10	3
Fabulous French Toast Platter, 13 oz.	1261	79	110	3	44
French Toast Slam®(2 sl.), 14 oz.	1180	75	74	2	49
Grand Slam Slugger ™ w/hash brown, 24 oz.	1040	57	95	4	38
• Grits, 4 oz.	80	0	18	0	2
H.B.'s w/Onions, Cheese, Gravy, 8 oz.	493	25	54	3	14
Ham & Cheddar Omel w/eggbeaters, 10 oz.	468	32	5	0	37
Ham & Cheddar Omelette, 10 oz.	595	47	5	0	41
Ham and Jalapeño Scramble, 25 oz.	1080	53	117	7	52
Hashed Browns w/ Cheddar Cheese, 6 oz.	280	19	21	2	7
Hashed Browns, 4 oz.	197	12	20	2	2
Heartland Scramble, 24 oz.	1190	59	118	7	43
Lumberjack Slam w/ hash browns, 22 oz.	1140	53	108	4	52
Meat Lover's Breakfast, 22 oz.	1230	66	109	5	50
Meat Lover's Scramble, 23 oz.	1280	71	103	4	54
Moons Over My Hammy ®, 13 oz.	760	40	52	2	46
Original Grand Slam ®, 13 oz.	740	43	56	2	33
• Smoked Sausage Scramble, 26 oz.	1480	88	118	7	55
Steakhouse Strip & Eggs, 11 oz.	560	37	3	0	57
T-bone Steak & Eggs, 14 oz.	991	77	1	1	73
Ultimate Omelette® w/hash browns, 16 oz.	830	62	26	3	40
Veggie-Cheese Omel w/eggbeaters, 12 oz.	346	22	11	3	25
Veggie-Cheese Omel w/hashbrowns, 17 oz.	670	48	28	4	30
Breakfast Menu - a la carte					
Bacon, 4 strips, 1 oz.	162	18	1	0	12
Bagel, dry (1), 4 oz.	310	1	65	2	11

(• = most healthy • = least healthy) **RESTAURANTS & FAST-FOOD • 141**

RESTAURANTS & FAST-FOOD CHAINS

Denny's (cont.)

	Cal	Fat	Cbs	Fbr	Prtn
Breakfast Menu - a la carte (cont.)					
Banana, whole, 4 oz.	110	0	29	4	1
Biscuit, 2 oz.	192	10	22	0	3
Cherry Topping, 3 oz.	86	0	21	0	0
Cinnamon Apple Filling, 3 oz.	90	2	19	1	0
Cream Cheese, 1 oz.	100	10	1	0	2
• Egg Beaters ® Egg Substitute, 4 oz.	56	0	2	0	11
English Muffin, dry (1), 2 oz.	150	2	27	2	5
Grapefruit, 5 oz.	60	0	16	6	1
Grapes, 3 oz.	55	1	15	1	1
Ham, grilled slice, Honey Smoked, 3 oz.	85	3	6	0	15
Maple-Flavored Syrup, 2 oz.	143	0	36	0	0
One Egg, 2 oz.	120	10	1	0	6
Sausage Patties (2) patties, 3 oz.	295	28	1	0	9
Sausage, 4 links, 3 oz.	354	32	0	0	16
Sugar-Free Maple-Flavored Syrup, 2 oz.	23	0	9	0	0
Toast, dry, (1), 1 oz.	90	1	17	1	3
• Two Eggs and More Breakfast, 11 oz.	630	47	21	2	31
Whipped Cream, dollop, 0.5 oz.	23	2	2	0	0
Whipped Margarine, 0.5 oz.	87	10	0	0	0
Condiments & Beverages					
BBQ Sauce, 2 oz.	47	1	11	0	0
Blue Cheese Dressing, 1 oz.	163	18	1	0	1
Butter Roll, 2 pcs.	260	9	38	1	5
Caesar Dressing, 1 oz.	133	14	1	0	1
Cherry Limeade, 15 oz.	240	0	62	0	0
Croutons, 1 oz.	112	6	12	1	2
• Fat Free Italian, 1 oz.	15	1	3	0	0
Fat Free Ranch Dressing, 1 oz.	25	0	6	0	0
French Dressing, 1 oz.	106	10	3	0	0
Garlic Dinner Bread, 2 pieces	170	11	15	1	2
Honey Mustard Dressing, 1 oz.	160	15	20	0	0
Island Fizz, 15 oz.	250	0	64	0	0
OJ Mango, 14 oz.	240	0	60	0	0
Pico de Gallo, 3 oz.	21	0	5	1	1
Pineapple Dream, 15 oz.	180	0	64	0	0
Ranch Dressing, 1 oz.	129	14	1	0	0
Razzdango, 15 oz.	220	0	59	1	0
Sour Cream, 2 oz.	91	9	2	0	1
Strawberry Mango Pucker, 15 oz.	200	0	51	1	0
Thousand Island Dressing, 1 oz.	118	11	5	0	0
• Very Double Berry, 14 oz.	280	0	69	0	0
Desserts					
Apple Crisp, a la mode, 12 oz.	723	21	133	6	6
Apple Pie, 7 oz.	470	21	68	3	4
Banana Split, 19 oz.	894	43	121	6	15
Carrot Cake, 8 oz.	799	45	99	2	9
Cheesecake, 7 oz.	580	38	51	0	8
Coconut Cream Pie, 7 oz.	701	32	100	4	4
Double Scoop/Sundae, 6 oz.	375	27	29	0	6
• Floats (Root beer or Cola), 12 oz.	280	10	47	0	3
French Silk Pie, 7 oz.	737	56	58	2	5
Hershey's Chocolate Cake, 5 oz.	631	33	79	2	5
• Hot Fudge Brownie a la mode, 10 oz.	997	42	147	6	12

RESTAURANTS & FAST-FOOD CHAINS

Denny's (cont.)	Cal	Fat	Cbs	Fbr	Prtn
Desserts (cont.)					
Malted Milkshake (van/choc), 12 oz.	583	26	82	1	12
Milkshake (van/choc), 12 oz.	560	26	76	1	11
Neutron Brownie (kids), 3 oz.	344	16	49	2	4
Oreo Blender Blast Off (Kids), 10 oz.	580	29	72	1	11
Oreo Blender Blaster, 15 oz.	895	46	112	2	16
Pecan Pie, 6 oz.	740	41	88	2	9
Pumpkin Pie, 7 oz.	499	11	77	2	8
Single Scoop/Sundae (Delicious Dip), 5 oz.	290	16	35	0	4
Fit Fare					
2% Milk, 5 oz.	87	5	7	0	5
Bagel, dry, 4 oz.	310	1	65	2	11
Baked Potato, plain w/skin, 7 oz.	220	0	51	5	5
Banana (1), 4 oz.	110	0	29	4	1
• Boca Burger w/ sm fruit bowl, 15 oz.	570	11	83	23	34
Cereal (average), 1 oz.	100	0	23	1	2
Chicken Noodle, 12 oz.	170	9	14	0	10
Choice: Oatmeal, 4 oz.	100	2	18	3	5
Corn, 4 oz.	110	2	23	3	3
English Muffin, dry, 2 oz.	150	2	27	2	5
Fruit Medley, 4 oz.	80	0	20	2	1
Grapes, 5 oz.	55	1	15	1	1
Grilled Chicken Breast Dinner w/ Vegetables, 11 oz.	390	11	12	2	57
Grilled Chicken Breast Salad, 16 oz.	320	13	15	4	36
Grits, 4 oz.	80	0	18	0	2
Mashed Potatoes, 5 oz.	170	7	23	2	3
Side Garden Salad (w/o dressing), 7 oz.	113	7	6	2	7
Skinny Moons w/ fruit, 14 oz.	560	12	73	3	37
Sliced Tomatoes, 2 oz.	13	0	3	1	1
Slim Slam ™ (w/ fruit topping), 15 oz.	530	9	76	3	33
Tilapia, w/ Rice & Vegetables., 14 oz.	420	13	40	5	34
Toast, dry, 1 oz.	92	1	17	1	3
Vegetable Beef, 12 oz.	140	5	11	3	7
• Vegetable Blend, 4 oz.	60	3	5	1	1
Veggie EB Omelette w/Eng. Muffin, 14 oz.	340	9	37	5	25
Kid's					
• Anti-Gravity Grapes, 3 oz.	60	0	15	1	0
Astronaut Applesauce, 3 oz.	84	0	19	1	0
Big Dipper French Toastix ™, 7 oz.	627	71	71	1	18
Cosmic Cheeseburger™, 4 oz.	341	20	24	1	15
Deep-Sea Salad™ w/ Ranch, 4 oz.	240	20	13	1	3
Delicious Dip Sundae, 5 oz.	413	19	59	2	6
Flying Saucer Pizza ™, 4 oz.	331	14	38	2	13
Galactic Grilled Cheese, 3 oz.	334	20	28	2	9
Goldfish® Galaxy, 2 oz.	284	3	0	0	0
Junior Grand Slam ®, 5 oz.	400	21	38	1	16
Little Dippers w/Applesauce & Marinara, 10 oz.	566	27	50	5	27
• Little Dippers w/ Marinara & Fries, 12 oz.	860	43	80	8	32
Macaroni & Cheese, 7 oz.	353	13	48	2	12
Moon Crater Mashed ™ w/ Gravy, 5 oz.	145	6	20	2	3
Moons & Stars Chicken Nuggets, 2 oz.	190	13	9	0	9
Neutron Brownie, 3 oz.	344	16	49	2	4
Smiley-Alien Hotcakes w/ Meat, 6 oz.	340	12	49	1	9
Smiley-Alien Hotcakes w/o Meat, 4 oz.	230	3	47	1	5

Denny's (cont.)	Cal	Fat	Cbs	Fbr	Prtn
Promotionals					
Apple Strudel French Toast Slam, 18 oz.	1060	54	92	3	50
Cherry Danish French Toast Slam, 18 oz.	1070	54	96	3	50
• Grilled Chicken (2 pcs.), 10 oz.	280	4	4	0	55
Grilled Shrimp Skewers w/ rice pilaf, 11 oz.	450	18	39	2	27
Mushroom Swiss Chopped Steak 4, 13 oz.	930	76	13	1	46
Slam Burger, 17 oz.	720	40	69	3	24
Southwestern Chicken Sandwich, 15 oz.	1020	50	81	4	59
Steak & Cheese Omelette w/ Hash Brown, 24 oz.	1190	56	107	4	61
• Supreme French Toast 1, 18 oz.	1380	84	113	4	45
Sandwiches/Salads/Soups					
Bacon Cheddar Burger, 13 oz.	970	70	33	4	56
Bacon, Lettuce & Tomato, 7 oz.	570	37	36	5	20
Boca Burger®, 11 oz.	510	16	64	9	31
Broccoli & Cheddar, 12 oz.	270	17	17	3	10
Chef's Salad 3, 18 oz.	360	17	17	5	37
Chicken Noodle, 12 oz.	170	9	14	0	10
Chicken Ranch Melt, 13 oz.	920	42	79	4	53
Clam Chowder, 12 oz.	170	11	13	0	4
Classic Burger w/ Cheese, 13 oz.	940	59	56	5	49
Classic Burger, 11 oz.	780	45	56	5	39
Club Sandwich, 11 oz.	658	34	55	4	29
Coleslaw, 5 oz.	260	22	15	3	2
Crispy Onion Burger w/ Fries, 21 oz.	1820	119	127	11	59
Fish Sandwich, 12 oz.	589	30	30	3	22
French Fries, unsalted, 5 oz.	423	20	57	5	6
Fried Chicken Strip Salad, 15 oz.	438	26	26	4	33
Grilled Chicken Breast Salad, 13 oz.	259	11	10	4	32
Grilled Chicken Sandwich w/o Dressing, 12 oz.	490	13	57	4	39
Jalapeño Burger w/ Fries, 19 oz.	1560	104	99	10	60
• Mini Burgers (6) w/ Onion Rings, 25 oz.	2180	133	173	9	78
Mushroom Swiss Burger, 16 oz.	900	55	62	5	46
Onion Rings, 4 oz.	381	23	38	1	5
Philly Melt, 17 oz.	740	43	51	3	40
Seasoned Fries, 5 oz.	460	28	46	4	4
Side Caesar (w/ dressing), 6 oz.	362	26	20	3	11
• Side Garden Salad (w/o dressing), 7 oz.	113	7	6	2	7
Spicy Buffalo Chicken Melt 1, 14 oz.	930	46	79	4	46
The Super Bird® Sandwich, 10 oz.	570	27	43	2	38
Turkey Breast Salad w/o dressing, 13 oz.	248	8	12	4	31
Vegetable Beef, 12 oz.	140	5	17	3	7
Western Burger w/ Fries, 21 oz.	1580	95	122	10	61
Seniors					
Grilled Cheese Sandwich, 7 oz.	540	30	50	2	17
Senior Belgian Waffle Slam ®, 9 oz.	580	41	29	1	23
Senior Chicken Strip Dinner, 5 oz.	285	10	31	0	19
Senior Club, 10 oz.	570	33	40	3	27
Senior Country Fried Steak, 5 oz.	341	23	18	6	14
Senior French Toast Slam, 7 oz.	591	43	37	1	22
• Senior Fried Shrimp Dinner, 4 oz.	149	6	14	1	10
Senior Grilled Chicken Breast, 6 oz.	200	5	15	1	25
Senior Grilled Tilapia, 6 oz.	248	10	0	0	39
Senior Lemon Pepper Tilapia, 9 oz.	509	41	6	1	33
Senior Pot Roast w/ Vegetables, 7 oz.	180	8	8	2	18

RESTAURANTS & FAST-FOOD CHAINS

Denny's (cont.)	Cal	Fat	Cbs	Fbr	Prtn
Seniors (cont.)					
• Senior Scram. Egg & Cheddar, 13 oz.	790	46	56	2	39
Senior Turkey & Stuffing, 9 oz.	430	12	58	3	20
Sr. Bacon Cheddar Burger w/ Fries, 7 oz.	433	25	27	2	24
Sr. Fish & Chips w/ Slaw & Fries 13 oz.	756	47	64	6	20
Sr. Omelette w/ Hashbrowns, 12 oz.	760	55	36	4	32
Sr. Starter w/ Biscuit, 8 oz.	410	42	23	2	16
Toppings					
Cherry Topping, 2 oz.	57	0	14	0	0
Chocolate Topping, 2 oz.	133	1	34	1	2
• Fudge Topping, 2 oz.	201	10	30	1	1
Strawberry Topping, 2 oz.	77	1	17	1	1
• Whipped Cream (2 tbsp.), 0.5 oz.	23	2	2	0	0

Dippin' Dots	Cal	Fat	Cbs	Fbr	Prtn
Cups: Flavored Ice					
Cherry Berry Ice, 75 g	90	0	23	0	0
Liberty Ice, 75 g	90	0	23	0	0
Pink Lemonade Ice, 75 g	90	0	23	0	0
Rainbow Ice, 75 g	90	0	23	0	0
Watermelon Ice, 75 g	90	0	23	0	0
Cups: Ice Cream					
Banana Split, 85 g	170	10	16	0	3
Bubble Gum, 85 g	165	10	15	0	3
Candy Bar Crunch, 85 g	208	13	34	0	3
Caramel Brownie Sundae, 85 g	170	10	16	0	3
Chocolate Chip Cookie Dough, 85 g	213	11	26	0	3
Chocolate, 85 g	165	10	15	0	3
Cookies 'n Cream w/ Oreo, 85 g	203	11	22	5	3
Cotton Candy, 85 g	170	10	16	0	3
Horchata, 85 g	170	10	16	0	3
Java Delight, 85 g	170	10	16	0	3
Mint Chocolate, 85 g	165	10	15	0	3
• Moose Tracks, 85 g	218	13	21	0	4
Peanut Butter Chip, 85 g	165	10	15	0	3
• Root Beer Float, 85 g	111	3	20	0	1
Strawberry, 85 g	170	10	16	0	3
Tropical Tie Dye, 85 g	170	10	16	0	3
Vanilla, 85 g	170	10	16	0	3
Cups: No Sugar Added					
No Sugar Added Fat Free Fudge, 85 g	92	0	18	0	4
No Sugar Added Reduced Fat Vanilla, 85 g	123	6	13	0	3
Cups: Sherbet					
Lemon Lime Sherbet, 85 g	97	1	22	0	1
Orange Sherbet, 85 g	97	1	22	0	1
Raspberry Sherbet, 85 g	97	1	22	0	1
Yogurt					
Strawberry Cheesecake, 85 g	100	0	21	0	4

Domino's Pizza	Cal	Fat	Cbs	Fbr	Prtn
12" Medium Feast Pizzas					
America's Favorite Feast, 59 g	130	10	4	1	6
Bacon Cheeseburger Feast, 55 g	140	11	3	1	9
Barbecue Feast, 51 g	130	8	8	0	7

(• = most healthy • = least healthy) **RESTAURANTS & FAST-FOOD • 145**

RESTAURANTS & FAST-FOOD CHAINS

Domino's Pizza (cont.)

	Cal	Fat	Cbs	Fbr	Prtn
12" Medium Feast Pizzas (cont.)					
Cheese Deep Dish, 23 g	60	5	2	0	4
• Cheese HT & TC, 18 g	45	4	1	0	3
Classic Hand-Tossed, 55 g	160	3	28	1	6
Crunchy Thin Crust, 22 g	80	4	12	1	2
Deluxe Feast, 56 g	100	8	4	1	5
Extra Cheese, 9 g	25	2	1	0	2
ExtravaganZZa, 81 g	160	12	5	1	9
Hawaiian Feast, 58 g	90	6	5	1	6
MeatZZa Feast, 65 g	150	11	4	1	8
Pepperoni Feast, 54 g	130	11	4	1	7
Philly Cheese Steak Feast, 44 g	100	7	1	0	7
Pizza Sauce, 15 g	10	1	1	0	0
• Ultimate Deep Dish, 56 g	160	6	24	3	4
Vegi Feast, 58 g	80	6	4	1	5
12" Medium, 1 topping pizza					
American Cheese, 11 g	40	3	0	0	2
Anchovies, 2 g	0	0	0	0	0
Bacon, 9 g	40	3	0	0	4
Banana Peppers, 8 g	0	0	0	0	0
Beef, 12 g	40	3	0	0	2
Black Olives, 8 g	10	1	1	0	0
Cheddar Cheese, 7 g	30	3	0	0	2
Cheese Deep Dish, 23 g	60	5	2	0	4
Cheese HT & TC, 18 g	45	4	1	0	3
Chicken Grilled, 12 g	15	0	0	0	2
Classic Hand-Tossed, 55 g	160	3	28	1	6
Crunchy Thin Crust, 22 g	80	4	12	1	2
Extra Cheese, 9 g	25	2	1	0	2
Garlic, 4 g	10	0	1	0	0
Green Chile Peppers, 8 g	0	0	0	0	0
Green Olive, 8 g	15	2	0	0	0
Green Peppers, 8 g	0	0	0	0	0
Ham, 10 g	10	0	0	0	2
Jalapeño, 8 g	0	0	0	0	0
• Mushrooms, 12 g	0	0	0	0	0
Onions, 8 g	0	0	1	0	0
Pepperoni, 8 g	40	4	0	0	2
Philly Meat, 9 g	10	0	0	0	2
Pineapple, 12 g	10	0	2	0	0
Pizza Sauce, 15 g	5	0	1	0	0
Provolone Cheese, 12 g	45	4	0	0	3
Sausage, 12 g	45	4	1	0	2
Tomatoes, 18 g	5	0	1	0	0
• Ultimate Deep Dish, 56 g	160	6	24	3	4
12" Medium, 2-3 topping pizza					
American Cheese, 11 g	40	3	0	0	2
Anchovies, 2 g	0	0	0	0	0
Bacon, 6 g	25	2	0	0	3
Banana Peppers, 5 g	0	0	0	0	0
Beef, 9 g	25	3	0	0	1
Black Olives, 5 g	5	1	1	0	0
Cheddar Cheese, 7 g	30	3	0	0	2
Cheese Deep Dish, 23 g	60	5	2	0	4

RESTAURANTS & FAST-FOOD CHAINS

Domino's Pizza (cont.)	Cal	Fat	Cbs	Fbr	Prtn
12" Medium, 2-3 topping pizza (cont.)					
Cheese HT & TC, 18 g	45	4	1	0	3
Chicken Grilled, 9 g	10	0	0	0	2
Classic Hand-Tossed, 55 g	160	3	28	1	6
Crunchy Thin Crust, 22 g	80	4	12	1	2
Extra Cheese, 9 g	25	2	1	0	2
Garlic, 3 g	10	0	1	0	0
Green Chile Peppers, 5 g	0	0	0	0	0
Green Olive, 5 g	10	1	0	0	0
• Green Peppers, 5 g	0	0	0	0	0
Ham, 7 g	10	0	0	0	1
Jalapeño, 5 g	0	0	0	0	0
Mushrooms, 9 g	0	0	0	0	0
Onions, 5 g	0	0	0	0	0
Pepperoni, 8 g	40	4	0	0	2
Philly Meat, 9 g	10	0	0	0	2
Pineapple, 9 g	5	0	1	0	0
Pizza Sauce, 15 g	10	1	1	0	0
Provolone Cheese, 12 g	45	4	0	0	3
Sausage, 9 g	30	3	0	0	1
Tomatoes, 12 g	0	0	1	0	0
• Ultimate Deep Dish, 56 g	160	6	24	3	4
14" Large Feast Pizzas					
America's Favorite Feast, 82 g	170	14	6	1	9
Bacon Cheeseburger Feast, 77 g	200	15	4	1	12
Barbecue Feast, 70 g	170	11	11	0	9
Cheese Deep Dish, 32 g	80	7	2	0	5
• Cheese HT & TC, 25 g	60	5	2	0	4
Classic Hand-Tossed, 75 g	220	4	38	2	8
Crunchy Thin Crust, 30 g	110	5	16	1	3
Deluxe Feast, 76 g	130	10	5	1	7
Extra Cheese, 12 g	30	3	1	0	2
ExtravaganZZa, 107 g	200	16	7	1	12
Hawaiian Feast, 82 g	130	8	7	1	8
MeatZZa Feast, 94 g	210	17	6	1	12
Pepperoni Feast, 74 g	180	15	5	1	10
Philly Cheese Steak Feast, 58 g	130	9	2	0	9
Pizza Sauce, 21 g	10	0	2	1	0
• Ultimate Deep Dish, 83 g	230	7	36	4	6
Vegi Feast, 79 g	120	8	6	1	7
14" Large, 1 topping pizza					
American Cheese, 12 g	45	4	0	0	2
Anchovies, 2 g	0	0	0	0	0
Bacon, 13 g	60	4	0	0	6
Banana Peppers, 11 g	0	0	1	0	0
Beef, 18 g	50	5	0	0	3
Black Olives, 7 g	10	1	1	0	0
Cheddar Cheese, 9 g	35	3	0	0	2
Cheese Deep Dish, 32 g	80	7	2	0	5
Cheese HT & TC, 25 g	60	5	2	0	4
Chicken Grilled, 18 g	20	1	0	0	3
Classic Hand-Tossed, 75 g	220	4	38	2	8
Crunchy Thin Crust, 30 g	110	5	16	1	3
Extra Cheese, 12 g	30	3	1	0	2

RESTAURANTS & FAST-FOOD CHAINS

Domino's Pizza (cont.)	Cal	Fat	Cbs	Fbr	Prtn
14" Large, 1 topping pizza (cont.)					
Garlic, 4 g	15	0	1	0	0
Green Chile Peppers, 11 g	0	0	0	0	0
Green Olive, 11 g	20	2	1	0	0
Green Peppers, 11 g	0	0	1	0	0
Ham, 13 g	15	1	0	0	2
• Jalapeño, 11 g	0	0	0	0	0
Mushrooms, 18 g	0	0	1	0	0
Onions, 11 g	0	0	1	0	0
Pepperoni, 11 g	50	5	0	0	2
Philly Meat, 12 g	15	1	0	0	2
Pineapple, 18 g	15	0	3	0	0
Pizza Sauce, 21 g	10	0	2	1	0
Provolone Cheese, 18 g	60	5	0	0	5
Sausage, 18 g	60	6	2	1	3
Tomatoes, 21 g	0	0	1	0	0
• Ultimate Deep Dish, 83 g	230	7	36	4	6
14" Large, 2-3 topping pizza					
American Cheese, 12 g	45	4	0	0	2
• Anchovies, 2 g	0	0	0	0	0
Bacon, 10 g	40	3	0	0	4
Banana Peppers, 7 g	0	0	0	0	0
Beef, 12 g	35	3	0	0	2
Black Olives, 7 g	10	1	1	0	0
Cheddar Cheese, 9 g	35	3	0	0	2
Cheese Deep Dish, 32 g	80	7	2	0	5
Cheese HT & TC, 25 g	60	5	2	0	4
Chicken Grilled, 12 g	15	0	0	0	2
Classic Hand-Tossed, 75 g	220	4	38	2	8
Crunchy Thin Crust, 30 g	110	5	16	1	3
Extra Cheese, 12 g	30	3	1	0	2
Garlic, 4 g	10	0	1	0	0
Green Chile Peppers, 7 g	0	0	0	0	0
Green Olive, 7 g	10	1	0	0	0
Green Peppers, 7 g	0	0	0	0	0
Ham, 11 g	10	1	0	0	2
Jalapeño, 7 g	0	0	0	0	0
Mushrooms, 12 g	0	0	0	0	0
Onions, 7 g	0	0	0	0	0
Pepperoni, 11 g	50	5	0	0	2
Philly Meat, 12 g	15	1	0	0	2
Pineapple, 12 g	10	0	2	0	0
Pizza Sauce, 21 g	10	0	2	1	0
Provolone Cheese, 18 g	60	5	0	0	5
Sausage, 12 g	45	4	1	0	2
Tomatoes, 16 g	0	0	1	0	0
• Ultimate Deep Dish, 83 g	230	7	36	4	6
Brooklyn Style Pizza					
• 14" Brooklyn Style w/ Pepperoni, 127 g	330	17	30	2	16
14" Brooklyn Style w/ Sausage, 136 g	350	18	31	2	16
16" Brooklyn Style w/ Pepperoni, 174 g	460	22	43	3	22
• 16" Brooklyn Style w/ Sausage, 187 g	480	25	44	3	22
Crispy Melt Pizza					
12" Plain Crispy Melt Pizza, 95 g	310	18	25	2	13

RESTAURANTS & FAST-FOOD CHAINS

Domino's Pizza (cont.)

	Cal	Fat	Cbs	Fbr	Prtn
Crispy Melt Pizza (cont.)					
14" Plain Crispy Melt Pizza, 129 g	430	24	35	2	17
Dessert Pizza					
10" OREO® Dessert Pizza, 44 g	120	4	20	1	2
Side Items					
Barbecue Buffalo Wings, 87 g	230	14	6	0	17
Blue Cheese Dipping Cup, 43 g	210	22	2	0	1
Blue Cheese Dressing, 43 g	230	24	2	0	2
Breadsticks, 33 g	130	7	14	1	3
Buffalo Chicken Kickers™, 50 g	90	3	6	1	9
Buttermilk Ranch Dressing, 43 g	220	24	2	0	1
Cheesy Bread, 38 g	140	7	14	1	4
Cinna Stix, 35 g	140	7	17	1	3
Creamy Caesar Dressing, 43 g	210	22	2	0	1
• Garlic Dipping Sauce, 50 g	440	49	0	0	0
Golden Italian Dressing, 43 g	220	23	2	0	0
Hot Buffalo Wings, 84 g	210	14	5	0	16
Hot Buffalo Cup, 43 g	120	12	3	0	0
• Light Italian Dressing, 43 g	20	1	2	0	0
Marinara Dipping Sauce, 57 g	25	0	5	1	1
Ranch Dipping Cup, 43 g	190	21	2	0	1
Salad, Garden Fresh, 120 g	70	4	5	2	4
Salad, Grilled Chicken Caesar, 159 g	100	5	6	2	10
Sweet Icing Dipper Cup, 71 g	250	3	57	0	0

Don Pablo's

	Cal	Fat	Cbs	Fbr	Prtn
Appetizers					
• Beef Taquitos, 6 taquitos	561	34	36	5	29
Chicken Flautas, 6 flautas	507	31	39	5	23
Single Flauta, 1 flauta	65	4	6	1	3
• Single Taquito, 1 taquito	63	3	5	1	4
Carnitas					
Carnitas Cold Set	187	14	19	9	3
Traditional Pork Carnitas	1050	38	118	12	59
Classic Fajitas					
7" Flour Tortilla, each	124	4	20	1	3
Chicken	851	29	90	6	56
Lettuce Wraps, 3-4 wraps	0	0	1	0	0
• Onions and Peppers, 7 oz.	186	13	17	4	3
• Steak	1174	68	106	6	34
Steak and Chicken Combo	1013	48	98	6	45
Classic Quesadillas					
Cheese - Large, 8 slices	1597	99	105	4	71
Cheese - Small, 4 slices	812	50	52	2	36
Mesquite Grilled Chicken - Large, 8 slices	1332	65	110	4	73
• Mesquite Grilled Chicken - Small, 4 slices	665	32	55	2	37
Mesquite Grilled Steak - Large, 8 slices	1561	91	122	4	61
Mesquite Grilled Steak - Small, 4 slices	780	45	61	2	30
• The Don's Sampler, 1 order	2002	118	129	13	103
Cool Amigos					
Chicken Nachos	745	46	42	8	44
Chicken Sandwich	1068	52	108	9	42
Cool Amigo Chicken Quesadilla	1507	85	137	10	47
Cool Amigo Fajitas - Beef	1272	63	134	15	42

Don Pablo's (cont.)

	Cal	Fat	Cbs	Fbr	Prtn
Cool Amigos (cont.)					
Cool Amigo Fajitas - Chicken	1099	44	125	15	51
• Cool Amigo Steak Quesadilla	1622	98	143	10	41
• Fried Ice Cream (Small)	424	18	58	1	6
Hamburger	1145	57	106	9	51
Steak Nachos	859	59	48	8	37
Create Your Own Combo					
Beef Enchilada, 1 enchilada	263	18	4	1	16
Beef Relleno, 1 relleno	299	17	20	1	16
Cheese Enchilada, 1 enchilada	232	16	5	1	11
• Cheese Relleno, 1 relleno	396	26	19	1	20
• Chicken Enchilada, 1 enchilada	210	13	9	1	8
Chicken Relleno, 1 relleno	235	11	21	1	12
Chicken Tamale, 1 tamale	222	10	25	4	7
Crispy Beef Taco, 1 taco	291	18	21	2	13
Crispy Chicken Taco, 1 taco	257	14	22	3	12
Pork Tamale, 1 tamale	270	14	24	3	11
Soft Beef Taco, 1 taco	327	18	29	2	15
Soft Chicken Taco, 1 taco	293	14	30	2	13
Spinach & Poblano Enchilada, 1 enchilada	258	13	30	2	5
Desserts					
Chocolate Volcano Cake	1380	77	161	2	11
• Fried Ice Cream, adult serving	827	35	116	2	12
• Sopapillas	1402	78	160	3	14
Dos Tacos					
Don Diego	758	38	58	12	35
• Dos Beef Tacos - Soft	851	37	92	12	40
Dos Beef Tacos -Crispy	820	41	81	14	37
Dos Chicken Tacos - Crispy	766	34	83	14	36
Dos Chicken Tacos - Soft	780	29	94	13	37
• Mamma's Skinny Enchiladas	476	14	51	10	25
Rico's Lunch	794	39	70	13	38
Fajita Cold Set					
• Combo Cheese Topping, 1 oz.	108	8	0	0	8
Guacamole (optional), 1 oz.	52	5	2	1	1
Pico de Gallo, 1 oz.	8	0	2	0	0
• Shredded Lettuce, 1 oz.	0	0	0	0	0
Sour Cream, 1 oz.	77	7	2	0	1
Fajita Enchiladas					
Chicken, 3 enchiladas	872	51	21	4	62
• Mama's Skinny Enchiladas, 3 enchiladas	368	14	18	4	24
• Steak, 3 enchiladas	1101	77	33	4	49
Three Amigos, 3 enchiladas	697	46	18	3	36
Fajita Nachos					
Chicken Nacho	1396	87	73	14	83
Steak Nacho	1430	99	71	15	72
Little Amigos					
• Beef Taco Dinner	483	24	50	8	21
Cheese Enchilada Dinner	515	29	33	7	25
Chicken Stix	739	46	75	5	13
Corn Dog	724	40	80	8	15
• Dogs in a Blanket	1248	78	98	7	41
Grilled Cheese Crisp	884	48	92	6	24

Don Pablo's (cont.)	Cal	Fat	Cbs	Fbr	Prtn
Lunch					
Don Pablo's Lunch	755	39	54	12	36
Dos Beef Enchiladas	754	39	53	11	39
Dos Cheese Enchiladas	755	39	55	12	33
• Dos Chicken Enchiladas	729	35	63	12	30
• El Favorito	982	52	81	12	40
Lunch-Sized Fajitas					
• Classic Chicken	600	20	74	4	31
• Classic Steak	772	39	83	4	21
Combo Fajita	685	29	78	4	26
Nachos					
Cheese	1317	98	48	7	63
Taco Beef	1625	113	85	14	70
Numero Uno Favorito					
• Chicken	1168	56	93	11	50
• Conquistador	1893	88	156	18	99
El Matador	1409	76	110	18	63
Steak and Chicken	1200	63	90	10	44
Quesadillas & Salads					
• Cheese	903	55	61	4	42
• Mesquite-Grilled Chicken	773	39	63	4	42
Mesquite-Grilled Steak	888	52	69	4	36
Salad Dressing					
Bleu Cheese, 3 oz.	451	48	3	0	3
• Cilantro Ranch Dressing, 3 oz.	494	46	20	1	3
• Don's House Vinaigrette, 3 oz.	357	31	10	3	6
Honey Mustard, 3 oz.	315	27	17	0	0
• Low Fat French, 3 oz.	150	4	30	1	34
Ranch, 3 oz.	318	34	3	0	2
Salads					
Caesar Salad (Plain)	1388	114	79	11	21
Chicken Caesar Salad	1563	118	85	11	49
Flour Tortilla Taco Shell	486	27	50	3	8
• Steak Caesar Salad	1792	144	97	11	37
• Tortilla Salad	549	29	59	7	14
Sides, Sauces & Garnishes					
Black Beans, 4 oz.	119	2	20	7	7
Charro Beans, 5 oz.	96	2	16	6	5
Chile-Mashed Potatoes, 3 oz.	108	6	12	1	1
• Chips and Salsa	338	17	43	5	5
Combo Cheese Topping, 1/4 oz.	27	2	0	0	2
Combo Cheese, 1 oz.	109	9	0	0	7
Guacamole, 1 oz.	52	5	2	1	1
Mexican Rice, 3 oz.	107	1	21	1	2
Pico de Gallo, 1 oz.	8	0	2	0	0
Ranchero Sauce, 5 oz.	44	0	9	1	1
Red Sauce, 2 oz.	17	0	4	1	0
Refritos, 5 oz.	262	10	31	11	13
Salsa, Spicy Chili Macho, 2 oz.	14	0	3	1	1
• Salsa, 1 oz.	6	0	1	0	0
Seasoned Vegetables, 6 oz.	98	5	13	3	3
Seasoned Vegetables, 6 oz.	98	5	13	3	3
Side Salad	108	7	8	2	5
Sour Cream Sauce, 2 oz.	66	4	5	0	1

(•= most healthy •= least healthy) **RESTAURANTS & FAST-FOOD • 151**

RESTAURANTS & FAST-FOOD CHAINS

Don Pablo's (cont.)

	Cal	Fat	Cbs	Fbr	Prtn
Sides, Sauces & Garnishes (cont.)					
Sour Cream, 1.5 oz.	77	7	2	0	1
Sour Crema, 1 oz.	57	5	1	0	1
Spoon Bread, 4 oz.	250	12	32	2	2
Sizzling Fajitas & Enchilada Combos					
Chicken Fajitas & Chicken Enchilada	986	34	105	6	55
• Shrimp Fajitas & Shrimp Enchilada	981	63	65	7	41
• Steak Fajitas & Steak Enchilada	1255	66	119	6	37
Soup					
• Tortilla Soup - Bottomless Bowl, 12 oz.	258	12	26	3	13
• White Chicken Chili - Bottomless Bowl, 12 oz.	541	32	48	8	23
White Chicken Chili - Cup, 6 oz.	234	13	23	4	11
The Don's Dips					
• Dip Sampler, 4 dips, 2 oz.	519	39	27	6	20
• Guacamole, 2 oz.	83	8	4	2	1
Prairie Fire Bean Dip, 2 oz.	126	8	8	3	6
Queso Blanco, 2 oz.	113	9	4	0	4
Queso, 2 oz.	105	8	3	0	6
Prairie Fire Bean Dip Cup, 6 oz.	378	25	23	8	17
Queso Blanco Cup, 6 oz.	339	27	13	1	12
Queso Cup, 6 oz.	315	23	10	1	19
Traditional Favorites					
• Chicken Burrito, 1 burrito	878	48	70	5	43
Chicken Chimichanga, 1 burrito	1099	42	114	8	64
• Spicy Ground Beef and Bean Burrito, 1 burrito	1389	73	123	19	66
Spicy Ground Beef Chimi De Oro, 1 burrito	1349	68	131	8	52

Donatos Pizza

	Cal	Fat	Cbs	Fbr	Prtn
Desserts					
Apple Dessert Thin Crust Pizza, 368 g	773	21	134	6	14
• Cherry Dessert Thin Crust Pizza, 368 g	799	21	140	1	14
• Chocolate Chunk Cookie, 85 g	430	21	57	2	6
Dressings & Croutons					
Apple Cider Vinaigrette, 2 oz.	140	12	8	0	0
Blue Cheese, 2 oz.	230	24	2	0	2
Buttermilk Ranch, 2 oz.	230	24	2	0	1
• Chicken Bacon Ranch Pizza Dip, 3 oz.	450	47	4	0	1
Dijon Honey Mustard, 2 oz.	200	18	8	1	1
Fat Free Ranch, 2 oz.	45	0	10	1	0
Honey French, 2 oz.	220	18	14	0	0
House Italian, 2 oz.	230	24	1	0	0
• Light Italian, 2 oz.	20	1	2	0	0
Roasted Red Pepper Croutons, 0.5 oz.	50	3	5	0	1
Thousand Island, 2 oz.	220	21	7	0	0
Tuscan Caesar, 2 oz.	180	18	3	0	1
Oven Baked Subs					
Big Don Italian, 318 g	720	34	67	3	36
w/Pizza Sauce, 325 g	654	26	69	3	36
Big Don Sausage Italian, 417 g	1000	56	68	3	54
w/Pizza Sauce, 424 g	934	48	70	3	54
• Big Ham and Cheese, 316 g	620	22	68	3	36
Big Steak Hoagie w/ Mushroom Gravy, 337 g	800	39	68	2	45
Big Steak Hoagie w/ Pizza Sauce, 340 g	804	39	68	3	45
Grilled Chicken Club, 414 g	899	44	71	3	53

RESTAURANTS & FAST-FOOD CHAINS

‣ Donatos Pizza (cont.)	Cal	Fat	Cbs	Fbr	Prtn
Oven Baked Subs (cont.)					
• Meatball, 407 g	1137	64	78	5	59
Roasted Vegy, 355 g	731	37	74	5	26
Steak and Cheese, 340 g	778	34	69	3	45
Pizza No Dough					
Chicken Spinach Mozzarella, 212 g	574	42	16	2	36
Chicken Vegy Medley™, 285 g	495	29	20	3	41
Classic Trio®, 220 g	532	37	18	3	34
Founder's Favorite®, 238 g	558	38	18	3	38
Hawaiian™, 200 g	436	26	22	4	30
Margherita, 231 g	589	46	16	2	32
Mariachi™ Beef, 283 g	528	34	23	4	35
Mariachi™ Chicken, 287 g	495	30	21	4	38
Pepperoni Zinger, 217 g	584	42	17	3	37
Pepperoni™, 175 g	499	35	17	2	31
Philly Cheesesteak, 224 g	521	33	19	2	38
Serious Cheese, 170 g	457	31	17	2	31
• Serious Meat™, 256 g	653	46	19	3	47
The Works™, 260 g	547	37	21	4	34
• Vegy™, 261 g	418	25	23	4	25
Pizza Thicker Crust					
BBQ Chicken, 325 g	810	31	90	3	40
Chicken Spinach Mozzarella, 307 g	791	38	73	3	41
Chicken Vegy Medley, 328 g	657	24	75	3	37
Classic Trio, 336 g	832	41	78	5	40
Founder's Favorite®, 349 g	858	42	78	4	44
Hawaiian, 318 g	758	32	82	5	38
Margherita, 294 g	766	39	72	3	35
Mariachi Beef, 362 g	796	36	81	5	37
Mariachi Chicken, 373 g	806	35	81	4	40
Pepperoni Zinger, 308 g	827	41	76	4	40
Pepperoni, 285 g	798	39	76	4	37
Philly Cheesesteak, 296 g	728	31	74	3	38
Serious Cheese, 291 g	798	38	77	4	40
• Serious Meat, 348 g	907	47	78	4	50
The Works, 375 g	847	41	81	6	40
• Vegy, 374 g	715	29	83	6	32
Pizza Thin Crust					
• BBQ Chicken, 270 g	792	26	66	2	34
Chicken Spinach Mozzarella, 253 g	631	33	49	2	36
• Chicken Vegy Medley™, 273 g	497	20	51	3	31
Classic Trio®, 288 g	674	37	52	3	35
Founder's Favorite®, 302 g	702	38	52	2	39
Hawaiian™, 265 g	588	27	56	4	32
Margherita, 239 g	606	35	48	2	30
Mariachi™ Beef, 312 g	630	32	55	3	32
Mariachi™ Chicken, 324 g	639	30	56	3	35
Pepperoni Zinger, 254 g	656	36	50	2	34
Pepperoni, 230 g	627	34	50	2	32
Philly Cheesesteak, 255 g	596	29	51	2	34
Serious Cheese™, 237 g	627	34	51	2	34
Serious Meat™, 293 g	736	42	52	3	44
Spinach, 256 g	611	34	51	2	29
The Works™, 329 g	689	37	56	4	35

RESTAURANTS & FAST-FOOD CHAINS

Donatos Pizza (cont.)

	Cal	Fat	Cbs	Fbr	Prtn
Pizza Thin Crust (cont.)					
Vegy™, 319 g	544	24	57	4	26
White, 217 g	690	42	49	1	34
Salads					
Caesar Side Salad, 104 g	87	6	3	1	7
• Entree Chicken Harvest Salad, 336 g	514	32	29	5	32
Italian Chef Entree Salad, 362 g	314	22	10	4	22
Italian Garden Side Salad, 142 g	108	8	4	2	7
Tuscan Chicken Caesar Entree Salad, 296 g	198	8	6	3	28
Starters					
3 Cheese Garlic Bread, 51 g	174	9	16	1	8
Breadsticks w/Nacho Cheese Sauce, 154 g	398	22	39	2	13
Breadsticks w/Pizza Sauce, 113 g	261	9	38	3	7
Buffalo Wings - BBQ, 232 g	595	43	10	0	34
Buffalo Wings - Garlic, 222 g	669	56	12	0	34
Buffalo Wings - Hot, 232 g	597	48	11	0	34
Buffalo Wings - Mild, 232 g	618	48	13	0	34
Buffalo Wings - Plain, 204 g	552	43	10	0	34
• Buffalo Wings - Spicy Garlic, 251 g	713	60	23	0	34
Buffalo Wings, 204 g	429	31	4	0	33
• Chicken Breast Strips, 74 g	125	4	12	0	11
Wedge Fries, 159 g	261	13	34	6	4
Stromboli					
3 Meat, 309 g	689	31	67	5	34
Cheese, 299 g	693	31	66	5	35
Deluxe, 304 g	613	25	68	5	28
• Pepperoni, 300 g	716	34	67	5	34
• Vegy, 310 g	606	24	69	5	27

Dunkin' Donuts

	Cal	Fat	Cbs	Fbr	Prtn
Bagels					
Blueberry Bagel, 1 bagel	330	3	66	2	10
Cinnamon Raisin Bagel, 1 bagel	330	3	65	3	10
Everything Bagel, 1 bagel	370	6	67	3	14
Multigrain Bagel, 1 bagel	380	6	68	5	14
Onion Bagel, 1 bagel	320	4	61	3	12
• Plain Bagel, 1 bagel	320	3	62	2	12
Poppyseed Bagel, 1 bagel	370	7	65	3	14
• Reduced Carb Bagel with Cheese, 1 bagel	380	12	45	14	25
Salt Bagel, 1 bagel	320	3	62	2	12
Sesame Bagel, 1 bagel	380	8	64	3	14
Wheat Bagel, 1 bagel	330	4	62	4	12
Bakery: Cookies					
Chocolate Chunk Cookie, 5 oz.	540	23	80	3	7
• Oatmeal Raisin Cookie, 5 oz.	480	14	83	5	8
• Peanut Butter Cup Cookie, 5 oz.	590	29	73	3	11
Bakery: Danish					
Apple Danish, 1 danish	330	20	32	1	4
Cheese Danish, 1 danish	340	22	30	1	4
• Strawberry Cheese Danish, 1 danish	320	20	31	1	4
Bakery: Muffins					
Banana Walnut Muffin, 1 muffin	540	25	69	3	10
Blueberry Muffin, 1 muffin	470	17	73	2	8
• Chocolate Chip Muffin, 1 muffin	630	26	89	2	10

RESTAURANTS & FAST-FOOD CHAINS

Dunkin' Donuts (cont.)	Cal	Fat	Cbs	Fbr	Prtn
Bakery: Muffins (cont.)					
Coffee Cake Muffin, 1 muffin	580	19	78	1	9
Corn Muffin, 1 muffin	510	18	77	1	8
Cranberry Orange Muffin, 1 muffin	440	17	66	3	8
• English Muffin, 3 oz.	160	2	31	2	6
Honey Bran Raisin Muffin, 1 muffin	480	15	79	5	8
Lemon Raspberry Muffin, 1 muffin	460	15	75	3	6
Pumpkin Muffin, 1 muffin	560	24	82	3	6
Reduced Fat Blueberry Muffin, 1 muffin	400	5	78	3	8
Bakery: Other					
• Biscuit, 1 biscuit	440	22	51	2	7
• Plain Croissant, 1 croissant	270	14	30	1	6
Breakfast Flat Bread					
• Ham & Swiss Flat Bread	350	12	41	2	20
• Three Cheese Flat Bread	460	24	42	2	20
Turkey Cheddar & Bacon Flat Bread	360	13	41	2	20
Breakfast Sandwiches					
Bacon Egg Cheese Bagel Sandwich	540	18	69	2	18
Bacon Egg Cheese Croissant Sandwich	440	25	33	1	19
Bacon Egg Cheese English Muffin Sandwich	360	16	36	1	17
Bacon Lover's Supreme Breakfast Sandwich	640	43	36	2	26
Egg Cheese Bagel Sandwich	470	15	65	2	20
Egg Cheese Biscuit Sandwich	540	29	53	2	16
Egg Cheese Croissant Sandwich	430	26	33	1	14
Egg Cheese English Muffin Sandwich	280	9	34	1	15
Ham Egg Cheese Bagel Sandwich	510	16	65	2	26
Ham Egg Cheese Croissant Sandwich	460	27	33	1	20
Ham Egg Cheese English Muffin Sandwich	310	10	34	1	21
• Hash Browns, 9 pieces	180	9	22	3	2
Sausage Egg Cheese Bagel Sandwich	660	35	63	3	28
• Sausage Egg Cheese Biscuit Sandwich	800	52	54	2	24
Sausage Egg Cheese Croissant Sandwich	630	45	34	1	24
Sausage Egg Cheese English Muffin Sandwich	530	32	37	1	23
Supreme Omelet on a Croissant	530	33	35	2	21
Coffee					
Coffee, 10 fl.oz.	15	0	3	0	1
• with Cream and Sugar, 10 fl.oz.	120	6	15	0	1
with Cream, 10 fl.oz.	70	6	3	0	1
with Milk and Sugar, 10 fl.oz.	80	1	16	0	2
with Milk, 10 fl.oz.	35	1	4	0	2
with Skim Milk and Sugar, 10 fl.oz.	70	0	16	0	2
with Skim Milk, 10 fl.oz.	25	0	4	0	2
with Sugar, 10 fl.oz.	60	0	15	0	1
Coolatta®					
Cherry Lime SoBe® Coolatta®, 16 fl.oz.	250	0	62	2	0
Coffee Coolatta® with 2% Milk, 16 fl.oz.	190	2	41	0	4
with Cream, 16 fl.oz.	350	22	40	0	3
with Milk, 16 fl.oz.	210	4	42	0	4
• with Skim Milk, 16 fl.oz.	170	0	41	0	4
Lemonade Coolatta®, 16ozs.	240	0	59	0	0
Strawberry Fruit Coolatta®, 16 fl.oz.	290	0	72	1	0
Tropicana Orange Coolatta®, 16 fl.oz.	370	0	92	3	1
• Vanilla Bean Coolatta®, 16 fl.oz.	500	17	85	2	1

(•= most healthy •= least healthy) **RESTAURANTS & FAST-FOOD • 155**

RESTAURANTS & FAST-FOOD CHAINS

Dunkin' Donuts (cont.)

	Cal	Fat	Cbs	Fbr	Prtn
Cream Cheese					
Chive Cream Cheese, 2oz.	170	17	4	2	4
Garden Vegetable Cream Cheese, 2oz.	170	15	4	0	2
Lite Cream Cheese, 2oz.	120	9	5	0	4
• Lite Garden Vegetable Cream Cheese, 2oz.	100	8	5	0	3
Plain Cream Cheese, 2oz.	190	17	4	0	4
Salmon Cream Cheese, 2oz.	170	17	2	0	4
• Strawberry Cream Cheese, 2oz.	190	17	9	0	4
Deli Classics: Sandwiches					
• Ham and Swiss Sandwich	360	11	44	4	23
Roast Beef and Swiss Sandwich	530	25	45	4	31
Tuna (Albacore) Sandwich	550	26	49	4	29
Turkey and Cheese Sandwich	510	22	45	4	35
Vegetarian Sandwich	420	21	51	8	9
Donuts					
Apple Crumb Donut, 1 donut	320	13	46	2	4
Apple N' Spice Donut, 1 donut	260	11	35	2	4
Bavarian Kreme Donut, 1 donut	250	11	35	1	4
Black Raspberry Donut, 1 donut	270	10	40	1	4
Blueberry Cake Donut, 1 donut	290	16	35	1	3
Blueberry Crumb Donut, 1 donut	330	13	48	2	4
Boston Kreme Donut, 1 donut	270	12	38	1	4
• Chocolate Coconut Cake Donut, 1 donut	370	21	42	3	3
Chocolate Frosted Cake Donut, 1 donut	330	19	36	2	4
Chocolate Frosted Donut, 1 donut	230	11	29	2	4
Chocolate Glazed Cake Donut, 1 donut	340	19	39	2	3
Chocolate Kreme Filled Donut, 1 donut	300	14	39	2	4
Cinnamon Cake Donut, 1 donut	310	18	34	2	4
Double Chocolate Cake Donut, 1 donut	340	20	36	3	3
• French Cruller, 1 donut	150	8	17	1	2
Glazed Cake Donut, 1 donut	330	18	38	2	3
Glazed Donut Jelly Filled Donut, 1 donut	270	10	39	1	4
Glazed Donut, 1 donut	230	10	30	1	4
Maple Frosted Donut, 1 donut	240	10	31	1	4
Marble Frosted Donut, 1 donut	230	11	30	1	4
Old Fashioned Cake Donut, 1 donut	280	18	26	2	3
Powdered Cake Donut, 1 donut	310	18	34	2	3
Pumpkin Glazed Donut, 1 donut	280	6	52	1	4
Strawberry Frosted Donut, 1 donut	240	10	32	1	4
Sugar Raised Donut, 1 donut	210	10	27	1	4
Vanilla Kreme Filled Donut, 1 donut	320	16	39	1	4
Wheat Glazed Cake Donut, 1 donut	310	19	32	1	4
Donuts: Fancies					
Apple Fritter, 1 fritter	290	13	35	2	4
Bow Tie Donut, 1 donut	300	17	34	1	4
• Chocolate Frosted Coffee Roll, 1 roll	340	20	36	1	4
Chocolate Iced Bismark, 1 donut	340	15	50	1	3
Coffee Roll, 1 roll	340	20	33	1	4
Eclair, 1 donut	300	15	39	1	3
• Glazed Fritter, 1 fritter	250	13	31	1	4
Maple Frosted Coffee Roll, 1 donut	340	20	36	1	4
Vanilla Frosted Coffee Roll, 1 donut	340	20	36	1	4
Donuts: Munchkins					
Cinnamon Cake Munchkin, 4 munchkins	260	15	29	2	3

Dunkin' Donuts (cont.)	Cal	Fat	Cbs	Fbr	Prtn
Donuts: Munchkins (cont.)					
Glazed Cake Munchkin, 4 munchkins	300	15	38	2	3
• Glazed Chocolate Cake Munchkin, 4 munchkins	300	15	39	2	2
Glazed Munchkin, 4 munchkins	300	15	38	2	3
Jelly Filled Munchkin, 5 munchkins	240	8	37	1	3
Plain Cake Munchkin, 4 munchkins	230	15	21	2	3
Powdered Cake Munchkin, 4 munchkins	260	15	29	2	3
• Sugar Raised Munchkin, 5 munchkins	190	8	26	1	3
Donuts: Sticks					
Cinnamon Cake Stick, 1 stick	340	20	36	2	4
Glazed Cake Stick, 1 stick	360	20	41	2	4
Glazed Chocolate Cake Stick, 1 stick	370	21	41	2	3
• Jelly Stick, 1 stick	420	20	53	2	4
• Plain Cake Stick, 1 stick	310	20	29	2	4
Powdered Cake Stick, 1 stick	340	20	37	2	4
Dunkin' Deli: Cravings Sandwiches					
Chicken Bruschetta Sandwich	580	25	48	4	42
Chipotle Chicken Sandwich	620	26	49	4	49
• Pastrami Supreme Sandwich	760	42	47	5	48
• Turkey Pesto Sandwich	530	23	46	4	33
Dunkin' Deli: Favorites Sandwiches					
• Avocado and Turkey Sandwich	500	22	49	8	38
Chicken Cordon Bleu Sandwich	550	19	51	4	45
Steak and Cheese Sandwich	510	23	45	4	30
• Toasted Italian Sandwich	630	34	49	5	35
Turkey and Bacon Club Sandwich	510	22	44	4	35
Dunkin' Deli: Salads					
Caesar Salad, 8 oz.	390	33	14	3	10
Chicken Caesar Salad, 11 oz.	520	36	16	3	34
Garden Salad, 14 oz.	240	12	24	5	12
• Mediterranean Salad, 15 oz.	220	11	23	5	10
• Oriental Salad, 14 oz.	580	35	39	4	30
Dunkin' Deli: Soups					
Broccoli Cheese Soup, 240 ml	180	13	10	1	7
• Chicken Noodle Soup, 240 ml	140	4	20	1	8
Clam Chowder, 240 ml	230	11	20	1	10
• Lasagna Soup, 240 ml	250	13	21	2	11
Timberline Chili with Beans, 240 ml	230	8	26	8	15
Flavored Coffee					
• Blueberry Coffee, 10 fl.oz.	20	0	4	0	1
Caramel Cinnamon Coffee, 10 fl.oz.	20	0	4	0	1
Caramel Coffee, 10 fl.oz.	20	0	4	0	1
Chocolate Coffee, 10 fl.oz.	20	0	4	0	1
Cinnamon Coffee, 10 fl.oz.	20	0	4	0	1
Coconut Coffee, 10 fl.oz.	20	0	4	0	1
French Vanilla Coffee, 10 fl.oz.	20	0	4	0	1
Hazelnut Coffee, 10 fl.oz.	20	0	4	0	1
• Pumpkin Spice Coffee Medium, 14 fl.oz.	240	8	39	0	4
Raspberry Coffee, 10 fl.oz.	20	0	4	0	1
Toasted Almond Coffee, 10 fl.oz.	20	0	4	0	1
Hot Espresso Drinks					
Cappuccino with Soy Milk, 10 fl.oz.	70	3	6	1	4
with Soy Milk and Sugar, 10 fl.oz.	120	3	20	1	4
Cappuccino, 10 fl.oz.	80	5	7	0	4

RESTAURANTS & FAST-FOOD CHAINS

Dunkin' Donuts (cont.)

	Cal	Fat	Cbs	Fbr	Prtn
Hot Espresso Drinks (cont.)					
with Sugar, 10 fl.oz.	130	5	21	0	4
Caramel Creme Hot Latte, 10 fl.oz.	260	9	40	0	8
Caramel Swirl Latte w/ Soy Milk, 10 fl.oz.	210	4	34	1	8
Caramel Swirl Latte, 10 fl.oz.	230	6	36	0	8
• Espresso, 2 fl.oz.	0	0	1	0	0
with Sugar, 2 fl.oz.	30	0	7	0	0
• Gingerbread Latte, 10 fl.oz.	400	9	68	0	10
Hot Latte Lite, 10 fl.oz.	70	0	10	0	6
Latte with Soy Milk, 10 fl.oz.	90	4	8	1	6
with Soy Milk and Sugar, 10 fl.oz.	150	4	22	1	6
Latte, 10 fl.oz.	120	4	0	9	0
with Sugar, 10 fl.oz.	160	6	22	0	6
Mocha Almond Hot Latte, 10 fl.oz.	290	10	46	1	8
Mocha Swirl Latte with Soy Milk, 10 fl.oz.	210	5	35	2	7
Mocha Swirl Latte, 10 fl.oz.	230	7	37	1	6
Pumpkin Spice Latte Medium, 16 fl.oz.	340	9	52	0	12
Turbo Hot™, 10 fl.oz.	130	6	20	0	1
Vanilla Latte Lite, 10 fl.oz.	80	0	12	0	7
Iced Coffee					
Berry Berry Iced Coffee, 16 fl.oz.	120	6	16	0	2
• Iced Coffee, 16 fl.oz.	15	0	3	0	1
with Cream and Sugar, 16 fl.oz.	120	6	16	0	2
with Cream, 16 fl.oz.	70	6	4	0	2
with Milk and Sugar, 16 fl.oz.	80	1	16	0	2
with Milk, 16 fl.oz.	35	1	4	0	2
with Skim Milk and Sugar, 16 fl.oz.	70	0	16	0	2
with Skim Milk, 16 fl.oz.	25	0	4	0	2
with Sugar, 16 fl.oz.	60	0	15	0	1
• Pumpkin Spice Iced Coffee, 24 fl.oz.	240	8	37	0	4
Turbo Ice™, 16 fl.oz.	120	7	14	0	1
Vanilla Iced Latte Lite, 16 fl.oz.	80	0	13	0	7
Iced Espresso Drinks					
Caramel Creme Iced Latte, 16 fl.oz.	260	9	40	0	8
Iced Caramel Swirl Latte, 16 fl.oz.	240	7	37	0	8
with Skim Milk, 16 fl.oz.	180	0	36	0	8
Iced Latte Lite, 16 fl.oz.	80	0	13	0	7
Iced Latte, 16 fl.oz.	120	7	11	0	6
Skim Milk and Sugar, 16 fl.oz.	120	0	23	0	7
• with Skim Milk, 16 fl.oz.	70	0	11	0	7
with Sugar, 16 fl.oz.	170	7	23	0	6
Iced Mocha Swirl Latte, 16 fl.oz.	240	8	38	1	7
with Skim Milk, 16 fl.oz.	180	1	37	1	7
Mocha Almond Iced Latte, 16 fl.oz.	290	10	46	1	8
• Pumpkin Spice Iced Latte, 24 fl.oz.	340	9	52	0	12
Turbo Ice™, 16 fl.oz.	120	7	14	0	1
Other Beverages					
Dunkaccino®, 10 fl.oz.	230	11	35	0	2
• Hot Chocolate, 10 fl.oz.	230	7	39	2	2
Vanilla Chai, 10ozs.	230	8	40	0	1
• White Hot Chocolate, 14 fl.oz.	340	13	55	0	3
Personal Pizza					
• Cheese Pizza, 1 pizza	400	19	46	2	18
Pepperoni Pizza, 1 pizza	410	19	45	2	19

Dunkin' Donuts (cont.)

	Cal	Fat	Cbs	Fbr	Prtn
Personal Pizza (cont.)					
• Supreme Pizza, 1 pizza	430	21	46	2	17
Smoothie					
• Mango Passion Fruit Smoothie, 24 fl.oz.	550	4	118	3	10
Strawberry Banana Smoothie, 24 fl.oz.	550	4	118	3	10
• Tropical Fruit Smoothie, 24 fl.oz.	540	4	117	2	11
Wildberry Smoothie, 24 fl.oz.	550	4	118	2	10

Dunn Bros. Coffee

	Cal	Fat	Cbs	Fbr	Prtn
Brewed Coffee					
• Brewed Coffee, 16 oz.	10	0	2	N/A	0
• Coffee with Steamed 2% Milk, 16 oz.	70	3	8	N/A	5
Coffee with Steamed Skim Milk, 16 oz.	55	0	8	N/A	5
Coffee with Steamed Soy Milk, 16 oz.	60	2	7	N/A	4
Depth Charge, 16 oz.	10	0	2	N/A	0
Chai Tea Latte					
• Chai Tea Latte, 16 oz.	165	4	27	N/A	7
• Skim Milk Chai Tea Latte, 16 oz.	140	0	27	N/A	7
Soy Milk Chai Tea Latte, 16 oz.	140	0	27	N/A	7
Espresso Drinks					
• Americano, 16 oz.	0	0	0	N/A	0
Caffe Latte, 16 oz.	142	5	14	N/A	9
Caramel Latte Macchiato, 16 oz.	230	5	38	N/A	8
Caramel Mocha Latte, 16 oz.	275	5	50	N/A	9
Mocha Latte, 16 oz.	275	5	50	N/A	10
Skim Milk Caffe Latte, 16 oz.	110	0	17	N/A	10
Skim Milk Cappuccino, 16 oz.	80	0	13	N/A	5
Skim Milk Caramel Latte Macchiato, 16 oz.	240	1	48	N/A	9
Skim Milk Caramel Mocha Latte, 16 oz.	240	1	50	N/A	9
Skim Milk Mocha Latte, 16 oz.	260	3	50	N/A	10
Skim Milk Vanilla Latte, 16 oz.	170	0	31	N/A	9
Skim White Mocha Latte, 16 oz.	260	5	46	N/A	8
Soy Cappuccino, 16 oz.	90	2	12	N/A	4
Soy Milk Caffe Latte, 16 oz.	140	4	16	N/A	9
Soy Milk Caramel Latte Macchiato, 16 oz.	260	4	47	N/A	8
Soy Milk Mocha Latte, 16 oz.	280	6	49	N/A	9
Soy Milk Vanilla Latte, 16 oz.	180	4	28	N/A	7
• Soy Milk White Mocha Latte, 16 oz.	290	8	45	N/A	7
Vanilla Latte, 16 oz.	210	5	30	N/A	9
White Mocha Latte, 16 oz.	270	9	52	N/A	8
Whole Milk Cappuccino, 16 oz.	110	5	12	N/A	5
Favorites					
Chocolate Steamed Nirvana, 16 oz.	325	5	63	N/A	8
• Hot Chocolate, 16 oz.	380	6	71	N/A	12
• Hot Spiced Apple Cider, 16 oz.	215	0	51	N/A	0
Skim Chocolate Steamed Nirvana, 16 oz.	290	3	61	N/A	7
Skim Hot Chocolate, 16 oz.	340	3	68	N/A	12
Soy Chocolate Steamed Nirvana, 16 oz.	300	5	60	N/A	7
Fruit Smoothies					
Mango, 16 oz.	250	0	58	1	0
• Strawberry Pink Freeze, 16 oz.	360	7	70	N/A	3
• Strawberry, 16 oz.	250	0	58	0	0
Wildberry, 16 oz.	250	0	58	0	0

Dunn Bros. Coffee (cont.)

	Cal	Fat	Cbs	Fbr	Prtn
IceCremas™					
Caramel IceCrema, 16 oz.	450	11	65	N/A	1
• Caramel Mocha IceCrema, 16 oz.	400	11	74	N/A	2
Chai IceCrema, 16 oz.	410	11	74	N/A	2
Coffee IceCrema, 16 oz.	260	10	41	N/A	1
Mocha IceCrema, 16 oz.	420	10	79	N/A	4
Skim Caramel Mocha IceCrema, 16 oz.	370	5	77	N/A	4
Skim Milk Caramel Mocha IceCrema, 16 oz.	370	5	77	N/A	4
Skim Milk Chai IceCrema, 16 oz.	350	4	75	N/A	4
• Skim Milk Coffee IceCrema, 16 oz.	210	3	41	N/A	3
Skim Milk Mocha IceCrema, 16 oz.	370	3	80	N/A	6
Soy Milk Chai IceCrema, 16 oz.	360	5	75	N/A	3
Iced Drinks					
• Cold Press Coffee, 16 oz.	10	0	2	N/A	0
Iced Caramel Latte Macchiato, 16 oz.	200	4	35	N/A	7
Iced Chai, 16 oz.	130	6	23	N/A	4
Iced Latte, 16 oz.	90	4	9	N/A	6
Iced Mocha, 16 oz.	230	3	45	N/A	6
Iced White Mocha, 16 oz.	230	7	47	N/A	5
Italian Cream Soda, 16 oz.	190	2	42	N/A	0
Italian Soda, 16 oz.	170	0	42	N/A	0
Skim Milk Iced Chai, 16 oz.	140	0	30	N/A	4
Skim Milk Iced Latte Macchiato, 16 oz.	170	1	35	N/A	7
Skim Milk Iced Latte, 16 oz.	80	0	12	N/A	6
Skim Milk Iced Mocha, 16 oz.	220	3	45	N/A	7
Skim Milk Iced White Mocha, 16 oz.	210	5	47	N/A	5
Soy Milk Iced Chai, 16 oz.	150	2	30	N/A	4
Soy Milk Iced Latte, 16 oz.	100	3	11	N/A	6
• Soy Milk Iced Mocha, 16 oz.	240	5	45	N/A	6
Soy Milk Iced White Mocha, 16 oz.	210	6	46	N/A	4
Vanilla Iced Nirvana, 16 oz.	210	16	17	N/A	4

Eat N' Park

	Cal	Fat	Cbs	Fbr	Prtn
Appetizers					
Breaded Zucchini	415	23	39	3	13
Buffalo Chicken Tenders	434	21	24	2	35
Cheese Sticks	411	25	17	0	30
• Onion Rings	209	13	19	1	4
• Southwest Quesadilla	853	50	56	7	48
Stuffed Mushrooms	217	15	7	1	14
Bakery					
Bagel (Plain), 1 piece	312	2	61	3	12
Bagel (Raisin), 1 piece	320	2	65	4	11
• Bear Claw, 1 piece	515	24	66	2	9
Biscuit (Cheese), 1 piece	127	6	15	1	3
Biscuit, 1 piece	214	13	22	1	3
Boston Brown Bread, 2 slices	279	9	43	1	7
Bun (Hoagie), 1 piece	178	2	34	2	6
Bun (Hot Dog), 1 piece	128	3	21	1	4
Bun (Superburger), 1 piece	183	3	32	2	5
Bun (Three Cheese Hoagie), 1 piece	470	26	44	2	15
Cookie (Chocolate Chip), 1 piece	207	9	28	1	3
Cookie (Christmas), 1 piece	250	8	42	0	2
Cookie (Easter), 1 piece	251	8	42	0	2

▶ Eat N' Park (cont.)	Cal	Fat	Cbs	Fbr	Prtn
Bakery (cont.)					
Cookie (Halloween), 1 piece	250	8	42	0	2
Cookie (Macadamia Nut), 1 piece	240	16	22	1	2
Cookie (Shamrock), 1 piece	250	8	42	0	2
Cookie (Smiley®), 1 piece	250	8	42	0	2
Cookie (Steeler/Penguin/Pirate), 1 piece	250	8	42	0	2
Cookie (Valentine), 1 piece	250	8	42	0	2
Cornbread, 1 piece	108	4	16	1	2
Croissant, 1 piece	258	15	27	1	5
Crumby Buns, 1 piece	193	9	24	1	3
English Muffin, 1 piece	133	1	26	2	4
Garlic Toast, 1 slice	465	19	61	3	11
Honey Bun, 1 piece	172	8	22	1	3
• Italian Bread, 1 slice	54	1	10	1	2
Muffin (Apple Raisin), 1 piece	249	7	43	2	4
Muffin (Banana Nut), 1 piece	284	13	39	2	5
Muffin (Blueberry), 1 piece	242	8	39	1	4
Muffin (Chocolate Nut), 1 piece	313	13	45	2	6
Muffin (Corn), 1 piece	212	8	31	1	4
Muffin (Cranberry), 1 piece	266	10	41	1	4
Muffin (Mocha Java), 1 piece	222	9	34	2	2
Muffin (Oat Bran Apple Raisin), 1 piece	296	10	46	2	6
Muffin (Oat Bran), 1 piece	333	13	47	2	8
Muffin (Pumpkin Raisin), 1 piece	259	8	44	2	5
Muffin (Strawberry Créme), 1 piece	273	9	43	1	5
Muffin (Strawberry Filled), 1 piece	280	9	45	1	5
Pastry Bite, 1 piece	114	7	11	0	1
Raisin Bread, 1 slice	71	1	14	1	2
Roll (Kaiser), 1 piece	179	3	32	1	6
Rye Bread, 1 slice	83	1	15	2	3
SnoTop, 1 piece	111	4	16	1	2
Sourdough Bread, 1 slice	68	1	13	1	2
Sticky Loaf, 1 piece	293	13	40	1	5
Toast (Buttered), 1 slice	262	14	30	1	5
Toast (Dry), 1 slice	134	2	25	1	4
Toast (Raisin, Buttered), 1 slice	244	14	27	2	4
Toast (Rye, Buttered), 1 slice	267	14	31	4	6
Toast (Sourdough, Buttered), 1 slice	237	13	25	1	5
Toast (Whole Wheat, Buttered), 1 slice	259	14	30	4	6
White Bread, 1 slice	67	1	12	1	2
Whole Wheat, 1 slice	79	1	15	2	3
Yellow Bread, 1 slice	114	2	21	1	3
Breakfast					
• Bacon, 1 slice	37	3	0	0	2
Bacon, 2 Slices	73	6	0	0	4
Bacon, 3 Slices	111	9	0	0	6
Banana Foster French Toast, 1	598	18	96	5	15
Cereal (with Milk)	363	5	82	13	13
Cornbeef Hash, 7 1/2 oz.	341	23	16	1	16
Eat'n Smart Smile	230	3	32	5	22
Egg Beaters	76	0	6	2	13
Eggs (2 Poached w/toast & Promise®)	352	20	26	1	17
Eggs Benedict	590	34	37	2	28
Eggs, 1 Fried	102	8	1	0	6

RESTAURANTS & FAST-FOOD CHAINS

Eat N' Park (cont.)

	Cal	Fat	Cbs	Fbr	Prtn
Breakfast (cont.)					
Eggs, 1 Poached	77	5	1	0	6
French Toast	128	5	14	1	7
Fruit Cup	60	0	15	1	1
Ham, 3 oz.	110	4	1	0	16
Hash Browns, 6 oz.	237	12	28	3	5
Homefries, 6 oz.	208	12	24	2	2
Oatmeal (Plain)	154	3	27	4	6
Oatmeal (with Bananas)	317	6	58	7	12
Oatmeal (with Fruit)	424	10	68	7	19
Oatmeal (with Milk)	224	5	34	5	11
Omelette (Bacon and Cheese)	500	39	2	0	33
Omelette (Cheese)	390	30	2	0	27
Omelette (Ham and Cheese)	463	32	3	63	38
Omelette (Meat Lovers)	716	55	4	0	49
Omelette (Supreme)	418	30	9	2	28
Omelette (Western)	344	21	7	1	30
Pancake (Blueberry), 1 pancake	286	4	55	2	7
Pancake, 1 pancake	223	3	43	2	6
Sausage, 1 link	132	12	0	0	5
Scrambler	619	29	55	2	34
• Strawberry Waffle, 1 waffle	724	29	100	3	16
Waffles (Belgian), 1 waffle	623	32	69	2	16
Burgers					
American Grill Burger, 6 oz.	617	37	32	3	38
Bacon Cheeseburger	591	31	33	2	42
BBQ Bacon Cheddar Burger, 6 oz.	886	55	53	2	45
• Black Angus Superburger®	1086	73	28	2	75
Cheeseburger, 6 oz.	522	26	33	2	37
• Classic Gardenburger	250	6	41	5	10
Hamburger, 6 oz.	477	22	32	2	34
Mushroom and Onion Burger	706	40	45	2	40
Original Superburger®	707	49	38	3	28
Condiments					
Butter (Whipped Blend)	96	11	0	0	0
Butter, 5 g	36	4	0	0	0
Cheese (Cream)	99	10	1	0	2
• Cheese (Mozzarella)	226	17	2	0	15
Honey	43	0	12	0	0
Honey Mustard	81	6	7	0	1
Jelly	34	0	9	0	0
Ketchup	23	0	6	0	0
• Lettuce (Leaf)	1	0	0	0	0
Lettuce (Shredded)	3	0	1	0	0
Margarine (Promise®)	32	4	0	0	0
Mayonnaise, 3/4 oz.	201	22	1	0	0
Mustard, 3/4 oz.	23	1	2	1	1
Onions (Grilled), 1 oz.	21	1	2	1	0
Onions (Raw)	11	0	2	1	0
Pickle Chips, 3 chips	3	0	1	0	0
Pickle Spear	4	0	1	0	0
Relish, 3/4 oz.	40	0	11	0	0
Salsa, 2 oz.	14	0	3	1	1
Sauce (BBQ), 2 oz.	84	0	22	0	0

Eat N' Park (cont.)	Cal	Fat	Cbs	Fbr	Prtn
Condiments (cont.)					
Sauce (Cheese), 2 oz.	151	12	4	0	7
Sauce (Chipotle BBQ), 2 oz.	170	1	41	1	1
Sauce (Cocktail), 2 oz.	71	0	19	1	1
Sauce (Lite Soy), 1 tbsp.	8	0	1	0	1
Sauce (Supreme), 2 oz.	151	16	2	0	0
Sauce (Sweet'n Sour), 2 oz.	81	2	16	1	0
Sauce (Teriyaki), 2 tbsp.	15	0	3	0	1
Sour Cream, 2 oz.	40	2	4	0	2
Syrup (Maple), 2 oz.	221	0	60	0	0
Syrup (Reduced Maple), 2 oz.	34	0	9	1	0
Syrup (Sugar-Free), 2 oz.	43	0	11	1	0
Tomatoes, 2 slices	6	0	1	0	0
Tomatoes, 2 wedges	5	0	1	0	0
Desserts					
Cheesecake (with Strawberries), 1 piece	751	36	105	1	8
Cheesecake, 1 piece	507	36	40	0	8
Dulce de Leche Cheesecake, 1 piece	720	49	64	1	10
Grilled Stickies à la Mode Loaf, 1 piece	487	28	53	2	6
Grilled Stickies à la Mode, 1 piece	728	39	81	2	9
Ice Cream, 2 Scoops	285	16	33	0	5
NSA Lactose-Free Lo-Carb Vanilla Ice Cream, 4 oz.	130	8	15	3	3
Pie (Apple Cranberry), 1 slice	655	36	78	3	5
Pie (Apple), 1 slice	489	24	66	3	4
Pie (Apple, No Sugar Added), 1 slice	341	10	61	4	3
Pie (Banana Crème), 1 slice	439	22	55	1	6
Pie (Blackberry), 1 slice	510	23	73	5	4
Pie (Blueberry), 1 slice	439	23	55	3	4
Pie (Cherry), 1 slice	457	24	58	3	5
Pie (Chocolate Peanut Butter), 1 slice	566	39	49	2	9
Pie (Coconut Crème), 1 slice	480	26	55	1	7
Pie (Dutch Apple), 1 slice	528	26	73	3	4
Pie (Lemon Meringue), 1 slice	262	13	31	1	4
Pie (Orchard Fresh), 1 slice	500	24	67	2	4
Pie (Oreo Cream), 1 slice	495	28	60	2	5
Pie (Peach, No Sugar Added), 1 slice	298	10	50	2	3
Pie (Peachberry), 1 slice	389	19	52	4	4
Pie (Pecan), 1 slice	679	40	79	2	7
Pie (Pumpkin), 1 slice	395	19	49	3	8
Pie (Shell, Baked), 1 piece	195	14	16	1	2
Pie (Strawberry), 1 slice	360	18	49	5	3
Pumpkin Cranberry Cheesecake, 1 piece	450	24	53	2	7
• Sherbet (Plain), 1 piece	98	1	22	0	1
Sundae (Apple), 1 piece	569	21	96	2	6
Sundae (Apple, Junior), 1 piece	305	12	50	1	3
Sundae (Chocolate), 1 piece	525	22	85	2	7
Sundae (Chocolate, Junior), 1 piece	283	12	44	1	4
Sundae (Hot Fudge), 1 piece	625	31	85	2	9
Sundae (Hot Fudge, Junior), 1 piece	333	17	45	1	5
Sundae (Oreo), 1 piece	503	21	73	3	7
Sundae (Strawberry), 1 piece	606	21	106	2	6
• Sundae (Turtle), 1 piece	935	49	111	8	23
Dinners					
Baked Lemon Sole	282	17	11	1	21

RESTAURANTS & FAST-FOOD CHAINS

Eat N' Park (cont.)

	Cal	Fat	Cbs	Fbr	Prtn
Dinners (cont.)					
• Breaded Fish	926	45	56	2	69
Chargrilled Chicken, 10 oz.	350	9	0	0	62
Chargrilled Chicken, 5 oz.	175	5	0	0	31
Chesapeake Crab Stuffed Cod	286	9	20	1	30
Chicken Broccoli Alfredo	604	19	61	4	45
Chicken Fillets, 5	529	26	28	1	43
Chicken Parmigiana Marinara	842	33	90	6	47
Chicken Parmigiana Meat Sauce	898	38	86	5	52
Chicken Stir-Fry	554	25	47	8	38
Ground Sirloin	422	25	0	0	45
Liver	283	12	12	1	32
Nantucket Cod	290	17	7	1	27
Pork Chops (Sesame)	320	18	2	0	34
Rosemary Chicken, 10 oz.	370	10	2	1	67
Salisbury Steak	442	24	28	1	28
Salmon (Alaskan Stockeye)	287	15	0	0	36
Scrod (Baked), 8 oz.	434	25	6	0	44
• Scrod (Floridian), 4 oz.	120	2	4	0	22
Scrod (Floridian), 8 oz.	240	3	8	6	44
Scrod (Maryland)	445	32	11	1	29
Spaghetti (Marinara)	621	8	120	7	19
Spaghetti (Meat Sauce)	820	19	140	8	26
T-Bone	568	39	1	1	50
Turkey	433	18	31	1	34
Dressing					
Bleu Cheese, 2 tbsp.	92	7	7	0	1
• Caesar, 2 tbsp.	245	25	8	0	0
French Fat-Free, 2 tbsp.	70	0	17	0	0
Fruit Salad, 2 tbsp.	143	14	5	0	0
House, 2 tbsp.	115	11	2	0	1
• Italian Fat-Free, 2 tbsp.	12	0	3	0	0
Italian, 2 tbsp.	122	12	4	0	0
Poppyseed, 2 tbsp.	240	16	24	0	0
Thousand Island, 2 tbsp.	95	9	3	0	0
Kids Menu					
Burger	285	15	21	1	16
• Cereal (Milk)	615	16	115	15	15
Cheeseburger	365	21	22	1	21
Chicken (Fillet)	317	16	17	1	26
Fish Plank	315	15	20	1	24
French Toast (Bacon)	355	16	35	1	17
French Toast (Sausage)	546	34	35	1	23
Giggle (Bacon)	380	27	20	1	13
Giggle (Sausage)	571	45	20	1	20
Grilled Cheese	524	39	21	1	22
Hot Dog	361	24	24	1	12
• Macaroni & Cheese	171	3	31	1	6
Peanut Butter & Jelly Sandwich	439	20	55	4	14
Pizza	413	13	49	2	15
Spaghetti	355	5	69	4	10
Salads					
• Buffalo Chicken	606	42	42	7	34
Chicken and Strawberry	216	6	13	6	29

▶ Eat N' Park (cont.)	Cal	Fat	Cbs	Fbr	Prtn
Salads (cont.)					
Chicken Portabella	320	11	23	5	34
Fruit with Sherbet	308	3	73	7	5
• Garden	95	3	16	4	3
Grilled Chicken	439	19	30	5	37
Napa Valley	504	25	18	8	47
Spinach and Chicken	376	17	9	3	47
Sandwiches					
Buffalo Chicken Sandwich	786	41	71	5	36
Chicken (Chargrilled), 5 oz.	350	7	39	4	33
Chicken (Fiesta), 5 oz.	430	13	41	3	37
Chicken Portabella Hoagie	836	55	46	3	40
Croissant (Tuna)	582	39	35	2	24
Grilled Cheese	507	36	26	1	21
• Hot Turkey	260	5	27	1	24
Pot Roast Melt	972	53	66	4	54
Reuben	720	49	31	4	38
Santa Fe Turkey and Bacon	854	60	44	2	37
Shredded Pot Roast	532	30	28	1	35
• Steak and Cheese	1011	71	38	2	53
Turkey Club	769	44	49	3	40
Whale of a Cod Sandwich	866	40	76	3	49
Seniors					
Baked Lemon Sole	141	9	6	1	11
• Banana Foster French Toast	495	15	82	4	10
Breaded Fish, 4 oz.	463	23	28	1	35
Chargrilled Chicken, 5 oz.	175	5	0	0	31
Chicken Fillet, 4 Pieces	423	21	22	1	34
French Toast	399	12	79	0	1
Hot Turkey Sandwich	175	5	18	1	15
Pork Chop (Sesame), 4 oz.	160	9	1	0	16
Pot Roast Sandwich	262	15	13	1	18
Rosemary Chicken, 5 oz.	196	6	2	1	33
Scrod (Baked), 4 oz.	330	24	6	0	22
• Scrod (Floridian), 4 oz.	119	2	4	0	22
Spaghetti (Marinara)	311	4	60	4	10
Spaghetti (Meat Sauce)	410	9	70	4	13
Sides					
Applesauce	108	0	28	2	0
Banana (Medium)	109	1	28	3	1
Bean Soup, 1 cup	145	4	18	4	10
Beef Noodle Soup, 1 cup	111	5	11	1	5
Broccoli (Steamed)	40	1	8	4	3
Broccoli Soup, 1 cup	197	11	22	1	4
Buttered Noodles	247	14	26	1	6
Cheese Soup, 1 cup	215	11	27	0	3
Chicken Noodle Soup, 1 cup	130	5	16	1	6
Chicken Rice Soup, 1 cup	76	1	11	1	4
Chili, 1 cup	132	5	13	4	9
Clam Chowder, 1 cup	159	8	19	0	3
Coleslaw	200	18	10	2	2
Cottage Cheese	114	2	5	0	18
• French Fries	347	18	44	4	4
• Gravy (Beef)	21	0	3	0	1

RESTAURANTS & FAST-FOOD CHAINS

Eat N' Park (cont.)

Sides (cont.)	Cal	Fat	Cbs	Fbr	Prtn
Gravy (Turkey)	32	1	3	0	2
Harvest Grain Soup, 1 cup	225	9	35	5	6
Minestrone Soup, 1 cup	85	2	15	2	4
Mushroom Barley Soup, 1 cup	69	1	13	3	3
Onion Rings, 10 pcs.	105	6	10	1	2
Potato (Baked)	190	0	44	3	4
Potato (Scalloped)	230	8	34	2	6
Potato (Whipped)	280	23	17	1	3
Potato Soup, 1 cup	214	10	32	1	2
Rice (Mexican)	111	2	22	1	3
Rice (White)	148	2	28	0	3
Rice Pilaf	137	4	23	1	4
Rice Pudding	163	2	31	0	5
Strawberries, Fresh Cup	51	1	12	4	1
Sugar Snap Peas	29	0	7	3	2
Vegetable Beef Barley Soup, 1 cup	103	3	13	3	6
Vegetarian Pasta Soup, 1 cup	44	1	9	1	1
Wedding Soup, 1 cup	110	3	12	1	5

Edo Japan

Bento Boxes	Cal	Fat	Cbs	Fbr	Prtn
Beef Yakisoba Bento, 575 g	830	30	102	3	43
Chicken and Beef Bento, 566 g	880	26	120	4	40
• Chicken Yakisoba Bento, 582 g	800	25	102	3	45
Seafood Grill Bento, 652 g	860	16	129	4	37
Sizzling Shrimp Bento, 625 g	800	16	122	4	40
• Sukiyaki Beef Bento, 571 g	900	28	120	4	39
Teriyaki Chicken Bento, 578 g	870	24	120	4	41
Edo Extras					
6 Extra Shrimp, 65 g	80	3	2	0	11
California Roll, 216 g	430	17	61	1	9
Extra Beef, 132 g	260	15	3	0	24
Extra Chicken, 139 g	220	11	3	0	26
• Rice Side Dish, 297 g	480	1	106	1	9
• Teriyaki Sauce, 60 ml	45	0	11	0	1
Tofu, 106 g	90	5	5	1	8
Vegetable Spring Roll, 45 g	120	6	14	2	3
Yakisoba Side Dish, 340 g	430	4	89	0	17
Teriyaki Dishes					
• Beef and Shrimp, 486 g	690	19	82	3	43
Beef Yakisoba, 425 g	540	18	62	2	36
Chicken and Beef, 416 g	590	14	80	3	32
Chicken and Shrimp, 493 g	660	15	82	3	45
Chicken Yakisoba, 432 g	510	14	62	2	37
• Curry Chicken Bowl, 375 g	500	21	27	3	17
Fresh Grilled Vegetables, 342 g	380	1	81	4	10
Ginger Pork, 414 g	650	23	82	3	26
Hawaiian Chicken, 440 g	590	12	85	3	33
Seafood Grill, 502 g	570	4	89	3	30
Sizzling Shrimp, 475 g	510	5	82	3	32
Sukiyaki Beef, 421 g	610	16	80	3	32
Teriyaki Chicken, 428 g	580	12	80	3	33
Tropical Teriyaki, 505 g	670	15	87	3	44

RESTAURANTS & FAST-FOOD CHAINS

Edo Japan (cont.)

	Cal	Fat	Cbs	Fbr	Prtn
Udon Soup					
• Beef Udon, 947 g	580	17	72	7	34
Chicken Udon, 953 g	550	13	72	7	36
Shrimp Udon, 964 g	480	5	74	8	34
• Vegetable Udon, 909 g	370	2	77	9	13

Einstein Bros. Bagels

	Cal	Fat	Cbs	Fbr	Prtn
Bagel Pretzels					
Asiago Cheese Bagel Pretzel, 116 g	300	5	57	2	12
• Cinnamon Sugar Bagel Pretzel, 123 g	330	3	71	3	9
• Plain Bagel Pretzel, 109 g	270	3	57	2	9
Salt Bagel Pretzel, 112 g	270	3	57	2	9
Bagel Dogs					
Add Cheddar Cheese, 8 oz.	660	32	64	2	30
• Add Cheddar Cheese, 8 oz.	670	33	64	2	32
Original Asiago Bagel Dog, 7 oz.	590	26	64	2	27
• Original Bagel Dog, 7 oz.	570	25	64	2	25
Bagels					
Asiago Cheese Bagel, 120 g	320	5	58	2	15
Blueberry Bagel, 115 g	290	2	64	3	9
Chocolate Chip Bagel, 113 g	290	3	60	3	10
Cinnamon Raisin Swirl Bagel, 115 g	290	1	64	3	10
Cinnamon Sugar, Chicago Style, 117 g	310	3	66	3	9
Cranberry Bagel, 115 g	290	1	64	3	9
Egg Bagel, 108 g	300	6	52	2	12
Everything Bagel, 112 g	290	2	60	2	10
Garlic Dip'd Bagel, 112 g	280	1	60	2	9
Good Grains Bagel, 112 g	290	3	62	4	10
Honey Whole Wheat Bagel, 108 g	270	1	61	3	9
Onion Bagel, 108 g	270	2	59	2	9
Onion Dip'd Bagel, 112 g	290	1	63	2	9
Plain Bagel, 108 g	270	1	59	2	9
Poppy Dip'd Bagel, 112 g	290	3	60	2	10
• Potato Bagel, 107 g	260	1	58	2	9
• Power Bagel, Fruit & Nut, 120 g	380	6	72	5	13
Pumpernickel Bagel, 108 g	270	2	58	3	10
Sesame Dip'd Bagel, 110 g	310	3	62	2	11
Sundried Tomato Bagel, 108 g	270	2	58	3	10
Bread, Specialty					
Braided Challah Roll, 78 g	220	4	41	1	8
• Ciabatta Bread, 113 g	290	3	60	2	10
• Multi Grain Bread, 49 g	130	3	23	2	5
Breakfast Sandwiches					
• Bacon & Spinach Panini, 13 oz.	860	49	69	7	40
Egg Way with Bacon, 10 oz.	610	25	63	3	35
Egg Way with Black Forest Ham, 11 oz.	580	21	63	2	39
Egg Way with Sausage, 11 oz.	610	24	64	2	38
Egg Way, Original, 9 oz.	540	20	63	3	30
• Egg Way, Spinach, Mshrm & Swiss, 11 oz.	540	20	65	3	29
Sausage Ranchero Panini, 12 oz.	690	28	65	5	44
Vegetable Breakfast Panini, 15 oz.	730	35	70	4	37
Breakfast Wraps					
• Sante Fe, 13 oz.	720	37	59	6	38
• Spicy Elmo, 12 oz.	730	41	56	6	36

RESTAURANTS & FAST-FOOD CHAINS

Einstein Bros. Bagels (cont.)

	Cal	Fat	Cbs	Fbr	Prtn
Coffee Extras					
Half & Half, 1 fl.oz.	40	3	1	N/A	1
Light Whipped Cream, 30 ml	35	3	2	0	0
On Top Reduced Fat Topping, 8 g	20	2	2	0	0
Skim Milk, 8 fl.oz.	80	0	15	0	7
Syrup, Blackberry, 30 ml	100	0	25	0	0
Syrup, Caramel, 1 fl.oz.	100	0	25	0	0
Syrup, Cherry, 30 ml	100	0	25	0	0
Syrup, Chocolate, 30 ml	0	0	4	0	0
Syrup, Hazelnut, 1 fl.oz.	100	0	25	0	0
Syrup, Vanilla, 1 fl.oz.	100	0	25	0	0
• Syrup, Vanilla, Sugar Free, 1 fl.oz.	0	0	4	0	0
Whole Milk, 8 fl.oz.	150	8	11	0	8
Coffee, Specialty (Medium)					
• Americano Regular, 8 fl.oz.	1	0	0	0	0
Cafe Latte Nonfat, 16 fl.oz.	140	1	20	0	14
Café Latte Whole milk, 16 fl.oz.	250	12	21	0	12
Café Latte, 16 fl.oz.	200	8	20	0	13
Cappuccino Nonfat Milk, 15 fl.oz.	130	1	19	0	13
Cappuccino Whole Milk, 16 fl.oz.	190	9	17	0	9
Cappuccino, 16 fl.oz.	190	7	19	0	12
Espresso, Regular, 2 fl.oz.	1	0	0	0	0
Low Fat Mocha, 15 fl.oz.	350	15	42	1	10
• Mocha Whole Milk, 16 fl.oz.	400	10	67	1	10
Mocha, 15 fl.oz.	390	20	42	1	9
Condiments & Spreads					
Ancho Lime Salsa, 1 oz.	10	1	1	0	0
Ancho Mayo, 16 g	50	5	1	0	0
Creamy Mustard Spread, 2 oz.	270	29	1	0	0
Deli Mustard, 5 g	5	0	0	0	0
Feta Pinenut Spread, 1 oz.	70	5	2	0	4
Honey Butter, 28 g	170	18	0	0	0
Hummus, 2 oz.	110	7	9	2	3
• Peanut Butter, Creamy, 2 oz.	330	28	12	4	14
Roasted Garlic Horseradish Spread, 28 g	15	0	4	1	0
Spicy Roasted Tomato Spread, 30 g	140	14	3	1	0
Whole Kosher Pickle, 50 g	5	0	1	1	0
• Yellow Mustard, 5 g	0	0	0	0	0
Cream Cheese					
Whipped Garden Vegetable Red. Fat, 20 g	60	5	3	0	1
Whipped Garlic Herb Reduced Fat, 20 g	60	5	3	0	1
Whipped Honey Almond Red. Fat, 20 g	70	5	6	0	1
Whipped Jalapeño Salsa Reduced Fat, 20 g	60	5	3	0	1
Whipped Onion and Chive, 20 g	70	6	3	0	1
• Whipped Plain Reduced Fat, 20 g	60	5	2	0	1
• Whipped Plain, 20 g	70	7	1	0	1
Whipped Smoked Salmon, 20 g	60	6	2	0	1
Whipped Strawberry Reduced Fat, 20 g	70	5	5	0	1
Deli Melts					
Ham Deli Melt, 10 oz.	540	18	62	3	38
Pastrami Deli Melt, 10 oz.	560	19	64	3	40
Tuna Salad Deli Melt, 11 oz.	610	25	64	3	40
• Turkey Deli Melt, 10 oz.	530	17	62	3	40
• Veggie Deli Melt, 13 oz.	660	30	76	5	25

RESTAURANTS & FAST-FOOD CHAINS

Einstein Bros. Bagels (cont.)	Cal	Fat	Cbs	Fbr	Prtn
Deli Sandwiches					
Deli Bacon, 9 oz.	830	52	52	4	39
• Deli Chicken Salad, 10 oz.	970	79	51	4	16
Deli Ham, 11 oz.	590	32	45	2	32
Deli Pastrami, 11 oz.	650	34	53	5	36
• Deli Tuna Salad, 10 oz.	440	15	50	4	29
Deli Turkey & Swiss, 11 oz.	700	42	49	4	37
Frozen Blended Drinks					
Wildberry, 18 fl.oz.	270	0	63	5	4
Gourmet Bagels					
Dutch Apple Bagel, 142 g	350	4	71	3	9
• Green Chile Bagel, 163 g	370	9	60	2	16
• Six-Cheese Bagel, 127 g	340	6	58	2	15
Spinach Florentine Bagel, 141 g	360	9	59	3	16
Iced Specialty Coffee					
Iced Latte, 16 fl.oz.	120	5	12	0	8
Iced Mocha, 16 fl.oz.	210	6	33	0	7
• Iced Non Fat Latte, 16 fl.oz.	90	0	12	0	8
Low Fat Iced Mocha, 16 fl.oz.	180	5	32	0	7
Low Fat Mocha, 12 fl.oz.	190	3	34	0	8
Whole Milk Iced Latte, 16 fl.oz.	190	9	17	0	9
• Whole Milk Iced Mocha, 16 fl.oz.	390	9	66	0	9
Other Hot Beverages (Medium)					
Chai Tea Latte 2% Milk, 16 fl.oz.	290	3	63	0	4
• Chai Tea Latte Skim Milk, 16 fl.oz.	270	0	63	0	4
• Chai Tea Latte Whole Milk, 16 fl.oz.	310	4	63	0	4
Hot Chocolate, 12 fl.oz.	290	11	39	0	9
• Hot Chocolate, Whole Milk, 12 fl.oz.	320	14	39	0	9
Pizza Bagels					
Andouille Sausage, 7 oz.	480	14	66	2	25
• Cheese, 6 oz.	440	11	66	2	23
Cheesy Garlic & Herb, 6 oz.	520	18	68	2	24
Pepperoni, 7 oz.	480	15	66	2	25
• Spinach and Mushroom, 10 oz.	620	26	73	4	27
Salad Dressings					
Caesar Dressing, 30 g	150	16	1	0	1
• Chile Lime Dressing, 32 g	60	4	5	0	1
• Raspberry Vinaigrette Dressing, 32 g	160	14	8	0	0
Salads (and Half Salads)					
• Bros Bistro Salad with Chicken, 15 oz.	960	72	39	7	39
Bros Bistro Salad, 11 oz.	820	68	38	7	14
Chicken Chipotle Salad, 14 oz.	670	41	53	10	25
Chipotle Salad, 12 oz.	600	39	53	10	13
Half Bros Bistro Salad with Chicken, 7 oz.	480	36	19	3	19
Half Bros Bistro Salad, 5 oz.	410	34	19	3	7
Half Caesar Salad with Chicken, 7 oz.	340	27	9	2	18
• Half Caesar Salad, 5 oz.	270	25	8	2	6
Half Chicken Chipotle Salad, 8 oz.	370	22	27	5	19
Half Chipotle Salad, 6 oz.	300	19	26	5	7
Sandwich Fillings					
Cheese Provolone, 1 oz.	80	6	0	0	5
Cheese, American, 1 oz.	80	6	1	0	4
Cheese, Gorgonzola, 1 oz.	100	9	0	0	7
Cheese, Medium Cheddar, 1 oz.	90	7	0	0	7

(• = most healthy • = least healthy) **RESTAURANTS & FAST-FOOD • 169**

RESTAURANTS & FAST-FOOD CHAINS

Einstein Bros. Bagels (cont.)

	Cal	Fat	Cbs	Fbr	Prtn
Sandwich Fillings (cont.)					
Cheese, Monterey Jack w/ Jalapeños, 1 oz.	80	6	1	0	5
Cheese, Monterey Jack, 1 oz.	80	6	0	0	5
Cheese, Swiss, 1 oz.	80	7	0	0	6
Chicken Breast, 4 oz.	140	5	1	0	24
• Chicken Salad, 4 oz.	700	74	2	0	5
Cold Smoked Salmon, 2 oz.	80	5	0	0	12
Ham, 3 oz.	100	4	0	0	16
Pastrami, 3 oz.	120	4	2	0	18
Thick Cut Bacon, 0.5 oz.	70	5	1	0	5
Tuna Salad, 4 oz.	170	10	2	1	18
• Turkey Sausage, 1 oz.	70	4	1	0	8
Sandwiches, Panini					
• Italian Chicken Panini, 13 oz.	830	42	67	5	50
• Turkey Club Panini, 14 oz.	790	39	68	7	47
Sides					
Bagel Croutons, 1 oz.	100	4	16	1	2
Fruit and Yogurt Parfait, 12 oz.	180	1	36	4	9
Fruit Salad, 11 oz.	140	0	36	3	2
• Kettle Classic Natural Potato Chips, 1 oz.	100	10	11	1	1
• Traditional Potato Salad, 140 g	355	29	20	2	3
Soups					
• Chicken Noodle (Cup), 9 oz.	120	4	14	1	5
Corn Crab Chowder (Cup), 9 oz.	280	18	18	1	8
Seafood Minestrone (Cup), 9 oz.	130	5	16	2	8
Turkey Chili (Cup), 9 oz.	220	7	24	5	20
• Vegetarian Broccoli Cheese (Cup), 9 oz.	290	20	16	2	14
Specialty Sandwiches					
Club Mex on Challah, 11 oz.	600	30	48	2	38
Grilled Chicken, Bacon and Swiss, 11 oz.	770	48	45	2	41
Lox & Bagel, 10 oz.	520	21	6	3	24
• Rachel (Overstuffed Size), 14 oz.	1050	71	53	2	55
Rachel (Regular Size), 10 oz.	930	66	51	2	37
Reuben (Overstuffed Size), 14 oz.	800	44	49	3	55
Reuben (Regular Size), 10 oz.	670	40	47	3	37
Roasted Turkey and Swiss, 11 oz.	700	42	49	4	37
Tasty Turkey on Asiago Bagel, 13 oz.	570	20	68	3	38
Turkey Rachel (Overstuffed Size), 14 oz.	970	65	50	1	59
Turkey Rachel (Regular Size), 10 oz.	890	64	50	1	39
Turkey Reuben (Overstuffed Size), 14 oz.	720	39	45	3	59
Turkey Reuben (Regular Size), 10 oz.	630	37	45	3	39
• Veg Out on Sesame Seed Bagel, 10 oz.	450	14	70	4	17
Sweets					
Apple Cinnamon Coffee Cake, 7 oz.	700	28	108	1	5
Blueberry Muffin, 5 oz.	480	22	65	2	6
Chocolate Chip Coffee Cake, 6 oz.	760	34	110	2	6
Chocolate Mudslide Cookie, 3 oz.	320	17	46	1	4
Cinnamon Stix, 4 oz.	370	21	41	2	5
Cinnamon Walnut Strudel, 5 oz.	630	42	56	4	9
English Toffee Snickerdoodle Cookie, 3 oz.	420	18	59	1	3
Fudge Brownie, 4 oz.	510	25	74	2	6
Heavenly Chocolate Chunk Cookie, 3 oz.	360	18	48	2	4
Iced Chocolate Hazelnut Croissant, 3 oz.	430	21	49	3	9
Iced Lemon Croissant, 3 oz.	371	17	46	2	8

RESTAURANTS & FAST-FOOD CHAINS

Einstein Bros. Bagels (cont.)

	Cal	Fat	Cbs	Fbr	Prtn
Sweets (cont.)					
Iced Sugar Cookie, 3 oz.	460	15	76	1	4
Lemon Pound Cake, 5 oz.	440	16	69	1	7
• Marshmallow Crispy Treat, 2 oz.	220	4	48	0	3
• Mixed Berry Coffee Cake, 7 oz.	710	29	109	2	5
Oatmeal Raisin Cookie, 3 oz.	320	11	54	2	5
Strawberry White Chocolate Muffin, 6 oz.	550	25	78	1	7
Wraps					
• California Chicken Wrap, 13 oz.	630	29	63	8	32
• Chipotle Turkey Wrap, 13 oz.	740	37	70	9	36

El Pollo Loco

	Cal	Fat	Cbs	Fbr	Prtn
Bowls & Salads					
Caesar Bowl, 12 oz.	520	25	45	4	28
Caesar Pollo Salad, 11 oz.	520	38	17	4	27
Caesar Pollo Salad, w/o dressing, 9 oz.	220	7	15	4	25
Chicken Tostada without Shell, 15 oz.	410	11	42	5	33
Chicken Tostada, 17 oz.	840	40	76	7	40
Garden Salad, 5 oz.	120	7	9	2	5
Loco Salad with Creamy Cilantro Dressing, 3 oz.	170	14	7	1	3
The Original Pollo Bowl®, 18 oz.	540	4	85	11	37
• Ultimate Pollo Bowl®, 24 oz.	880	26	90	12	67
Burritos					
BRC Burrito, 8 oz.	390	10	61	6	14
Classic Chicken Burrito®, 10 oz.	500	14	63	6	30
Pollo Asado Burrito, 12 oz.	600	23	58	5	41
• Twice Grilled Burrito™, 15 oz.	830	37	58	5	66
Ultimate Grilled Burrito, 14 oz.	650	20	80	8	38
Desserts					
Caramel Flan, 6 oz.	290	12	41	0	5
Churros, 2 each	300	18	32	2	3
• Vanilla Kid Cone, 1 each	200	5	33	0	5
• Vanilla Large Cone, 1 each	510	14	84	0	14
Vanilla Regular Cone, 1 each	330	8	55	0	8
Vanilla Soft Serve - cup, 5 oz.	300	8	48	0	8
Dining					
BRC Burrito, 8 oz.	390	10	61	6	14
Caesar Pollo Salad w/o dressing, 9 oz.	220	7	15	4	25
Chicken Breast, Skinless, 4 oz.	180	4	0	0	35
Chicken Tortilla Soup (w/o Tortilla Strips), 10 oz.	140	6	8	2	15
Chicken Tortilla Soup, 11 oz.	210	9	18	2	16
Chicken Tostada w/o Shell, 15 oz.	410	11	42	5	33
• Fresh Vegetables (w/o margarine), 4 oz.	35	0	8	3	2
Garden Salad (w/o Tortilla Strips), 5 oz.	80	5	5	1	5
Garden Salad, 5 oz.	120	7	9	2	5
Pinto Beans, 6 oz.	140	0	25	7	9
Skinless Breast Meal, 12 oz.	310	12	17	5	35
Skinless Breast Meal, Special Request, 12 oz.	270	10	12	5	34
Spanish Rice, 5 oz.	160	1	34	1	3
Taco al Carbon, 3 oz.	150	5	17	1	11
• The Original Pollo Bowl®, 18 oz.	540	4	85	11	37
Dressings					
Creamy Cilantro, 2 oz.	220	23	1	0	1
Light Creamy Cilantro, 1 pkt.	70	5	6	0	1

(•= most healthy •= least healthy) **RESTAURANTS & FAST-FOOD • 171**

RESTAURANTS & FAST-FOOD CHAINS

El Pollo Loco (cont.)

	Cal	Fat	Cbs	Fbr	Prtn
Dressings (cont.)					
• Light Italian, 1 pkt.	20	1	2	0	0
• Ranch, 1 pkt.	230	24	2	0	1
Thousand Island, 1 pkt.	220	21	6	0	0
Flame Grilled Chicken					
• Chicken Breast, 4 oz.	220	9	0	0	36
Chicken Breast, Skinless, 4 oz.	180	4	0	0	35
Chopped Breast Meat, 3 oz.	100	2	0	0	21
• Leg, 2 oz.	90	4	0	0	12
Thigh, 3 oz.	220	15	0	0	21
Wing, 1 oz.	90	5	0	0	11
Kids Meal					
BBQ Sauce, 1 oz.	44	0	11	0	1
• Cheese Quesadilla, 5 oz.	420	23	35	2	19
French Fries - Kid Size, 3 oz.	240	11	31	3	3
• Leg, 2 oz.	90	4	0	0	12
Popcorn Chicken, 3 oz.	200	12	10	3	14
Loco Value Menu					
BRC Burrito, 8 oz.	390	10	61	6	14
• Cheese Quesadilla, 5 oz.	420	23	35	2	19
Chicken Taquito, 1 each	190	9	18	1	10
• Leg, 2 oz.	90	4	0	0	12
Loco Nachos, 3 oz.	310	18	31	3	6
Loco Salad w/ Creamy Cilantro Dressing, 3 oz.	170	14	7	1	3
Taco al Carbon, 3 oz.	150	5	17	1	11
Two Churros, 2 each	300	18	32	2	3
Mexican Favorites					
Chicken Soft Taco, 5 oz.	270	13	19	2	17
Chicken Tortilla Soup (with Tortilla Strips), 11 oz.	210	9	18	2	16
Chicken Verde Quesadilla, 9 oz.	590	27	53	4	40
• Crunchy Chicken Taco, 3 oz.	190	8	16	2	12
• Grilled Chicken Nachos, 17 oz.	1090	55	99	14	47
Salsas & More					
Avocado Salsa (Hot), 1 oz.	30	3	1	1	0
Chipotle Salsa (Hot), 1 oz.	5	0	1	0	0
Fried Serrano Pepper, 0 oz.	15	2	0	0	0
Guacamole, 1 oz.	45	4	4	1	1
• House Salsa (Mild), 1 oz.	5	0	1	0	0
• Jack & Poblano Queso, 2 oz.	100	8	4	0	3
Jalapeño Hot Sauce (Packet), 0 oz.	5	0	1	0	0
Ketchup (Packet), 0 oz.	10	0	2	0	0
Pico de Gallo (Medium), 1 oz.	10	1	1	0	0
Sour Cream, 1 oz.	60	5	1	0	1
Sides					
BBQ Black Beans, 6 oz.	200	3	36	4	7
Cole Slaw, 6 oz.	120	9	8	2	1
Corn Cobbette, 5 oz.	90	1	19	2	2
• French Fries, 6 oz.	440	21	57	6	6
• Fresh Vegetables (w/o margarine), 4 oz.	35	0	8	3	2
Fresh Vegetables (with margarine), 4 oz.	60	3	8	3	2
Garden Salad, 5 oz.	120	7	9	2	5
Gravy, 1 oz.	10	0	2	0	0
Macaroni & Cheese, 6 oz.	280	17	28	0	11
Mashed Potatoes, 5 oz.	100	1	20	2	2

RESTAURANTS & FAST-FOOD CHAINS

El Pollo Loco (cont.)

	Cal	Fat	Cbs	Fbr	Prtn
Sides (cont.)					
Pinto Beans, 6 oz.	140	0	25	7	9
Refried Beans (with Cheese), 6 oz.	270	7	36	10	14
Spanish Rice, 5 oz.	160	1	34	1	3
Tortillas & Chips					
6.5" Flour Tortillas, 2 each	210	7	30	2	5
• 6" Corn Tortillas, 2 each	120	2	24	2	2
• Tortilla Chips, 2 oz.	210	10	28	3	3

Famous Dave's

	Cal	Fat	Cbs	Fbr	Prtn
Entrees					
Char-Grilled Chicken Sandwich	510	10	53	3	54
• Dave's Sassy BBQ Chicken Salad	540	25	50	4	33
Georgia Chopped Pork Sandwich	510	15	62	3	37
• Sweet and Sassy Grilled Salmon Platter	450	26	11	1	43
Side Dish					
Drunkin' Apples, 4 oz.	140	5	26	2	1
• Firecracker Green Beans, 6 oz.	60	3	7	3	4
• Wilbur Beans, 4 oz.	150	4	26	4	8

Fatburger

	Cal	Fat	Cbs	Fbr	Prtn
Add-Ons					
American Cheese, 19 g	70	6	1	0	4
• Bacon, 15 g	70	6	0	0	4
Cheddar Cheese, 28 g	110	9	0	0	7
Chili Cup, 217 g	270	15	13	3	21
Fat Fries, 226 g	550	26	72	8	8
Homemade Onion Rings, 158 g	510	29	57	4	7
• Skinny Fries, 158 g	490	20	71	6	6
Shakes					
• Chocolate Shake, 495 g	880	38	120	4	14
• Strawberry Shake, 439 g	700	32	91	5	12
Vanilla Shake, 453 g	730	30	103	0	12
Signature Items					
Baby Fat, 155 g	300	15	24	0	18
• Fat Salad Wedge, 156 g	70	5	4	111	5
Fatburger, 255 g	520	29	32	7	30
Grilled Chicken Sandwich, 209 g	360	13	32	4	29
Hot Dog, 126 g	380	22	31	2	14
• Kingburger, 400 g	820	41	64	7	49
Sausage & Egg Sandwich, 155 g	620	44	33	3	23
Turkeyburger, 261 g	550	31	38	5	30
Veggieburger, 276 g	430	12	45	12	35

Fazoli's

	Cal	Fat	Cbs	Fbr	Prtn
Choose A Topping					
• Broccoli	25	0	5	3	3
Broccoli and Tomatoes	30	0	6	3	3
Garlic Shrimp	160	12	3	1	10
Italian Sausage	240	21	3	1	10
• Meatballs	250	18	6	1	13
Peppery Chicken	70	1	1	0	14
Desserts					
• Chocolate Chunk Cookie	510	26	68	3	5

(•= most healthy •= least healthy) **RESTAURANTS & FAST-FOOD • 173**

RESTAURANTS & FAST-FOOD CHAINS

Fazoli's (cont.)

	Cal	Fat	Cbs	Fbr	Prtn
Desserts (cont.)					
• Original Cheesecake	290	22	17	0	6
Turtle Cheesecake	450	28	43	2	6
Drinks					
Lemon Ice - Peach	360	0	90	0	0
Lemon Ice - Pomegranate	360	0	90	0	0
Lemon Ice - Strawberry	320	0	81	0	0
• Lemon Ice - Triple Berry	360	0	91	0	0
• Original Lemon Ice - Regular	180	0	45	0	0
Extras					
Breadstick, Dry, 1 each	100	2	20	0	3
Garlic Breadstick, 1 each	150	7	20	1	3
Kids Meals					
Cheese Pizza	270	11	31	2	13
Fettuccine Alfredo	290	5	50	2	9
Meat Lasagna	260	13	21	2	14
Pepperoni Pizza	310	14	31	2	14
Ravioli with Marinara Sauce	290	7	43	3	13
Ravioli with Meat Sauce	300	8	42	3	15
Spaghetti with Marinara Sauce	270	2	53	4	9
Spaghetti with Meat Sauce	300	4	53	4	11
• Spaghetti with Meatballs	350	7	55	4	14
• Ziti with Meat Sauce	190	6	25	3	9
Oven-Baked Pastas					
Baked Spaghetti	680	22	90	7	32
Baked Spaghetti with Meatballs	940	40	100	9	46
Chicken Parmesan	960	33	117	9	56
Meat Lasagna	510	25	43	5	27
Rigatoni Romano	1090	54	101	11	51
Panini					
• Four Cheese & Tomato	510	22	53	3	28
Grilled Chicken	540	18	56	3	35
• Smoked Turkey	620	29	54	3	35
Pasta Bowls					
• Fettuccine with Alfredo - Regular	780	18	125	5	24
Fettuccine with Alfredo - Small	520	12	83	4	16
• Fettuccine with Marinara - Small	450	3	88	7	15
Fettuccine with Marinara- Regular	670	4	132	10	23
Fettuccine with Meat Sauce - Regular	750	10	131	10	29
Fettuccine with Meat Sauce - Small	500	7	87	7	20
Penne with Alfredo - Regular	780	18	125	5	24
Penne with Alfredo - Small	520	12	83	4	16
Penne with Marinara - Small	450	3	88	7	15
Penne with Marinara- Regular	670	4	132	10	23
Penne with Meat Sauce - Regular	750	10	131	10	29
Penne with Meat Sauce - Small	500	7	87	7	20
Ravioli with Marinara Sauce	500	15	71	7	22
Ravioli with Meat Sauce	550	20	71	7	26
Spaghetti with Alfredo - Regular	780	18	125	5	24
Spaghetti with Alfredo - Small	520	12	83	4	16
Spaghetti with Marinara - Small	450	3	88	7	15
Spaghetti with Marinara- Regular	670	4	132	10	23
Spaghetti with Meat Sauce - Regular	750	10	131	10	29
Spaghetti with Meat Sauce - Small	500	7	87	7	20

RESTAURANTS & FAST-FOOD CHAINS

Fazoli's (cont.)

Fazoli's (cont.)	Cal	Fat	Cbs	Fbr	Prtn
Pasta Bowls (cont.)					
Ziti with Meat Sauce - Regular	700	22	95	10	34
Ziti with Meat Sauce - Small	480	15	65	6	23
Pizza					
• Cheese, 1 slice	270	11	31	2	13
• Pepperoni, 1 slice	310	14	31	2	14
Salad Dressings & Croutons					
• Caesar, 2 oz.	230	25	1	0	1
Croutons, pack	70	3	8	0	2
Fat Free Honey Mustard, 2 oz.	60	0	15	1	0
• Fat Free Italian, 2 oz.	25	0	6	0	0
Honey French, 2 oz.	220	18	14	0	0
Italian, 2 oz.	160	14	7	0	0
Lite Ranch, 2 oz.	120	12	2	0	1
Ranch, 2 oz.	220	24	2	0	1
Salads					
Caesar Side Salad	40	2	4	2	4
Chicken & Fruit	220	2	28	4	23
• Chicken & Pasta Caesar	440	15	41	4	35
Chicken BLT Ranch	270	10	13	4	31
• Garden Side Salad	25	0	4	3	2
Parmesan Chicken	360	15	31	4	31
Pasta Side Salad	320	12	41	1	11
Sampler Platters					
Classic Sampler	810	25	110	8	34
Ultimate Sampler	980	29	134	11	43
Submarinos					
Club	730	34	65	3	37
Ham n' Swiss	680	30	65	3	34
• Italian Beef	660	24	68	3	46
• Original	940	58	68	4	35

Firehouse Subs

Firehouse Subs	Cal	Fat	Cbs	Fbr	Prtn
Chili & Salads					
• Chief's Salad w/ Chicken Salad, 16 oz.	690	54	16	3	31
Chief's Salad w/ Grilled Chicken, 16 oz.	340	15	12	3	36
Chief's Salad w/ Ham, 16 oz.	360	8	16	3	26
• Chief's Salad w/Turkey, 16 oz.	300	15	12	3	34
Chiefs Salad w/Tuna Salad, 16 oz.	540	35	16	3	36
Chili, 8 oz.	320	18	20	6	20
Desserts					
• Brownies, 4 oz.	420	18	63	1	5
• Chocolate Chip Cookie, 3 oz.	290	14	37	2	5
Oatmeal Raisin Cookie, 3 oz.	310	16	35	3	5
Peanut Butter Cookie, 3 oz.	360	26	25	3	10
Large Subs					
• Chicken Salad (10 oz), 20 oz.	1380	90	99	4	50
Club on a Sub, 19 oz.	810	23	94	4	58
Corned Beef, 16 oz.	600	25	84	4	51
Engine Company, 18 oz.	670	19	88	4	62
Engineer, 20 oz.	620	26	94	4	50
Grilled Chicken (8 oz), 18 oz.	680	12	90	4	60
Ham, 16 oz.	630	10	94	4	43
Hero, 18 oz.	680	15	93	4	57

(• = most healthy • = least healthy) **RESTAURANTS & FAST-FOOD • 175**

RESTAURANTS & FAST-FOOD CHAINS

Firehouse Subs (cont.)

	Cal	Fat	Cbs	Fbr	Prtn
Large Subs (cont.)					
Hook & Ladder, 18 oz.	660	18	94	4	50
Italian, 9 oz.	1000	45	98	4	54
Meatball, 7 oz.	1220	69	98	5	54
NY Steamer, 14 oz.	750	38	86	2	59
Pastrami, 16 oz.	640	13	88	4	47
Roast Beef, 16 oz.	600	11	85	4	61
Steak, 17 oz.	830	27	93	6	58
Tuna Salad (10 oz), 20 oz.	1090	53	98	4	60
Turkey, 16 oz.	560	8	88	4	40
• Veggie (no meat), 14 oz.	500	20	92	5	17
Medium Subs					
Chicken Salad (5 oz.), 12 oz.	760	46	63	2	27
Club on A Sub, 11 oz.	490	13	60	2	32
Corned Beef, 11 oz.	400	17	55	2	34
Engine Company, 11 oz.	410	11	57	2	33
Engineer, 12 oz.	380	14	61	2	27
Grilled Chicken, 11 oz.	410	7	58	2	32
Ham, 11 oz.	430	7	62	2	28
Hero (6 oz. meat), 13 oz.	460	12	61	2	42
Hook & Ladder, 11 oz.	400	10	60	2	27
Italian, 11 oz.	660	33	60	2	29
• Meatball, 11 oz.	800	45	65	3	35
NY Steamer, 8 oz.	520	20	56	1	32
Pastrami, 11 oz.	420	9	58	2	31
Roast Beef, 11 oz.	400	8	56	2	40
Steak, 10 oz.	490	15	60	3	31
Tuna Salad (5 oz), 12 oz.	610	28	62	2	32
• Turkey, 11 oz.	370	4	58	2	26
Veggie (no meat), 10 oz.	370	11	60	3	11

Five Guys Famous Burgers and Fries

	Cal	Fat	Cbs	Fbr	Prtn
Famous Burgers					
• Bread, 77 g	260	9	39	2	7
Hamburger Beef, 94 g	280	19	0	N/A	26
• Hebrew National Hotdog, 90 g	285	26	1	0	11
Sides					
Five Guys Fries, 122 g	310	15	39	3	5
Toppings					
A.1. Original Steak Sauce, 17 g	15	0	3	0	0
Cattlemen's BBQ Sauce, 17 g	60	0	16	0	0
Frank's Original Hot Sauce, 5 g	0	0	0	0	0
• French's Yellow Mustard, 17 g	0	0	0	0	0
Green Peppers, 25 g	5	0	2	1	0
Jalapeños, 11 g	3	0	1	0	0
Ketchup, 17 g	15	0	4	0	0
Kraft American Cheese, 19 g	70	6	1	0	4
Lettuce, 30 g	4	0	1	1	0
• Mayonnaise, 14 g	100	11	N/A	N/A	0
Mt. Olive Fresh Kosher Dill Pickles, 28 g	5	0	1	0	0
Mt. Olive Special Sweet Green Relish, 15 g	15	0	4	0	0
Onions, 26 g	10	0	3	1	0
Patrick Cudahy Bacon, 14 g	80	7	0	0	4
Sautéed Mushrooms, 25 g	10	0	1	1	0

RESTAURANTS & FAST-FOOD CHAINS

Five Guys Famous Burgers and Fries (cont)	Cal	Fat	Cbs	Fbr	Prtn
Toppings (cont.)					
Tomatoes, 52 g	9	0	2	1	1

Fox's Pizza Den	Cal	Fat	Cbs	Fbr	Prtn
Pizza					
12 Cheese Pizza, 1 pizza	1244	37	170	6	55
12 Pepperoni Pizza, 1 pizza	1420	53	170	6	63
• 14 sq. Cheese Slice, 1 slice	155	5	21	1	7
14 sq. Pepperoni Slice, 1 slice	178	7	21	1	8
16 Cheese Pizza, 1 pizza	2214	66	302	11	98
• 16 Pepperoni Pizza, 1 pizza	2484	90	302	11	110
16" Round Pizza, 1 slice	226	7	31	116	10
20 sq. Cheese Slice, 1 slice	221	7	30	1	10
20 sq. Pepperoni Slice, 1 slice	248	9	30	1	11

Freshens	Cal	Fat	Cbs	Fbr	Prtn
Smoothie					
All That Razz, 21 oz.	360	0	79	3	12
Berry Breeze, 21 oz.	306	0	77	3	1
Blueberry Bay, 21 oz.	376	0	81	4	12
Caribbean Craze, 21 oz.	288	0	73	2	1
Jamaican Jammer, 21 oz.	355	0	78	2	12
Mango Beach, 21 oz.	90	0	48	1	0
Maui Mango, 21 oz.	292	0	74	2	1
Mystic Mango, 21 oz.	357	3	82	2	3
Orange Shooter, 21 oz.	334	3	77	1	3
Orange Sunrise, 21 oz.	353	3	81	2	3
Peach Passion, 21 oz.	152	0	32	1	10
Peach Sunset, 21 oz.	268	0	67	2	1
Peachy Pineapple, 21 oz.	327	0	69	2	11
• Pina Collider, 21 oz.	429	4	88	2	12
Pineapple Paradise, 21 oz.	331	4	77	1	0
Raspberry Royale, 21 oz.	270	0	67	3	1
• Strawberry Oasis, 21 oz.	89	0	49	1	1
Strawberry Shooter, 21 oz.	246	0	64	1	1
Strawberry Squeeze, 21 oz.	313	0	68	1	11
Strawberry Sunrise, 21 oz.	153	0	35	1	10

Fuddruckers	Cal	Fat	Cbs	Fbr	Prtn
Extras					
American Cheese, 1 slice	50	5	1	0	3
• Cheese Sauce, 2 fl.oz.	40	3	6	0	1
• Fuddruckers Spud Spice, 100 g	267	5	49	14	8
Mild Cheddar Cheese, 1 slice	80	7	0	0	5
Monterey Jack w/ Peppers, 1 slice	110	9	1	0	6
Monterey Jack, 1 slice	80	7	0	0	5
Signature Spread, Garlic & Herb, 1 tbsp.	90	10	0	0	0
Swiss, 1 slice	80	6	1	0	6
Hamburger Bun					
• Bun Dough, 3 oz.	240	5	40	1	7
• Bun Mix, 100 g	410	10	67	2	10
Meat Products					
• Ground Beef 76/24, 4 oz.	330	28	0	0	18
Turkey Patty, Approx. 1/3 lb.	240	17	0	0	21

(•= most healthy •= least healthy) **RESTAURANTS & FAST-FOOD • 177**

RESTAURANTS & FAST-FOOD CHAINS

Fuddruckers (cont.)

	Cal	Fat	Cbs	Fbr	Prtn
Meat Products (cont.)					
• Veggie Patty, Approx. 1/4 lb.	150	4	22	3	8
Sides					
Beer Battered Onion Rings, 4 pcs.	150	8	18	1	2
Potato Wedges, 3 oz.	120	3	20	2	2

Giordano's

	Cal	Fat	Cbs	Fbr	Prtn
• Small Cheese Stuffed Pizza, 7 oz.	550	25	57	4	25
Small Spinach Stuffed Pizza, 7 oz.	500	21	54	6	24
• Small Vegetarian Stuffed Pizza, 7 oz.	470	19	55	6	21

Gloria Jean's

	Cal	Fat	Cbs	Fbr	Prtn
Blended Tea Lattes (Regular)					
• Chai Tea Latte, 24 oz.	174	3	31	0	5
• Green Tea Latte, 24 oz.	359	14	54	0	9
Mango Tea Latte, 24 oz.	316	12	55	0	2
Chillers (Regular)					
Chai Chiller, 24 oz.	416	14	66	0	6
• Crème Brulee Espresso Chiller, 24 oz.	319	9	52	0	6
Mocharetto Espresso Chiller, 24 oz.	405	13	66	1	7
Swiss Orange Mocha Espresso Chiller, 24 oz.	365	13	57	1	7
Vanilla Caramel Chiller, 24 oz.	634	21	100	0	12
• Very Vanilla Chiller, 24 oz.	839	38	114	0	11
White Caramel Oreo Chiller, 24 oz.	821	26	133	1	14
White Chocolate Oreo Chiller, 24 oz.	666	26	95	1	13
Cold Coffee Drinks (Regular)					
• Butter Rum Chiller, 24 oz.	656	19	112	0	12
Iced Café au Lait, 24 oz.	65	2	6	0	4
Iced Café Mocha, 24 oz.	397	17	51	1	12
Iced Cappuccino Chiller, 24 oz.	484	16	66	0	18
Iced Coffee, 24 oz.	5	0	0	0	1
Iced Latte, 24 oz.	200	8	19	0	13
• Iced Toddy, 24 oz.	2	0	0	0	0
Iced Toddy Supreme, 24 oz.	537	47	19	0	12
Iced White Chocolate Mocha, 24 oz.	410	19	50	0	11
Cold Drinks (Regular)					
Bulk Iced Tea, 24 oz.	5	0	1	0	0
• Italian Cream Soda, 24 oz.	441	13	83	0	3
Italian Cream Soda, Sugar-Free Syrup, 24 oz.	145	13	6	0	3
Italian Soda, 24 oz.	296	0	77	0	0
• Italian Soda, Sugar-Free Syrup, 24 oz.	0	0	0	0	0
Fruit Chillers (Regular)					
• Banana Chiller, 24 oz.	371	0	91	7	0
Banana Cream Chiller, 24 oz.	394	1	87	5	5
• Bananaberry Split Chiller, 24 oz.	709	26	123	6	8
Raspberries 'N Cream Chiller, 24 oz.	394	1	87	5	5
Raspberry Fruit Chiller, 24 oz.	371	0	91	7	0
Strawberries 'N Cream Chiller, 24 oz.	394	1	87	5	5
Strawberry Fruit Chiller, 24 oz.	371	0	91	7	0
Wildberries 'N Cream Fruit Chiller, 24 oz.	394	1	87	5	5
Wildberry Fruit Chiller, 24 oz.	371	0	91	7	0
Holiday Drinks (Regular)					
Butter Rum Latte, 16 oz.	580	17	100	0	10
• Noel Nog, 16 oz.	516	29	52	0	15

Gloria Jean's (cont.)	Cal	Fat	Cbs	Fbr	Prtn
Holiday Drinks (cont.)					
• Sleigh Ride Chiller, 16 oz.	586	19	92	0	11
Sleigh Ride Mocha, 16 oz.	538	17	87	0	10
White Chocolate Sleigh Ride, 16 oz.	582	19	91	0	13
Hot Coffee Drinks (Regular)					
Cafe Americano, 16 oz.	2	0	0	0	0
Cafe au Lait, 16 oz.	109	4	10	0	7
Cafe Breve, 16 oz.	314	28	10	0	7
Cafe Latte, 16 oz.	154	6	14	0	10
Cafe Mocha, 16 oz.	388	16	51	1	12
Cappuccino, 16 oz.	124	5	11	0	8
Creme Brulee Latte, 16 oz.	352	11	54	0	10
Espresso Con Pana, Double	21	2	1	0	0
Espresso Con Pana, Single	20	2	1	0	0
Espresso Macchiato, Double	9	0	1	0	1
Espresso Macchiato, Single	9	0	1	0	1
Espresso, Double	2	0	0	0	0
• Espresso, Single	1	0	0	0	0
Mocha Truffle, 16 oz.	320	13	43	2	12
• Mocharetto, 16 oz.	506	16	81	1	12
Swiss Orange Mocha, 16 oz.	447	16	66	1	12
Vanilla Caramelatte, 16 oz.	376	10	64	0	9
White Chocolate Mocha, 16 oz.	401	18	49	0	11
Hot Drinks (Regular)					
Hot Chai, 16 oz.	213	3	40	0	5
Hot Chocolate, 16 oz.	431	18	55	1	14
• Hot Tea, 16 oz.	0	0	0	0	0
Irish Nut Crème, 16 oz.	403	13	60	0	10
Mocha Caramelatte, 16 oz.	416	12	65	1	11
• Mon Cheri Mocha, 16 oz.	450	14	70	1	11
Steamers, 16 oz.	358	11	56	0	11
Steamers, Sugar-Free Syrup, 16 oz.	210	11	17	0	11
White Hot Chocolate, 16 oz.	445	20	54	0	14
Kids Drinks					
• BananaBerry Chiller	330	13	47	0	7
• Grapple Fruit Chiller	330	13	45	0	7
Strawbical Fruit Chiller	330	13	47	0	7
WaterBerry Chiller	330	13	47	0	7
Mocha Chillers (Regular)					
Banana Ana Mocha Chiller, 24 oz.	619	13	118	3	11
Banana Split Mocha Chiller, 24 oz.	701	13	138	5	11
• Coco Loco Mocha Chiller, 24 oz.	536	13	97	2	11
Cookies 'N Cream Mocha Chiller, 24 oz.	588	19	94	1	11
Cookies 'N Mint Mocha Chiller, 24 oz.	756	20	135	3	13
• English Toffee Twist Mocha Chiller, 24 oz.	776	27	124	2	11
Malted Mocha Chiller, 24 oz.	722	17	131	2	16
Mint Choco Bomb Mocha Chiller, 24 oz.	596	13	112	2	11
Nutty Mocha Frost Chiller, 24 oz.	750	22	130	3	13
Raspberry Dazzle Mocha Chiller, 24 oz.	619	13	118	3	11
Strawberry Supreme Mocha Chiller, 24 oz.	619	13	118	3	11
Promotional Drinks (Regular)					
• Chocolate Fudge Chiller, 24 oz.	664	28	108	4	17
• Iced Chai with Skim Milk, 24 oz.	193	0	41	0	6
Java Chiller, 24 oz.	459	18	70	1	5

(• = most healthy • = least healthy) **RESTAURANTS & FAST-FOOD • 179**

RESTAURANTS & FAST-FOOD CHAINS

Gloria Jean's (cont.)

	Cal	Fat	Cbs	Fbr	Prtn
Promotional Drinks (cont.)					
Java Light Chiller, 24 oz.	255	6	41	1	9
Lite Mocha Chiller, 24 oz.	195	3	42	20	14
Madagascar Vanilla Chiller, 24 oz.	662	35	91	0	8
Strawberry Vanilla Chiller, 24 oz.	550	13	101	5	6

Godfather's Pizza

	Cal	Fat	Cbs	Fbr	Prtn
Desserts					
Apple Dessert (Alum Pan), 1/6	139	2	28	1	3
Apple Dessert (Large), 1/10	229	5	42	1	5
Apple Dessert (Medium), 1/8	206	4	39	1	4
Apple Dessert (Small), 1/6	202	5	37	1	4
• Breadsticks, 1 piece	80	2	14	1	2
Cheesesticks, 1/6	130	4	18	1	5
Cherry Dessert (Alum Pan), 1/6	142	2	29	1	3
Cherry Dessert (Large), 1/10	233	5	44	1	5
Cherry Dessert (Medium), 1/8	210	4	40	1	4
Cherry Dessert (Small), 1/6	206	5	38	1	4
Chocolate Chip Cookie, 1/6	195	8	30	0	2
Cinnamon Streusel (Alum Pan), 1/6	161	3	30	1	3
Cinnamon Streusel (Large), 1/10	258	7	45	1	5
Cinnamon Streusel (Medium), 1/8	228	6	40	1	5
Cinnamon Streusel (Small), 1/6	226	6	39	1	4
M&M Streusel Dessert (Alum Pan), 1/6	173	4	31	1	4
• M&M Streusel Dessert (Large), 1/10	300	8	51	1	5
M&M Streusel Dessert (Medium), 1/8	263	7	45	1	5
M&M Streusel Dessert (Small), 1/6	249	7	42	1	5
Monkey Bread (Alum Pan), 1/6	120	2	23	1	3
Potato Wedges, 4 oz.	192	9	24	4	3
Jumbo Original					
All Meat Combo, 1/10 pizza	610	27	56	3	29
Bacon Cheeseburger, 1/10 pizza	580	27	55	3	28
• Cheese, 1/10 pizza	430	13	53	2	20
Combo, 1/10 pizza	580	24	57	4	28
Hawaiian, 1/10 pizza	460	13	58	2	22
Hot Stuff, 1/10 pizza	590	26	56	3	28
Humble Pie, 1/10 pizza	620	30	56	3	27
Pepperoni, 1/10 pizza	490	18	54	2	22
Super Combo, 1/10 pizza	630	28	58	4	32
Super Hawaiian, 1/10 pizza	500	18	57	2	23
• Super Taco, 1/10 pizza	640	31	57	4	31
Taco, 1/10 pizza	590	27	56	3	30
Veggie, 1/10 pizza	450	14	56	3	21
Large Golden					
All Meat Combo, 1/10 pizza	350	17	29	2	16
Bacon Cheeseburger, 1/10 pizza	330	16	29	1	15
• Cheese, 1/10 pizza	250	9	28	1	11
Combo, 1/10 pizza	330	15	30	2	15
Hawaiian, 1/10 pizza	270	10	31	1	12
Hot Stuff, 1/10 pizza	340	17	29	1	15
Humble Pie, 1/10 pizza	350	18	29	1	15
Pepperoni, 1/10 pizza	290	13	28	1	12
Super Combo, 1/10 pizza	370	18	31	2	18
Super Hawaiian, 1/10 pizza	291	12	30	1	13

Godfather's Pizza (cont.)	Cal	Fat	Cbs	Fbr	Prtn
Large Golden (cont.)					
• Super Taco, 1/10 pizza	380	20	30	2	17
Taco, 1/10 pizza	350	17	30	2	17
Veggie, 1/10 pizza	260	10	30	2	11
Large Original					
All Meat Combo, 1/10 pizza	410	18	38	2	20
Bacon Cheeseburger, 1/10 pizza	390	18	36	2	19
• Cheese, 1/10 pizza	290	9	38	1	14
Combo, 1/10 pizza	390	16	39	3	12
Hawaiian, 1/10 pizza	310	9	38	1	15
Hot Stuff, 1/10 pizza	400	18	38	2	19
Humble Pie, 1/10 pizza	420	20	38	2	18
Pepperoni, 1/10 pizza	330	12	36	1	15
Super Combo, 1/10 pizza	430	19	39	3	22
Super Hawaiian, 1/10 pizza	340	12	38	2	16
• Super Taco, 1/10 pizza	450	22	38	3	22
Taco, 1/10 pizza	420	19	38	2	22
Veggie, 1/10 pizza	310	10	38	2	14
Large Thin					
All Meat Combo, 1/10 pizza	310	17	20	1	14
Bacon Cheeseburger, 1/10 pizza	290	17	20	1	13
• Cheese, 1/10 pizza	220	10	19	1	9
Combo, 1/10 pizza	290	16	21	2	14
Hawaiian, 1/10 pizza	240	10	22	1	11
Hot Stuff, 1/10 pizza	300	17	20	1	13
Humble Pie, 1/10 pizza	310	19	20	1	13
Pepperoni, 1/10 pizza	250	13	19	1	11
Super Combo, 1/10 pizza	330	19	22	2	16
Super Hawaiian, 1/10 pizza	250	12	21	1	11
• Super Taco, 1/10 pizza	340	21	21	2	16
Taco, 1/10 pizza	310	18	21	1	15
Veggie, 1/10 pizza	230	10	21	1	10
Medium Golden					
All Meat Combo, 1/8 pizza	300	14	27	1	14
Bacon Cheeseburger, 1/8 pizza	270	12	26	1	13
• Cheese, 1/8 pizza	220	8	26	1	10
Combo, 1/8 pizza	290	13	28	2	13
Hawaiian, 1/8 pizza	240	8	29	1	11
Hot Stuff, 1/8 pizza	290	14	27	1	13
Humble Pie, 1/8 pizza	310	15	27	1	13
Pepperoni, 1/8 pizza	260	11	26	1	11
Super Combo, 1/8 pizza	320	15	28	2	16
Super Hawaiian, 1/8 pizza	250	10	27	1	11
• Super Taco, 1/8 pizza	330	17	28	2	15
Taco, 1/8 pizza	300	14	27	2	15
Veggie, 1/8 pizza	230	8	27	1	10
Medium Original					
All Meat Combo, 1/8 pizza	370	16	35	2	18
Bacon Cheeseburger, 1/8 pizza	330	13	35	2	16
• Cheese, 1/8 pizza	260	7	34	1	12
Combo, 1/8 pizza	350	14	37	3	17
Hawaiian, 1/8 pizza	280	8	38	1	13
Hot Stuff, 1/8 pizza	360	6	35	2	17
Humble Pie, 1/8 pizza	380	18	35	2	16

RESTAURANTS & FAST-FOOD CHAINS

Godfather's Pizza (cont.)

	Cal	Fat	Cbs	Fbr	Prtn
Medium Original (cont.)					
Pepperoni, 1/8 pizza	290	10	34	1	13
Super Combo, 1/8 pizza	390	17	37	3	19
Super Hawaiian, 1/8 pizza	280	8	37	1	13
• Super Taco, 1/8 pizza	390	18	36	2	19
Taco, 1/8 pizza	360	16	36	2	18
Veggie, 1/8 pizza	270	9	36	2	12
Medium Thin					
All Meat Combo, 1/8 pizza	280	15	20	1	13
Bacon Cheeseburger, 1/8 pizza	250	13	20	1	11
• Cheese, 1/8 pizza	180	8	16	1	8
Combo, 1/8 pizza	250	13	18	1	11
Hawaiian, 1/8 pizza	200	9	19	1	9
Hot Stuff, 1/8 pizza	270	15	20	1	12
Humble Pie, 1/8 pizza	270	16	17	1	11
Pepperoni, 1/8 pizza	220	11	16	1	9
Super Combo, 1/8 pizza	300	16	21	2	14
Super Hawaiian, 1/8 pizza	230	11	21	1	10
• Super Taco, 1/8 pizza	310	18	21	2	14
Taco, 1/8 pizza	260	15	17	1	13
Veggie, 1/8 pizza	190	9	18	1	8
Mini Original					
All Meat Combo, 1/4 pizza	220	10	21	1	10
Bacon Cheeseburger, 1/4 pizza	210	10	21	1	10
• Cheese, 1/4 pizza	150	4	20	1	7
Combo, 1/4 pizza	210	8	22	2	10
Hawaiian, 1/4 pizza	160	4	23	1	7
Hot Stuff, 1/4 pizza	210	9	21	1	10
• Humble Pie, 1/4 pizza	230	11	21	1	10
Pepperoni, 1/4 pizza	160	5	20	1	7
Super Combo, 1/4 pizza	220	9	22	1	11
Super Hawaiian, 1/4 pizza	180	6	21	1	8
Super Taco, 1/4 pizza	230	10	22	2	11
Taco, 1/4 pizza	210	9	22	1	11
Veggie, 1/4 pizza	160	5	21	1	7

Gold Star Chili

	Cal	Fat	Cbs	Fbr	Prtn
Burritos					
Chili Beef Burrito with Topper, 383 g	710	32	78	8	30
• Chili Beef Burrito, 292 g	570	20	75	8	23
Crispy Chicken Burrito with Topper, 334 g	790	36	84	5	32
• Crispy Chicken Burrito, 277 g	840	22	62	5	27
Grilled Chicken Burrito with Topper, 325 g	730	33	72	4	37
Grilled Chicken Burrito, 268 g	580	19	59	4	33
Chili by the Bowl					
Chili, 8 oz.	213	12	8	3	18
Veggie Chili Bowl, 255 g	160	2	29	6	8
Fries and Garlic Bread					
Cheese Fries, 184 g	520	32	42	5	15
Chili Cheese Fries, 269 g	596	36	46	6	22
Fries, 149 g	366	19	44	5	5
Garlic Bread w/ Cheese, 68 g	271	18	19	1	8
• Garlic Bread, 54 g	213	13	19	1	5

RESTAURANTS & FAST-FOOD CHAINS

Gold Star Chili (cont.)

	Cal	Fat	Cbs	Fbr	Prtn
Gold Star Chili					
Regular 2-Way bean, 425 g	489	12	71	8	25
Regular 2-Way onion bean, 468 g	505	12	75	9	25
Regular 2-Way onion, 383 g	436	11	62	6	21
Regular 2-Way, 340 g	420	11	58	5	21
Regular 3-Way, 397 g	648	30	59	5	35
Regular 4-Way, 439 g	665	30	63	6	35
Regular 5-Way, 525 g	733	30	76	9	40
• Super 5-Way, 794 g	1141	51	109	13	63
Gold Star Coney					
Cheese Coney, 160 g	343	18	31	2	15
Chili Cheese Sandwich, 132 g	288	12	30	2	14
• Chili Sandwich, 132 g	211	5	32	3	9
Coney, 146 g	286	14	30	2	12
• Low Carb Coney Bowl, 298 g	570	47	7	2	34
Sensational Entree Sized Salads					
• Caesar Salad, 105 g	90	5	6	1	7
Cafe Salad, 134 g	110	7	8	2	5
Crispy Chicken Caesar Salad, 238 g	280	11	22	2	23
Crispy Chicken Cafe Salad, 238 g	210	8	12	2	25
• Grilled Chkn Spring Harvest Salad, 315 g	300	13	23	3	25
Half Cafe Salad, 238 g	280	11	22	2	23
Low Carb Chili Salad, 230 g	160	7	23	3	5

Golden Corral

	Cal	Fat	Cbs	Fbr	Prtn
Brass Bell Bakery®					
Apple Pie, 1/10 pie	320	13	49	2	3
• Banana Pudding, 1/2 cup	466	19	70	N/A	3
Bread Pudding, 1/2 cup	200	5	37	1	4
Brownies, 1	240	9	40	1	2
Carrot Cake, 4 oz.	390	19	52	1	3
Cherry Pie, 1/10 pie	310	13	46	2	3
Chocolate Chip Cookies, 1	100	5	13	0	1
Chocolate White Chip Cookies, 1	100	5	13	1	1
Cinn-a-Gold Rolls®, 1	320	10	52	3	5
Coconut, 1	100	5	13	0	1
Key Lime Cheesecake, 1/10 pie	360	19	42	1	4
• Oatmeal Raisin Cookies, 1	90	4	14	1	1
Peanut Butter with Nuts Cookies, 1	100	6	12	0	2
Breads/Muffins					
• Corn Muffins, 3 oz.	204	5	32	N/A	4
Kaiser Rolls, 1	160	2	31	1	6
• Skillet Cornbread, 1 Portion	120	3	22	1	2
Yeast Rolls (without butter), 1	195	2	42	1	5
Cold Buffet					
• Cajun Potato Salad, 1 cup	330	23	22	2	9
Carrot & Raisin Salad, 1/2 cup	113	5	17	N/A	1
Chicken Salad, 1/2 cup	210	15	9	1	11
Coleslaw, 1 cup	250	19	19	4	2
Macaroni Salad, 1/2 cup	190	8	26	N/A	3
Marinated Mushroom, 1/2 cup	103	7	6	N/A	2
• Marinated Vegetables, 1/2 cup	47	2	5	N/A	1
Seafood Salad, 1 cup	270	17	18	2	11
Sliced Yellow Peaches, 1/2 cup	70	0	17	1	0

RESTAURANTS & FAST-FOOD CHAINS

Golden Corral (cont.)	Cal	Fat	Cbs	Fbr	Prtn
Cold Buffet (cont.)					
Tuna Salad, 1/2 cup	237	12	8	N/A	22
Condiments					
Cocktail Sauce, 1/4 cup	70	2	13	0	1
• Honey Butter (indiv. cup), 10 g	60	6	2	0	0
• Tartar Sauce, 2 tbsp.	150	16	1	0	0
Hot Buffet					
Asian Pork Roast, 1 cup	510	34	10	4	42
Awesome Pot Roast, 4 oz.	206	12	1	0	24
Barbecue Chicken (Leg Quarter), 1	480	22	20	2	50
Barbecue Pork Spareribs, 82 g	230	16	3	1	19
Barbecue Pork, 3 oz.	170	8	5	1	18
Bourbon Street Chicken, 4 oz.	210	11	5	1	23
Broccoli & Rice, 1/2 cup	220	5	36	N/A	6
Brown Gravy, 1 oz.	100	4	16	0	0
Buttered Noodles, 1/2 cup	163	4	24	N/A	4
Chicken & Pastry Noodles, 4 oz.	94	4	9	1	6
Chicken Breast Fillet, Marinated, 5 oz.	120	2	2	0	24
Chicken Tenders, 3 oz.	190	9	7	1	22
Country Fried Steak, 3 oz.	152	7	12	0	11
Creamy Chicken & Pasta, 1 cup	210	6	25	2	14
Fresh Fried Chicken (Leg/Thigh), 3 oz.	250	19	2	0	16
Grilled Pork Chop or Loin Slices, 3 oz.	119	4	0	N/A	19
Grilled Pork Chops (with bone), 1	200	13	0	N/A	20
Ham (Pit Style, Smoked), 2 oz.	80	2	1	N/A	10
Macaroni & Beef, 1 cup	260	11	26	3	13
Macaroni & Cheese, 1 cup	400	18	42	2	17
Mashed Potatoes (Scratch), 4 oz.	120	6	14	1	2
Meatloaf, 4 oz.	190	10	10	3	16
Pizza, 1 slice	230	8	28	2	10
Pork Roast, 3 oz.	220	17	0	1	17
Pork Steaks, 3.5 oz.	250	14	0	N/A	31
Potato Casserole, 1 cup	280	9	40	1	9
Poultry Gravy, 1 oz.	104	3	16	0	3
Roast Beef, 3 oz.	180	10	1	N/A	23
Roasted Herb Pork Chop, 3 oz.	334	17	6	N/A	34
Rotisserie Chicken (Breast/Wing), 6 oz.	320	15	1	0	44
Sirloin Steak, 3 oz.	219	13	0	N/A	24
Spaghetti Pasta, 2 oz.	210	1	42	2	7
Spaghetti Sauce, 1/2 cup	110	0	25	2	2
• Steakburgers, 6 oz.	859	55	0	N/A	55
Tamales, Beef, 85 g	240	16	18	3	6
Tortillas, 2	325	7	56	N/A	9
• Turkey Breast w/ Wing, 2 oz.	70	3	1	N/A	10
White Rice, 1/2 cup	178	5	27	N/A	2
Ice Cream/Toppings					
Caramel Topping, 100 g	318	4	67	0	3
Chocolate Soft Serve, 1/2 cup	100	2	18	1	3
Chocolate Syrup, 100 g	249	1	62	2	1
Hot Fudge Topping, 100 g	320	10	54	2	4
Sherbet, 1/2 cup	90	1	23	0	1
Strawberry Topping, 100 g	192	0	49	1	1
• Turtle Coating, 100 g	633	50	46	2	2
Vanilla Soft Serve, 1/2 cup	100	2	17	0	3

RESTAURANTS & FAST-FOOD CHAINS

Golden Corral (cont.)	Cal	Fat	Cbs	Fbr	Prtn
No Sugar Added/Sugar Free					
Blueberry Pie, 1/10 pie	270	8	48	2	4
Cheesecake, 1	220	14	18	1	4
Chocolate Chocolate Chip Cookies, 1	90	5	12	1	1
Oatmeal Bar, 1 Square	90	3	11	0	2
• Red Gelatin, 1/2 cup	10	0	0	N/A	1
Vanilla Cake, 7 oz.	130	7	19	0	1
Salad Bar Meats					
• Turkey - Dark, Julienne, 2 oz.	70	2	2	0	10
• Turkey - White, Julienne, 2 oz.	90	5	2	0	9
Salad Dressing					
Blue Cheese Dressing, 2 tbsp.	190	20	4	1	1
Creamy Caesar Dressing, 2 tbsp.	110	11	2	0	1
Dijon Honey Mustard Dressing, 2 tbsp.	130	11	7	0	0
• Fat Free Ranch Dressing, 2 tbsp.	35	0	2	0	0
Fat Free Red French Dressing, 2 tbsp.	40	0	10	1	0
Fat Free Thou Island Dressing, 2 tbsp.	40	0	9	1	0
French Dressing, 2 tbsp.	120	11	5	0	0
Hot Bacon Dressing, 2 tbsp.	140	14	5	0	0
Lite Olive Oil Vinaigrette, 2 tbsp.	60	6	3	0	0
Poppy Seed Dressing, 2 tbsp.	130	10	8	0	0
Ranch Dressing, 2 tbsp.	120	12	2	0	1
Red French Dressing, 2 tbsp.	120	11	7	0	0
Sesame Oriental Dressing, 2 tbsp.	160	15	6	0	0
Thousand Island Dressing, 2 tbsp.	130	11	6	2	0
Seafood					
Battered Pollock Fish Fillet, 4 oz.	210	9	18	1	14
Breaded Butterflied Shrimp, 4 oz.	210	2	37	1	12
• Breaded Jumbo Shrimp, 4 oz.	230	2	36	1	16
Breaded Shrimp, 4 oz.	200	2	32	1	15
Cajun Style Fish Fillet, 3.5 oz.	210	9	19	N/A	13
Cajun Whitefish, 3 oz.	110	7	0	N/A	10
Cracker Crumb Fish Fillet, 3.5 oz.	229	13	17	N/A	13
Hot Steamed Shrimp, 1 cup	160	2	0	N/A	37
Kentucky Style Fish Fillet, 4 oz.	130	5	14	2	13
Salmon Fillet, Carved, 2 oz.	138	9	0	N/A	11
Salmon Steaks w/Lemon Hrb Bttr, 3.5 oz.	208	14	4	1	17
• Steamed Whitefish, 3 oz.	82	3	0	N/A	10
Soup & Potato Bar					
Baked Potato (small, plain), 1	109	0	25	N/A	2
Broccoli Florets with Cheese, 1/2 cup	140	9	8	1	4
• Chicken Gumbo, 1/2 cup	70	2	10	1	5
Chicken Noodle, 1/2 cup	100	3	12	1	6
Clam Chowder, 1/2 cup	140	6	17	1	4
Potato with Bacon, 1/2 cup	120	5	17	3	2
Sweet Potato (Small), 1	137	0	32	N/A	2
• Timberline Chili, 1 cup	270	12	23	5	19
Vegetable Beef, 1/2 cup	100	2	17	2	5
Sunrise Breakfast Buffet					
• Bacon, 1 piece	60	5	1	0	4
• Corned Beef Hash, 1 cup	420	30	22	6	19
Creamed Chipped Beef, 1/2 cup	75	11	9	0	8
Eggs, Scrambled, 4 oz.	160	11	2	0	12
French Toast, 1 slice	241	8	23	N/A	12

RESTAURANTS & FAST-FOOD CHAINS

Golden Corral (cont.)

	Cal	Fat	Cbs	Fbr	Prtn
Sunrise Breakfast Buffet (cont.)					
Hash Brown Casserole, 1/2 cup	155	7	17	N/A	5
Hash Browns, 1/2 cup	102	7	8	N/A	1
Sausage Gravy, 1 oz.	41	3	2	0	2
Sausage Links, 3 Links	160	14	1	N/A	9
Sausage Patties, 1	247	21	0	0	15
Split Smoked Sausage, 1	250	23	2	0	9
Vegetables					
Asian Beans, 1 cup	140	2	26	6	4
Black-eyed Peas, 1/2 cup	149	1	28	N/A	10
Brussels Sprouts, 6 g	35	0	5	3	3
Cheese Sauce, Cheddar, 1/4 cup	110	9	4	N/A	3
Collard Greens, 3.5 oz.	60	4	4	2	2
Corn-on-the-Cob, 1	106	2	22	N/A	3
Creamed Corn, 3.5 oz.	90	1	20	1	2
Creamed Spinach, 1/2 cup	180	13	11	2	4
• Cut Corn, 1 cup	310	9	52	N/A	6
Escalloped Apples, 2/3 cup	180	2	40	3	1
Fresh Steamed Broccoli, 1/2 cup	25	1	5	N/A	3
Fresh Steamed Cabbage, 1/2 cup	60	5	1	N/A	0
Fresh Steamed Carrots, 1/2 cup	79	5	6	N/A	0
• Fresh Steamed Cauliflower, 1/2 cup	13	0	2	N/A	1
Fresh Vegetable Trio, 1/2 cup	25	0	5	N/A	1
Glazed Sesame Carrots, 1 cup	260	16	27	5	2
Green & Yellow Beans, 1/2 cup	71	5	9	N/A	1
Green Beans, 1/2 cup	34	0	6	N/A	1
Green Peas, 1/2 cup	109	6	10	N/A	3
Northern Beans, 1/2 cup	149	1	28	N/A	10
Pinto Beans, 1/2 cup	149	1	28	N/A	10
Ranch Style BBQ Beans, 1/2 cup	130	3	20	6	6
Southern Style Cabbage, 1/2 cup	26	1	4	N/A	1
Spinach, 1/3 cup	20	0	2	2	2
Squash Medley, 1/2 cup	66	5	3	N/A	0
Steamed Zucchini, 1/2 cup	60	5	1	N/A	0
Turnip Greens, 2/3 cup	18	0	3	2	2
Yams & Apples, 1/2 cup	160	2	35	1	1

Great Steak & Potato

	Cal	Fat	Cbs	Fbr	Prtn
Baked Potatoes					
Broccoli & Cheese, 238 g	295	12	35	4	13
Cheese & Bacon, 209 g	427	23	29	3	25
Potato Skins, 202 g	438	30	26	2	17
• Single, 6 g	158	0	36	4	4
Sour Cream & Chive, 170 g	198	7	31	3	4
• The Great Potato - Chicken, 360 g	519	24	37	4	32
The Great Potato - Ham, 360 g	503	26	43	4	29
The Great Potato - Steak, 374 g	542	29	37	4	35
The Great Potato - Turkey, 360 g	473	23	39	4	31
The King, 241 g	497	30	31	3	26
Breads/Tortillas					
• Bread, 12" White, 170 g	420	4	82	6	18
Bread, 7" Wheat, 113 g	310	4	56	5	13
Bread, 7" White, 113 g	290	3	55	4	11
• Pita, serving, 79 g	220	5	38	3	7

RESTAURANTS & FAST-FOOD CHAINS

Great Steak & Potato (cont.)	Cal	Fat	Cbs	Fbr	Prtn
Breads/Tortillas (cont.)					
Tortilla, Low-Carb, Whole Wheat, 102 g	273	6	42	30	11
Cheese					
• Cheese, Mild Cheddar, serving, 2 oz.	223	18	0	N/A	14
Cheese, Provolone, serving, 2 oz.	202	16	2	N/A	14
• Cheese, Swiss, serving, 2 oz.	200	16	2	0	16
Kids Meals					
Nuggets, Kids, 78 g	165	9	10	1	11
Meats					
Chicken, serving, 4 oz.	138	3	0	0	19
Corned Beef, serving, 3 oz.	137	8	0	0	15
• Gyro Meat, serving, 4 oz.	205	12	5	1	21
Ham, serving, 4 oz.	122	4	6	N/A	16
Steak, serving, 5 oz.	160	7	0	0	22
Turkey, serving, 4 oz.	91	1	2	N/A	18
Salads					
Chef, 398 g	244	11	13	3	27
• Garden, 256 g	37	0	8	3	2
Grilled Chicken, 464 g	389	21	13	4	32
Grilled Ham, 464 g	371	22	20	4	29
• Grilled Steak, 464 g	395	25	13	4	32
Grilled Turkey, 464 g	336	19	15	4	31
Sandwiches					
Buffalo Chicken Sandwich, Regular, 467 g	841	41	67	6	48
• Chicken Bacon Ranch, Regular - LTO, 432 g	995	56	66	6	55
Chicken Philly, Regular, 417 g	938	53	63	5	47
Chicken Philly, Wrap, 406 g	921	57	50	31	47
Chicken Teriyaki, Regular, 446 g	962	53	66	5	49
Chicken Teriyaki, Wrap, 435 g	945	57	53	31	49
Great Steak, Regular, 432 g	963	58	63	5	49
Great Steak, Wrap, 421 g	946	62	50	31	49
Ham Delight, Regular, 417 g	929	55	72	5	44
Ham Delight, Wrap, 406 g	912	58	58	31	44
Ham Explosion, Regular, 460 g	931	55	71	6	45
Ham Explosion, Wrap, 449 g	914	58	58	32	46
Reuben, Regular, 383 g	848	48	64	6	43
Reuben, Wrap, 372 g	831	51	51	32	43
Super Steak, Regular, 474 g	972	58	65	6	49
Super Steak, Wrap, 463 g	955	62	52	32	50
Turkey Philly, Regular, 417 g	892	52	65	5	46
Turkey Philly, Wrap, 406 g	875	55	52	31	47
Veggie Delight, Regular, 389 g	831	53	67	6	28
• Veggie Delight, Wrap, 378 g	814	56	54	33	29
Sauces/Dressings					
Dressing, Ranch, 1 oz.	171	12	1	N/A	1
Dressing, Thousand Island, 1 oz.	125	0	4	0	0
• Mayonnaise, Dijon, 28 g	205	22	0	0	0
Mayonnaise, Regular, 28 g	202	18	0	0	0
Oil, serving, 0.5 oz.	80	9	0	0	0
• Sauce, Buffalo, 1 oz.	10	0	2	0	0
Sauce, Dipping - Tomato, 2 oz.	14	0	3	0	1
Sauce, Teriyaki, 1 oz.	24	4	3	0	2
Sauce, Tzatziki, 1 oz.	46	0	2	0	0

RESTAURANTS & FAST-FOOD CHAINS

Great Steak & Potato (cont.)

	Cal	Fat	Cbs	Fbr	Prtn
Sides					
Cheese Sticks, Small, 97 g	286	17	23	1	13
Fresh Style Fry, Regular, 397 g	668	37	80	9	9
Fried Onion Petals, 86 g	190	11	22	2	2
Toppings - Baked Potato					
Bacon, 1 oz.	76	18	0	0	7
• Cheddar Cheese, 2 oz.	223	12	0	N/A	14
Cheese Sauce, 2 oz.	155	0	3	0	9
• Chives, 1 oz.	0	4	0	0	0
Ham, 4 oz.	122	7	6	N/A	16
Sour Cream, 32 g	69		1	0	1
Steak, 5 oz.	160	1	0	0	22
Turkey, 4 oz.	91	7	2	N/A	18
Toppings - Sandwich					
Broccoli, serving, 4 ea.	12	0	2	1	1
• Cucumber, serving, 1 oz.	4	0	1	0	0
Dill Pickle, serving, 1 ea.	5	0	1	N/A	0
Green Pepper, serving, 1 oz.	4	0	1	0	0
Lettuce, serving, 2 oz.	9	0	2	1	1
Mushrooms, serving, 1 oz.	5	2	1	0	1
Olives, serving, 1 oz.	16	0	1	0	0
Onion, serving, 2 oz.	19	0	4	1	1
• Pineapple, serving, 2 oz.	26	5	7	1	0
Sauerkraut, serving, 2 oz.	11	0	2	2	1
Tomato, serving, 1 oz.	5	0	1	0	0

Great Wraps

	Cal	Fat	Cbs	Fbr	Prtn
Breads					
• Croutons, 1 oz.	75	10	9	N/A	N/A
• Flour Tortilla, 12 oz.	320	10	47	N/A	10
Pita, 7 oz.	220	3	43	N/A	7
Spinach Tortilla, 12 oz.	290	9	43	N/A	10
Tomato Basil Tortilla, 12 oz.	320	9	49	N/A	10
Cheese					
• Cheddar Mix, 2 oz.	220	18	2	N/A	14
Crumbled Feta, 1 oz.	120	5	2	N/A	10
• Parmesan, 1 oz.	20	2	0	N/A	N/A
Pepper Jack, 2 oz.	220	18	2	N/A	12
Provolone, 2 oz.	200	16	2	N/A	14
Swiss, 2 oz.	160	12	2	N/A	12
Dressings					
• Balsamic Vinaigrette, 1 oz.	60	5	4	N/A	0
• Caesar, 2 oz.	300	32	4	N/A	0
Cuban Sauce, 1 oz.	170	16	2	N/A	0
Feta, 2 oz.	160	16	4	N/A	2
Lite Ranch, 2 oz.	200	3	2	N/A	2
Mayo, 1 oz.	100	11	2	N/A	0
Zeke, 2 oz.	90	10	4	N/A	2
Fresh Veggies					
• Black Olives, 1 oz.	60	3	1	N/A	0
Chopped Cucumber, 1 oz.	3	0	1	N/A	0
Chopped Onion, 1 oz.	10	0	2	N/A	1
Chopped Pepperoncini, 1 oz.	5	0	0	N/A	0
Chopped Tomatoes, 2 oz.	10	0	0	N/A	0

Great Wraps (cont.)

	Cal	Fat	Cbs	Fbr	Prtn
Fresh Veggies (cont.)					
Jalapeños, 1 oz.	17	1	1	N/A	0
Red Pepper, 1 oz.	20	1	2	N/A	1
Romaine, 2 oz.	10	N/A	1	N/A	1
• Shredded Lettuce, 2 oz.	0	0	0	N/A	0
Spinach, 2 oz.	5	0	1	N/A	1
Sprouts, 1 oz.	2	0	0	N/A	0
Meats					
Bacon, 2 Slices	80	7	0	N/A	4
Chicken, 4 oz.	79	1	N/A	N/A	16
• Gyro, 4 oz.	350	32	4	N/A	11
Ham, 2 oz.	80	2	2	N/A	9
Large Chicken Tenderloin, 4 oz.	90	3	N/A	N/A	18
• Pork, 2 oz.	73	3	0	N/A	11
Steak, 4 oz.	110	4	1	N/A	19
Tuna, 4 oz.	105	2	0	N/A	23
Turkey, 4 oz.	80	0	4	N/A	18
Roasted Veggies					
Garlic Mushrooms, 1 oz.	5	2	1	N/A	1
• Green Pepper, 1 oz.	4	0	1	N/A	1
• Portabella Mushrooms, 3 oz.	81	14	5	N/A	4
Sauteed Onion, 1 oz.	27	1	3	N/A	1

Green Burrito

	Cal	Fat	Cbs	Fbr	Prtn
Burritos					
• Bean & Cheese Burrito - Chicken, 340 g	660	28	67	10	42
Bean & Cheese Burrito - Grnd Beef, 340 g	760	39	69	12	39
Bean & Cheese Burrito - Steak, 340 g	690	30	70	10	41
Bean & Cheese Burrito, 407 g	830	38	99	18	37
Carne Asada Burrito, 333 g	690	31	65	4	37
Grilled Chicken Burrito, 506 g	1080	54	91	3	57
The Green Burrito™ - Chicken, 633 g	920	33	120	14	45
The Green Burrito™ - Steak, 633 g	950	35	122	14	45
Sides					
Chips & Cheese, 142 g	690	40	65	4	17
Chips, 57 g	300	15	37	2	4
• Guacamole, 40 g	45	4	3	2	1
Pinto Beans & Cheese, 241 g	320	16	43	16	17
Rice, 198 g	340	10	58	1	4
Sour Cream, 40 g	50	4	3	0	2
Specialities					
Enchiladas (2) - Cheese, 220 g	430	28	30	4	13
Super Nachos - Chicken, 454 g	1020	55	96	14	44
• Super Nachos - Ground Beef, 465 g	1150	68	99	16	43
Super Nachos - Steak, 456 g	1050	58	99	14	45
Taco Salad - Chicken, 587 g	820	44	73	14	44
Taco Salad - Ground Beef, 587 g	940	57	75	16	40
Taco Salad - Steak, 587 g	850	47	76	14	44
• Taquitos (2) - Chicken, 92 g	150	7	16	3	6
Taquitos (5) - Chicken, 208 g	350	15	39	6	15
Tacos					
Fish Taco, 171 g	300	12	36	3	10
• Hard Taco - Chicken, 110 g	200	10	14	1	12
Hard Taco - Ground Beef, 110 g	250	15	15	2	12

RESTAURANTS & FAST-FOOD CHAINS

Green Burrito (cont.)

	Cal	Fat	Cbs	Fbr	Prtn
Tacos (cont.)					
Hard Taco - Steak, 110 g	220	11	15	1	14
Soft Taco - Chicken, 123 g	210	7	18	1	15
Soft Taco - Ground Beef, 123 g	260	13	19	2	13
Soft Taco - Steak, 123 g	260	13	19	2	13

Hardee's

	Cal	Fat	Cbs	Fbr	Prtn
Breakfast					
Bacon Biscuit, 120 g	430	28	35	0	8
Bacon, Egg & Cheese Biscuit, 174 g	560	38	37	0	16
Big Country Brkfast - Bacon, 355 g	980	56	90	3	28
Big Country Brkfast - Chicken, 458 g	1140	61	105	4	44
Big Country Brkfast - Ham, 377 g	970	53	90	3	33
• Big Country Brkfast - Pork Chop, 455 g	1220	68	102	4	48
Big Country Brkfast - Sausage, 374 g	1060	64	91	4	30
Big Country Brkfast - Steak, 412 g	1150	68	98	4	36
Biscuits 'N' Gravy, 251 g	530	34	47	0	8
Breaded Chicken Fillet Biscuit, 226 g	600	34	50	1	24
Breaded Country Steak Biscuit, 180 g	620	41	44	0	16
Breaded Pork Chop Biscuit, 222 g	690	42	48	1	29
Country Ham Biscuit, 144 g	440	26	36	0	14
Country Steak & Egg Biscuit, 223 g	690	47	44	0	22
Egg Biscuit, 152 g	450	29	35	0	11
Frisco Breakfast Sandwich, 185 g	420	20	37	2	24
Ham, Egg & Cheese Biscuit, 220 g	560	35	37	0	16
Hash Rounds - medium, 114 g	350	22	34	3	4
Hash Rounds - small, 83 g	260	16	25	2	3
Loaded Biscuit 'N' Gravy Breakfast Bowl, 326 g	770	54	49	1	20
Loaded Breakfast Burrito, 258 g	780	51	38	2	40
Loaded Omelet Biscuit, 198 g	640	44	37	0	21
Loaded Omelet, 89 g	270	21	2	0	16
Low Carb Breakfast Bowl, 208 g	620	50	6	2	36
Made from Scratch Biscuit, 109 g	370	23	35	0	5
Monster Biscuit, 212 g	710	51	37	0	24
Pancake Platter, 135 g	300	5	55	2	8
Sausage & Egg Biscuit, 185 g	610	44	36	0	17
Sausage Biscuit, 142 g	530	38	36	0	11
Sunrise Croissant with Bacon, 138 g	450	29	28	0	19
Sunrise Croissant with Ham, 164 g	430	26	28	0	23
Sunrise Croissant with Sausage, 161 g	550	38	29	0	22
• Sunrise Croissant, 57 g	210	10	26	0	4
Desserts					
Apple Turnover, 85 g	290	15	36	1	2
Chocolate Chip Cookie, 68 g	290	11	44	0	4
• Chocolate Malt (Hand-Dipped), 16 fl.oz.	780	35	97	2	17
Chocolate Shake (Hand-Dipped) (reg), 16 fl.oz.	700	34	85	1	15
• Single Scoop Ice Cream Bowl, 113 g	235	13	27	0	5
Single Scoop Ice Cream Cone, 126 g	285	13	37	0	6
Strawberry Malt (Hand-Dipped), 16 fl.oz.	775	33	98	0	17
Strawberry Shake (Hand-Dipped) (reg), 16 fl.oz.	700	33	86	0	14
Vanilla Malt (Hand-Dipped), 16 fl.oz.	770	35	97	0	17
Vanilla Shake (Hand-Dipped) (reg), 16 fl.oz.	710	33	87	0	14
Kids Meal					
• 2 Chicken Strips, 175 g	501	25	50	3	19

Hardee's (cont.)	Cal	Fat	Cbs	Fbr	Prtn
Kids Meal (cont.)					
• Cheeseburger, 210 g	600	27	68	4	21
Hamburger, 197 g	560	24	67	4	18
Lunch & Dinner (Sandwiches & Burger)					
1/2 lb. Grilled Sourdough Thickburger, 381 g	1030	77	42	3	42
1/2 lb. Six Dollar Burger, 412 g	1060	73	58	3	40
1/3 lb. Bacon Cheese Thickburger, 334 g	910	64	50	3	33
1/3 lb. Cheeseburger, 254 g	680	39	52	2	29
1/3 lb. Low Carb Thickburger, 245 g	420	32	5	2	30
1/3 lb. Mushroom 'N' Swiss Thickburger, 276 g	720	42	48	2	35
1/3 lb. Thickburger, 349 g	910	64	53	3	30
1/4 lb. Double Cheeseburger, 186 g	510	26	38	1	28
1/4 lb. Double Hamburger, 161 g	420	19	37	1	23
2/3 lb. Double Bacon Cheese Thickburger, 463 g	1300	97	50	3	54
2/3 lb. Double Thickburger, 471 g	1250	90	54	3	51
• 2/3 lb. Monster Thickburger, 413 g	1420	108	46	2	60
3 Piece Chicken Strips, 145 g	380	21	27	1	22
5 Piece Chicken Strips, 241 g	630	34	45	2	37
Big Chicken Fillet Sandwich, 351 g	800	37	76	3	41
Big Hot Ham 'N' Cheese, 244 g	520	24	40	2	40
Big Roast Beef, 199 g	470	23	38	2	29
Charbroiled BBQ Chicken Sandwich, 242 g	340	4	40	3	33
Charbroiled Chicken Club Sandwich, 277 g	560	30	32	3	39
Cheeseburger, 131 g	350	16	36	1	17
• Hamburger, 118 g	310	12	36	1	14
Hot Dog, 152 g	420	30	22	1	16
Hot Ham 'N' Cheese, 191 g	420	18	39	2	30
Low Carb Charbroiled Chkn Club Sandwich, 250 g	370	21	10	2	35
Regular Roast Beef, 137 g	330	16	29	2	19
Spicy Chicken Sandwich, 159 g	470	25	46	2	13
Sides					
American Cheese slice (large), 16 g	60	5	1	0	3
Au Jus Sauce, 85 g	10	0	2	0	0
Bacon - 2 strips, 9 g	45	4	0	0	3
BBQ Sauce Dipping Sauce, 28 g	45	0	10	1	1
Chicken Gravy, 43 g	20	1	3	0	0
Cole Slaw small, 113 g	170	10	20	2	1
Crispy Curls - Medium, 132 g	410	20	52	4	5
French Fries-Medium, 166 g	520	24	67	5	8
Fried Chicken Breast, 148 g	370	15	29	0	29
Fried Chicken Leg, 69 g	170	7	15	0	13
Fried Chicken Thigh, 121 g	330	15	30	0	19
Fried Chicken Wing, 66 g	200	8	23	0	10
Honey Mustard Dipping Sauce, 28 g	110	9	6	0	0
Horseradish Sauce, 7 g	25	2	1	0	0
• Hot Sauce, 7 g	0	0	0	0	0
Ketchup, 9 g	10	0	2	0	0
Mashed Potatoes small, 142 g	90	2	17	0	1
Mayonnaise, 12 g	90	9	1	0	0
Peach Cobbler, 180 g	280	7	56	1	3
Ranch Dressing Dipping Sauce, 28 g	160	16	2	0	0
Sweet N Sour Dipping Sauce, 28 g	45	0	10	0	0
Swiss Cheese slice, 16 g	50	4	0	0	4

(• = most healthy • = least healthy)   **RESTAURANTS & FAST-FOOD** •

RESTAURANTS & FAST-FOOD CHAINS

Harvey's	Cal	Fat	Cbs	Fbr	Prtn
Breakfast					
• Bacon (3 Strips), 8 g	38	2	0	0	5
• Breakfast Club Deluxe, 264 g	478	24	33	2	34
Breakfast Club, 256 g	440	22	33	2	29
Extra Egg, 50 g	90	6	0	0	12
Homefries, 116 g	300	19	29	3	3
Sausage, 45 g	130	9	3	0	9
Toast (2 Slices White), 71 g	180	2	35	1	6
Toast (2 Slices Whole Wheat), 71 g	170	2	32	3	7
Dipping Sauces					
Creamy Caesar Dressing, 43 g	90	0	21	1	1
• Creamy Garlic Peppercorn Ranch Dressing, 43 g	160	12	13	0	1
Fat Free Honey Dijon Dressing, 43 g	80	1	17	0	0
• Light Italian Dressing, 43 g	80	0	21	0	0
Garnishes					
Bacon (Approx. 2 Slices), 5 g	25	2	0	0	3
Barbecue Sauce, 28 g	50	0	12	0	0
• Hot Peppers, 14 g	0	0	1	1	0
Ketchup, 8ml	10	0	0	0	0
Lettuce, 28 g	4	0	1	0	0
Light Mayonnaise, 15 g	45	5	1	0	0
Mustard, 7ml	5	0	0	0	0
Onions, 50 g	10	0	5	0	1
Pickle (Approx. 2 Slices), 40 g	5	0	0	0	0
• Real Canadian Cheddar Cheese Slice, 14 g	60	5	0	0	3
Relish, 20 g	20	0	5	0	0
Spicy Buffalo Sauce, 28 g	50	4	5	1	0
Tomato (Approx. 2 Slices), 50 g	10	0	2	0	0
Kids Combos					
• Cheeseburger Meal	830	35	112	4	25
• Chicken Strip Meal – 3 pcs.	610	21	92	3	16
Hamburger Meal	780	28	110	4	21
Hot Dog Meal	720	24	110	4	8
Main Menu Items					
Angus Burger w/ Cheese, 160 g	430	20	36	1	24
Angus Burger w/ Cheese, bacon, 183 g	540	29	36	1	29
Angus Burger, 146 g	370	16	36	1	21
Angus Patty only, 91 g	200	13	4	0	16
Chicken Strips – 3 Pieces, 114 g	310	16	24	1	19
Entrée Chicken Salad, 429 g	140	2	16	5	19
Entrée Garden Salad, 366 g	70	1	16	5	4
Grilled Chicken only, 117 g	170	4	1	2	32
Grilled Chicken, 183 g	340	6	32	1	37
Hot Dog only, 57 g	160	12	3	1	5
Hot Dog with Bun, 117 g	320	14	34	2	8
• Original Bacon Cheeseburger, 175 g	540	31	36	2	26
Original Cheeseburger, 160 g	440	23	35	2	21
Original Hamburger, 146 g	380	18	35	2	18
Original Patty only, 80 g	210	16	4	1	13
• Side Garden Salad, 198 g	40	0	8	3	2
Veggieburger, patty only, 73 g	150	7	7	4	15
Veggieburger, 142 g	317	9	39	5	20
Salad Dressings					
• Creamy Caesar Dressing, 29 ml	140	14	2	0	1

RESTAURANTS & FAST-FOOD CHAINS

Harvey's (cont.)

	Cal	Fat	Cbs	Fbr	Prtn
Salad Dressings (cont.)					
Creamy Garlic Peppercorn Ranch Dressing, 29 ml	140	14	2	0	0
• Fat Free Honey Dijon Dressing, 28 ml	50	0	12	0	0
Light Italian Dressing, 28 ml	60	4	6	0	0
Side Orders					
Fries – Regular, 120 g	320	13	46	3	3
Gravy, 92 g	35	1	5	0	1
Onion Rings – Regular, 81 g	280	14	34	1	3
• Poutine, 284 g	630	37	52	2	22

Heavenly Ham

	Cal	Fat	Cbs	Fbr	Prtn
Bone-In Hams					
• All Glaze and Visible Signs of Fat Removed, 3 oz.	159	3	4	N/A	17
• Glazed, 3 oz.	190	11	4	N/A	17
Boneless Hams					
• All Glaze and Visible Signs of Fat Removed, 3 oz.	89	1	4	N/A	17
• Glazed, 3 oz.	120	4	4	N/A	17
Classic Sandwiches					
Dill-ectable Tuna	830	50	67	6	27
Heavenly's Famous Ham Salad	620	13	94	6	27
Perfect Turkey Salad	670	37	59	6	28
Swiss Philly	640	39	44	3	34
The Classic Roast Beef	650	39	52	4	35
The Divine Chicken Salad	790	62	36	2	22
The Heavenly Original	810	46	63	2	29
The Turkey Classic	790	36	86	6	31
• Veggie Heaven	610	37	48	3	23
Desserts					
Chocolate Chip, 1 cookie	270	12	40	1	3
• Fudge Brownie, 1 brownie	430	23	50	2	5
Heath Bar Crunch, 1 cookie	280	14	37	1	2
• Oatmeal Raisin Nut, 1 cookie	260	12	35	2	3
Peanut Butter, 1 cookie	290	18	29	2	7
White Chocolate Macadamia Nut, 1 cookie	290	15	35	1	3
Extras					
• Spinach Dip, 2 tbsp	130	14	2	0	1
• Tomato & Cucumber, 1/2 cup	60	5	5	1	1
Signature Sandwiches					
• Paradise Club	860	51	65	2	29
The Smokehouse	760	46	53	3	35
The Turkey Bistro	730	47	50	3	29
Turkey Ranch Wrangler	730	41	56	3	36
• Zesty Roast Beef	590	30	53	3	36
Soups & Salads					
Chef Salad	170	6	10	3	20
Chicken Salad	210	15	7	0	10
Chicken Salad Salad	260	17	14	3	14
• Garden Delight	35	0	6	3	3
Ham Salad	240	6	26	0	14
Ham Salad Salad	300	8	35	3	18
Heavenly Seven Bean Soup	150	2	24	5	9
• Taste of Italy Salad	490	35	14	4	31
Tuna Salad	290	25	0	0	18
Tuna Salad Salad	360	29	6	3	18

RESTAURANTS & FAST-FOOD CHAINS

Heavenly Ham (cont.)

	Cal	Fat	Cbs	Fbr	Prtn
Soups & Salads (cont.)					
Turkey Salad	330	26	15	3	12
Spreads					
That Mustard, 1 tsp.	25	0	5	N/A	0
Turkeys					
Breast Whole Smoked Turkey, 3 oz.	146	8	1	N/A	18
• Glazed Boneless Smoked Turkey, 3 oz.	60	0	3	N/A	12
• Whole Roasted Turkey, 3 oz.	160	10	0	N/A	17

High Tech Burrito

	Cal	Fat	Cbs	Fbr	Prtn
Asian Pan Seared Shrimp	325	13	N/A	6	N/A
Braised Tofu	467	10	N/A	6	N/A
California	475	11	N/A	9	N/A
Fresh Veggie	460	6	N/A	6	N/A
• Grilled Chicken Breast	237	8	N/A	6	N/A
Grilled Steak Fiesta	259	12	N/A	6	N/A
• Low Fat Chicken	532	10	N/A	6	N/A
Yellow Curry Shrimp	399	6	N/A	4	N/A

Hometown Buffet

	Cal	Fat	Cbs	Fbr	Prtn

For nutritional information please see Country Buffet on pg. 122

Hooters

	Cal	Fat	Cbs	Fbr	Prtn
Entrees					
Dozen Raw Oysters	115	4	7	0	12
• Garden Salad	115	2	22	4	4
• Grilled Big Fish Sandwich	435	5	46	3	52
Grilled Chicken Garden Salad	265	4	23	4	33
Grilled Chicken Sandwich	420	4	51	3	45
Snow Crab Legs, 1 lb	300	4	1	0	61
Steamed Shrimp	230	3	1	0	48
Side Dish					
Baked Beans	115	1	24	3	4
• Coleslaw	120	9	9	1	0
• Side Garden Salad	60	1	12	2	2

Hot Dog On A Stick

	Cal	Fat	Cbs	Fbr	Prtn
Cheese on a Stick					
American Cheese on a Stick, 1 pc	240	13	22	1	9
Pepper Jack Cheese on a Stick, 1 pc	240	13	21	1	9
French Fries					
Fries, 7 oz.	700	37	83	6	9
Fresh Lemonade					
Cherry Lemonade, 18 oz.	230	0	58	0	0
• Lime Lemonade, 18 oz.	250	0	63	0	0
Original Lemonade, 18 oz.	210	0	52	0	0
• Sugar Free Lemonade, 18 oz.	15	0	3	0	0
Hot Dogs					
• Hot Dog on a Bun	470	26	41	2	18
Hot Dog on a Stick™	250	14	23	1	9
• Veggie Dog	180	3	24	2	13

RESTAURANTS & FAST-FOOD CHAINS

Hungry Howie's Pizza	Cal	Fat	Cbs	Fbr	Prtn
Chicken Tenders					
Chicken Tenders, 2 pcs	140	5	11	0	13
Dressings					
Blue Cheese, 1 oz.	150	3	1	0	1
Creamy Italian, 1 oz.	120	2	2	0	0
Fat Free Italian, 2 oz.	25	0	5	0	0
Fat Free Ranch, 2 oz.	45	0	10	1	0
• French Style, 1 oz.	30	0	7	0	0
Greek, 1 oz.	110	2	2	0	0
Italian, 1 oz.	80	1	2	0	0
• Ranch, 1 oz.	180	3	1	0	0
Thousand Island, 1 oz.	140	2	4	0	0
Large Pizza					
Cheese Only Large Pizza, 1 slice	208	5	25	1	12
• Anchovies Topping only, 1 slice	55	3	0	0	9
• Bacon Topping only, 1 slice	42	1	1	0	8
Banana Peppers Topping only, 1 slice	8	0	1	0	0
Beef Topping only, 1 slice	29	2	0	0	1
Black Olives Topping only, 1 slice	10	0	1	0	0
Green Olives Topping only, 1 slice	10	0	1	0	0
• Green Peppers Topping only, 1 slice	2	0	1	0	0
Ham Topping only, 1 slice	7	0	0	0	1
Mushroom Topping only, 1 slice	2	0	0	0	0
Onions Topping only, 1 slice	3	1	0	1	0
Pepperoni Topping only, 1 slice	22	2	0	0	1
Pineapple Topping only, 1 slice	5	1	1	1	1
Sausage Topping only, 1 slice	26	2	0	0	2
Large Thin Pizza					
Cheese Only Large Thin Pizza, 1 slice	124	6	11	1	8
• Anchovies Topping only, 1 slice	55	3	0	0	9
• Bacon Topping only, 1 slice	42	1	1	0	8
Banana Peppers Topping only, 1 slice	8	0	1	0	0
Beef Topping only, 1 slice	29	2	0	0	1
Black Olives Topping only, 1 slice	10	0	1	0	0
Green Olives Topping only, 1 slice	10	0	1	0	0
• Green Peppers Topping only, 1 slice	2	0	1	0	0
Ham Topping only, 1 slice	7	0	0	0	1
Mushroom Topping only, 1 slice	2	0	1	0	0
Onions Topping only, 1 slice	3	1	1	0	1
Pepperoni Topping only, 1 slice	22	2	0	0	1
Pineapple Topping only, 1 slice	5	1	1	1	1
Sausage Topping only, 1 slice	26	2	0	0	2
Medium Pizza					
Cheese Only Medium Pizza, 1 slice	191	6	23	1	11
• Anchovies Topping only, 1 slice	44	3	0	0	7
• Bacon Topping only, 1 slice	32	1	0	0	6
Banana Peppers Topping only, 1 slice	6	0	1	0	0
Beef Topping only, 1 slice	30	0	0	0	2
Black Olives Topping only, 1 slice	7	0	0	0	0
Green Olives Topping only, 1 slice	7	0	0	0	1
Green Peppers Topping Only, 1 slice	2	1	0	0	0
Ham Topping only, 1 slice	7	0	0	0	1
Mushroom Topping only, 1 slice	2	0	0	0	0
Onions Topping only, 1 slice	2	1	0	0	1

Hungry Howie's Pizza (cont.)	Cal	Fat	Cbs	Fbr	Prtn
Medium Pizza (cont.)					
Pepperoni Topping only, 1 slice	22	2	0	0	1
Pineapple Topping only, 1 slice	5	1	2	1	1
Sausage Topping only, 1 slice	27	2	0	0	2
Medium Thin Pizza					
Cheese Only Medium Thin Pizza, 1 slice	111	5	10	0	7
Anchovies Topping only, 1 slice	44	3	0	0	7
Bacon Topping only, 1 slice	32	1	0	0	6
Banana Peppers Topping only, 1 slice	6	0	1	0	0
Beef Topping only, 1 slice	30	2	0	0	2
Black Olives Topping only, 1 slice	7	0	0	0	0
Green Olives Topping only, 1 slice	7	0	0	0	0
Green Peppers Topping only, 1 slice	2	1	0	0	1
Ham Topping only, 1 slice	7	0	0	0	1
Mushroom Topping only, 1 slice	2	0	0	0	0
Onions Topping only, 1 slice	2	1	0	0	1
Pepperoni Topping only, 1 slice	22	2	0	0	1
Pineapple Topping only, 1 slice	5	1	2	1	1
Sausage Topping only, 1 slice	27	2	0	0	2
Oven Baked Subs					
Deluxe Italian Sub, 1/2 sub	506	18	61	2	24
Ham & Cheese Sub, 1/2 sub	475	15	61	2	26
Pizza Special Sub, 1/2 sub	606	24	68	3	29
Pizza Sub, 1/2 sub	689	34	67	3	30
Steak & Cheese Sub, 1/2 sub	491	15	64	2	27
Turkey Club Sub, 1/2 sub	556	15	63	2	42
Turkey Sub, 1/2 sub	466	13	63	2	25
Vegetarian Sub, 1/2 sub	530	21	64	3	22
Salads					
Large Antipasto, 1/4 salad	101	7	3	1	8
Large Chef, 1/4 salad	99	6	4	2	8
Large Garden, 1/4 salad	17	0	3	2	1
Large Greek, 1/4 salad	109	7	7	2	6
Small Antipasto, 1/2 salad	115	7	3	2	9
Small Chef, 1/2 salad	114	7	4	2	9
Small Garden, 1/4 salad	20	0	3	2	1
Small Greek, 1/2 salad	126	7	8	2	7
Sauces					
Blue Cheese Dressing, 1 oz.	152	16	1	0	1
Dipping Sauce, 3 oz.	45	1	9	1	3
Ranch Dressing, 1 oz.	175	19	1	0	0
Small Pizza					
Cheese Only Pizza, 1 slice	161	4	20	1	10
Anchovies Topping only, 1 slice	34	3	0	0	5
Bacon Topping only, 1 slice	23	0	0	0	4
Banana Peppers Topping only, 1 slice	5	0	0	0	0
Beef Topping only, 1 slice	21	1	0	0	1
Black Olives Topping only, 1 slice	5	0	0	0	0
Green Olives Topping only, 1 slice	5	0	0	0	0
Green Peppers Topping only, 1 slice	1	0	0	0	0
Ham Topping only	6	0	0	0	1
Mushroom Topping only	2	0	0	0	0
Onions Topping only	1	0	0	0	0
Pepperoni Topping only	20	2	0	0	1

RESTAURANTS & FAST-FOOD CHAINS

Hungry Howie's Pizza (cont.)

	Cal	Fat	Cbs	Fbr	Prtn
Small Pizza (cont.)					
Pineapple Topping only, 1 slice	4	0	1	1	0
Sausage Topping only, 1 slice	20	1	0	0	1
Wings					
Howie Wings, 5 wings	180	13	0	0	14
X-Large Pizza					
Cheese Only Extra Large Pizza, 1 slice	395	9	395	2	23
Anchovies Topping only, 1 slice	88	5	88	0	14
Bacon Topping only, 1 slice	52	1	52	0	10
Banana Peppers Topping only, 1 slice	12	0	12	0	0
Beef Topping only, 1 slice	37	3	37	0	2
Black Olives Topping only, 1 slice	11	1	11	0	0
Green Olives Topping only, 1 slice	11	1	11	0	0
Green Peppers Topping only, 1 slice	2	0	2	0	0
Ham Topping only, 1 slice	8	1	8	0	2
Mushroom Topping only, 1 slice	3	0	3	0	0
Onions Topping only, 1 slice	3	1	3	0	1
Pepperoni Topping only, 1 slice	26	2	26	0	1
Pineapple Topping only, 1 slice	6	1	6	1	0
Sausage Topping only, 1 slice	33	2	33	0	2

In-N-Out Burger

	Cal	Fat	Cbs	Fbr	Prtn
Burgers					
Cheeseburger w/Onion, 268 g	480	27	39	3	22
Protein® Style (no bun), 300 g	330	25	11	3	18
with mustard & ketchup, no spread, 268 g	400	18	41	3	22
Double-Double® w/ Onion, 330 g	670	41	39	3	37
Protein® Style (no bun), 362 g	520	39	11	3	33
with mustard & ketchup, no spread, 330 g	590	32	41	3	37
Hamburger w/ Onion, 243 g	390	19	39	3	16
Protein® Style (no bun), 275 g	240	17	11	3	13
with mustard & ketchup, no spread, 243 g	310	10	41	3	16
Shakes					
Chocolate Shake, 15 oz.	690	36	83	0	9
Strawberry Shake, 15 oz.	690	33	91	0	9
Vanilla Shake, 15 oz.	680	37	78	0	9
Sides					
French Fries, 125 g	400	18	54	2	7

Islands Restaurants

	Cal	Fat	Cbs	Fbr	Prtn
Appetizers					
Cheddar Fries, 4 oz.	310	20	27	N/A	N/A
Chips & Salsa, 4 oz.	290	12	43	N/A	N/A
Island Fries, 5 oz.	420	31	32	N/A	N/A
Nachos, 4 oz.	400	29	20	N/A	N/A
Onion Rings, 4 oz.	380	15	55	N/A	N/A
Quesadilla, 4 oz.	290	20	18	N/A	N/A
Spinach-Artichoke Dip w/ Chips, 4 oz.	290	19	25	N/A	N/A
Tiki Tenders, 5 oz.	360	21	15	N/A	N/A
Wings - Buffalo Style, 11 oz.	780	60	10	N/A	N/A
Burgers					
Big Wave w/ Cheese, 17 oz.	1220	75	69	N/A	N/A
Big Wave, 15 oz.	990	57	63	N/A	N/A
Bleunami, 16 oz.	1290	88	65	N/A	N/A

Islands Restaurants (cont.)

	Cal	Fat	Cbs	Fbr	Prtn
Burgers (cont.)					
Hawaiian, 19 oz.	1450	91	85	N/A	N/A
Hula, 20 oz.	1390	90	70	N/A	N/A
• Kilauea, 20 oz.	1650	115	80	N/A	N/A
Maui, 18 oz.	1430	96	72	N/A	N/A
Pipeline, 20 oz.	1430	91	72	N/A	N/A
Sunset, 18 oz.	1250	75	75	N/A	N/A
• Veggie, 11 oz.	630	24	90	N/A	N/A
Dessert					
Chocolate Lava Dessert, 5 oz.	480	29	50	N/A	N/A
Kona Pie, 4 oz.	350	23	34	N/A	N/A
Gremmie					
Gremmie Fries, 4 oz.	290	17	32	N/A	N/A
Jr. Quesadilla w/ applesauce/carrots, 10 oz.	560	26	72	N/A	N/A
• Jr. Sundae, 3 oz.	220	15	17	N/A	N/A
Jr. Tiki Tenders w/ applesauce/carrots, 12 oz.	630	24	69	N/A	N/A
Jr. Wave w/chz, w/ applesauce/carrots, 14 oz.	760	40	65	N/A	N/A
• Lil Chili Chz Dogger w/ applesauce/carrots, 16 oz.	1050	71	66	N/A	N/A
Lil Dogger w/ applesauce/carrots, 11 oz.	630	36	62	N/A	N/A
Sandcastle w/ applesauce/carrots, 10 oz.	520	21	66	N/A	N/A
Salads					
• Caesar - small, 5 oz.	270	20	14	N/A	N/A
China Coast, 25 oz.	1130	73	75	N/A	N/A
Garden salad, 8 oz.	300	27	3	N/A	N/A
Jungle Caesar - w/ chicken, 18 oz.	760	43	25	N/A	N/A
• Kaanapali Kobb, 30 oz.	1520	116	21	N/A	N/A
Wiqui Waqui, 29 oz.	960	53	47	N/A	N/A
Sandwiches & Other Items					
Moa kai (Tuna), 14 oz.	1310	101	65	N/A	N/A
• Rotisserie Chicken, 35 oz.	1650	80	148	N/A	N/A
Sandpiper, 18 oz.	1020	51	70	N/A	N/A
• Shorebird, 14 oz.	990	50	69	N/A	N/A
Toucan, 15 oz.	1050	52	79	N/A	N/A
Wedge, 12 oz.	1320	100	62	N/A	N/A
Soup					
Tortilla Soup - bowl, 12 oz.	320	20	20	N/A	N/A
Tortilla Soup - Large, 23 oz.	630	39	40	N/A	N/A
Tacos					
Baja, 23 oz.	870	35	70	N/A	N/A
• Cabo Loco, 19 oz.	1480	104	65	N/A	N/A
Islands Fish, 19 oz.	1320	84	100	N/A	N/A
• Northshore, 19 oz.	790	30	67	N/A	N/A
Yaki, 19 oz.	960	34	85	N/A	N/A

Jack in the Box

	Cal	Fat	Cbs	Fbr	Prtn
Breakfast					
Bacon Breakfast Jack®, 113 g	300	14	29	1	16
Bacon, Egg & Cheese Biscuit, 149 g	430	25	34	1	17
Blueberry French Toast Sticks, 121 g	450	20	59	3	8
Breakfast Jack®, 125 g	290	12	29	1	17
Chicken Biscuit, 154 g	450	24	42	2	15
Ciabatta Breakfast Sandwich, 278 g	710	36	63	3	36
Extreme Sausage® Sandwich, 213 g	670	48	31	2	29
• Hash Brown, 57 g	150	10	13	2	1

Jack in the Box (cont.)

	Cal	Fat	Cbs	Fbr	Prtn
Breakfast (cont.)					
Meaty Breakfast Burrito, 183 g	480	29	29	2	25
Original French Toast Sticks, 121 g	470	23	58	4	7
Sausage Biscuit, 131 g	440	29	32	2	12
Sausage Breakfast Jack®, 154 g	450	28	29	1	20
Sausage Croissant, 174 g	580	39	37	2	21
Sausage, Egg & Cheese Biscuit, 234 g	740	55	35	2	27
Sirloin Steak & Egg Burrito no Salsa, 289 g	790	48	52	6	37
• Sirloin Steak & Egg Burrito w/ Salsa, 312 g	790	48	54	6	37
Spicy Chicken Biscuit, 169 g	460	22	44	2	21
Supreme Croissant, 151 g	450	25	36	1	20
Ultimate Breakfast Sandwich, 249 g	570	27	49	2	34
Burgers & More					
Bacon 'n' Cheese Ciabatta Burger, 395 g	1120	76	66	4	45
Bacon Ultimate Cheeseburger, 338 g	1090	77	53	2	46
BBQ Bacon Sirloin Burger, 336 g	1010	49	91	4	52
Hamburger deluxe, 169 g	370	21	31	2	17
with Cheese, 194 g	460	28	33	2	21
• Hamburger, 118 g	310	14	30	1	16
with Cheese, 131 g	350	17	31	1	18
Jumbo Jack®, 261 g	600	35	51	3	21
with Cheese, 286 g	690	42	54	3	25
Junior Bacon Cheeseburger, 131 g	430	25	30	1	20
• Sirloin Bcn Chz Burger w/ Onions, 422 g	1160	76	61	4	58
Sirloin Chz Brgr w/ Grilled Onions, 421 g	1070	71	61	4	53
Sirloin Steak Melt, 277 g	640	40	34	2	36
Sngle Bacon Chz Ciabatta Burger, 308 g	870	54	66	4	31
Sourdough Jack®, 245 g	710	51	36	3	27
Sourdough Ultimate Cheeseburger, 291 g	950	73	36	2	38
Ultimate Cheeseburger, 323 g	1010	71	53	2	40
Chicken & Fish					
Bacon Chicken Sandwich, 152 g	440	24	39	2	1
Chicken Breast Strips (4), 201 g	500	25	36	3	3
• Chicken Fajita Pita - no salsa, 185 g	280	9	30	2	2
Chicken Sandwich, 145 g	400	21	38	2	1
Chipotle Chkn Ciabatta™ with Grilled Chkn, 312 g	690	28	65	4	4
w/ Spicy Crispy Chkn, 297 g	750	34	75	5	3
Fish & Chips - medium, 250 g	660	34	70	5	1
Jack's Spicy Chicken®, 270 g	620	31	61	4	2
w/ Cheese, 294 g	700	37	62	4	2
• Sirloin Steak 'n' Cheddar Ciabatta, 325 g	770	38	65	4	4
Sourdough Grilled Chicken Club, 266 g	530	28	34	3	3
Kids Meal					
• Applesauce (1 portion cup), 113 g	100	0	25	1	0
Chicken Breast Strips (2), 100 g	250	12	18	2	17
Grilled Cheese, 94 g	330	18	31	2	11
Hamburger, 118 g	310	14	30	1	16
• w/ cheese, 131 g	350	17	31	1	18
Natural Cut Fries - kids portion, 82 g	220	11	27	3	3
Salads					
Asian Chkn Salad (w/ Grilled Chkn), 365 g	160	2	18	5	22
(w/ Crispy Chicken), 394 g	330	13	34	7	21
Chkn Club Salad (w/ Grilled Chkn), 373 g	320	16	11	4	34
(w/ Crispy Chicken), 402 g	480	27	28	6	33

(• = most healthy • = least healthy) **RESTAURANTS & FAST-FOOD • 199**

Jack in the Box (cont.)

	Cal	Fat	Cbs	Fbr	Prtn
Salads (cont.)					
• Side Salad, 123 g	50	3	5	2	3
SW Chkn Salad (w/ Grilled Chkn), 430 g	320	12	27	7	31
(w/ Crispy Chicken), 459 g	480	23	44	9	30
Sauces & Dressings					
Asian Sesame Dressing, 71 g	230	17	20	0	1
Bacon Ranch Dressing, 71 g	320	33	4	0	2
Barbecue Dipping Sauce, 28 g	45	0	11	0	0
Buttermilk House Dipping Sauce, 25 g	130	13	3	0	0
Creamy Southwest Dressing, 71 g	270	27	4	0	1
Franks® Red Hot® Buffalo Dipping Sauce, 28 g	10	0	2	0	0
Lite Ranch Dressing, 71 g	190	18	3	0	1
Log Cabin® Syrup, 62 g	190	0	49	0	0
Low Fat Balsamic Dressing, 71 g	40	2	6	0	0
Mayo-Onion Sauce (0.5 oz), 14 g	90	10	1	0	0
• Ranch Dressing, 71 g	390	41	4	0	1
Soy Sauce, 9 g	5	0	1	0	1
Sweet & Sour Dipping Sauce, 28 g	45	0	11	0	0
• Taco Sauce, 9 g	0	0	0	0	0
Tartar Sauce, 43 g	210	22	2	0	0
Zesty Marinara Dipping Sauce, 25 g	15	0	4	0	0
Shakes & Desserts					
Cheesecake, 103 g	310	16	34	0	7
Chocolate Ice Cream Shake, 16 oz.	880	45	107	1	14
• Chocolate Overload Cake, 93 g	300	7	57	0	4
Egg Nog Shake, 16 oz.	870	44	103	0	13
• OREO® Cookie Ice Cream Shake, 16 oz.	910	49	102	1	14
Strawberry Ice Cream Shake, 16 oz.	880	44	105	0	13
Vanilla Ice Cream Shake, 16 oz.	790	44	83	0	13
Snacks & Extras					
Bacon Cheddar Potato Wedges, 257 g	720	48	52	4	21
Beef Monster Taco®, 112 g	240	14	20	3	8
Egg Roll (1), 57 g	130	6	15	2	5
Egg Rolls (3), 170 g	400	19	44	6	14
• Fruit Cup, 198 g	90	0	22	2	1
Mozzarella Cheese Sticks (3), 71 g	240	12	21	1	11
Natural Cut Fries - medium, 166 g	450	23	54	6	6
Onion Rings (8), 119 g	500	30	51	3	6
Regular Beef Taco, 76 g	160	8	15	2	5
• Sampler Trio, 236 g	750	39	65	5	35
Seasoned Curly Fries - medium, 125 g	400	23	45	5	6
Spicy Chicken Bites (7), 93 g	290	14	21	3	18
Stuffed Jalapeños (3), 72 g	230	13	22	2	7

Jack's

	Cal	Fat	Cbs	Fbr	Prtn
Breakfast Items					
Bacon Biscuit	290	15	31	10	8
Biscuit	250	11	31	10	5
Biscuit w/butter	350	23	31	10	5
• Egg and Cheese Biscuit	550	34	35	10	26
• Eggs	190	13	3	10	14
Sausage Biscuit	400	25	31	10	13
Chicken & Sides					
Chicken Breast	321	19	9	0	28

RESTAURANTS & FAST-FOOD CHAINS

Jack's (cont.)

	Cal	Fat	Cbs	Fbr	Prtn
Chicken & Sides (cont.)					
• Chicken Fingers, 3 Pieces	470	24	33	0	30
Chicken Leg	150	10	5	0	11
Chicken Thigh	260	19	9	0	13
Chicken Wings	170	12	6	0	9
• Mashed Potatoes, 4 oz.	70	1	15	2	0
Healthy Choice					
• Crispy Chicken	430	26	22	2	27
Grilled Chicken	260	12	7	2	30
Grilled Chicken Sandwich	410	15	44	6	25
Grits	100	8	8	2	1
• Side Salad	70	5	3	1	4
Spring Salad	170	11	7	2	11
Low Carb Items					
4 oz. Burger Patty w/cheese & 4 oz. green beans	670	48	10	3	50
• Eggs & Bacon Platter w/ 2 eggs & 3 slices bacon	250	18	3	0	19
Grilled Chkn w/ 4 oz. Green Beans & Cole Slaw	320	16	22	10	21
Sandwiches & Fries					
Big Bacon	700	42	45	18	36
Big Jack	500	27	40	4	25
Cheeseburger	380	17	35	4	22
• Double Big Jack Cheese	930	60	43	4	56
Double Cheeseburger	590	33	37	4	38
• Hamburger	270	9	35	4	15

Jamba Juice

	Cal	Fat	Cbs	Fbr	Prtn
All Fruit					
Mega Mango, 24 fl.oz.	340	1	85	6	4
Peach Perfection, 24 fl.oz.	320	1	78	6	2
• Pomegranate Paradise, 24 fl.oz.	340	1	86	5	2
• Strawberry Whirl, 24 fl.oz.	310	1	76	6	2
Baked Goods					
Apple Cinnamon Pretzel, 5 oz.	380	4	76	4	11
Blueberry Oatcake, 3 oz.	280	10	42	7	6
• Omega-3 Choc. Brownie Cookie, 1.5 oz.	150	4	30	2	N/A
Omega-3 Oatmeal Cookie, 2 oz.	150	6	26	3	2
Reduced-Fat Blueberry Lemon Loaf, 3 oz.	290	8	53	2	2
Reduced-Fat Cranberry Orange Loaf, 3 oz.	310	9	52	4	6
• Sourdough Parmesan Pretzel, 5 oz.	410	10	67	3	14
Zucchini Walnut Loaf, 3 oz.	270	9	43	4	5
Blended with A Purpose					
3 g Energizer, 24 fl.oz.	470	2	110	6	3
Acai Super-Antidoxidant, 24 fl.oz.	420	6	86	5	7
Coldbuster, 24 fl.oz.	410	3	95	5	5
• Fit n' Fruitful, 24 fl.oz.	370	4	84	6	3
Pomegranate Heart Defender, 24 fl.oz.	440	1	103	4	6
Protein Berry w/ Soy Protein, 24 fl.oz.	430	2	88	5	19
Protein Berry w /Whey, 24 fl.oz.	390	1	80	5	19
Boosts					
3 g Charger Super Boost, 3 g	5	0	2	2	N/A
Green Caffeine Boost, 2.7 g	5	0	2	2	N/A
Omega-3 Super Boost, 10 g	30	2	7	1	1
Soy Protein Boost, 8.9 g	30	N/A	N/A	N/A	8
Weight Burner Super Boost, 3.5 g	30	3	N/A	N/A	N/A

(• = most healthy • = least healthy) **RESTAURANTS & FAST-FOOD • 201**

RESTAURANTS & FAST-FOOD CHAINS

Jamba Juice (cont.)

	Cal	Fat	Cbs	Fbr	Prtn
Boosts (cont.)					
• Whey Protein Super Boost, 12 g	45	0	1	N/A	10
Creamy Indulgences					
• Matcha Green Tea Blast, 24 fl.oz.	440	1	97	1	10
Orange Dream Machine, 24 fl.oz.	490	2	107	1	11
• Peanut Butter Moo'd, 24 fl.oz.	840	21	139	7	25
Fresh Squeezed Juices					
Carrot Juice, 16 fl.oz.	90	1	22	0	4
Orange Juice, 16 fl.oz.	220	1	52	1	3
Jamba Classic					
Aloha Pineapple, 24 fl.oz.	470	2	111	4	8
Banana Berry, 24 fl.oz.	450	2	106	5	4
Caribbean Passion, 24 fl.oz.	420	2	97	4	3
Citrus Squeeze, 24 fl.oz.	440	2	104	4	5
Mango-a-go-go, 24 fl.oz.	470	2	110	4	3
• Orange a Peel, 24 fl.oz.	400	1	93	4	8
Peach Pleasure, 24 fl.oz.	440	2	104	4	4
Razzmatazz, 24 fl.oz.	440	2	102	4	3
Strawberries Wild, 24 fl.oz.	400	1	94	4	5
• Strawberry Surf Rider, 24 fl.oz.	490	2	119	4	3
Jamba Light					
Berry Fulfilling, 24 fl.oz.	260	1	57	8	8
• Mango Mantra, 24 fl.oz.	280	1	64	5	9
• Strawberry Nirvana, 24 fl.oz.	250	1	55	6	8
Juices					
Orange Carrot Banana, 16 fl.oz.	170	1	40	1	3
Orange Mango Passion, 16 fl.oz.	180	1	43	1	2
Shots					
Matcha Green Tea Shot-OJ, 4 fl.oz.	60	0	13	1	1
• Matcha Green Tea Shot-Soy Milk, 4 fl.oz.	80	0	16	1	3
• Wheatgrass Shot, 1 fl.oz.	5	0	1	0	1
Wheatgrass Shot, 2 fl.oz.	15	0	1	0	1
Smoothies with Organic Granola					
• Berry Topper, 16 fl.oz.	490	10	89	10	13
• Chunky Strawberry, 16 fl.oz.	570	17	91	9	17
Mango Peach Topper, 16 fl.oz.	500	10	95	9	13
Yogurt & Fruit Blends					
• Bright Eyed & Blueberry, 16 fl.oz.	220	1	43	2	11
Bright Eyed & Blueberry, 24 fl.oz.	350	1	70	4	16
Sunrise Strawberry, 16 fl.oz.	240	1	49	2	11
• Sunrise Strawberry, 24 fl.oz.	380	1	78	4	17

Jimboy's Tacos

	Cal	Fat	Cbs	Fbr	Prtn
Burritos					
• Bean, 255 g	530	28	55	6	16
Chicken, 213 g	590	29	45	3	37
• Ground Beef, 213 g	610	32	50	2	29
Shredded Beef, 213 g	540	24	45	3	36
Combo Burritos					
• Chicken, 284 g	580	28	52	5	28
• Ground Beef, 284 g	620	33	57	5	25
Shredded Beef, 284 g	580	28	53	6	29
Dessert					
ChocoTaco, 113 g	390	21	47	1	5

Jimboy's Tacos (cont.)

	Cal	Fat	Cbs	Fbr	Prtn
Dinner Plates					
Bean Burrito, 255 g	530	28	55	6	16
Bean Taco, 112 g	190	12	16	3	6
Cheese Enchilada, 168 g	390	27	16	2	22
Chicken Combo Burrito, 284 g	580	28	52	5	28
Chicken Enchilada, 168 g	320	18	16	2	22
Chicken Taco, 106 g	200	11	12	2	12
Chile Relleno, 128 g	300	24	8	2	14
Combination Plate Base, 354 g	470	15	71	7	12
• Ground Beef Combo Burrito, 284 g	620	33	57	5	25
Ground Beef Enchilada, 168 g	330	20	19	2	19
Ground Beef Taco, 106 g	220	14	15	2	10
Shredded Beef Combo Burrito, 284 g	580	28	53	6	29
Shredded Beef Enchilada, 168 g	300	17	16	2	22
• Shredded Beef Taco, 106 g	190	11	13	2	13
El Gordos					
Chicken, 208 g	400	20	29	2	26
• Ground Beef, 208 g	460	25	35	2	23
Shredded Beef, 208 g	400	19	30	3	27
• Steak, 222 g	400	18	33	3	29
Enchiladas					
Cheese (Includes Rice), 168 g	350	20	28	2	16
Chicken (Includes Rice), 253 g	460	21	42	2	25
• Ground Beef (Includes Rice), 253 g	470	23	45	2	21
• Shredded Beef (Includes Rice), 168 g	300	17	16	2	22
Kid's Meals					
• Cheese Quesadilla & Chips, 166 g	690	40	63	5	21
Ground Beef Taco & Chips, 170 g	510	29	51	5	14
• Kid-Size Bean Burrito & Chips, 179 g	480	25	54	6	11
Quesadillas					
• Cheese, 109 g	400	25	27	2	18
Chicken, 144 g	450	26	28	2	24
• Ground Beef, 144 g	480	29	31	2	23
Shredded Beef, 144 g	450	26	28	2	25
Side Orders					
6" Corn Tortilla, 27 g	60	1	12	1	0
8" Flour Tortilla, 52 g	170	4	28	2	0
Corn Chips, 69 g	280	15	36	4	0
• French Fries, 250 g	700	34	89	8	0
Side Cheese Sauce, 2 oz.	70	4	7	0	0
Side Guacamole, 2 oz.	90	8	4	2	0
• Side Salsa Cruda, 2 oz.	10	0	2	1	0
Side Sour Cream, 2 oz.	110	11	2	0	0
Super Burritos					
Chicken, 406 g	630	31	58	8	29
• Ground Beef, 392 g	670	35	63	8	27
Shredded Beef, 392 g	610	29	58	8	31
• Steak, 401 g	600	28	59	8	32
Super Nachos					
• Chicken, 420 g	830	45	86	9	26
• Ground Beef, 393 g	780	40	78	12	29
Shredded Beef, 420 g	830	44	87	9	27
Taco Salads					
Bean, 513 g	530	29	50	10	18

(• = most healthy • = least healthy)   **RESTAURANTS & FAST-FOOD • 203**

RESTAURANTS & FAST-FOOD CHAINS

Jimboy's Tacos (cont.)

	Cal	Fat	Cbs	Fbr	Prtn
Taco Salads (cont.)					
• Ground Beef, 584 g	660	37	56	10	30
Chicken, 584 g	610	31	50	10	33
Shredded Beef, 584 g	610	31	51	10	35
Tacoburger					
Ground Beef (Patty), 183 g	370	27	17	2	15
Tacos					
Bean, 112 g	190	12	16	3	6
Chicken, 106 g	200	11	12	2	12
Ground Beef, 106 g	220	14	15	2	10
• Jimboy's Fish Taco, 129 g	233	15	16	inc	10
Shredded Beef, 106 g	190	11	13	2	13
• Steak, 134 g	190	10	15	2	14
Taquitos					
Ground Beef (3 in a serving), 90 g	230	17	16	3	5
The Works					
• Guacamole & Sour Cream, 61 g	90	8	4	1	1
• Guacamole, 34 g	35	3	2	1	0
Sour Cream, 42 g	50	5	2	0	1
Tostadas					
• Bean, 241 g	290	20	23	5	8
Chicken, 276 g	330	21	23	5	15
• Ground Beef, 276 g	360	24	26	5	14
Shredded Beef, 276 g	330	21	23	5	16
Vegetarian					
Bean Burrito, 255 g	530	28	55	6	16
Bean Taco, 112 g	190	12	16	3	6
Bean Tostada, 241 g	290	20	23	5	8
Cheese Enchilada & Rice, 168 g	350	20	28	2	16
Cheese Quesadilla, 109 g	400	25	27	2	18
• Chile Relleno & Rice, 304 g	530	32	40	2	20
Reg.Nachos (Chips & Cheese), 162 g	360	19	43	4	6
• Side Pinto Beans, 213 g	180	11	16	5	6
Side Spanish Rice, 164 g	260	5	48	1	5
Veggie Burrito, 354 g	500	17	72	7	15

Jimmy John's

	Cal	Fat	Cbs	Fbr	Prtn
8" Sub Sandwiches					
Big John®, 270 g	564	27	54	1	24
J.J.B.L.T.™, 238 g	662	35	54	1	29
• Pepe®, 298 g	684	37	55	1	30
• Totally Tuna™, 357 g	507	20	58	3	23
Turkey Tom®, 282 g	555	26	54	1	24
Vegetarian, 302 g	640	36	57	2	21
Vito®, 289 g	579	25	56	1	32
Giant Club Sandwiches					
Beach Club®, 409 g	796	37	78	2	37
Billy Club®, 416 g	867	40	77	1	48
• Bootlegger Club®, 377 g	720	28	74	1	40
Club Lulu™, 339 g	790	34	74	1	42
Club Tuna®, 429 g	724	29	79	3	35
Country Club®, 405 g	840	38	75	1	47
Gourmet Smoked Ham Club, 399 g	851	37	76	1	45
Gourmet Veggie Club®, 374 g	856	46	77	2	33

RESTAURANTS & FAST-FOOD CHAINS

Jimmy John's (cont.)	Cal	Fat	Cbs	Fbr	Prtn
Giant Club Sandwiches (cont.)					
Hunter's Club®, 411 g	854	38	76	1	49
• Italian Night Club®, 422 g	975	52	77	1	47
Low-Carb Options					
Hunter's Club® Unwich, 357 g	520	38	8	2	35
The J.J. Gargantuan™ Unwich, 488 g	769	55	11	2	57
Low-Fat Options					
Slim 4 Turkey Breast, 207 g	407	1	70	0	27
Turkey Tom®, 282 g	555	26	54	1	24
Plain Slims					
Slim 1 Ham & Cheese, 235 g	539	12	72	0	34
Slim 2 Roast Beef, 207 g	419	2	71	0	27
Slim 3 Tuna Salad, 272 g	582	19	74	1	25
• Slim 4 Turkey Breast, 207 g	407	1	70	0	27
Slim 5 Salami, Capicola, Cheese, 232 g	624	21	72	0	35
Slim 6 Double Provolone, 206 g	588	19	71	0	32
• The J.J. Gargantuan™, 504 g	1008	55	60	1	67
Side Items					
BBQ Jimmy Chips, 30 g	160	9	17	0	2
• Chocolate Chunk Cookie, 99 g	421	18	62	1	5
Jalapeño Chips, 30 g	150	7	18	1	2
• Pickle, Spear, 25 g	4	0	1	0	0
Pickle, Whole, 100 g	15	0	3	1	0
Raisin Oatmeal Cookie, 105 g	421	16	65	4	7
Regular Chips, 30 g	160	8	18	0	2
Sea Salt & Vinegar Chips, 30 g	140	8	16	0	2

Johnny Rockets	Cal	Fat	Cbs	Fbr	Prtn
Chicken & Salads					
• Chicken Club Sandwich, 371 g	1068	39	126	3	63
Chicken Tenders, 213 g	520	22	47	2	35
Crispy Chicken Club Salad, 434 g	651	40	46	4	42
• Garden Salad, 305 g	271	19	21	3	17
Grilled Chicken Breast Sandwich, 271 g	632	33	52	4	34
Grilled Chicken Club Salad, 420 g	529	33	23	5	51
Desserts					
• A La Mode, 113 g	260	16	26	0	3
• Apple Pie, 293 g	930	59	88	6	9
Hot Fudge Sundae, 290 g	830	47	93	0	2
Fountain					
Add Malt, 14 g	60	2	10	0	2
• Big Apple Shake, 670 g	1585	90	175	5	20
Butterfinger® Shake, 517 g	1020	58	114	2	16
Chocolate Peanut Butter Shake, 510 g	1000	62	80	2	14
• Float, 411 g	420	26	42	0	5
Hershey's® Chocolate Shake, 574 g	1100	60	120	4	16
Mocha Fudge Shake, 488 g	870	52	89	0	6
Oreo® Cookies & Cream Shake, 517 g	1040	60	114	2	16
Strawberry Shake, 574 g	810	48	82	0	14
Strawberry-Banana Shake, 573 g	890	49	102	2	15
Vanilla Shake, 574 g	1120	60	131	2	15
Kids Fountain					
Add Malt, 8 g	36	1	6	0	1
• Big Apple, 402 g	951	36	79	1	9

(• = most healthy • = least healthy)   **RESTAURANTS & FAST-FOOD • 205**

RESTAURANTS & FAST-FOOD CHAINS

Johnny Rockets (cont.)

	Cal	Fat	Cbs	Fbr	Prtn
Kids Fountain (cont.)					
Butterfinger® Shake, 310 g	612	35	68	1	10
Chocolate Peanut Butter Shake, 306 g	600	37	48	1	8
• Float, 247 g	252	16	25	0	3
Hershey's® Chocolate Shake, 344 g	660	36	72	2	10
Kids Jr. Sundae, 226 g	580	32	65	1	6
Mocha Fudge Shake, 293 g	522	31	53	0	4
Oreo® Cookies & Cream Shake, 310 g	624	36	68	1	10
Strawberry Shake, 344 g	486	29	49	0	8
Strawberry-banana Shake, 344 g	534	29	61	1	9
Vanilla Shake, 344 g	672	36	79	1	9
Kids Menu					
American Fries, 114 g	266	12	39	5	4
• Kids Chicken Tenders, 107 g	260	11	24	1	18
Kids Grilled Cheese, 87 g	386	18	40	0	14
Kids Hamburger, 121 g	378	17	38	1	18
Kids Hot Dog, 133 g	422	24	38	1	12
• Kids Peanut Butter & Jelly, 138 g	457	17	64	1	13
Original Hamburgers					
#12, 349 g	880	57	58	3	35
• Chili, 464 g	1254	84	67	6	60
Patty Melt, 261 g	786	48	48	3	39
Rocket Double®, 406 g	1192	79	58	3	62
Rocket Single®, 296 g	832	52	57	3	35
Route 66, 301 g	911	63	53	3	35
Smoke House, 294 g	972	60	60	3	49
St. Louis, 313 g	991	68	53	3	43
• Streamliner®, 299 g	422	11	60	8	26
The Original, 322 g	790	50	57	3	30
Turkey Single, 287 g	732	42	56	3	34
Other Favorites					
Bacon, Lettuce & Tomato, 201 g	491	30	42	1	19
• Chili Dog, 289 g	815	55	46	3	32
Egg Salad Sandwich, 313 g	688	49	41	3	26
Grilled Cheese, 151 g	542	30	40	0	21
Grilled Ham & Cheese, 243 g	514	24	40	0	16
• Hot Dog, 133 g	422	24	38	1	12
Philly Cheese Steak, 361 g	715	30	58	3	50
Tuna Melt, 300 g	754	45	40	3	48
Tuna Salad Sandwich, 313 g	708	46	41	3	39
Starters					
American Fries, 227 g	531	23	77	9	7
Cheese Fries, 284 g	759	42	78	9	21
• Chili Bowl, 369 g	872	69	24	5	39
Half Fries & Half Rings, 264 g	720	36	92	9	9
Onion Rings, 193 g	500	34	22	4	29
Rocket Wings® – Large Order, 276 g	538	20	33	0	50
• Rocket Wings® – Regular Order, 138 g	323	10	17	0	25

Kentucky Fried Chicken

	Cal	Fat	Cbs	Fbr	Prtn
Chicken					
• Extra Crispy Breast, 162 g	440	27	15	0	34
Extra Crispy Drumstick, 60 g	160	10	6	0	12
Extra Crispy Thigh, 114 g	370	28	12	0	18

RESTAURANTS & FAST-FOOD CHAINS

Kentucky Fried Chicken (cont.)	Cal	Fat	Cbs	Fbr	Prtn
Chicken (cont.)					
Extra Crispy Whole Wing, 52 g	170	11	6	1	12
Original Breast w/o skin, breading, 108 g	140	2	1	0	29
Original Breast, 161 g	360	21	7	0	37
• Original Drumstick, 59 g	130	8	2	0	12
Original Thigh, 126 g	330	24	8	0	20
Original Whole Wing, 47 g	130	8	4	0	11
Desserts					
Apple Pie Mini's (3), 114 g	370	20	44	2	2
Double Choc. Chip Cake, 76 g	330	16	41	1	4
Lil' Bucket™ Chocolate Cream, 113 g	280	13	38	3	3
Lil' Bucket™ Lemon Crème, 127 g	410	15	61	2	7
Lil' Bucket™ Strawberry Short Cake, 99 g	210	7	33	1	2
Sweet Life Chocolate Chip Cookie, 35 g	160	7	23	1	2
Sweet Life Oatmeal Raisin Cookie, 35 g	150	5	24	1	2
Sweet Life Sugar Cookie, 35 g	160	6	23	0	2
• Teddy Grahams®, Cinnamon, 21 g	90	3	15	1	1
Popcorn Chicken					
Popcorn Chicken-Individual, 116 g	400	26	22	3	21
• Popcorn Chicken-Kids, 85 g	290	19	16	2	16
Popcorn Chicken-Large, 160 g	550	35	30	3	29
Pot Pie / Bowls					
• Chicken and Biscuit Bowl, 481 g	870	44	88	7	29
Chicken Pot Pie, 423 g	770	40	70	5	33
KFC Bowls™-Mshd Potato w/ Gravy, 531 g	740	35	80	7	27
• KFC Bowls™-Rice w/ Gravy, 384 g	620	28	67	6	26
Salads & More					
Caesar Side Salad w/o Dressing/croutons, 82 g	50	3	2	1	4
Crispy BLT Salad w/o Dressing, 360 g	330	17	18	4	28
• Crspy Caesar Salad w/o Dressing/croutons, 315 g	350	19	16	3	29
Hidden Valley® Ranch Dressing, 57 g	200	20	3	0	1
Hidden Valley® Golden Italian Light Dressing, 43 g	45	3	6	0	0
Hidden Valley® Ranch Fat Free Dressing, 43 g	35	0	8	0	1
• House Side Salad w/o Dressing, 90 g	15	0	2	1	1
KFC® Creamy Parmesan Caesar Dressing, 57 g	260	26	4	0	2
KFC® Parmesan Garlic Croutons Pouch, 14 g	60	3	8	0	2
Roasted BLT Salad w/o Dressing, 347 g	200	6	8	4	29
Rsted Caesar Salad w/o Dressing/croutons, 301 g	220	8	6	3	30
Sandwiches					
• Crispy Twister®, 252 g	550	28	49	3	26
Double Crunch Sandwich, 213 g	470	23	38	2	27
Honey BBQ Sandwich, 147 g	280	4	40	3	22
KFC Snacker®, 119 g	290	13	29	2	15
Buffalo, 118 g	260	8	31	1	15
Fish w/o Sauce, 108 g	290	12	29	1	17
Fish, 120 g	330	15	31	1	17
• Honey BBQ, 101 g	210	3	32	2	14
Ultimate Cheese, 120 g	280	11	30	1	15
Oven Roasted Twister®, 269 g	420	17	40	3	28
w/o Sauce, 247 g	330	7	39	3	28
Tender Roast® Sandwich, 236 g	380	13	29	2	37
w/o Sauce, 217 g	300	5	28	2	37
Sides (Individual)					
Baked Beans, 136 g	220	1	45	7	8

(• = most healthy • = least healthy)   **RESTAURANTS & FAST-FOOD • 207**

Kentucky Fried Chicken (cont.)

	Cal	Fat	Cbs	Fbr	Prtn
Sides (Individual) (cont.)					
Biscuit, 57 g	220	11	24	1	4
Cole Slaw, 130 g	180	10	22	3	1
Corn on the Cob (3"), 82 g	70	2	13	3	2
Corn on the Cob (5.5"), 162 g	150	3	26	7	5
• Green Beans, 96 g	50	2	7	2	2
Macaroni and Cheese, 136 g	180	8	18	0	8
Mashed Potatoes with Gravy, 151 g	140	5	20	1	2
Mashed Potatoes without Gravy, 108 g	110	4	17	1	2
Potato Salad, 128 g	180	9	22	2	2
• Potato Wedges, 102 g	260	13	33	3	4
Seasoned Rice, 99 g	150	1	32	2	4
Strips					
Crispy Strips, 2 strips	240	13	11	0	20
Crispy Strips, 3 strips	350	19	16	0	29
Wings					
Boneless Fiery Buffalo Wings, 5 wings	420	20	33	3	28
Boneless Honey BBQ Wings, 5 wings	450	20	41	4	28
Boneless Sweet & Spicy Wings, 5 wings	440	19	38	3	27
• Boneless Teriyaki Wings, 5 wings	500	21	50	3	28
• Fiery Buffalo Wings, 5 wings	380	24	19	2	21
HBBQ Wings, 5 wings	390	24	23	3	21
Hot Wings®, 5 wings	350	24	14	2	20
Sweet & Spicy Wings, 5 wings	400	24	24	2	21
Teriyaki Wings, 5 wings	480	25	40	2	22

Kilwin's

	Cal	Fat	Cbs	Fbr	Prtn
Almond Bark, Milk Chocolate, 40 g	221	14	22	1	3
Almond Bark, White Chocolate, 40 g	221	13	24	1	3
Almond Butter Brickle, 40 g	218	14	23	1	2
Almond Cluster - Dark Chocolate, 40 g	221	16	18	3	4
Almond Cluster - Milk Chocolate, 40 g	226	16	18	2	4
Almond Toffee Crunch Bar, 40 g	192	13	18	1	2
Almond Toffee Crunch, 40 g	220	15	20	1	3
Almonds rstd & salted, 40 g	210	12	23	2	2
Almonds, Dark Chocolate, 40 g	225	16	19	1	4
Almonds, Milk Chocolate, 40 g	219	15	20	3	3
Amaretto Truffle, 40 g	237	17	21	1	3
Apricots, Dark Chocolate, 40 g	140	5	24	1	1
Apricots, Milk Chocolate, 40 g	142	5	24	1	1
Bavarian Cream, 40 g	167	6	28	0	1
Black Licorice Twist, 40 g	143	0	39	0	0
Bombe' Truffle, 40 g	230	17	21	2	2
Brugg Truffle, 40 g	230	17	21	2	2
Butter Pecan Fudge, 40 g	242	17	22	1	1
Caramel Assortment, 40 g	184	9	26	1	1
Caramel Assortment, 40 g	233	16	22	1	2
Caramel Corn, 40 g	207	13	22	1	2
Caramel Sucker, 40 g	163	9	20	0	1
Caramel Topping, 40 g	107	5	15	1	1
Caramellows, Dark Chocolate, 40 g	173	9	23	1	1
Caramellows, Milk Chocolate, 40 g	178	8	24	0	2
Caramels, Dark Chocolate, 40 g	182	9	26	1	1
Caramels, Milk Chocolate, 40 g	185	8	27	0	1

RESTAURANTS & FAST-FOOD CHAINS

Kilwin's (cont.)	Cal	Fat	Cbs	Fbr	Prtn
Cashew Brittle, 40 g	195	10	28	1	1
Cashew Cluster - Milk Chocolate, 40 g	228	17	16	1	5
Cashew Cluster, Dark Chocolate, 40 g	225	17	16	2	5
Cashew Tuttles, Dark Chocolate, 40 g	205	13	21	1	3
Cashew Tuttles, Milk Chocolate, 40 g	207	13	21	1	4
Cashews, Dark Chocolate, 40 g	252	21	15	2	3
Cashews, Milk Chocolate, 40 g	222	16	18	2	4
Cashews, rstd & salted, 40 g	246	23	9	2	6
Chausse' Truffle, 40 g	240	17	20	0	2
Cherri Suisse Truffle, 40 g	232	16	21	1	2
Cherry Coins, 40 g	205	9	16	3	4
Cherry Cordial Assortment, 40 g	175	7	28	1	1
Cherry Cordial Assortment, 40 g	184	9	26	1	1
Cherry Cordial, Dark Chocolate, 40 g	173	7	28	1	1
Cherry Cordials, Milk Chocolate, 40 g	177	7	28	1	1
Chocolate Berryblues, 40 g	170	9	21	1	2
Chocolate Blackberries, 40 g	220	16	18	2	3
Chocolate Bon Bon, 40 g	167	6	29	0	1
Chocolate Card "Thank You", 40 g	153	9	17	1	2
Chocolate Coffee Beans, 40 g	178	7	29	1	1
Chocolate Cream, Dark Chocolate, 40 g	166	6	28	1	1
Chocolate Cream, Milk Chocolate, 40 g	168	6	28	1	1
Chocolate Espresso Beans, 40 g	200	12	23	2	3
Chocolate Fudge, 40 g	174	5	31	0	1
Chocolate Ice Cream Suckers, 40 g	135	4	26	0	0
Chocolate Jordan Almonds, 40 g	220	15	18	2	5
Chocolate Peanut Butter Fudge, 40 g	176	6	29	1	1
Chocolate Pecan Fudge, 40 g	169	5	31	0	1
Chocolate Star Pop, 40 g	231	14	23	1	2
Chocolate Toffee Almonds, 40 g	220	15	18	2	5
Chocolate Walnut Fudge, 40 g	175	6	31	0	0
Cinnamon Roasted Almond, 40 g	137	0	34	0	1
Coconut Cluster, Dark Chocolate, 40 g	204	12	24	3	2
Coconut Cluster, Milk Chocolate, 40 g	209	12	24	2	2
Coconut Macaroon, Dark Chocolate, 40 g	233	13	28	3	2
Coffee Truffle, 40 g	233	16	21	1	2
Custom Coin Dark Mint Chocolate, 40 g	350	21	37	2	5
Custom Gold Coins Milk Chocolate, 40 g	229	14	25	1	3
Custom Silver Coins Milk Chocolate, 40 g	221	14	25	3	2
Dark Chocolate Almonds, 40 g	210	13	21	2	4
Dark Chocolate Bar, 40 g	310	21	28	2	6
Dark Chocolate Break-up, 40 g	210	13	23	3	2
Dark Chocolate Heart, 40 g	221	14	25	3	2
Dark Chocolate Sea Foam, 40 g	130	0	32	0	1
Family Assortment, 40 g	209	13	23	1	2
Family Assortment, 40 g	206	12	24	1	2
Family Assortment, 40 g	209	13	23	1	2
Family Assortment, 40 g	204	12	23	1	2
• Flavored Swizzle Stick, 40 g	50	0	14	0	0
Fontineau Truffle, 40 g	229	16	21	1	2
French Chocolate, 40 g	198	11	24	1	2
French Mint Truffle, 40 g	226	15	23	1	1
Gourmet Chocolate Nut Mix, 40 g	220	16	18	2	3
Gourmet Nut Mix, 40 g	220	15	18	2	5

RESTAURANTS & FAST-FOOD CHAINS

Kilwin's (cont.)	Cal	Fat	Cbs	Fbr	Prtn
Gummi Bears, 40 g	140	0	34	0	0
Gummi Pet Crocodile, 40 g	130	0	32	0	2
Gummy Bears, 40 g	158	0	40	0	0
Hazelnut Truffle, 40 g	233	17	21	1	2
Heavenly Hash, 40 g	183	8	26	2	3
Holland Mints, 40 g	160	5	32	1	1
Irish Cream Truffle, 40 g	233	16	21	1	2
Jamaican Truffle, 40 g	232	16	21	1	2
Jaw Breaker 2.25", 40 g	160	0	40	0	0
Katy Cream Assort, 40 g	174	7	28	1	1
Katy Cream Assort, 40 g	182	8	28	1	1
Katy Kiss Cluster, 40 g	218	14	21	1	4
Kilwin's Dome Milk Chocolate, 40 g	231	14	24	1	3
Kilwin's Fudge Topping, 40 g	232	14	26	1	3
Kilwin's Square Mint, 40 g	231	14	24	1	3
Le Gran Truffle, 40 g	233	17	21	1	2
Licorice Bridge Mix, 40 g	130	1	31	0	1
Macadamia Nuts rstd & salted, 40 g	286	30	5	4	4
Macadamia Tuttles, Milk Chocolate, 40 g	222	16	20	1	2
Macadamia Tuttles, White Chocolate, 40 g	216	15	21	1	2
Maple Cream, Dark Chocolate, 40 g	163	6	29	1	1
Maple Walnut Fudge, 40 g	168	4	32	0	0
Marshmallow, Dark Chocolate, 40 g	181	9	25	2	2
Marshmallow, Milk Chocolate, 40 g	186	9	25	1	2
Marzipan Bar, 40 g	150	3	30	3	3
Marzipan Fruits, 40 g	196	0	48	0	1
Milk Chocolate Alligator, 40 g	223	13	25	1	2
Milk Chocolate Almond Bar, 40 g	336	21	37	4	3
Milk Chocolate Almonds, 40 g	200	15	19	3	4
Milk Chocolate Bar, 40 g	153	9	17	1	2
Milk Chocolate Bar, 40 g	153	9	17	1	2
Milk Chocolate Bar, 40 g	229	14	25	1	3
Milk Chocolate Bar, 40 g	330	18	39	2	5
Milk Chocolate Break-up, 40 g	218	13	24	1	2
Milk Chocolate Caramel Apple, 40 g	220	12	25	0	2
Milk Chocolate Cigar, 40 g	179	7	29	1	3
Milk Chocolate Cigar, 40 g	231	14	24	1	3
Milk Chocolate Cigar, 40 g	231	14	24	1	3
Milk Chocolate Coins, 40 g	153	9	17	1	2
Milk Chocolate Crayons, 40 g	76	5	8	0	1
• Milk Chocolate Crisp Rice Bar, 40 g	350	22	34	2	6
Milk Chocolate Doctor Kit, 40 g	229	14	25	1	3
Milk Chocolate Fish, 40 g	229	14	25	1	3
Milk Chocolate Golf Set, 40 g	218	13	24	1	2
Milk Chocolate Hairdresser, 40 g	218	13	24	1	2
Milk Chocolate Heart, 40 g	229	14	25	1	3
Milk Chocolate Malt Balls, 40 g	190	9	28	1	2
Milk Chocolate Maltballs, 40 g	190	9	26	1	3
Milk Chocolate Mini Car, 40 g	229	14	25	1	3
Milk Chocolate Pansie, 40 g	229	14	25	1	3
Milk Chocolate Peanut Dino, 40 g	240	16	22	1	4
Milk Chocolate Peanuts, 40 g	220	15	18	2	5
Milk Chocolate Peanuts, 40 g	180	12	23	3	3
Milk Chocolate Raisins, 40 g	181	8	26	1	2

RESTAURANTS & FAST-FOOD CHAINS

Kilwin's (cont.)	Cal	Fat	Cbs	Fbr	Prtn
Milk Chocolate Raisins, 40 g	190	9	26	3	2
Milk Chocolate Sea Foam, 40 g	180	10	26	2	1
Milk Chocolate Tool Kit, 40 g	218	13	24	1	2
Milk Moose Sucker, 40 g	150	8	18	0	1
Mint Cookie Malt Balls, 40 g	140	1	31	0	2
Mint Smoothie Assortment, 40 g	180	8	26	1	2
Mint Smoothies, Dark Chocolate, 40 g	226	16	22	2	2
Mint Smoothies, Milk Chocolate, 40 g	229	16	22	1	2
Mixed Nuts, rstd & salted, 40 g	271	20	13	4	9
Molasses Chips, Dark Chocolate, 40 g	191	9	29	2	1
Molasses Chips, Milk Chocolate, 40 g	191	8	30	1	2
Natural Pistachios, 40 g	286	30	5	3	3
Nutcracker Sweets, 40 g	181	8	26	1	4
Orange Cream, Dark Chocolate, 40 g	161	5	30	1	1
Orange Cream, Milk Chocolate, 40 g	161	5	30	0	1
Orange Jellies, Dark Chocolate, 40 g	182	7	29	2	1
Orange Jellies, Milk Chocolate, 40 g	187	7	30	1	1
Orange Peel, Dark Chocolate, 40 g	167	8	26	2	1
Orange Peel, Milk Chocolate, 40 g	171	7	27	1	1
Oreo Cookie, White Chocolate, 40 g	209	11	27	0	2
Oreo Cookies, Milk Chocolate, 40 g	210	11	25	1	2
Pastel Chocolate Cherries, 40 g	200	10	26	1	2
Peanut Butter Cup, 40 g	180	5	33	1	2
Peanut Butter Fudge, 40 g	168	4	32	0	0
Peanut Cluster, Dark Chocolate, 40 g	217	15	18	3	5
Peanut Cluster, Milk Chocolate, 40 g	223	15	18	2	5
Peanut Corn, 40 g	166	4	32	1	1
Peanuts, Roasted & Salted, 40 g	243	22	7	4	9
Pecan Bark, Dark Chocolate, 40 g	219	15	21	2	2
Pecan Bark, Milk Chocolate, 40 g	226	15	22	1	3
Pecan Brittle, 40 g	152	8	19	0	1
Pecan Cluster, Dark Chocolate, 40 g	235	18	17	2	3
Pecan Cluster, Milk Chocolate, 40 g	240	18	18	2	3
Pecan Streakers, 40 g	212	13	24	2	3
Pecan Turtle Assortment, 40 g	175	7	28	1	2
Pecan Tuttles, Dark Chocolate, 40 g	223	16	19	2	2
Pecan Tuttles, Milk Chocolate, 40 g	226	16	19	1	2
Pecans rstd & salted, 40 g	232	20	4	4	11
Pecans, Dark Chocolate, 40 g	232	19	12	1	7
Pecans, Milk Chocolate, 40 g	247	21	15	2	3
Peppermint Patties Dark Chocolate, 40 g	177	8	28	1	1
Peppermint Patty, 40 g	200	9	33	2	3
Peanut Brittle, 40 g	186	14	21	3	2
Pnt Butter Cruncher Dark Chocolate, 40 g	214	13	23	2	3
Pnt Butter Cruncher Milk Chocolate, 40 g	218	13	23	1	3
Pnt Butter Smoothie, Dark Chocolate, 40 g	218	14	22	2	2
Pnt Butter Smoothie, Milk Chocolate, 40 g	222	14	22	1	3
Pretzels, Milk Chocolate, 40 g	199	9	27	1	3
Pretzels, White Chocolate, 40 g	199	9	28	0	2
Raisin Cluster, Dark Chocolate, 40 g	180	9	26	2	2
Raisin Cluster, Milk Chocolate, 40 g	186	9	27	1	2
Rasp & Blackberries, 40 g	190	10	25	1	2
Raspberry & Blackberry 10# case, 40 g	152	2	35	0	0
Raspberry Cream, Dark Chocolate, 40 g	159	5	29	1	1

RESTAURANTS & FAST-FOOD CHAINS

Kilwin's (cont.)

	Cal	Fat	Cbs	Fbr	Prtn
Raspberry Cream, Milk Chocolate, 40 g	162	5	30	0	1
Raspberry Jellies, Dark Chocolate, 40 g	184	8	29	2	1
Raspberry Jellies, Milk Chocolate, 40 g	187	7	30	1	1
Raspberry Truffle, 40 g	230	17	21	2	2
Red Licorice Ropes, 40 g	160	0	39	0	0
Red Licorice Twist, 40 g	140	0	36	0	0
Royal Nut Assortment, 40 g	231	17	18	2	4
Royal Nut Assortment, 40 g	245	19	18	2	4
Salt Water Taffy, 40 g	130	8	15	2	1
Salt Water Taffy, bulk 27# case, 40 g	232	17	21	1	2
Sanded Lemon Drops, 40 g	166	0	42	0	0
Sour Gummi Bears, 40 g	136	0	32	0	2
Star of David, 40 g	180	11	20	2	2
Strawberry Bon Bon, 40 g	161	4	31	0	1
Sugar Free Caramel Corn, 40 g	224	15	20	2	4
Sugar Free Chocolate Fudge, 40 g	160	10	27	1	2
Sugar Free Chocolates, 40 g	147	9	27	2	2
Sugar Free Dark Pnut Cluster, 40 g	199	17	16	8	6
Sugar Free Festival Mints, 40 g	180	15	22	8	2
Sugar Free Hard Candy, 40 g	138	3	35	1	1
Sugar Free Milk Cashew Tuttle, 40 g	190	14	22	1	2
Sugar Free Milk Pecan Turtles, 40 g	190	14	21	2	3
Sugar Free Milk Pnut Cluster, 40 g	187	16	16	8	6
Sugar Free Milk Squares, 40 g	159	14	21	10	2
Sugar Free Pnt Brittle, 40 g	154	4	36	0	2
Sugar Free Pnut Butter Fudge, 40 g	150	9	26	0	2
Sugar Free Pnut Cluster Asst, 40 g	190	16	18	6	5
Sugar Free Taffy, 40 g	160	0	40	0	0
Sugar Free Toffee Crunch, 40 g	164	8	27	1	4
Sugar Free Vanilla Fudge, 40 g	150	9	28	0	1
Sugar Free White Pnut Cluster, 40 g	197	15	18	1	5
Sugar Free White Squares, 40 g	175	13	26	0	2
Swedish Fish, 40 g	160	3	37	0	0
Tart Cherry Cluster, Milk Chocolate, 40 g	194	9	27	1	2
Truffle Assortment, 40 g	226	16	19	1	2
Tuxedo Espresso Beans, 40 g	190	9	26	1	3
Vanilla Butter Cream, Dark Chocolate, 40 g	166	6	28	1	1
Vanilla Butter Cream, Milk Chocolate, 40 g	168	6	28	1	1
White Chocolate Break-up, 40 g	218	12	26	0	1
White Chocolate Popcorn, 40 g	220	16	18	1	2
White Golf Ball, 40 g	223	12	27	0	1
White Golf Ball, 40 g	129	6	19	0	1
White Moose Sucker, 40 g	164	10	18	1	2

Kohr Bros.

	Cal	Fat	Cbs	Fbr	Prtn
• Chocolate, 80 g	140	6	18	0	4
• Orange Sherbet, 87 g	104	2	21	1	1
Vanilla, 80 g	130	6	16	0	4

Kolache Factory

	Cal	Fat	Cbs	Fbr	Prtn
Croissants					
• Fruit (Average), 5 oz.	510	24	67	1	8
• Ham & Cheese, 7 oz.	620	39	45	0	23
Ham & Egg, 7 oz.	610	38	46	0	22

RESTAURANTS & FAST-FOOD CHAINS

Kolache Factory (cont.)	Cal	Fat	Cbs	Fbr	Prtn
Croissants (cont.)					
Italian Chicken, 8 oz.	550	32	46	0	20
Kolaches					
Bacon & Cheese, 2 oz.	180	7	23	0	6
Bacon, Egg & Cheese, 5 oz.	360	16	35	0	15
BBQ Beef, 3 oz.	180	6	18	0	13
Club, 5 oz.	260	9	35	0	10
Cream Cheese, 3 oz.	180	7	25	0	5
Fruit (Average), 4 oz.	180	3	38	1	3
Ham & Cheese, 3 oz.	180	7	23	0	7
Italian Chicken, 3 oz.	190	7	23	0	9
Jalapeño & Cheese, 3 oz.	180	7	25	0	5
Pizza, 3 oz.	200	9	24	0	7
• Polish, 6 oz.	510	29	47	0	17
Ranchero, 6 oz.	380	18	35	0	18
Sausage & Cheese, 3 oz.	240	11	29	0	7
• Sausage, 2 oz.	130	5	17	0	3
Sausage, Egg & Cheese, 5 oz.	400	20	35	0	18
Specialties					
Cinnamon Roll, 5 oz.	460	14	74	1	9
Cinnamon Twist, 4 oz.	450	29	45	4	6
• Mini-Cinnamon Roll, 4 oz.	230	7	37	0	4
• Raisin Nut Roll, 3 oz.	600	24	89	2	10
Sticky Bun, 5 oz.	440	20	61	1	6

Koo Koo Roo	Cal	Fat	Cbs	Fbr	Prtn
Buffalo Wings (w/o Sauce)					
• 12 Buffalo Wings	1212	55	84	4	88
6 Buffalo Wings	606	28	42	2	44
Burritos					
• California Chicken Burrito	810	41	60	4	46
Fajita Chicken Burrito	750	33	70	4	40
• Original Chicken Burrito	709	28	71	5	41
Chicken Bowls (w/o Sauce)					
Chargrilled Chicken Bowl	569	19	57	4	41
• Southwest Bowl	570	19	67	8	37
• Spicy Ginger Garlic Bowl	485	6	63	2	42
Tostada Bowl (w/o shell)	528	22	45	7	40
Cold Side Dishes					
Cantaloupe & Honeydew, 5 oz.	50	0	12	1	1
• Creamy Coleslaw, 5 oz.	238	20	14	2	1
Cucumber Salad, 5 oz.	41	0	9	2	1
Tangy Tomato Salad, 5 oz.	60	4	6	1	1
• Tossed Salad (w/o dressing), 3 oz.	16	0	3	1	1
Dessert					
Chewy Chocolate Chip Cookie, 3 oz.	360	15	53	1	3
Chewy Oat Raisin Cookie, 3 oz.	370	15	54	3	6
Kellogg's® Rice Krispies Treats®, 3 oz.	340	7	68	0	3
• Peanut Butter Cup Cookie, 3 oz.	460	22	58	2	8
• Snickerdoodle Cookie, 3 oz.	330	16	43	1	4
Triple Chocolate Brownie, 3 oz.	334	9	57	0	5
Extras					
BBQ Vinaigrette Dressing, 2 oz.	101	4	14	0	0
Caesar Dressing, 2 oz.	235	26	1	0	0

RESTAURANTS & FAST-FOOD CHAINS

Koo Koo Roo (cont.)

	Cal	Fat	Cbs	Fbr	Prtn
Extras (cont.)					
• Celery Sticks, 6 pcs	8	0	2	1	0
Chinese Salad Dressing, 3 oz.	325	26	26	0	0
Chipotle Sauce, 1 oz.	130	14	0	0	0
Cilantro Ranch Dressing, 2 oz.	200	21	2	0	0
Cranberry Sauce, 1 oz.	45	0	11	0	0
• Curry Sauce, 3 oz.	630	69	3	0	0
Fruit by the Foot ®, 1	80	2	17	0	0
Gravy, 2 oz.	50	4	3	0	1
House Salad Dressing, 2 oz.	90	6	6	0	0
Lahvash, 1	60	0	12	0	3
Pico De Gallo, 2 oz.	8	0	2	0	0
Ranch Dressing, 1 oz.	140	15	1	0	0
Rudi Roll, Half	150	2	29	1	6
Salsa, 2 oz.	11	0	2	1	1
Sour Cream, 1 oz.	60	6	1	0	1
Spicy Ginger & Garlic Sauce, 4 oz.	320	28	8	0	4
Tostada Shell, 1	403	34	21	1	3
Wing Sauce, 1 oz.	28	2	2	0	0
Fresh Roasted Turkey					
Hand Carved Turkey Sandwich	599	32	31	5	46
• Sliced Turkey Breast	182	8	0	0	25
Traditional Turkey Dinner	692	29	67	8	42
• Turkey Pot Pie	883	44	83	6	37
Hot Side Dishes					
Baked Yam, 6 oz.	197	0	47	7	3
Black Beans, 6 oz.	125	3	23	6	8
Butternut Squash, 6 oz.	66	0	17	3	2
Creamed Spinach, 5 oz.	100	6	10	3	4
Green Beans, 4 oz.	62	3	9	4	2
Italian Vegetable, 6 oz.	47	2	7	2	1
Kernel Corn, 5 oz.	105	1	26	3	4
• Macaroni & Cheese, 6 oz.	340	17	32	1	15
Mashed Potatoes, 7 oz.	186	5	32	3	4
Roasted Garlic Potatoes, 5 oz.	133	5	21	2	2
Saffron Rice, 4 oz.	175	7	25	1	2
Spanish Rice, 5 oz.	145	3	27	1	3
• Steamed Vegetables, 4 oz.	38	0	8	3	2
Sticky Rice, 5 oz.	155	0	34	0	3
Stuffing, 5 oz.	111	7	11	1	3
Original Chicken					
1 Original Breast, 4 oz.	187	6	0	0	34
3 Piece Original Dark, 5 oz.	320	16	5	0	39
Rotisserie Chicken					
• Breast & Wing, 7 oz.	355	16	1	0	49
• Half Rotisserie Chicken, 11 oz.	655	34	2	0	80
Leg & Thigh, 5 oz.	300	18	1	0	31
Salads (w/o Dressing)					
BBQ Chicken Salad	365	14	22	6	38
Chicken Caesar Salad	286	11	13	4	34
• Chinese Chicken Salad	550	29	39	10	40
• House Salad	113	4	16	5	6
Sandwiches					
• BBQ Chicken Sandwich	562	12	71	3	45

RESTAURANTS & FAST-FOOD CHAINS

Koo Koo Roo (cont.)	Cal	Fat	Cbs	Fbr	Prtn
Sandwiches (cont.)					
• Chicken Caesar Sandwich	781	36	63	2	56
Original Chicken Sandwich	661	29	63	3	41
Soups					
• Chicken Noodle Soup, 5 oz.	71	3	4	0	6
• Chicken Tortilla Soup, 5 oz.	112	6	7	1	8
Ten Vegetable Soup, 5 oz.	94	2	16	4	3
Wraps					
Caesar Chicken Wrap	757	39	59	4	42
Chipotle Chicken Wrap	924	43	89	6	42

Krispy Kreme Doughnuts	Cal	Fat	Cbs	Fbr	Prtn
Chillers					
Berries & Kreme Chiller, 20 oz.	960	40	150	1	3
• Chocolate Chiller, 20 oz.	1050	42	170	4	6
Lemon Sherbert Chiller, 20 oz.	980	40	155	1	3
Lotta Latte Chiller, 20 oz.	1050	40	79	1	5
Mocha Dream Chiller, 20 oz.	1050	41	171	2	5
Orange You Glad Chiller, 20 oz.	300	0	71	0	0
Oranges & Kreme Chiller, 20 oz.	970	40	150	1	3
• Very Berry Chiller, 20 oz.	290	0	71	0	0
Doughnut Holes					
• Glazed Blueberry Donut Holes, 56 g	220	12	27	1	3
Glazed Cake Donut Holes, 56 g	210	10	29	1	2
Glazed Chocolate Cake Donut Holes, 56 g	210	10	29	1	2
Glazed Pumpkin Spice Donut Holes, 56 g	210	10	29	1	2
• Original Glazed Donut Holes, 54 g	200	11	25	1	2
Doughnuts					
• Apple Fritter, 101 g	380	20	47	2	4
Caramel Kreme Crunch, 98 g	380	19	49	1	4
Chocolate Glazed Cruller, 69 g	290	15	37	1	3
Chocolate Iced Cake, 71 g	280	14	36	1	3
Chocolate Iced Custard Filled, 86 g	300	17	35	1	3
Chocolate Iced Glazed, 66 g	250	12	33	1	3
Chocolate Iced Kreme Filled, 86 g	350	20	39	1	3
Chocolate Iced w/Sprinkles, 71 g	270	12	38	1	3
Cinnamon Apple Filled, 81 g	290	16	32	1	3
Cinnamon Bun, 67 g	260	16	28	1	3
Cinnamon Twist, 59 g	240	15	23	1	3
Dulce De Leche, 75 g	300	18	31	1	3
Glazed Chocolate Cake, 80 g	300	15	42	2	3
Glazed Cinnamon, 54 g	210	12	24	1	2
Glazed Cruller, 54 g	240	14	26	1	2
Glazed Kreme Filled, 86 g	340	20	39	1	3
Glazed Lemon Filled, 85 g	290	16	35	1	3
Glazed Pumpkin Spice, 80 g	300	14	42	1	2
Glazed Raspberry Filled, 85 g	300	16	36	1	3
Glazed Sour Cream, 80 g	300	13	43	1	2
Maple Iced Glazed, 66 g	240	12	32	1	3
New York Cheesecake, 90 g	340	20	34	1	4
Original Glazed, 52 g	200	12	22	1	2
Powdered Cake, 71 g	290	14	37	1	3
Powdered Strawberry Filled, 81 g	290	16	33	1	3
• Sugar, 49 g	200	12	21	0	2

(• = most healthy • = least healthy)   **RESTAURANTS & FAST-FOOD • 215**

RESTAURANTS & FAST-FOOD CHAINS

Krispy Kreme Doughnuts (cont.)	Cal	Fat	Cbs	Fbr	Prtn
Doughnuts (cont.)					
Traditional Cake, 57 g	230	13	25	1	3

Krystal	Cal	Fat	Cbs	Fbr	Prtn
B.A. Burger					
• BA Double Bacon Cheese, 305 g	800	53	41	2	44
BA w/ Cheese, 218 g	530	32	40	2	25
BA, 202 g	470	27	39	2	22
Breakfast					
4 Carb Scrambler (bacon), 6 oz.	370	29	4	1	24
4 Carb Scrambler (sausage), 8 oz.	600	51	3	2	32
Bacon Egg Cheese Biscuit, 137 g	390	23	33	0	11
Biscuit & Gravy, 200 g	280	14	34	0	5
Chik Biscuit, 137 g	360	15	40	0	13
• Country Breakfast, 230 g	660	42	46	8	24
• Kryspers, 51 g	190	13	17	2	1
Krystal Sunriser, 94 g	240	14	14	2	12
Plain Biscuit, 87 g	270	13	33	0	5
Sausage Biscuit, 144 g	480	33	33	0	12
Scrambler, 312 g	440	26	33	3	20
Chiks					
Krystal Chik, 81 g	240	11	24	2	11
Dessert					
Blueberry Freeze, 454 g	230	0	58	0	0
Cherry Freeze, 454 g	230	0	58	0	0
Fried Apple Turnover, 81 g	220	10	31	2	3
Grape Freeze, 454 g	230	0	57	0	0
Green Apple Freeze, 454 g	230	0	57	0	0
• Lemon Icebox Pie, 99 g	260	9	41	2	5
• Orange Freeze, 454 g	220	0	54	0	0
Pomegranate Freeze, 454 g	230	0	57	0	0
Pups					
Chili Cheese Pup, 76 g	210	12	17	2	9
• Corn Pup, 68 g	260	19	19	1	5
• Plain Pup, 57 g	170	9	15	1	6
Sides					
Chik'n Bites (sm), 113 g	310	19	16	1	17
Chik'n Bites Salad, 262 g	290	20	12	4	20
Chili Cheese Fries, 207 g	540	28	59	6	13
• Krystal Chili, 217 g	200	7	22	7	13
Regular Fries, 119 g	470	20	53	7	4
The Famous Krystal					
Bacon Cheese Krystal, 65 g	190	10	16	2	10
Cheese Krystal, 68 g	180	9	17	2	9
• DBL Cheese Krystal, 121 g	310	16	26	1	16
Double Krystal, 108 g	260	13	24	2	13
• Krystal, 60 g	160	7	17	1	7

L&L Hawaiian Barbecue	Cal	Fat	Cbs	Fbr	Prtn
• BBQ Beef, 5 oz.	330	11	25	0	33
BBQ Chicken, 5 oz.	380	20	22	N/A	29
BBQ Short Ribs, 5 oz.	460	37	5	0	27
Chicken Katsu, 5 oz.	350	24	12	N/A	43
Katsu Sauce, 2 oz.	45	0	11	0	0

RESTAURANTS & FAST-FOOD CHAINS

L&L Hawaiian Barbecue (cont.)

	Cal	Fat	Cbs	Fbr	Prtn
• Macaroni Salad, 5 oz.	520	30	57	N/A	5

LaRosa's Pizzeria

	Cal	Fat	Cbs	Fbr	Prtn
Appetizers					
Barbecue Wings (12 wings), 549 g	1257	77	48	3	102
Barbecue Wings (18 wings), 823 g	1884	115	71	5	153
Blue Cheese Dipping Cup, 42 g	230	24	2	0	2
Chicken Tenders, 243 g	541	31	30	0	35
Diablo Sauce, 64 g	206	15	17	0	0
Four Taste Sampler, 669 g	1569	99	82	3	83
French Fry Basket w/ Provolone, 385 g	862	56	73	7	31
Garlic Sauce Dipping Sauce, 51 g	360	40	0	0	0
Mozzarella Cheese Sticks, 181 g	636	43	36	0	18
Onion Twists (Regular), 207 g	462	27	48	2	7
Pizza Sauce Dipping Cup, 57 g	50	2	7	1	1
Ranch Dipping Cup, 42 g	230	24	2	0	1
• Seasoned Kitchen Chips (Regular), 170 g	433	26	47	6	4
Special Recipe Wings (12 wings), 549 g	1261	87	21	3	101
Special Recipe Wings (18 wings), 823 g	1890	130	32	4	152
Spicy Hot Wings (12 wings), 542 g	1247	85	26	3	101
Spicy Hot Wings (18 wings), 811 g	1864	128	38	4	152
Calzones					
• 3 Meat & 3 Cheese, 441 g	1080	55	102	5	46
• 3 Veggie & 3 Cheese, 438 g	860	34	105	6	35
Cheese & Pepperoni, 375 g	960	45	101	5	39
Cheese, 364 g	840	34	101	5	34
Philly Cheesesteak Calzone, 348 g	872	39	90	3	38
• Philly Chicken Calzone, 341 g	745	24	90	3	40
Pizza Sauce Dipping Cup, 57 g	50	2	7	1	1
Ranch Dipping Cup, 42 g	230	24	2	0	1
Sausage Pelucci Calzone, 425 g	1042	52	92	5	50
Desserts					
Greater's Big Scoop cup, 210 g	600	42	56	2	6
Hot Fudge Brownie, 1/2 portion	758	40	99	1	9
Italian Crème Cake, 257 g	998	57	112	3	11
• Pizza Frite, 1/2 portion	342	6	64	2	8
Focaccia Style Pizza (Medium)					
• Cheese (1/10 pizza), 42 g	230	12	23	1	7
• Florentine (1/10 pizza), 94 g	240	13	24	1	7
• Roma (1/10 pizza), 94 g	300	18	23	1	10
Fresh Baked Breads					
Breadsticks (5 pcs.), 309 g	998	13	190	5	35
• Breadsticks w/ Provolone (5 pcs.), 389 g	1293	35	193	5	56
• Garlic Bread (2 pcs.), 66 g	240	9	35	1	5
Garlic Bread w/ Provolone (2 pcs.), 104 g	390	21	35	1	16
Garlic Sauce Dipping Sauce, 51 g	360	40	0	0	0
Pizza Sauce Dipping Cup, 57 g	50	2	7	1	1
Fresh Salads and Soup					
Baked Onion Soup, 272 g	304	16	28	1	13
Grilled Chicken Salad, 318 g	296	12	11	3	35
JoJo BLT w/ Chkn Antipasto, 271 g	317	21	12	3	19
• JoJo's BLT Salad w/ dressing, 257 g	505	35	9	2	39
• Minestrone Soup, 336 g	130	2	22	3	9
• Tossed Salad, 205 g	163	9	10	3	9

RESTAURANTS & FAST-FOOD CHAINS

▶ LaRosa's Pizzeria (cont.)

	Cal	Fat	Cbs	Fbr	Prtn
Fresh Salads and Soup (cont.)					
Tuna Salad, 350 g	458	30	19	3	29
Hand Tossed Pizzas (Medium)					
Blanca, 86 g	251	10	27	1	12
Buddy Topper, 124 g	309	14	29	1	15
• Cheese, 96 g	230	8	29	1	10
Deluxe Topper, 123 g	291	12	29	1	15
• Meat Topper, 122 g	320	15	29	1	17
Pelucci Topper, 120 g	288	13	29	1	14
Pepperoni Topper, 111 g	298	14	29	1	14
Veggie Topper, 120 g	264	10	30	1	13
Hoagies					
Baked Buddy Hoagy, 248 g	665	28	62	2	39
Baked Royal Hoagy, 254 g	601	22	62	2	37
Fillet of Haddock Hoagy, 302 g	630	15	81	2	38
Link Sausage Hoagy, 273 g	621	24	64	3	36
Meatball Hoagy, 334 g	689	26	77	4	36
• Original Steak Hoagy, 321 g	727	35	65	3	39
• Philly Chicken Hoagy, 264 g	451	4	64	2	40
Philly Steak Hoagy, 263 g	621	25	64	2	34
Ingredients and Dressings for Hoagies					
Italian Dressing, 57 g	320	34	3	0	0
Kitchen Chips, 28 g	150	9	15	2	2
• Mushroom Sauce Mayonnaise, 57 g	400	11	0	0	0
• Pickle Chips, 39 g	5	0	1	0	0
Pizza Sauce, 57 g	50	2	7	1	1
Provolone, 28 g	103	7	1	0	7
Red Onion Slices, 14 g	6	0	1	0	0
Sharp White Cheddar, 26 g	92	8	1	0	5
Tartar Sauce, 57 g	260	24	11	0	1
Tomato Slices, 51 g	11	0	2	1	1
Kid's Meals (values include all components of kids meal)					
Cheese Sticks & Potatoes, 286 g	536	28	55	3	11
Chicken Tenders & Potatoes, 299 g	492	26	49	3	16
• Mac 'n Cheese, 310 g	378	12	58	3	11
Smiley Pizza – Cheese, 382 g	726	30	79	4	32
• Smiley Pizza – Pepperoni, 396 g	796	36	79	4	35
Spaghetti and Meatball, 311 g	515	10	86	6	18
Lite and Low Fat Menu Items					
Large Lite Deluxe Pizza, 1 slice	300	9	42	2	11
• Low Fat Grilled Chicken Hoagy, 347 g	520	9	56	3	54
Low Fat Grilled Chicken Salad Meal, 349 g	380	10	40	3	31
Medium Lite Deluxe Pizza, 1 slice	190	6	27	1	7
• Minestrone Soup, 1 bowl	80	1	15	2	4
Small Lite Deluxe Pizza, 1 slice	170	5	25	1	6
Pan Crust Pizzas (Medium)					
Blanca, 100 g	350	22	28	1	12
Buddy Topper, 126 g	312	14	29	1	16
Cheese, 105 g	300	16	30	1	10
Deluxe Topper, 134 g	370	21	31	2	15
• Meat Topper, 132 g	400	23	30	1	16
• Pelucci Topper, 123 g	295	12	29	2	15
Pepperoni Topper, 121 g	370	22	30	1	14
Veggie Topper, 141 g	320	16	32	2	11

RESTAURANTS & FAST-FOOD CHAINS

LaRosa's Pizzeria (cont.)

	Cal	Fat	Cbs	Fbr	Prtn
Pasta Dinners					
Add Chicken Strips w/ Trad. Sauce, 283 g	284	10	21	4	29
Add Link Sausage w/ Trad. Sauce, 283 g	416	26	21	5	25
Add Meatballs (3) w/ Trad. Sauce, 264 g	381	23	25	4	19
Cheese Ravioli, 496 g	661	26	80	6	30
Lasagna w/ Meat Sauce, 599 g	735	38	61	7	40
Meat Ravioli, 496 g	621	22	102	8	30
• Minestrone Soup, 336 g	130	2	22	3	5
Spaghetti & Meatballs, 640 g	870	28	119	11	35
Spaghetti or Ziti w/ Alfredo Sauce, 546 g	976	50	104	4	24
Spaghetti or Ziti w/ Meat Sauce, 546 g	698	18	104	10	6
Spaghetti or Ziti w/ Trad. Sauce, 546 g	640	12	113	10	20
Tossed Salad w/o dressing, 205 g	163	9	10	3	9
• Ziti Chicken Alfredo, 596 g	982	42	102	4	44
Ziti Sausage Pelucci, 624 g	766	20	115	11	30
Salad Dressing (one packet)					
Blue Cheese, 43 g	220	24	2	0	2
Caesar, 29 g	160	17	1	0	1
Fat Free Honey Dijon, 43 g	70	0	16	1	0
• Fat Free Italian, 43 g	20	0	4	0	0
Fat Free Ranch, 43 g	40	0	10	1	0
Honey French, 43 g	210	18	14	0	0
LaRosa's Creamy Garlic, 43 g	250	26	3	0	1
LaRosa's Italian, 43 g	230	26	2	0	0
• Ranch, 43 g	260	29	1	0	0
Thousand Island, 43 g	220	21	7	0	0
Stuffed Pizza Pie					
• Cheese, 114 g	339	14	40	2	13
• Meat, 239 g	790	53	44	2	33
Veggie, 167 g	393	18	43	2	14
Traditional Crust Pizzas (Medium)					
Blanca, 73 g	260	16	17	1	11
Buddy Topper, 105 g	275	15	20	1	14
• Cheese, 76 g	200	10	19	1	9
Deluxe Topper, 105 g	270	16	20	1	13
• Meat Topper, 102 g	300	18	20	1	15
Pelucci Topper, 102 g	258	13	20	1	13
Pepperoni Topper, 94 g	280	16	20	1	13
Veggie Topper, 113 g	220	11	21	2	10

LaMar's

	Cal	Fat	Cbs	Fbr	Prtn
Donuts					
Apple Fritter	650	26	91	N/A	N/A
Apple Spice Cake Donut	340	17	44	N/A	N/A
Bavarian Cream Bizmark	620	22	101	N/A	N/A
Blueberry Cake Donut	350	17	47	N/A	N/A
Blueberry Filled Bizmark	520	20	81	N/A	N/A
Caramel Iced LaMar's Bar (Unfilled)	430	18	59	N/A	N/A
Cherry Filled Bizmark	550	19	88	N/A	N/A
Chocolate Iced Bar (Chocolate Fluff Filled)	800	35	118	N/A	N/A
Chocolate Iced Bar (Bavarian Cream Filled)	600	22	96	N/A	N/A
Chocolate Iced Bar (White Fluff Filled)	810	35	120	N/A	N/A
Chocolate Iced Cake Donut	330	18	37	N/A	N/A
Chocolate Iced LaMar's Bar (Unfilled)	540	22	81	N/A	N/A

(• = most healthy • = least healthy) **RESTAURANTS & FAST-FOOD • 219**

RESTAURANTS & FAST-FOOD CHAINS

LaMar's (cont.)

Donuts (cont.)	Cal	Fat	Cbs	Fbr	Prtn
Cinnamon Roll	690	25	106	N/A	N/A
Cinnamon Twist	770	26	120	N/A	N/A
German Chocolate Knot	480	27	54	N/A	N/A
Lemon Filled Bizmark	530	21	80	N/A	N/A
Old Fashioned Sour Cream Donut	420	18	60	N/A	N/A
• Raisin Nut Cinnamon Roll	850	27	137	N/A	N/A
Ray's Chocolate Glazed Donut	290	11	44	N/A	N/A
• Ray's Original Glazed Donut	220	10	31	N/A	N/A
White Iced Cake Donut	320	17	38	N/A	N/A

Little Caesar's

Caesar Dips®	Cal	Fat	Cbs	Fbr	Prtn
Buffalo Ranch, 43 g	230	24	3	0	0
• Buffalo, 43 g	140	14	4	0	0
• Buttery Garlic, 43 g	380	42	0	0	0
Cheezy, 43 g	210	21	3	0	1
Chipotle, 43 g	220	24	2	0	0
Ranch, 43 g	250	26	3	0	0
Pizza					
• 14" Hot-N-Ready® Pizza Cheese, 94 g	200	7	25	1	10
14" Hot-N-Ready® Pizza Pepperoni, 99 g	230	9	25	1	11
3 Meat Treat®, 113 g	280	14	25	1	14
Baby Pan! Pan! Cheese, 133 g	320	15	33	1	14
• Baby Pan!Pan! Cheese, Pepperoni, 140 g	360	18	33	1	16
Deep Dish Pizza Cheese, 138 g	320	13	38	1	14
Deep Dish Pizza Pepperoni, 145 g	360	16	38	1	16
Hula Hawaiian™, 123 g	230	8	28	1	12
Ultimate Supreme, 124 g	260	11	26	1	12
Vegetarian, 125 g	220	9	27	2	11
Specialty Items					
Barbecue Caesar Wings, 33 g	70	4	3	0	4
Chocolate Churro Sauce, 28 g	90	3	16	0	0
Churros, 42 g	150	4	25	1	2
Crazy Bread®, 38 g	100	3	15	1	3
Crazy Sauce®, 113 g	45	0	10	1	2
Dulce De Leche Churro Sauce, 28 g	90	3	16	0	0
Hot Caesar Wings, 33 g	60	5	1	0	4
Italian Cheese Bread®, 46 g	130	7	13	0	6
Mild Caesar Wings, 30 g	60	4	1	0	4
• Oven Roasted Caesar Wings®, 26 g	50	4	0	0	4
• Pepperoni Cheese Bread® 10 pcs, 49 g	150	8	13	0	7

Long John Silver's

Chicken	Cal	Fat	Cbs	Fbr	Prtn
Chicken Plank®, 52 g	140	8	9	1	8
Desserts					
Chocolate Cream Pie, 74 g	310	22	24	1	5
• Pecan Pie, 95 g	370	15	55	2	4
• Pineapple Cream Pie, 89 g	290	13	39	1	4
Dipping Sauces					
Cocktail Sauce, 1 oz.	25	0	6	0	0
Tartar Sauce, 1 oz.	101	9	4	0	0

RESTAURANTS & FAST-FOOD CHAINS

Long John Silver's (cont.)	Cal	Fat	Cbs	Fbr	Prtn
Fish and Seafood					
Alaskan Flounder, 104 g	250	11	26	2	12
Baked Cod, 101 g	120	5	1	0	22
Battered Fish, 92 g	260	16	17	1	12
• Battered Shrimp, 14 g	45	3	3	0	2
• Breaded Clams, 85 g	320	19	29	2	9
Buttered Lobster Bites, 99 g	250	9	27	2	14
Popcorn Shrimp, 83 g	270	16	23	1	9
Salads & Dressings					
• Crispy Chicken Club Salad, 390 g	510	30	35	5	28
Garden Ranch Dressing, 43 g	230	24	2	0	1
Lite Italian Dressing, 43 g	20	1	3	0	0
Shrimp & Seafood Salad, 356 g	260	12	22	4	18
Thousand Island Dressing, 43 g	220	21	7	0	0
Sandwiches					
• Chicken Sandwich, 137 g	360	15	40	3	14
Fish Sandwich, 177 g	470	23	48	3	18
Ultimate Fish Sandwich ®, 199 g	530	28	49	3	21
Sides					
Cole Slaw, 4 oz.	200	15	15	3	1
• Hushpuppies, 23 g	60	3	9	1	1
• Large Fries, 5 oz.	390	17	56	5	4
Lobster Stuffed Crab Cake, 62 g	170	9	16	1	6
Regular Fries, 3 oz.	230	10	34	3	3
Starters					
Cheesesticks, 45 g	140	8	12	1	4
Clam Chowder, 245 g	170	8	19	1	4
• Corn Cobbette, 95 g	90	3	14	3	3
Crumblies®, 1 oz.	170	12	14	1	1
• Rice, 4 oz.	180	4	34	3	3

Macaroni Grill	Cal	Fat	Cbs	Fbr	Prtn
Amore De La Grill					
Boursin Filet	930	63	39	5	52
Chicken Portobello	1020	66	61	5	46
Chicken Sorrentino	1050	46	85	6	72
Grilled Halibut	830	43	56	2	52
• Grilled Pork Chops	1940	111	93	8	114
Grilled Salmon (Teriyaki)	1230	74	79	5	56
Honey Balsamic Chicken	1190	59	94	10	68
• Pollo Magro "Skinny Chicken"	330	5	29	5	42
Simple Salmon	660	42	18	8	51
Tuscan Ribeye	1000	66	40	6	58
Antipasti					
Calamari Fritti	1210	78	66	4	62
Crab Stuffed Mushrooms	750	38	71	12	32
Mozzarella Fritta	880	63	54	3	24
Parmesan Crusted Artichokes	820	62	40	6	27
Peasant Bread, 1 Loaf	520	11	89	4	14
• Romano's Sampler (All 3)	1640	98	126	7	62
Fried Calamari only	670	29	59	3	39
Fried Mozzarella only	480	32	32	1	15
Tomato Bruschetta only	450	33	31	2	8
Garnish only	60	4	4	1	1

RESTAURANTS & FAST-FOOD CHAINS

Macaroni Grill (cont.)

	Cal	Fat	Cbs	Fbr	Prtn
Antipasti (cont.)					
Shrimp & Artichoke Dip w/ Croutons	980	52	88	7	43
Tomato Bruschetta	1000	70	75	6	17
Brick-Oven Pizzas					
• BBQ Chicken Pizza, whole pizza	970	24	135	6	48
• Pesto Chicken Pizza, whole pizza	1940	101	163	18	97
Pizza Margherita, whole pizza	1010	34	123	7	49
Sicilian Pizza, whole pizza	1450	70	124	7	75
Clasico Italian					
Chicken & Shrimp Scaloppine, Dinner	1380	97	68	6	45
Chicken & Shrimp Scaloppine, Lunch	1260	89	66	6	38
Chicken Marsala, Dinner	1090	66	76	4	33
Chicken Marsala, Lunch	980	59	73	4	26
Chicken Scaloppine, Dinner	1110	71	68	6	42
Chicken Scaloppine, Lunch	1010	64	65	6	35
Eggplant Parmesan, Dinner	1240	64	118	23	45
Eggplant Parmesan, Lunch	1080	57	102	17	40
Fettuccine Alfredo w/ Chicken, Lunch & Dinner	1370	97	68	4	51
Fettuccine Alfredo w/ Shrimp, Lunch & Dinner	1320	95	70	4	43
Fettuccine Alfredo, Lunch & Dinner	1130	81	68	4	28
Layers & Layers of Lasagna, Dinner	1680	87	120	9	100
Layers & Layers of Lasagna, Lunch	890	47	61	4	53
Mama's Trio, Lunch & Dinner	1290	69	81	4	86
Mushroom Ravioli, Lunch & Dinner	990	67	57	4	27
Primo Chicken Parmesan, Dinner	2220	148	126	5	90
Primo Chicken Parmesan, Lunch	1380	86	89	4	51
Spaghetti & Meat Sauce, Dinner	1110	63	87	8	44
• Spaghetti & Meat Sauce, Lunch	830	46	66	6	35
• Spaghetti & Mtballs w/ Meat Sauce, Dinner	2430	128	207	14	96
Spaghetti & Mtballs w/ Meat Sauce, Lunch	1290	79	84	8	59
Spaghetti & Mtballs w/Tom. Sauce, Dinner	1430	81	119	11	56
Spaghetti & Mtballs w/Tom. Sauce, Lunch	1080	63	89	8	40
Traditional Lasagna, Lunch & Dinner	1040	54	65	4	66
Twice Bkd Lasagna w/ Mtballs, Lunch & Dinner	1470	83	81	6	90
Veal Marsala, Lunch & Dinner	1320	66	132	4	39
Veal Parmesan, Lunch & Dinner	1270	64	116	6	56
Desserts					
Amaretto Apple Crispetti	1300	45	218	3	10
• Dessert Ravioli	1630	74	223	3	19
• Italian Sorbetto with Biscotti	330	4	71	0	2
Lemon Passion	1150	56	149	0	17
New York Cheesecake	980	69	75	0	16
New York Cheesecake w/ Caramel Fudge	1610	96	169	1	21
Smothered Chocolate Cake	1180	68	140	6	15
Tiramisu	1000	64	89	1	12
Dressings & Sauces					
Balsamic Vinaigrette Dressing, 1 fl.oz.	100	9	2	0	0
Basil Aioli Sauce, 1 fl.oz.	130	14	1	0	2
Caesar Dressing, 1 fl.oz.	160	16	1	0	1
Cider Vinaigrette Dressing, 1 fl.oz.	140	11	9	0	0
Creamy Italian Dressing, 1 fl.oz.	110	10	5	0	0
• Fat-Free Creamy Italian Dressing, 1 fl.oz.	30	0	5	1	0
Honey Mustard Dressing, 1 fl.oz.	130	12	6	0	0
Italian Dressing, 1 fl.oz.	90	8	2	0	0

RESTAURANTS & FAST-FOOD CHAINS

Macaroni Grill (cont.)

	Cal	Fat	Cbs	Fbr	Prtn
Dressings & Sauces (cont.)					
Low-Fat Caesar Dressing, 1 fl.oz.	30	2	4	0	1
Parmesan Peppercorn Ranch, 1 fl.oz.	90	9	1	0	2
Pizzaiola Sauce, 1 fl.oz.	30	2	2	0	0
Roasted Garlic Lemon Vinaigrette, 1 fl.oz.	170	17	4	0	0
Toscana Dressing, 1 fl.oz.	160	17	1	0	0
Insalata (Salads)					
Caesar della Casa (House)	260	21	13	2	6
w/o dressing	110	5	12	2	6
Chicken Caesar	920	69	24	6	54
w/o dressing	462	20	20	6	51
Chicken Florentine	840	53	62	7	33
w/o dressing	490	19	50	7	33
Garden della Casa (House)	240	15	20	3	6
w/o dressing	130	5	15	3	6
Insalata Blu	640	53	13	5	18
w/o chicken	760	56	13	5	41
w/o chicken, w/o dressing	570	38	9	5	41
w/o dressing	440	36	9	5	18
Mozzarella Alla Caprese, half order	260	21	5	1	11
Mozzarella Alla Caprese, full order	450	36	9	2	19
Parmesan-Crusted Chicken	1190	63	60	5	91
w/o dressing	1060	49	59	5	88
● Seared Sea Scallops	1320	91	40	6	80
w/o dressing	1050	68	22	6	81
Steak & Arugula	890	71	11	4	47
w/o dressing	570	37	9	3	47
Kid's - Lunch & Dinner					
Chicken Fingerias	650	45	39	1	23
● Double Macaroni 'n' Cheese	1200	62	108	6	68
Fettuccine Alfredo	580	30	53	3	23
● Grilled Chicken & Broccoli	390	5	51	6	33
Mona Lisa's Cheese Masterpizza	840	20	120	6	41
Mona Lisa's Pepperoni Masterpizza	920	27	120	6	44
Spaghetti & Meatballs w/ Meat Sauce	550	24	56	4	27
Spaghetti & Meatballs w/ Tomato Sauce	500	20	58	4	22
Kid's Sides					
Caesar della Casa w/ Caesar Dressing	170	12	11	2	4
Garden della Casa w/ Creamy Italian Dressing	120	8	9	1	3
● Grilled Asparagus	40	2	4	2	2
Grilled Broccoli	80	3	11	5	3
Macaroni 'n' Cheese	350	18	30	1	19
Shoestring Fries	250	15	27	2	3
● Vanilla Ice Cream w/ Chocolate Sauce, 1 Scoop	400	23	43	0	3
Oven Stuffed Pasta					
Chicken Cannelloni, Dinner	1080	58	62	4	73
● Chicken Cannelloni, Lunch	720	39	42	3	49
● Lobster Ravioli, Lunch & Dinner	1090	78	55	4	36
● Marsala Chicken Ravioli	1300	85	55	3	64
Mushroom Ravioli	820	59	42	3	18
Pasta Di Prima					
Carmela's Chicken Rigatoni, Dinner	1320	85	84	6	36
Carmela's Chicken Rigatoni, Lunch	1030	64	64	5	32
Pasta Milano, Dinner	1120	57	108	13	46

RESTAURANTS & FAST-FOOD CHAINS

Macaroni Grill (cont.)

Pasta Di Prima (cont.)	Cal	Fat	Cbs	Fbr	Prtn
• Pasta Milano, Lunch	920	48	83	10	40
• Penne Rustica, Dinner	1540	80	101	9	92
Penne Rustica, Lunch	1300	71	76	6	79
Penne with Oven Roasted Chicken	1330	80	83	8	60
Seafood Linguine	1130	71	79	6	38
Shrimp Portofino, Dinner	1110	78	66	5	35
Shrimp Portofino, Lunch	1070	78	66	5	29
Sizzling Shrimp Scampi	1380	97	94	7	20
Vodka Rustica, Lunch & Dinner	1160	58	77	6	59
Sandwiches					
• Brick-Oven Meatball Sandwich	1890	115	149	10	62
• Chicken Caesar Calzonetto	1540	88	124	8	65
Roasted Chicken & Cheese Sandwich	1630	91	128	8	68
Signature Sides					
Garlic Mashed Potatoes	280	14	35	3	3
• Grilled Asparagus	30	1	4	2	2
Pasta Salad	460	16	69	4	12
• Romano's Parmesan Chips	660	51	39	3	8
Sautéed Broccoli	260	22	12	5	4
Signature Soups					
Chicken Toscana Soup, 1 cup	260	16	18	1	11
Italian Sausage & Tomato Soup, 1 cup	180	7	22	3	8

Maggie Moo's Icecream

	Cal	Fat	Cbs	Fbr	Prtn
• Fat Free, 72 g	80	0	18	0	3
Low-Carb NSA, 64 g	130	9	10	0	2
Sorbet, 85 g	90	0	22	0	0
• Udderly Cream, 80 g	180	11	18	0	3

Manchu Wok

	Cal	Fat	Cbs	Fbr	Prtn
BBQ Pork, 5 oz.	427	26	21	0	26
Beef & Broccoli, 5 oz.	271	23	10	2	8
Black Mushroom, 5 oz.	159	10	11	1	8
Black Pepper Beef, 5 oz.	286	25	8	1	8
Butterfly Shrimp, 5 oz.	235	7	30	1	13
Chicken & Mushrooms, 5 oz.	254	22	8	1	7
Chicken Wings, 5 oz.	406	33	7	0	19
Chicken with Snow, 5 oz.	227	18	11	2	6
Dry Ribs, 5 oz.	339	22	18	0	15
Fried Rice, 8 oz.	310	14	39	2	7
• Garlic Green Bean, 5 oz.	117	7	12	3	3
General Tso's Chicken, 5 oz.	319	21	23	1	10
Ginger Beef, 5 oz.	318	16	31	1	13
Green Bean Chicken, 5 oz.	258	21	11	2	8
Honey Garlic Chicken, 5 oz.	326	15	39	1	32
Honey Garlic Ribs, 5 oz.	393	19	42	0	51
Hunan Beef, 5 oz.	290	24	13	1	8
Kung Pao Chicken, 5 oz.	242	19	10	1	6
Lemon Chicken, 5 oz.	331	23	21	0	11
Mixed Vegetables, 5 oz.	130	9	12	3	2
Noodles, 8 oz.	259	13	29	3	6
Orange Chicken, 5 oz.	279	15	29	1	8
Oriental Grilled, 5 oz.	255	9	21	0	19

RESTAURANTS & FAST-FOOD CHAINS

Manchu Wok (cont.)	Cal	Fat	Cbs	Fbr	Prtn
Pineapple Chicken, 5 oz.	253	17	20	1	5
Satay Chicken, 5 oz.	211	16	11	1	6
Sesame Chicken, 5 oz.	415	17	55	1	12
Spicy Beef, 5 oz.	287	25	9	1	8
• Sweet & Sour Chicken, 5 oz.	450	32	26	3	14
Sweet & Sour Pork, 5 oz.	271	16	24	1	8
Sweet & Sour Sauce, 4 oz.	115	0	30	0	0

Max & Erma's	Cal	Fat	Cbs	Fbr	Prtn
Appetizers					
Black Bean Rolls Up	577	10	95	10	29
Beverages					
Fruit Smoothie	124	0	29	1	1
Dressings					
• Bleu Cheese, 2 tbsp.	201	21	0	0	1
Fat-Free French, 2 tbsp.	126	0	31	2	0
Fat-Free Honey Mustard, 2 tbsp.	60	0	14	0	0
Italian, 2 tbsp.	110	12	1	0	0
• Low-Fat Tex Mex Dressings, 2 tbsp.	23	0	2	0	3
Ranch, 2 tbsp.	120	13	1	0	1
Entrees					
Caribbean Chicken, Lunch Portion	536	20	59	3	28
Salads					
• Baby Green Salad w/o breadstick	119	11	6	2	1
Half Hula Bowl	366	4	57	4	24
• Hula Bowl	576	7	79	6	46
Shrimp Stack Salad	322	12	33	3	20
Sides					
Fruit Salad, 5 oz.	54	0	17	1	1
Garlic Breadstick, 1 Bread	156	6	21	0	4

Mazzio's Pizza	Cal	Fat	Cbs	Fbr	Prtn
Deep Pan Pizza Choices: One Topping Pizzas					
• Canadian Bacon, 137 g	330	14	38	2	13
Cheese, 130 g	332	15	38	2	11
Chicken, 144 g	338	14	38	2	14
Hamburger (Beef), 144 g	359	17	38	2	14
Pepperoni, 131 g	352	17	37	2	12
• Sausage, 144 g	374	19	38	2	13
Deep Pan Pizza Choices: Pricebuster Pizzas					
• Cheesebuster, 130 g	348	16	38	2	13
• Meatbuster, 146 g	385	20	38	2	13
Supremebuster, 144 g	356	17	38	2	12
Deep Pan Pizza Choices: Specialty Pizzas					
4 Meat, 151 g	403	21	38	2	14
California Alfredo, 144 g	383	19	38	2	15
Chicken Club, 150 g	355	16	38	2	15
Combo, 160 g	381	19	39	2	13
• Greek, 142 g	414	24	38	2	15
Lucky 7 Pizza, 162 g	353	17	39	2	11
Mazzio's "Works", 171 g	406	21	39	2	14
Mexican, 183 g	413	21	42	3	15
Veggie, 152 g	331	15	39	2	10

RESTAURANTS & FAST-FOOD CHAINS

Mazzio's Pizza (cont.)

	Cal	Fat	Cbs	Fbr	Prtn
Dippin Zone: Calzone Rings & Quesapizza					
Chicken Quesapizza w/o Sauce, 113 g	317	13	33	1	16
Four Meat/Four Cheese Calzone w/o Sauce, 96 g	274	11	33	1	11
• Ham Bacon & Cheddar Calzone w/o Sauce, 90 g	244	8	32	1	11
Pepperoni Calzone w/o Sauce, 87 g	260	10	33	1	10
• Pepperoni Quesapizza w/o Sauce, 99 g	332	16	32	1	13
Dippin Zone: Dippin Ribs					
Rib Dippers (3/4 lb) Tossed w/ BBQ, 138 g	458	32	13	N/A	28
Dippin Zone: Dippin' Chicken					
• Boneless Dippin' Chicken (10 ct), 51 g	122	6	7	0	10
• Rstd & BBQ Tossed Wings (10 ct), 82 g	191	12	7	N/A	14
Wings of Fire (10 ct) w/o Sauce, 71 g	161	11	1	N/A	15
Dippin Zone: Dippin' Fries					
Cheese Fries, 179 g	432	26	35	3	14
• Fries w/ Sandwich, 266 g	558	29	67	7	6
• Full Order, 133 g	279	14	34	3	3
Dippin Zone: Dippin' Sauces					
BBQ, 2 oz.	140	N/A	34	N/A	N/A
Blue Cheese, 2 oz.	302	32	2	N/A	2
• Buffalo, 2 oz.	19	N/A	4	N/A	N/A
Chocolate, 2 oz.	177	1	43	1	N/A
• Cool Ranch, 2 oz.	372	39	2	0	1
Honey Mustard, 2 oz.	260	22	14	N/A	N/A
Ketchup, 2 oz.	50	N/A	13	N/A	N/A
Marinara, 2 oz.	29	1	5	1	1
Picante, 2 oz.	20	N/A	4	1	N/A
Southwestern Ranch, 2 oz.	321	34	2	0	1
Vanilla, 2 oz.	181	0	45	0	N/A
Dippin Zone: Italian Dippin'					
Toasted Ravioli w/o Sauce, 43 g	118	5	13	1	5
Artichoke Spin Dip w/ Bread, 87 g	245	16	18	2	6
• Breadsticks w/o Sauce, 52 g	150	3	26	1	5
• Cheese Dippers w/o Sauce, 128 g	405	18	47	2	13
• Garlic Cheese Toast w/o Sauce, 54 g	205	13	16	1	6
Garlic Toast w/o Sauce, 40 g	160	10	15	1	3
Mozzarella Sticks w/o Sauce, 57 g	181	12	10	N/A	9
Dippin Zone: Southwestern Dippin'					
• Cheese Nachos w/ Jalapeños, 113 g	423	30	19	2	20
Nachos (Beef w/ Jalapeños), 142 g	484	34	20	2	25
Nachos (Chicken w/ Jalapeños), 135 g	448	30	20	2	24
• Nachos (Sausage w/ Jalapeños), 142 g	504	37	20	2	23
Dippin Zone: Sweet Dippin'					
Cinnamon Sticks w/o Sauce, 145 g	626	36	70	2	5
French Bread					
Deli, 1 bread	480	20	60	3	18
• Greek, 1 bread	623	31	61	3	28
• Hawaiian, 1 bread	449	13	62	3	23
Pepperoni, 1 bread	495	21	58	3	22
Southwestern Chicken, 1 bread	532	20	61	3	28
Original Crust Pizza Choices: One Topping Pizzas					
• Canadian Bacon, 113 g	231	8	30	2	11
Cheese, 105 g	234	9	30	2	10
Chicken, 120 g	239	7	31	2	13
Hamburger (Beef), 120 g	260	10	31	2	13

RESTAURANTS & FAST-FOOD CHAINS

Mazzio's Pizza (cont.)

	Cal	Fat	Cbs	Fbr	Prtn
Original Crust Pizza Choices: One Topping Pizzas (cont.)					
Pepperoni, 106 g	254	10	30	2	11
Sausage, 120 g	276	12	31	2	12
Original Crust Pizza Choices: Pricebuster Pizzas					
Cheesebuster, 105 g	249	9	30	2	11
Meatbuster, 121 g	286	13	31	2	12
Supremebuster, 119 g	257	10	31	2	10
Original Crust Pizza Choices: Specialty Pizzas					
4 Meat, 126 g	305	15	31	2	13
California Alfredo, 119 g	285	13	30	1	14
Chicken Club, 125 g	257	9	31	2	14
Combo, 135 g	282	12	31	2	11
Greek, 117 g	315	17	30	1	14
Lucky 7 Pizza, 137 g	255	10	32	2	10
Mazzio's "Works", 146 g	307	14	31	2	13
Mexican, 158 g	314	14	35	3	14
Veggie, 127 g	232	8	31	2	9
Pasta Choices: Signature Pastas					
Chicken Parmesan, 614 g	947	27	135	9	65
Chicken Spinach Artichoke Pasta, 463 g	1005	38	113	10	49
Chicken-Fried Chicken Alfredo, 479 g	1290	69	120	5	70
Fettuccine Alfredo, 343 g	1061	56	107	4	33
Garlic Toast, 1 Piece	160	10	15	1	3
Greek Pasta, 458 g	1456	94	107	6	41
Lasagna Red & White, 669 g	984	62	64	5	46
w/ Alfredo, 598 g	1264	94	55	3	53
w/ Marinara, 740 g	704	30	73	8	39
w/ Meat Sauce, 712 g	949	52	64	8	57
Spaghetti w/ Marinara, 449 g	641	13	120	8	22
w/ Meat Sauce, 428 g	825	25	113	8	36
w/ Meatballs (4) & Marinara, 562 g	972	34	126	10	42
w/ Meatballs (4) & Meat Sauce, 541 g	1156	50	119	9	55
Sandwiches					
Chkn, Bacon & Swiss (Focaccia), 392 g	1021	70	48	2	48
Chkn, Bacon & Swiss (Hoagie), 510 g	1362	72	120	6	60
Ham & Cheddar (Focaccia), 351 g	747	47	47	1	36
Ham & Cheddar (Hoagie), 470 g	1088	50	119	5	49
Kosher Pickle Spear, 28 g	5	N/A	1	N/A	N/A
Mazzio's Sub (Focaccia), 344 g	768	49	45	1	37
Mazzio's Sub (Hoagie), 462 g	1109	52	117	5	49
Turkey & Swiss (Focaccia), 376 g	718	38	46	1	41
Turkey & Swiss (Hoagie), 494 g	1059	40	118	5	53
Tuscan Smash (Focaccia), 354 g	645	34	45	1	33
Tuscan Smash (Hoagie), 473 g	986	36	117	5	46
Thin Crust Pizza Choices: One Topping Pizzas					
Canadian Bacon, 91 g	179	8	18	1	10
Cheese, 84 g	182	9	18	1	9
Chicken, 98 g	187	8	18	1	12
Hamburger, 98 g	208	11	19	2	11
Pepperoni, 85 g	202	11	18	1	9
Sausage, 98 g	224	12	19	1	10
Thin Crust Pizza Choices: Pricebuster Pizzas					
Cheesebuster, 84 g	197	9	19	1	10
Meatbuster, 100 g	234	13	19	2	11

(• = most healthy • = least healthy) **RESTAURANTS & FAST-FOOD • 227**

RESTAURANTS & FAST-FOOD CHAINS

Mazzio's Pizza (cont.)

	Cal	Fat	Cbs	Fbr	Prtn
Thin Crust Pizza Choices: Pricebuster Pizzas (cont.)					
Supremebuster, 98 g	205	11	19	2	9
Thin Crust Pizza Choices: Specialty Pizzas					
4 Meat, 105 g	253	15	19	2	12
California Alfredo, 98 g	233	13	18	1	12
Chicken Club, 104 g	205	9	19	1	13
Combo, 114 g	231	13	19	2	10
• Greek, 96 g	263	17	19	1	12
Lucky 7 Pizza, 116 g	203	10	20	2	9
Mazzio's "Works", 125 g	255	15	20	2	11
Mexican, 136 g	262	14	23	3	12
• Veggie, 105 g	180	8	19	2	8

McDonald's

	Cal	Fat	Cbs	Fbr	Prtn
Breakfast					
Bacon, Egg, Cheese Biscuit, 5 oz.	450	25	36	2	18
Bacon, Egg, Cheese McGriddles®, 4 oz.	460	21	48	2	19
Big Breakfast® 9 oz.	720	46	49	3	27
Biscuit (Large), 3.2 oz.	320	16	39	3	5
Biscuit (Regular), 2.7 oz.	250	11	32	2	4
• Dlx Breakfast w/o Syrup/Margarine, 15 oz.	1070	55	109	6	36
• Egg McMuffin®, 5 oz.	300	12	30	2	18
English Muffin, 2 oz.	160	3	27	2	5
Grape Jam, 0.5 oz.	35	0	9	0	0
Hash Browns, 2 oz.	140	8	15	2	1
Hotcake Syrup, 60 g	180	0	45	0	0
Hotcakes & Sausage (w/o Syrup/Margarine), 7 oz.	520	24	61	3	15
Hotcakes (w/o Syrup/Margarine), 5 oz.	350	9	60	3	8
McSkillet Burrito w/ Sausage, 8 oz.	610	36	44	3	27
w/ Steak, 9 oz.	570	30	44	3	32
Sausage Biscuit w/ Egg, 6 oz.	500	32	35	2	17
Sausage Biscuit, 4 oz.	410	27	33	2	11
Sausage Burrito, 4 oz.	300	16	26	1	12
Sausage McGriddles®, 5 oz.	420	22	44	2	11
Sausage McMuffin®, 4 oz.	370	22	29	2	14
w/ Egg, 6 oz.	450	27	30	2	21
Sausage Patty, 1 oz.	170	15	1	0	7
Sausage, Egg, Cheese McGriddles®, 7 oz.	560	32	48	2	20
Scrambled Eggs (2), 3 oz.	170	11	1	0	15
Strawberry Preserves, 0.5 oz.	35	0	9	0	0
Whipped Margarine, 6 g	40	5	0	0	0
Chicken McNuggets®/Selects® Premium Breast Strips/Sauces					
Barbecue Sauce, 28 g	50	0	12	0	0
• Chicken McNuggets® (6 piece), 3 oz.	250	15	15	0	15
Creamy Ranch Sauce, 2 oz.	200	22	2	0	0
Honey, 14 g	50	0	12	0	0
Hot Mustard Sauce, 28 g	60	3	9	2	1
• Premium Breast Strips (3 pcs.), 5 oz.	380	20	28	0	23
Spicy Buffalo Sauce, 2 oz.	70	7	1	2	0
SW Chipotle Barbecue Sauce, 2 oz.	70	0	18	1	0
Sweet 'N Sour Sauce, 28 g	50	0	12	0	0
Tangy Honey Mustard Sauce, 2 oz.	70	3	13	0	1
Desserts/Shakes					
• Apple Dippers, 68 g	35	0	8	0	0

RESTAURANTS & FAST-FOOD CHAINS

McDonald's (cont.)	Cal	Fat	Cbs	Fbr	Prtn
Desserts/Shakes (cont.)					
Baked Apple Pie, 3 oz.	270	12	36	4	3
Chocolate Chip Cookie, 33 g	160	7	22	1	2
Chocolate Triple Thick® Shake, 16 fl.oz.	580	14	102	1	13
Cinnamon Melts, 4 oz.	460	19	66	3	6
Fruit 'n Yogurt Parfait, 5 oz.	160	2	31	1	4
w/o Granola, 5 oz.	130	2	25	0	4
Hot Caramel Sundae, 6 oz.	340	8	60	1	7
Hot Fudge Sundae, 6 oz.	330	10	54	2	8
Kiddie Cone, 1 oz.	45	1	8	0	1
Low Fat Caramel Dip, 1 oz.	70	1	15	0	0
McDonaldland® Choco Chip Cookies, 2 oz.	270	11	39	1	3
McDonaldland® Cookies, 2 oz.	250	8	42	1	4
• McFlurry® w/ M&M'S® Candies, 12 fl.oz.	620	20	96	1	14
McFlurry® w/ OREO® Cookies, 12 fl.oz.	560	16	88	0	14
Oatmeal Raisin Cookie, 33 g	150	6	22	1	2
Peanuts (for Sundaes), 0.5 oz.	45	4	2	1	2
Strawberry Sundae, 6 oz.	280	6	49	1	6
Strawberry Triple Thick® Shake, 16 fl.oz.	560	13	97	0	13
Sugar Cookie, 32 g	150	6	21	0	2
Vanilla Reduced Fat Ice Cream Cone, 3 oz.	150	4	24	0	4
Vanilla Triple Thick® Shake, 16 fl.oz.	550	13	96	0	13
French Fries					
Ketchup Packet, 10 g	15	0	3	0	0
• Large French Fries, 6 oz.	570	30	70	7	6
Medium French Fries, 4 oz.	380	20	47	5	4
Salt Packet, 1 g	0	0	0	0	0
• Small French Fries, 3 oz.	250	13	30	3	2
Iced Coffee					
Caramel (Medium), 24 fl.oz.	190	8	27	0	1
Hazelnut (Medium), 24 fl.oz.	190	8	29	0	1
Regular (Medium), 24 fl.oz.	200	8	30	0	1
Vanilla (Medium), 24 fl.oz.	190	8	29	0	1
Salad					
Asian Salad w/ Grilled Chicken, 13 oz.	300	10	23	5	32
w/ Crispy Chicken, 13 oz.	380	17	33	5	27
w/o Chicken, 9 oz.	150	7	15	5	8
Bacon Ranch Salad w/ Grilled Chkn, 11 oz.	260	9	12	3	33
w/ Crispy Chicken, 11 oz.	350	16	23	3	28
w/o Chicken, 8 oz.	140	7	10	3	9
Butter Garlic Croutons, 0.5 oz.	60	2	10	1	2
Caesar Salad w/ Grilled Chicken, 11 oz.	220	6	12	3	30
w/ Crispy Chicken, 11 oz.	300	13	22	3	25
w/o Chicken, 8 oz.	90	4	9	3	7
• Side Salad, 3 oz.	20	0	4	1	1
Snack Size Fruit & Walnut Salad, 163 g	210	8	31	2	4
Southwest Salad w/ Grilled Chkn, 12 oz.	320	9	30	7	30
• w/ Crispy Chicken, 12 oz.	400	16	41	7	25
w/o Chicken, 8 oz.	140	5	20	6	6
Salad Dressings: Newman's Own®					
• Creamy Caesar Dressing, 2 fl.oz.	190	18	4	0	2
Creamy Southwest Dressing, 2 fl.oz.	100	6	11	0	1
• Low Fat Balsamic Vinaigrette, 2 fl.oz.	40	3	4	0	1
Low Fat Family Recipe Italian, 2 fl.oz.	60	3	8	0	1

RESTAURANTS & FAST-FOOD CHAINS

McDonald's (cont.)

	Cal	Fat	Cbs	Fbr	Prtn
Salad Dressings: Newman's Own® (cont.)					
Low Fat Sesame Ginger Dressing, 2 fl.oz.	90	3	15	0	1
Ranch Dressing, 2 fl.oz.	170	15	9	0	1
Sandwiches					
Big Mac®, 8 oz.	540	29	45	3	25
Big N' Tasty®, 7 oz.	460	24	37	3	24
w/ Cheese, 8 oz.	510	28	38	3	27
Cheeseburger, 4 oz.	300	12	33	2	15
Chipotle BBQ Snack Wrap w/ Grilled Chkn, 4 oz.	260	8	28	1	18
Dble Cheeseburger, 6 oz.	440	23	34	2	25
• Dble Quarter Pounder® w/ Cheese, 10 oz.	740	42	40	3	48
Filet-O-Fish®, 5 oz.	380	18	38	2	15
• Hamburger, 4 oz.	250	9	31	2	12
Honey Mustard Snack Wrap w/ Crispy Chkn, 4 oz.	320	15	34	1	14
McChicken®, 5 oz.	360	16	40	1	14
McRib®†, 7 oz.	500	26	44	3	22
Premium Crispy Chkn Club Sandwich, 9 oz.	660	28	63	4	39
Premium Grilled Chkn Classic Sandwich, 8 oz.	420	10	51	3	32
Premium Grilled Chkn Ranch BLT Sandwich, 9 oz.	520	16	53	3	40
Ranch Snack Wrap® w/ Grilled Chkn, 4 oz.	270	10	26	1	18
Quarter Pounder®+, 6 oz.	410	19	37	3	24
w/ Cheese, 7 oz.	510	26	40	3	29

Mr. Goodcents

	Cal	Fat	Cbs	Fbr	Prtn
Bread					
• Gold, 106 g	189	3	26	17	17
Wheat Bread, 128 g	279	4	54	5	12
• White Bread, 128 g	288	2	58	2	10
Cold Subs (Half Sub)					
Centsable Sub Wheat Bread, 227 g	493	20	57	5	25
Centsable Sub White Bread, 227 g	502	19	61	2	23
Cheese Mix Wheat Bread, 213 g	571	26	57	5	30
Cheese Mix White Bread, 213 g	580	25	61	2	29
Ham & Cheese Wheat Bread, 227 g	410	10	58	5	26
Ham & Cheese White Bread, 227 g	419	9	62	2	24
Italian Sub Wheat Bread, 213 g	622	34	57	5	27
Italian Sub White Bread, 213 g	631	33	61	2	25
Original, Wheat Bread, 213 g	512	23	56	5	24
Original, White Bread, 213 g	520	22	60	2	22
Oven Rstd Chicken, Wheat Bread, 213 g	355	6	54	5	27
Oven Rstd Chicken, White Bread, 213 g	364	5	58	2	25
Penny Club Wheat Bread, 213 g	364	7	56	5	24
Penny Club White Bread, 213 g	373	5	60	2	22
Pepperoni & Cheese Wheat Bread, 227 g	709	43	57	5	29
• Pepperoni & Cheese White Bread, 227 g	718	41	61	2	28
Roast Beef Wheat Bread, 213 g	369	7	54	5	27
Roast Beef White Bread, 213 g	378	5	58	2	25
Tuna Salad Wheat Bread, 213 g	500	21	62	6	21
Tuna Salad White Bread, 213 g	509	20	66	3	19
Turkey Wheat Bread, 213 g	354	6	57	5	22
Turkey White Bread, 213 g	363	4	61	2	20
• Veggie Sub Wheat Bread, 212 g	295	4	57	7	13
Veggie Sub White Bread, 212 g	305	2	61	3	11

RESTAURANTS & FAST-FOOD CHAINS

Mr. Goodcents (cont.)

	Cal	Fat	Cbs	Fbr	Prtn
Desserts					
• Baked Brownie, 65 g	260	10	41	1	3
• Giant Chocolate Chip Cookie, 71 g	420	22	52	1	4
Giant Peanut Butter Cookie, 71 g	340	20	36	2	6
Dress Options					
American Cheese, 14 g	41	3	0	0	5
Bacon, 3 slices	61	5	0	0	4
Cheddar Cheese, 14 g	57	5	0	0	5
Jalapeños, 7 g	2	0	0	0	0
Mayonnaise, 7 g	51	6	0	0	0
Mozzarella, 14 g	40	3	0	0	3
• Mustard, 7 g	0	0	0	0	0
Olives, 7 g	28	2	2	0	0
Pepper Jack, 14 g	51	4	1	0	3
Pickles, 14 g	5	0	1	0	0
Provolone, 14 g	50	4	0	0	4
• Ranch Dressing, 14 g	83	9	1	0	0
Spicy Mustard, 7 g	7	0	0	0	0
Spicy Ranch, 14 g	67	7	1	0	0
Standard Dress, 21 g	26	2	2	1	1
Standard Dress, no oil, 14 g	11	0	2	1	1
Swiss, 14 g	53	4	0	0	4
Goodcents Gold "Premium" Sandwiches					
Cold Centsable Sub, 234 g	460	25	31	17	34
Cold Cheese Mix, 220 g	481	26	30	17	36
Cold Ham & Cheese, 234 g	350	11	32	17	36
Cold Italian Sub, 220 g	649	44	30	17	38
Cold Mr. Goodcent Original, 220 g	479	28	29	17	33
Cold Oven Roasted Chicken Breast, 220 g	290	6	26	17	38
Cold Penny Club, 220 g	304	7	29	17	34
• Cold Pepperoni & Cheese, 234 g	750	54	32	17	40
Cold Roast Beef, 220 g	309	7	26	17	37
Cold Tuna Salad, 220 g	410	21	34	17	27
Cold Turkey, 220 g	289	6	30	17	31
• Cold Veggie Sub, 181 g	205	3	30	18	18
Hot Chkn Bacon Ranch w/ Cheddar, 291 g	580	31	28	17	52
Hot Chkn Parmesan w/ Mozzarella, 305 g	436	15	33	17	47
Hot Meatball w/ Mozzarella, 291 g	624	33	38	17	45
Pastrami & Swiss, 284 g	440	18	28	17	46
Philly Jack 'n Cheese, 248 g	430	16	32	17	41
Roast Beef 'n Cheddar, 263 g	452	17	28	17	45
Hot Subs (Half Sub)					
Chken Parmesan Wheat Bread w/ Mzzrella, 326 g	526	15	61	6	41
Chken Parmesan White Bread w/ Mzzrella, 326 g	535	14	65	2	39
Chkn Bacon Ranch Wheat Bread w/ Chddr, 297 g	670	31	55	5	46
Chkn Bacon Ranch White Bread w/ Chddr, 297 g	679	30	59	2	44
Meatball Wheat Bread w/Mozzarella, 312 g	714	33	65	6	39
• Meatball White Bread w/ Mozzarella, 312 g	723	32	69	2	37
Pastrami & Swiss, Wheat, 305 g	530	18	56	6	40
Pastrami & Swiss, White, 305 g	539	17	60	2	38
• Philly Jack 'n Cheese, Wheat, 269 g	520	17	59	5	35
Philly Jack 'n Cheese, White, 269 g	529	15	63	2	33
Roast Beef 'n Cheddar, Wheat, 284 g	542	17	56	6	39
Roast Beef 'n Cheddar, White, 284 g	551	16	60	2	37

(• = most healthy • = least healthy) **RESTAURANTS & FAST-FOOD • 231**

RESTAURANTS & FAST-FOOD CHAINS

Mr. Goodcents (cont.)

	Cal	Fat	Cbs	Fbr	Prtn
Pastas					
Alfredo Sauce on Mostaccioli, 397 g	1290	80	106	4	29
• Chicken Alfredo on Mostaccioli, 510 g	1423	85	106	4	52
Chicken Parmesan on Mostaccioli, 525 g	695	12	100	5	42
Lasagna, 400 g	524	22	54	4	30
Red Sauce on Mastaccioli w/Mtball, 482 g	747	19	105	5	31
• Red Sauce on Mostaccioli, 397 g	522	4	100	5	17
Salads					
Chef Salad, 440 g	195	8	19	5	14
Garden Salad, 369 g	98	3	15	5	4
Grilled Chicken Salad, 482 g	232	8	15	5	27
• Side Salad, 212 g	52	2	8	3	2
• Tuna Salad, 454 g	320	21	23	6	14
Sides					
• Breadstick (1), 43 g	90	0	19	1	3
• Meatballs (2), 114 g	225	15	5	0	14
Pasta Salad, 142 g	213	6	35	1	5
Potato Salad, 142 g	192	7	28	2	2
Soups					
• Broccoli Cheese Soup, 8 oz.	360	22	32	4	10
• Chicken Noodle Soup, 8 oz.	120	1	22	0	6
Cream of Potato Soup, 8 oz.	320	14	42	4	8

Mr. Pita

	Cal	Fat	Cbs	Fbr	Prtn
12" Jumbo Size					
• Cranberry Turkey	597	2	104	4	39
Grilled Chicken & Broccoli	541	6	79	3	38
Grilled Chicken Caesar	514	7	70	1	37
Grilled Hawaiian Chicken	546	6	80	2	39
Grilled Raspberry Chicken	495	5	78	2	33
Ultra Combo (Chicken/Turkey)	514	4	77	3	38
Ultra Grilled Chicken	553	6	78	2	36
Ultra Supreme	510	5	77	2	37
• Ultra Turkey	495	2	77	3	39
7" Value Size					
• Cranberry Turkey	275	1	50	2	16
Grilled Chicken & Broccoli	235	2	36	1	16
Grilled Chicken Caesar	224	3	31	1	16
Grilled Hawaiian Chicken	232	2	35	1	16
Grilled Raspberry Chicken	214	2	35	1	14
Ultra Combo (Chicken/Turkey)	221	2	34	2	16
Ultra Grilled Chicken	229	3	34	2	15
Ultra Supreme	223	2	34	1	16
• Ultra Turkey	214	1	34	2	16
9" Regular Size					
• Cranberry Turkey	424	1	77	3	25
Grilled Chicken & Broccoli	373	4	57	2	24
Grilled Chicken Caesar	353	4	50	1	24
Grilled Hawaiian Chicken	375	4	57	1	25
• Grilled Raspberry Chicken	342	3	56	1	22
Ultra Combo (Chicken/Turkey)	354	3	56	2	24
Ultra Grilled Chicken	367	4	56	2	23
Ultra Supreme	350	3	56	1	23
Ultra Turkey	343	1	56	2	25

RESTAURANTS & FAST-FOOD CHAINS

Mr. Sub	Cal	Fat	Cbs	Fbr	Prtn
6" Classic Subs					
Albacore Tuna, 174 g	280	8	36	2	18
Assorted, 180 g	280	8	38	2	16
BBQ Rib, 141 g	360	16	34	1	20
BLT, 133 g	260	8	34	2	12
Breaded Chicken, 203 g	370	13	45	2	20
Great Canadian Club, 184 g	300	8	38	2	20
Grilled Chicken, 181 g	260	5	37	2	20
Italian Salami, 158 g	280	10	35	2	14
Louisiana Chicken, 161 g	280	8	34	1	19
Maple Baked Ham, 174 g	240	4	39	2	15
Meatball, 146 g	360	14	38	1	20
Mediterranean Vegetables, 182 g	220	4	40	3	8
w/ Cheese, 210 g	300	10	41	3	13
Montreal Style Corned Beef, 154 g	270	6	33	1	21
Pizza Supremo, 110 g	270	10	33	1	14
Philly Style Steak w/o Cheese, 133 g	250	5	34	1	18
w/ Cheese, 145 g	300	8	35	1	21
Roast Beef, 154 g	280	7	34	1	21
• Santa Fe Spicy Chicken, 230 g	370	13	45	2	20
Seafood w/ Crab, 154 g	290	10	42	1	11
Smoked Turkey Breast, 160 g	230	4	35	2	15
• Veggie, 118 g	180	2	34	2	7
6" Grilled Subs					
Classic Reuben, 182 g	280	6	34	2	21
Grilled Buffalo Chicken, 181 g	260	5	37	2	20
• Tuna Melt, 126 g	230	3	32	1	21
w/ Cheese, 156 g	330	10	33	1	29
Ultimate Club w/o Cheddar, 188 g	270	5	38	2	18
• w/ Cheese, 216 g	380	14	38	2	24
Breads: 12" Tortillas					
Cheese, 106 g	300	7	50	2	7
• Spinach w/ Pesto & Garlic, 106 g	300	7	50	2	8
Tomato w/ Basil, 106 g	300	7	50	2	7
• Whole Wheat, 106 g	290	7	47	5	10
Breads: 6" Buns					
Greek Sub Bun, 75 g	190	3	35	2	7
• Mozza-Cheddar Sub Bun, 77 g	190	4	32	2	8
• Multigrain Sub Bun, 70 g	170	2	32	2	7
White Sub Bun, 70 g	170	2	32	2	7
Whole Wheat Sub Bun, 70 g	170	2	32	2	7
Cheese					
• Cheddar Cheese for 6" Subs, 28 g	120	9	0	0	6
Cheese Shred for Salads, 22 g	75	5	1	0	6
Cheese Shred for Wraps, 15 g	50	4	1	0	4
Feta Cheese for Greek Salad, 30 g	85	7	1	0	5
Parmesan for Caesar Salad, 15 g	60	4	1	0	4
Process Slice for 6" Pizza Sub, 25 g	80	6	3	0	5
• Process Slice for 6" Subs, 12 g	40	3	2	0	3
Cookies					
Carnival, 37 g	170	7	24	1	2
Double Chocolate Chip, 37 g	170	8	23	1	2
Milk Chocolate Chunk, 37 g	170	8	23	1	2
• Oatmeal Raisin, 37 g	160	7	23	2	2

(• = most healthy • = least healthy)   **RESTAURANTS & FAST-FOOD** · 233

RESTAURANTS & FAST-FOOD CHAINS

Mr. Sub (cont.)

	Cal	Fat	Cbs	Fbr	Prtn
Cookies (cont.)					
• Triple Chocolate Chip, 37 g	170	8	23	1	2
Dressings					
• Caesar, 36 g	200	21	2	0	1
French, 36 g	130	13	5	0	0
Greek Feta, 36 g	170	17	4	0	1
• Lite Italian, 36 g	80	9	1	0	0
Ranch, 36 g	190	20	2	0	1
Renee's Dressings					
Balsamic, 45 g	170	16	6	0	0
Buttermilk Ranch, 45 g	180	18	3	0	2
• Greek Feta, 45 g	280	30	2	0	2
Mighty Caesar, 45 g	280	30	2	0	1
• Spring Herb and Garlic, 45 g	110	11	3	0	1
Salads					
Albacore Tuna, 240 g	140	6	8	2	13
Classic Caesar, 122 g	70	5	2	1	5
• Garden, 185 g	35	1	6	2	2
• Grilled Chicken Caesar, 185 g	160	7	6	1	18
Maple Baked Ham, 225 g	85	2	10	2	8
Mediterranean Greek, 225 g	70	3	8	2	3
Seafood w/ Crab, 240 g	150	8	15	2	6
Smoked Turkey Breast, 225 g	85	2	8	2	10
Sauces					
BBQ Sauce, 30 g	40	0	10	0	0
Buttermilk Ranch, 10 g	40	4	1	0	0
Honey Mustard, 10 g	20	0	4	0	0
• Hot Sauce, 10 g	4	0	0	0	0
Louisiana Sauce, 10 g	5	0	1	0	0
Mayo Lite, 10 g	35	4	2	0	0
Meatball Sauce, 30 g	15	0	9	1	2
• Mr Sub Secret Sauce, 10 g	40	5	0	0	0
Yellow Mustard, 10 g	5	0	1	0	0
Soups					
Chicken Noodle, 250 g	110	3	17	1	4
Chicken w/ Rice, 250 g	90	2	15	1	3
Chili W/ Beef, 250 g	198	1	34	10	13
Cream of Broccoli, 250 g	170	10	16	2	3
Cream of Mushroom, 250 g	170	10	16	1	4
Cream of Potato & Leek, 250 g	190	9	23	2	4
Cream of Tomato, 250 g	150	6	20	2	4
Creamy Tomato & Rstd Red Pepper, 250 g	110	3	19	2	4
• Garden Vegetable, 250 g	60	0	13	1	2
• Hearty Chili w/ Beef, 250 g	231	2	36	11	18
Italian Wedding, 250 g	140	4	24	1	4
Mediterranean Chicken, 250 g	110	4	15	1	4
Minestrone, 250 g	80	0	17	2	4
Pasta Fagioli, 250 g	150	2	28	6	7
Vegetable Beef & Barley, 250 g	90	1	18	2	3
Toppings					
Bacon, 2 strips	50	4	0	0	3
Banana Peppers, 10 g	2	0	0	0	0
• Croutons, 14 g	60	2	10	0	1

RESTAURANTS & FAST-FOOD CHAINS

Mr. Sub (cont.)	Cal	Fat	Cbs	Fbr	Prtn
Toppings (cont.)					
Cucumbers, 3 slices	2	0	0	0	0
• Dill Pickles, 3 slices	1	0	0	0	0
Green Olives, 10 g	10	1	1	0	0
Green Pepper, 10 g	2	0	1	0	0
Iceberg Lettuce, 28 g	15	0	3	1	1
Jalapeño Peppers, 10 g	2	0	0	0	0
Red Onions, 10 g	4	0	1	0	0
Sliced Mushrooms, 10 g	3	0	1	0	0
Tomatoes, 3 wheels	20	0	4	1	1
Wraps					
Albacore Tuna, 248 g	460	16	52	6	25
Louisiana Chicken, 190 g	430	15	48	5	25
Roast Beef, 218 g	440	14	50	5	29
Seafood w/ Crab, 218 g	470	19	61	5	15
Smoked Turkey Breast, 220 g	370	9	51	6	20
Veggie, 164 g	310	8	49	6	10

Mrs. Fields	Cal	Fat	Cbs	Fbr	Prtn
Bite-Size Nibbler® Cookies					
Cinnamon Sugar, 37 g	170	8	22	0	2
• Debra's Special Nibbler, 38 g	170	7	23	1	2
• Peanut Butter, 38 g	180	10	20	1	3
Semi-Sweet Chocolate, 38 g	170	8	24	1	2
Triple Chocolate, 38 g	170	9	23	1	2
White Chunk Macadamia, 38 g	180	9	23	0	110
Brownies					
Butterscotch Blondie, 76 g	350	14	52	0	3
Double Fudge, 76 g	360	20	45	2	4
• Pecan Fudge, 76 g	360	20	46	2	4
• Special Walnut Fudge & Blondie, 76 g	330	16	43	1	4
Toffee Fudge, 76 g	360	19	47	2	4
Walnut Fudge, 76 g	360	20	45	2	4
Cakes					
Chocolate Chip, 83 g	350	17	45	1	4
Cookies					
• Butter, 44 g	200	8	29	1	2
• Cut Out, 90 g	400	19	56	0	2
Debra's Special, 44 g	200	9	28	1	2
Peanut Butter, 44 g	210	12	24	1	4
Semi-Sweet Chocolate, 44 g	210	10	29	2	2
w/ Walnuts, 44 g	220	11	29	2	2
Triple Chocolate, 44 g	210	11	28	2	2
White Chunk Macadamia, 44 g	230	12	27	1	3
Muffins					
Blueberry, 21 g	70	3	10	0	1
• Chocolate Chip, 21 g	80	4	11	1	1
Mandarin Orange, 21 g	80	3	9	0	1
• Raspberry, 21 g	70	3	10	0	1

Noah's Bagels	Cal	Fat	Cbs	Fbr	Prtn
Bagel Dogs					
Artichoke & Grlc Sasge Bagel Dog, 229 g	530	11	81	3	29
Asiago Bagel Dog, 239 g	730	32	84	2	28

(• = most healthy • = least healthy) **RESTAURANTS & FAST-FOOD • 235**

Noah's Bagels (cont.)

	Cal	Fat	Cbs	Fbr	Prtn
Bagel Dogs (cont.)					
Cajun Andouille Sausage Bagel Dog, 225 g	600	21	78	3	28
• Chicken Portobello Bagel Dog, 229 g	510	12	78	5	29
Everything Bagel Dog, 237 g	660	27	76	4	29
• Plain Bagel Dog, 232 g	740	34	78	2	29
Polish Bagel Dog, 236 g	680	30	78	3	26
Bagel Sandwiches					
Chicken Salad on Plain Bagel, 312 g	740	36	77	4	32
Corned Beef on Plain Bagel, 382 g	910	45	94	4	39
Egg Salad on Plain Bagel, 312 g	750	40	77	4	23
• Hummus on Plain Bagel, 297 g	530	10	94	7	17
N.Y. Lox on Plain Bagel, 299 g	590	19	81	3	28
Pastrami on Plain Bagel, 382 g	910	45	94	4	39
• Rachel on Plain Bagel, 397 g	1010	51	100	3	45
Reuben on Plain Bagel, 397 g	910	40	95	3	44
Roast Beef on Plain Bagel, 382 g	750	31	78	4	44
Tuna Salad on Plain Bagel, 326 g	610	19	77	4	32
Turkey on Plain Bagel, 382 g	760	29	76	4	52
Veggie Sandwich, 283 g	560	18	85	3	17
Whitefish on Plain Bagel, 340 g	930	52	83	3	35
Bagels					
Asiago Cheese Topped Bagel, 134 g	410	5	78	2	17
Blueberry, 120 g	360	1	79	3	12
Candy Cane Bagel, 118 g	340	4	69	2	12
Cheddar Bagel, 113 g	300	2	63	2	11
Chocolate Chip Bagel, 120 g	400	5	80	3	12
Chopped Garlic Bagel, 124 g	360	1	78	2	12
Cinnamon Raisin Bagel, 120 g	360	1	80	2	11
Cinnamon Sugar Bagel, 149 g	520	21	78	2	12
Cracked Pepper Bagel, 120 g	390	5	78	3	12
Cranberry Orange Bagel, 120 g	360	1	80	3	11
Egg Bagel, 120 g	360	2	76	2	12
Everything Bagel, 124 g	360	2	77	2	12
• Good Grains Powerbagel, 114 g	280	5	53	9	13
Irish Soda Bagel, 113 g	360	6	69	4	11
Onion Bagel, 120 g	360	2	77	3	12
Plain Bagel, 120 g	350	1	77	2	12
Poppyseed Bagel, 124 g	370	1	78	2	13
Potato Bagel, 106 g	350	5	69	2	10
• Power Bagel w/ Peanut Butter, 117 g	750	34	92	7	27
Power Bagel, 120 g	410	5	81	4	13
Pumpernickel Bagel, 120 g	350	1	76	3	12
Pumpkin Bagel, 120 g	330	2	69	4	12
Salt Bagel, 124 g	350	1	77	2	12
Sesame Seed Bagel, 124 g	370	3	77	2	13
Sun-Dried Tomato Bagel, 120 g	360	2	77	3	12
Whole Wheat Bagel w/ Seeds, 124 g	350	3	74	4	13
Whole Wheat Bagel, 120 g	330	1	73	4	12
Bialies					
Artichoke Spinach & Asiago Bialy, 260 g	660	18	94	4	33
Artichoke Tomato Red Onion & Asiago Bialy, 323 g	670	18	98	5	33
Cheese Pizza Bialy, 248 g	600	12	97	5	28
• Four Cheese Tomato & Rosemary Bialy, 277 g	670	19	97	5	33
Mushroom & Four Cheese Bialy, 267 g	660	18	94	3	34

Noah's Bagels (cont.)	Cal	Fat	Cbs	Fbr	Prtn
Bialies (cont.)					
• Traditional Bialy, 177 g	450	5	91	3	14
Blended Drinks					
Frozen Café Caramel, 18 oz.	600	16	110	0	8
Frozen Café Latte, 18 oz.	460	18	72	0	9
Frozen Café Mocha, 18 oz.	570	14	107	0	7
• Frozen Strawberry, 18 oz.	440	19	73	3	6
Frozen Vanilla, 18 oz.	580	31	86	0	10
• Mudslide Smoothie, 18 oz.	690	36	101	1	11
Breads					
Braided Challah, 2 oz.	150	3	26	1	6
Challah Roll, 4 oz.	270	5	51	2	9
• Ciabatta Bread, 4 oz.	320	3	64	3	12
Corn Meal Rye Bread, 1 slice	170	1	35	2	6
• Focaccia Wedge, 1 oz.	110	3	17	0	4
Marble Rye Bread, 1 slice	160	1	34	1	6
Multigrain Bread, 1 slice	160	2	32	3	6
Potato Bread, 1 slice	220	3	44	2	6
Coffee Extras					
Light Whipped Cream, 30ml	30	2	2	0	0
On Top Reduced Fat Topping, 8 g	20	2	2	0	0
• Syrup, Almond, 30ml	90	0	23	0	0
Syrup, Hazelnut, 30ml	80	0	20	0	0
Syrup, Premium, Sugar Free Caramel, 30ml	0	0	0	0	0
• Syrup, Premium, Sugar Free Vanilla, 30ml	0	0	0	0	0
Syrup, Vanilla, 30ml	80	0	19	0	0
Condiments					
Deli Mustard, 5	4	0	0	0	0
• Mayo, 14	110	12	0	0	0
Whole Kosher Pickle, 50	5	0	1	1	0
• Yellow Mustard, 5	0	0	0	0	0
Deli Sandwich					
California Chicken, 365 g	520	19	56	4	43
Chicken Salad Deli, 262 g	590	36	41	3	28
Cornbeef Deli, 227 g	540	22	53	2	33
Deli Beef Roast, 296 g	390	8	41	3	39
• Double Decker Club Sandwich, 398 g	920	33	104	11	46
Egg Salad Deli, 262 g	600	41	41	3	18
Grilled Chicken Caesar Sandwich, 334 g	740	44	54	3	38
Pastrami Deli, 227 g	540	22	53	2	33
Rachel Sandwich, 347 g	860	51	64	3	40
Reuben Sandwich, 347 g	750	40	59	2	40
Spicy Chicken Sandwich, 331 g	530	22	52	3	36
Tuna Salad Deli, 276 g	450	20	41	4	27
• Turkey Deli, 296 g	390	6	39	3	46
Ultimate Grilled Cheese, 306 g	870	50	77	2	36
White Fish on Corn Meal Rye, 276 g	750	52	41	3	29
Egg Sandwiches					
• Egg Mit Artichoke & Tomato, 332 g	550	15	79	4	26
Egg Mit Cheese & Tomato, 336 g	800	39	83	3	33
Egg Mit Lox & Cheese, 281 g	610	23	74	2	29
Egg Mit Lox & Chi, 313 g	800	39	81	3	32
Egg Mit Plain, 265 g	710	34	81	2	25
Egg Mit Spinach Mushrm & Swiss, 315 g	840	43	82	3	35

RESTAURANTS & FAST-FOOD CHAINS

Noah's Bagels (cont.)

	Cal	Fat	Cbs	Fbr	Prtn
Egg Sandwiches (cont.)					
• Egg Mit Turkey Sausage, 353 g	900	46	82	3	44
Egg Mit w/Cheese, 294 g	790	39	81	2	32
Egg Spinach, Bacon Panini, 339 g	770	35	71	3	36
Egg, Vegetarian Omelet Panini, 311 g	670	26	75	4	36
Eggs Sensations					
Egg Sensation, 341 g	430	25	18	2	28
Gourmet Bagels					
• Dutch Apple Bagel (plain), 155 g	400	3	86	4	12
Jalapeño Cheddar Bagel, 141 g	420	6	78	2	18
• Roasted Red Pepper Bagel, 170 g	440	7	79	2	18
Six-cheese Bagel, 141 g	420	6	78	2	18
Spinach Florentine Bagel, 148 g	430	7	78	2	18
Iced Specialty Coffee					
Iced Americano, 8 oz.	1	0	0	0	0
• Iced Coffee, 12 oz.	0	0	0	0	0
Iced Latte, 16 oz.	120	5	12	0	8
Iced Mocha, 16 oz.	210	6	33	0	7
Iced Non Fat Latte, 16 oz.	90	0	12	0	8
Low Fat Iced Mocha, 16 oz.	180	3	32	0	7
Low Fat Mocha, Regular, 12 oz.	190	3	34	0	8
• Reg Macchiato, 12 oz.	240	6	36	0	9
Kosher Melts					
Hummus Ammmus Melt, 304 g	660	20	95	5	28
• Pizza Melt, 276 g	550	13	86	4	24
Tuna Melt, 304 g	680	24	82	3	36
• Veggie Melt, 311 g	700	33	83	3	24
Panini Sandwiches					
Italian Chicken Panini, 329 g	760	33	68	3	50
Kosher Vegetarian on Plain Bagel, 401 g	860	40	79	4	51
• Tuna Panini, 331 g	740	28	89	8	40
Turkey Club Panini, 318 g	760	27	86	8	50
Vegetarian Panini, 401 g	840	41	71	3	50
Salad Dressings					
Asian Sesame Dressing, 2 tbsp.	140	12	6	0	1
Caesar Dressing, 2 tbsp.	150	16	1	0	1
• Dressing, Raspberry Vinaigrette, 2 tbsp.	160	14	8	0	0
• Harvest Chicken, 2 tbsp.	90	8	3	0	1
Salad Extras					
Bagel Croutons, 1 oz.	25	1	4	0	1
Salads					
Coleslaw, 85 g	180	16	8	1	1
Traditional Potato Salad, 140 g	290	21	21	2	3
Salads					
Caesar Salad, 198 g	410	35	16	2	4
Chicken Caesar Salad, 376 g	660	50	24	4	31
Chinese Chicken Salad, 369 g	480	5	84	4	14
• City Salad, 326 g	810	68	37	4	16
• Tuna Salad, 326 g	260	15	10	3	19
Sandwich Fillings					
American Cheese, 1 oz.	70	6	1	0	4
Cheddar Cheese, 1 oz.	80	7	0	0	5
Provolone Cheese, 1 oz.	70	6	0	0	5
• Smoked Salmon, 2 oz.	110	6	2	0	12

RESTAURANTS & FAST-FOOD CHAINS

Noah's Bagels (cont.)	Cal	Fat	Cbs	Fbr	Prtn
Sandwich Fillings (cont.)					
Swiss Cheese, 1 oz.	80	6	1	0	6
Sides					
Egg Salad, 4 oz.	200	17	5	0	9
• Tuna Salad, 4 oz.	150	6	3	0	21
• White Fish Salad, 2 oz.	225	20	1	0	9
Soups					
Broccoli, Sharp Cheddar (Bowl), 14 oz.	540	35	31	3	26
Broccoli, Sharp Cheddar (Cup), 9 oz.	280	19	15	2	13
Chicken & Wild Rice (Bowl), 14 oz.	440	9	67	5	24
Chicken & Wild Rice (Cup), 9 oz.	150	4	23	1	9
Chicken Noodle (Bowl), 14 oz.	510	21	39	5	38
• Chicken Noodle (Cup), 9 oz.	100	5	9	1	3
Clam Chowda (Bowl), 14 oz.	370	25	25	1	13
Clam Chowda (Cup), 9 oz.	260	15	20	1	10
Cream of Asparagus Soup (bowl), 14 oz.	390	35	17	4	11
Cream of Asparagus Soup (cup), 9 oz.	240	22	10	3	7
Low Fat Minestrone (Bowl), 14 oz.	430	6	75	11	20
Low Fat Minestrone (Cup), 9 oz.	110	4	19	2	4
Split Pea Soup (Bowl), 14 oz.	210	13	14	4	11
Split Pea Soup (Cup), 9 oz.	130	8	9	2	7
Turkey Chili (Bowl, 14 oz.	330	11	34	6	24
Turkey Chili (Cup), 9 oz.	230	7	25	5	20
Specialty Coffee					
• Americano Regular, 8 oz.	1	0	0	0	0
Cafe Latte, Regular, 10 oz.	100	1	14	0	10
Caffe Latte Nonfat, Regular, 12 oz.	100	0	14	0	9
Cappuccino Nonfat, Regular, 12 oz.	60	0	9	0	6
Cappuccino, Regular, 12 oz.	90	4	9	0	6
Espresso, Regular, 15 oz.	1	0	0	0	0
Low Fat Mocha, Regular, 12 oz.	190	3	34	0	8
• Macchiato, Regular, 12 oz.	240	6	36	0	9
Mocha, Regular, 12 oz.	230	6	34	0	8
Spreads					
Butter, 14	100	11	0	0	0
Fruit Spread, Grape, 1 oz.	75	0	19	0	0
Hummus, 2 oz.	110	7	9	2	3
• Peanut Butter, Crunchy, 2 tbsp.	641	52	2	7	23
Raspberry Preserves, 1 oz.	71	0	18	1	0
• Strawberry Preserves, 1 oz.	71	0	18	0	0
Sweets					
Apple Cinnamon Coffee Cake, 7 oz.	660	25	106	2	5
Blueberry Coffee Cake, 6 oz.	610	25	97	2	6
Blueberry Muffin, 5 oz.	470	21	64	2	6
Cheesecake Brownie, 5 oz.	520	27	67	2	9
• Chocolate Chip Coffee Cake, 6 oz.	730	31	108	2	7
• Cinnamon Twists, 4 oz.	370	21	41	2	5
Trail Mix Cookie, 4 oz.	480	19	70	4	8
White Chocolate Raspberry Scone, 4 oz.	480	22	63	2	7
White Chocolate Walnut Cookie, 4 oz.	439	24	52	2	6
Whipped Cream Cheese					
Blueberry, 20 g	70	5	6	0	1
Cappuccino, 20 g	70	5	5	0	0
• Garden Vegetable, 20 g	60	5	2	0	1

(• = most healthy • = least healthy) **RESTAURANTS & FAST-FOOD • 239**

RESTAURANTS & FAST-FOOD CHAINS

Noah's Bagels (cont.)

	Cal	Fat	Cbs	Fbr	Prtn
Whipped Cream Cheese (cont.)					
Garlic Herb, 20 g	60	5	3	0	1
Gingerbread, 20 g	70	5	5	0	0
Honey Almond Red. Fat, 20 g	70	5	5	0	1
Jalapeño Salsa, 20 g	60	5	3	0	1
Maple Raisin Walnut, 20 g	60	5	4	0	1
Onion and Chive, 20 g	70	6	3	0	4
Plain Reduced Fat, 20 g	60	5	2	0	1
Plain, 20 g	70	7	1	0	1
• Pumpkin, 20 g	100	8	6	0	1
Smoked Salmon, 20 g	60	5	3	0	1
Strawberry, 20 g	70	5	5	0	1
Sundried Tomato & Basil, 20 g	80	5	2	0	1

Noodles & Company

	Cal	Fat	Cbs	Fbr	Prtn
American (Regular)					
Buttered Noodles	940	42	111	3	32
• Caesar Salad	310	27	10	2	10
Chicken Noodle Soup	350	11	35	2	27
House Marinara	660	17	102	6	24
Mushroom Stroganoff	920	47	96	3	29
• Wisconsin Mac & Cheese®	1050	47	113	5	40
Asian (Regular Size)					
Bangkok Curry	460	16	69	8	10
• Chinese Chop Salad	250	10	36	5	7
Indonesian Peanut Sauté	660	20	132	11	19
Japanese Pan Noodles®	630	9	125	9	17
• Pad Thai	750	17	136	8	13
Thai Curry Soup	400	19	49	4	8
Mediterranean (Regular Size)					
Pasta Fresca	720	18	106	6	25
Penne Rosa	810	37	91	6	25
• Pesto Cavatappi®	820	34	91	5	26
• The Med Salad	320	13	38	5	12
Tomato Basil Bisque	450	30	39	3	7
Whole Grain Tuscan Fettuccine	600	23	78	15	23

Nothing but Noodles

	Cal	Fat	Cbs	Fbr	Prtn
Add-Ons					
• Beef, 1/2 bowl	110	4	0	0	17
Chicken, 1/2 bowl	100	3	0	0	18
• Shrimp, 1/2 bowl	53	1	1	0	10
Tofu, 1/2 bowl	60	4	1	0	7
Desserts					
Cannoli, 1 bowl	374	17	44	1	10
• Cotton Candy, 1 bowl	65	0	17	0	0
Key Lime Pie, 1 bowl	590	33	67	1	11
• New York Cheesecake, 1 bowl	770	53	59	0	15
Triple Chocolate Cake, 1 bowl	710	33	106	4	6
Kids					
Alfredo, 1 bowl	719	55	39	2	19
• Buttery Noodles, 1 bowl	723	49	51	2	21
Macaroni & Cheese, 1 bowl	454	26	38	2	18
• Spaghetti, 1 bowl	291	6	47	5	13

RESTAURANTS & FAST-FOOD CHAINS

Nothing but Noodles (cont.)

	Cal	Fat	Cbs	Fbr	Prtn
Noodle Bowls - American					
Beef Stroganoff, 1/2 bowl	508	31	33	2	26
Buttery Noodles, 1/2 bowl	651	44	46	2	19
Santa Fe Pasta, 1/2 bowl	705	54	40	3	18
Southwest Chipotle, 1/2 bowl	713	58	41	4	11
Spicy Cajun Pasta, 1/2 bowl	660	50	44	4	9
Noodle Bowls - Asian					
Pad Thai Noodles, 1/2 bowl	602	10	118	4	14
Sesame Lo Mein, 1/2 bowl	411	11	64	4	5
Spicy Japanese Noodles, 1/2 bowl	419	8	74	4	10
Thai Peanut, 1/2 bowl	568	20	89	5	11
Noodle Bowls - Italian					
Basil Pesto, 1/2 bowl	574	42	36	3	14
Cappelini Primavera, 1/2 bowl	500	28	56	4	10
Fettuccini Alfredo, 1/2 bowl	723	56	36	2	20
Margherita Pasta, 1/2 bowl	474	31	36	3	9
Marinara Pasta, 1/2 bowl	487	11	77	8	23
Three-Cheese Macaroni, 1/2 bowl	446	21	45	2	20
Pasta-Less Bowls					
Cheesy Chicken & Vegetables, 1/2 bowl	318	21	6	2	29
Chicken Pomodoro, 1/2 bowl	452	34	7	2	28
Primavera Chkn & Vegetables, 1/2 bowl	318	15	26	2	22
Shrimp Pesto Florentine, 1/2 bowl	308	25	5	2	16
Thai Curry Beef & Vegetables, 1/2 bowl	443	30	16	4	32
Rice Dishes					
General Tso's Chicken, 1/2 bowl	760	44	69	1	24
Kung Pao Chicken, 1/2 bowl	935	51	89	5	31
Thai Peanut Stir Fry, 1/2 bowl	595	27	59	3	29
Salads					
BBQ Chicken Salad, 1/2 bowl	205	15	11	3	9
Caesar Salad, 1/2 bowl	247	19	14	2	7
Chopped Salad, 1/2 bowl	229	15	10	3	7
Cranberry Spinach Salad, 1/2 bowl	154	10	18	3	3
Garden Fresh Salad, 1/2 bowl	110	5	12	2	5
Greek Salad, 1/2 bowl	409	31	26	3	9
Hunk of Lettuce, 1/2 bowl	229	21	7	2	6
Mandarin Orange Salad, 1/2 bowl	205	14	13	2	2
Oriental Salad, 1/2 bowl	187	11	20	4	4
Pear & Balsamic Spinach Salad, 1/2 bowl	395	28	38	3	7
Spicy Cucumber & Chkn Salad, 1/2 bowl	284	15	10	3	28
Steak Salad, 1/2 bowl	135	19	7	2	11
Sun-Dried Tomato, 1/2 bowl	271	12	32	4	11
Soups					
Tomato Bisque, 1/2 bowl	253	23	9	1	2
Starters					
Cucumber Side Salad, 1 bowl	193	16	13	1	2
Fresh Mozzarella, 1 bowl	767	27	134	1	20
Garlic Breadsticks, 1 bowl	106	4	0	1	2
Mozzarella Cheese Bread, 1 bowl	633	17	86	3	33
Potstickers, 1 bowl	479	33	39	5	11
Thai Lettuce Wraps, 1/2 bowl	361	23	15	2	24

(• = most healthy • = least healthy) **RESTAURANTS & FAST-FOOD • 241**

RESTAURANTS & FAST-FOOD CHAINS

O'Charley's

	Cal	Fat	Cbs	Fbr	Prtn
Appetizers & Sides					
• Buffalo Kickin' Wings, 10 pcs.	1830	147	43	3	77
Chckn O' Tenders- Create Your Own Combo, 6 pcs.	850	57	34	1	50
Chicken O' Tenders, 6 pcs.	850	57	34	1	50
Chips and Salsa, full order	520	18	82	4	12
Chkn O' Tenders w/ Buffalo Sauce, 6 pcs.	810	53	31	2	51
Chkn O' Tenders w/ Chipotle BBQ Sauce, 6 pcs.	690	32	47	1	50
Chkn O' Tenders w/ Honey Mustard, 6 pcs.	850	57	34	1	50
French Fries, full order	300	18	30	2	3
Island Cole Slaw, 1 side	250	19	19	2	1
Loaded Baked Potato, 1 side	480	29	54	6	12
Onion Rings w/ Sauce, full order	1800	139	119	6	10
Over-Loaded Potato Skins, full order	1340	99	48	0	70
Plain Potato, 1 side	420	24	52	6	9
• Rice Pilaf, 1 side	200	5	31	1	4
Smashed Potatoes, 1 side	370	12	47	5	2
Southwstrn Chkn Quesadilla, full order	990	59	53	2	62
Spicy Jack Cheese Wedges, 7 pcs.	880	60	55	0	29
Spinach & Artichoke Dip, full order	940	51	107	7	18
Steak House Quesadilla, full order	1330	95	56	3	63
Three-Cheese Shrimp Dip, full order	870	49	85	10	32
Top Shelf Combo Appetizer, full order	1830	130	81	1	84
Brunch					
• Brunch Bread with Jelly	260	10	38	1	5
Cajun Chicken Omelette	870	63	13	0	60
• Cranberry Pecan Waffle	1380	61	189	6	15
Eggs & Bacon	820	53	56	1	28
Eggs & Sausage	890	60	56	1	31
Ham & Cheese Omelette	1140	78	59	1	48
Spanish Omelette	1180	80	66	1	47
Steak & Eggs	1260	78	57	1	78
Strawberry Chocolate Chip Waffle	1290	50	196	4	16
Ultimate Omelette	1180	79	68	2	48
Chicken & Ribs					
Chicken Parmesan	860	42	70	3	49
Chipotle BBQ Ribs, full rack	1540	95	89	3	78
Chipotle BBQ Ribs, half rack	780	47	48	2	39
• Grilled Chicken	460	13	26	3	47
Prime Time Prime Rib, 10 oz.	1020	79	3	0	70
• Prime Time Prime Rib, 16 oz.	1630	127	4	1	111
Signature Baby Back Ribs, full rack	1480	96	76	3	77
Signature Baby Back Ribs, half rack	750	48	39	2	39
Teriyaki Chicken	500	6	57	1	51
Desserts					
• Blueberry Muffin, 1 piece	60	4	8	0	1
Caramel Pie Ice Cream Scoop - 1 scoop	160	7	23	0	3
Key Lime Pie, 1 slice	610	23	90	0	10
Ooey Gooey Caramel Pie, 1 slice	720	27	106	0	12
• Ultimate Choc. Chocolate Cake, 1 slice	1080	59	152	6	12
Dressings					
Balsamic Dressing, 2 oz.	230	17	17	0	0
Bleu Cheese Dressing, 2 oz.	230	25	4	0	2
Greek Feta Vinaigrette, 2 oz.	620	64	7	2	4
Honey Mustard Dressing, 2 oz.	330	32	11	0	0

RESTAURANTS & FAST-FOOD CHAINS

O'Charley's (cont.)	Cal	Fat	Cbs	Fbr	Prtn
Dressings (cont.)					
Honey Mustard, Light, 2 oz.	120	4	21	0	0
• Italian Dressing, Light, 2 oz.	70	5	7	0	0
Ranch Dressing, 2 oz.	190	19	4	0	1
Ranch Dressing, Light, 2 oz.	70	5	7	0	0
Thousand Island Dressing, 2 oz.	210	19	8	0	0
Kid's Menu					
Jr. Brunch	600	36	55	1	13
Jr. Cheeseburger	650	35	48	2	34
Jr. Chicken Tenders	310	17	12	1	25
Jr. Corn Dogs	500	38	32	3	11
Jr. French Toast	1100	56	117	2	8
Jr. Hamburger	540	25	47	2	27
Jr. Macaroni and Cheese	360	23	27	0	14
• Jr. Pasta	230	4	42	2	7
Jr. Shrimp	310	18	25	1	12
• Jr. Waffle	1150	55	149	1	12
Sandwiches & Burgers					
Bacon & Cheese Trio Chkn Sandwich	800	40	53	3	55
Bacon & Cheese Trio Chkn Sandwich w/ Mayo	1110	75	54	3	55
Buffalo Kickin Sandwich	980	58	72	4	41
Club Sandwich	1020	59	83	5	44
Grilled Chicken Sandwich	610	27	52	3	37
Half-Club Sandwich-Lunch	510	30	42	2	22
• Mushroom Swiss Burger	1490	111	56	5	65
Whiskey Sirloin Sandwich	930	48	65	3	58
Seafood & Pasta					
Bayou Shrimp Pasta	1280	78	101	6	43
Blackened Rainbow Trout	690	52	5	2	48
Cajun Chicken Pasta	1260	69	88	5	68
Caribbean Coconut Shrimp	650	26	88	2	17
• Catfish Platter	1690	141	65	25	39
Catfish Platter - Lunch	1170	99	37	18	31
Cedar-Planked Salmon	590	35	2	1	63
Chipotle BBQ Salmon, 10 oz.	670	37	17	1	63
Fisherman's Platter	1410	85	108	5	49
• Fresh Atlantic Grilled Salmon - Lunch	370	22	2	1	38
• Fried Shrimp Dinner	490	30	27	1	29
Grilled Shrimp Dinner	600	41	33	1	22
Whiskey Salmon, 10 oz.	760	44	23	1	64
Signature Soups & Salads					
• Black & Bleu Caesar Salad	920	65	21	5	62
• Broccoli & Three Cheese Soup, 1 cup	100	5	10	1	3
Cajun Chicken Salad	740	49	17	4	57
California Chicken Salad	560	26	42	7	41
Chicken Harvest Soup, 1 cup	220	11	16	1	12
Chicken Tortilla Soup, 1 cup	120	7	11	1	4
Clam Chowder, 1 cup	170	10	11	1	7
Classic Chicken Caesar Salad	490	30	13	2	38
House Salad - Entree	230	11	19	3	11
House Salad - Side	210	11	15	2	10
O'riginal Southern Fried Chicken Salad	720	41	34	4	53
Pecan Chicken Tender Salad	840	54	46	7	43
Roasted Tomato Basil Soup, 1 cup	130	9	10	1	3

RESTAURANTS & FAST-FOOD CHAINS

O'Charley's (cont.)

	Cal	Fat	Cbs	Fbr	Prtn
Signature Soups & Salads (cont.)					
Southwestern Steak Soup, 1 cup	100	5	10	1	3
Steak					
• Butcher's Cut Steak, 5 oz.	260	14	0	0	30
Filet Mignon	500	30	0	0	52
Flame-Grilled Top Sirloin, 10 oz.	580	35	0	0	61
Flame-Grilled Top Sirloin, 7 oz.	430	28	0	0	43
Louisiana Sirloin	670	38	3	1	74
Our Favorite Ribeye Steak	810	55	0	0	72
• Steak Tips Monterey	1000	64	47	2	55

Old Spaghetti Factory

	Cal	Fat	Cbs	Fbr	Prtn
Appetizers					
Bay Shrimp Crostini, 8 oz.	630	19	86	3	26
• Garlic Cheese Bread Starter, 14 oz.	1220	85	105	5	17
Meatballs Starter	910	61	23	1	65
Portuguese Linguica, 17 oz.	840	37	85	11	40
Sausage Starter, 284 g	690	56	7	1	31
• Shrimp, Spinach & Artichoke Dip, 298 g	580	9	103	5	21
Tapenade of Black Olives, 10 oz.	810	37	99	5	18
Tortellini Starter, 340 g	930	56	82	2	25
Desserts					
• Caramel Turtle Pie Dessert, 9 oz.	660	29	93	0	7
Mud Pie Dessert, 9 oz.	680	32	90	3	9
• New York Cheese Cake w/ Berry Topping, 8 oz.	690	40	72	1	10
Dinner Menu Items					
Baked Chicken (Orzo Pilaf/Broccoli), 17 oz.	740	48	20	4	59
Baked Chicken, 447 g	880	47	55	4	58
Chicken Fettuccine, 517 g	960	56	74	6	43
Chicken Marsala, 498 g	960	44	55	4	81
Chicken Parmigiana, 554 g	840	34	84	5	46
Eggplant Parmigiana, 532 g	670	32	75	8	23
• Fettuccine Alfredo, 439 g	1130	83	71	4	31
Lasagna, 454 g	630	33	36	4	45
Pot Pourri, 461 g	710	30	84	6	26
Salmon Tuscany, 17 oz.	680	43	21	1	52
• Spaghetti w/ Tomato Sauce, 425 g	440	5	84	7	14
w/ Clam Sauce & Mizithra, 439 g	960	54	81	5	39
w/ Clam Sauce, 425 g	690	28	84	5	22
w/ Meat & Clam Sauce, 425 g	580	17	84	6	22
w/ Meat Sauce & Mizithra, 439 g	850	42	80	5	38
w/ Meat Sauce & Sausage, 539 g	830	35	85	6	43
w/ Meatballs, 20 oz.	840	33	86	5	47
w/ Mizithra, 384 g	1010	64	74	4	37
w/ Mushroom & Clam Sauces, 425 g	570	18	83	5	18
w/ Mushroom & Meat Sauces, 425 g	460	6	83	6	17
w/ Mushroom Sauce & Mizithra, 439 g	850	43	80	5	34
w/ Mushroom Sauce, 425 g	460	7	83	6	14
w/ Rich Meat Sauce, 425 g	470	5	83	6	21
w/ Tomato & Meat Sauces, 425 g	460	5	84	6	17
w/ Tomato & Mizithra, 439 g	840	42	81	5	34
w/ Tomato Sauce & Clam Sauce, 425 g	560	17	84	6	18
Spinach & Cheese Ravioli, 319 g	480	15	59	4	24
Spinach Tortellini w/ Alfredo Sauce, 342 g	930	56	82	2	25

Old Spaghetti Factory (cont.)

	Cal	Fat	Cbs	Fbr	Prtn
Dinner Specials					
Angel Hair Florentine, 454 g	600	21	73	6	29
Chicken Penne w/ Tomato Alfredo, 17 oz.	760	32	74	4	42
• Coconut Shrimp Curry, 516 g	860	45	76	6	39
Meatloaf w/ Eggplant & Broccoli, 16 oz.	720	48	34	4	37
Pesto Basil Cream Sauce, 411 g	790	47	73	5	20
Rigatoni Bolognese, 398 g	620	32	48	3	33
• Shrimp & Artichoke Linguini, 13 oz.	590	18	78	7	28
Spaghetti Vesuvius, 425 g	590	18	82	6	22
Kids Meals					
Grilled Cheese Sandwich, 102 g	360	22	28	1	11
Macaroni & Cheese, 284 g	350	9	57	2	11
• Spaghetti w/ Tomato Sauce & Meatballs, 333 g	440	13	59	4	20
• Spaghetti w/ Tomato Sauce, 284 g	300	4	56	4	9
Lunch Menu Items					
Chicken Fettuccine, 404 g	830	55	56	4	31
Chicken Parmigiana, 554 g	840	34	84	5	46
Fettuccine Alfredo, 312 g	780	55	53	3	21
Lasagna, 369 g	520	27	29	3	37
Pot Pourri, 284 g	480	22	54	4	16
• Spaghetti w/ Tomato Sauce, 284 g	300	4	56	4	9
w/ Brown Butter & Mizithra, 242 g	590	34	49	3	23
w/ Clam & Mizithra, 262 g	520	26	53	3	18
w/ Clam Sauce, 284 g	460	19	56	3	15
w/ Meat & Clam, 284 g	380	11	56	4	14
w/ Meat & Mizithra, 262 g	450	19	53	4	17
w/ Meat Sauce & Sausage, 390 g	620	29	57	4	28
w/ Meatballs, 383 g	610	24	62	4	35
w/ Mushroom & Clam, 284 g	380	12	56	4	12
w/ Mushroom & Meat, 284 g	310	4	55	4	12
w/ Mushroom & Mizithra, 262 g	450	19	52	3	15
w/ Mushroom Sauce, 284 g	310	5	55	4	9
w/ Rich Meat Sauce, 284 g	310	4	55	4	14
w/ Tomato & Clam Sauce, 284 g	380	11	56	4	12
w/ Tomato & Meat Sauce, 284 g	300	4	56	4	12
w/ Tomato & Mizithra, 262 g	440	18	53	4	15
Spinach & Cheese Ravioli, 319 g	480	15	59	4	24
• Spinach Tortellini w/ Alfredo Sauce, 342 g	930	56	82	2	25
Lunch Specials					
Angel Hair Florentine, 454 g	600	21	73	6	29
• Chicken Cacciatore, 19 oz.	1120	66	82	4	48
Manicotti, 326 g	510	21	55	3	26
• Shrimp & Artichoke Linguini, 354 g	440	14	58	6	21
Shrimp Newberg, 411 g	800	47	54	3	42
Platters					
• Hearty Platter #4 w/ Tomato Sauce, 709 g	740	9	140	11	23
w/ Clam Sauce, 709 g	1140	47	140	8	37
w/ Meat Sauce, 709 g	780	9	139	11	34
• w/ Mizithra, 624 g	1590	98	122	7	59
w/ Mushroom Sauce, 709 g	760	12	138	10	24
Lasagna & Chicken Marsala, 709 g	1000	42	42	4	104
Ravioli & Spaghetti w/ Meat Sauce, 602 g	790	19	115	8	38
Spaghetti w/ Sauce, Mtballs & Sausage, 687 g	1280	64	94	7	75

(• = most healthy • = least healthy)

RESTAURANTS & FAST-FOOD CHAINS

Old Spaghetti Factory (cont.)

	Cal	Fat	Cbs	Fbr	Prtn
Salad Dressings					
1000 Island, 2 oz.	150	15	4	0	1
Balsamic Vinaigrette, 28 g	170	18	2	0	0
Blue Cheese, 2 oz.	190	21	1	0	2
• Caesar, 57 g	320	34	1	0	2
Creamy Pesto, 2 oz.	200	21	1	0	1
• Fat Free Honey Mustard, 2 oz.	60	0	13	0	0
Reduced Calorie French, 2 oz.	100	6	13	0	0
Salads					
BLT Salad, 14 oz.	760	59	30	8	31
Cobb Salad (no dressing), 19 oz.	700	44	15	5	62
• Dinner Chicken Caesar Salad, 20 oz.	1050	83	29	6	47
House Salad w/Caesar Dressing, 6 oz.	190	15	8	2	5
Lunch Chicken Caesar Salad, 15 oz.	780	60	21	4	40
Mango Macadamia Chicken Salad, 20 oz.	850	51	70	6	34
• Orzo Salad, 4 oz.	80	3	11	1	2
Shrimp Louie Salad, 15 oz.	680	56	19	3	27
Small Caesar Salad, 7 oz.	380	34	11	3	8
Sandwiches					
Brie & Arugula Sandwich, 13 oz.	1350	102	61	4	46
• Factory Burger, 20 oz.	1380	89	39	2	100
Meatball Sandwich, 447 g	900	50	64	6	50
• Sausage Sandwich, 411 g	830	49	57	5	41
Seafood Cheddar Melt, 15 oz.	980	56	74	6	44
Tuscan Chicken Sandwich, 496 g	1110	67	55	6	74
Sides					
• Broccoli Salad Garnish, 71 g	120	11	5	2	2
• Large Side of Broccoli, 424 g	630	58	18	10	20
Small Side of Broccoli, 212 g	320	29	9	5	10
Soups					
Chicken Mulligatawny, 9 oz.	250	14	20	2	10
• Chicken Orzo, 9 oz.	90	3	9	1	8
• Clam Chowder, 9 oz.	380	29	25	2	6
Cream of Broccoli, 9 oz.	220	12	19	2	9
Mediterranean White Bean, 9 oz.	150	6	19	6	6
Minestrone, 10 oz.	120	5	15	3	5

Olive Garden

	Cal	Fat	Cbs	Fbr	Prtn
Appetizers					
Alfredo Dipping Sauce	380	N/A	N/A	N/A	N/A
Breadstick w/ Garlic-Butter Spread	150	N/A	N/A	N/A	N/A
Bruschetta	440	N/A	N/A	N/A	N/A
Calamari	890	N/A	N/A	N/A	N/A
Add Marinara Sauce	70	N/A	N/A	N/A	N/A
Add Parmesan-Peppercorn Sauce	300	N/A	N/A	N/A	N/A
Caprese Flatbread	600	N/A	N/A	N/A	N/A
Create a Sampler Italiano					
Add Marinara Sauce	70	N/A	N/A	N/A	N/A
Add Parmesan-Peppercorn Sauce	300	N/A	N/A	N/A	N/A
Add Tomato Sauce	45	N/A	N/A	N/A	N/A
Calamari	440	N/A	N/A	N/A	N/A
Chicken Fingers	330	N/A	N/A	N/A	N/A
Fried Mozzarella	370	N/A	N/A	N/A	N/A
Fried Zucchini	370	N/A	N/A	N/A	N/A

Olive Garden (cont.)	Cal	Fat	Cbs	Fbr	Prtn
Appetizers (cont.)					
Stuffed Mushrooms	410	N/A	N/A	N/A	N/A
Toasted Beef & Pork Ravioli	360	N/A	N/A	N/A	N/A
Grilled Chicken Flatbread	760	N/A	N/A	N/A	N/A
Hot Artichoke-Spinach Dip	660	N/A	N/A	N/A	N/A
Marinara Dipping Sauce	70	N/A	N/A	N/A	N/A
Mussels di Napoli	180	N/A	N/A	N/A	N/A
Sicilian Scampi	500	N/A	N/A	N/A	N/A
• Smoked Mozzarella Fondula	930	N/A	N/A	N/A	N/A
Stuffed Mushrooms	410	N/A	N/A	N/A	N/A
Beef & Pork					
Chianti Braised Short Ribs	1060	N/A	N/A	N/A	N/A
Mixed Grill	770	N/A	N/A	N/A	N/A
• Pork Filettino	640	N/A	N/A	N/A	N/A
• Steak Gorgonzola-Alfredo	1310	N/A	N/A	N/A	N/A
Steak Toscana	880	N/A	N/A	N/A	N/A
Beverages					
Bellini Peach-Raspberry Iced Tea	70	N/A	N/A	N/A	N/A
Caffe Latte	130	N/A	N/A	N/A	N/A
Caffe le Toscana Coffee	3	N/A	N/A	N/A	N/A
Caffe Mocha	180	N/A	N/A	N/A	N/A
Cappuccino	150	N/A	N/A	N/A	N/A
Caramel Hazelnut Macchiato	220	N/A	N/A	N/A	N/A
Cream Sodas	200	N/A	N/A	N/A	N/A
• Frozen Cappuchino	320	N/A	N/A	N/A	N/A
Herbal and Flavored Hot Tea	3	N/A	N/A	N/A	N/A
Italian Sodas	120	N/A	N/A	N/A	N/A
• Lavazza Espresso	2	N/A	N/A	N/A	N/A
Raspberry Lemonade	145	N/A	N/A	N/A	N/A
Sicilian Splash	100	N/A	N/A	N/A	N/A
Chicken					
Chicken & Gnocchi Veronese	1030	N/A	N/A	N/A	N/A
• Chicken & Shrimp Carbonara	1440	N/A	N/A	N/A	N/A
Chicken Alfredo	1430	N/A	N/A	N/A	N/A
Chicken Marsala	770	N/A	N/A	N/A	N/A
Chicken Scampi	1020	N/A	N/A	N/A	N/A
Garlic-Herb Chicken con Broccoli	960	N/A	N/A	N/A	N/A
Stuffed Chicken Marsala	800	N/A	N/A	N/A	N/A
• Venetian Apricot Chicken	380	N/A	N/A	N/A	N/A
Classic Recipes					
Capellini Pomodoro	840	N/A	N/A	N/A	N/A
Chicken Parmigiana	1090	N/A	N/A	N/A	N/A
Eggplant Parmigiana	850	N/A	N/A	N/A	N/A
Fettuccine Alfredo	1220	N/A	N/A	N/A	N/A
Five Cheese Ziti al Forno	1050	N/A	N/A	N/A	N/A
Lasagna Classico	850	N/A	N/A	N/A	N/A
• Linguine alla Marinara	430	N/A	N/A	N/A	N/A
Spaghetti & Italian Sausage	1270	N/A	N/A	N/A	N/A
Spaghetti & Meatballs	1110	N/A	N/A	N/A	N/A
Spaghetti w/ Meat Sauce	710	N/A	N/A	N/A	N/A
• Tour of Italy	1450	N/A	N/A	N/A	N/A
Filled Pastas					
• Braised Beef & Tortelloni	1020	N/A	N/A	N/A	N/A
Cheese Ravioli w/ Marinara Sauce	660	N/A	N/A	N/A	N/A

RESTAURANTS & FAST-FOOD CHAINS

Olive Garden (cont.)

	Cal	Fat	Cbs	Fbr	Prtn
Filled Pastas (cont.)					
w/ Meat Sauce	790	N/A	N/A	N/A	N/A
Manicotti Formaggio	940	N/A	N/A	N/A	N/A
• Ravioli di Portobello	610	N/A	N/A	N/A	N/A
Fish & Seafood					
Grilled Shrimp Caprese	900	N/A	N/A	N/A	N/A
Herb-Grilled Salmon	610	N/A	N/A	N/A	N/A
• Parmesan Crusted Tilapia	590	N/A	N/A	N/A	N/A
• Seafood Alfredo	1020	N/A	N/A	N/A	N/A
Seafood Portofino	800	N/A	N/A	N/A	N/A
Shrimp & Asparagus Risotto	620	N/A	N/A	N/A	N/A
Shrimp Primavera	730	N/A	N/A	N/A	N/A
Pizza					
• Chicken Alfredo Pizza	1180	N/A	N/A	N/A	N/A
Create Your Own Pizza					
Add Bell Peppers	10	N/A	N/A	N/A	N/A
Add Black Olives	45	N/A	N/A	N/A	N/A
Add Italian Sausage	140	N/A	N/A	N/A	N/A
Add Mushrooms	6	N/A	N/A	N/A	N/A
Add Onions	15	N/A	N/A	N/A	N/A
Add Pepperoni	120	N/A	N/A	N/A	N/A
Add Roma Tomatoes	10	N/A	N/A	N/A	N/A
• Cheese Only	910	N/A	N/A	N/A	N/A
Soups & Salads					
Garden-Fresh Salad w/ dressing	350	N/A	N/A	N/A	N/A
w/out Dressing	120	N/A	N/A	N/A	N/A
• Grilled Chicken Caesar	850	N/A	N/A	N/A	N/A
• Minestrone, 1 bowl	100	N/A	N/A	N/A	N/A
Pasta e Fagioli, 1 bowl	130	N/A	N/A	N/A	N/A
Zuppa Toscana, 1 bowl	170	N/A	N/A	N/A	N/A

On the Border Mexican Grill

	Cal	Fat	Cbs	Fbr	Prtn
Appetizers					
Border Sampler, full	1970	121	114	18	107
Chicken Flautas w/ Queso, full	1060	68	64	8	49
• Chile Con Queso, 1 bowl	390	29	14	1	25
Chips & Salsa, full	500	25	58	6	6
Dble-Stacked Club Quesadillas, full	1860	123	88	15	101
Empanadas - Beef, full	1150	81	68	5	37
Empanadas - Chicken, full	1090	74	68	3	34
Fajita Chicken Con Queso w/ Tortillas	1480	93	61	1	94
Grande Fajita Nachos - Chicken, full	1890	113	109	28	110
Grande Fajita Nachos - Combo, full	1940	121	109	28	103
Grande Fajita Nachos - Steak, full	1970	127	109	29	96
Guacamole Live!, full	520	60	23	11	10
Guacamole, full	170	13	12	7	3
Queso Live! - Fajita Chicken w/ Chips	1320	84	77	12	70
Queso Live! - Fajita Steak w/ Chips	1390	94	77	13	61
Queso Live! - Taco Beef w/ Chips	1390	95	80	15	59
• Stacked Border Nachos, full	2740	166	191	38	122
Stffd Jalapeños w/ Chili con Queso, full	980	56	70	4	58
Ultimate Loaded Queso	900	59	46	16	49
Border Smart					
Chicken Salsa Fresca, full order	520	9	60	12	50

RESTAURANTS & FAST-FOOD CHAINS

On the Border Mexican Grill (cont.)	Cal	Fat	Cbs	Fbr	Prtn
Border Smart (cont.)					
Grilled Fajita Chicken Tacos, full order	570	9	78	18	48
• Jalapeño-BBQ Salmon, full order	590	21	45	24	54
• Pico Shrimp Tacos, full order	490	5	78	17	34
Burritos & Chimis					
Beef Burrito w/ Chili con Carne Sauce	930	49	57	4	61
Big Beef Bordurrito w/ Side Salad	1600	103	119	9	46
Big Chicken Bordurrito w/ Side Salad	1420	87	121	8	42
Border Chimichanga - Fajita Chicken	1230	93	51	3	34
Border Chimichanga - Ground Beef	1310	98	49	4	41
Border Chimichanga- Spicy Chicken	1160	85	46	2	33
Chicken Burrito w/ Sour Cream Sauce	850	54	55	3	30
Three Sauce Fajita Chicken Burrito	870	45	59	3	51
Three Sauce Fajita Steak Burrito	1050	61	57	4	54
Create Your Own Combo					
Cheese Chile Relleno, 1 each	880	61	60	1	28
Chicken Flautas w/ Chili con Queso, 1 each	300	19	17	2	16
Crispy Taco - Beef, 1 each	330	20	19	4	18
• Crispy Taco - Chicken, 1 each	240	12	16	2	12
Crispy Taco - Veggie, 1 each	250	16	20	3	6
Dos XX® Fish Tacos, 1 serving	1590	113	100	5	40
Empanadas - Beef w/ Chili con Queso, 2 each	530	38	30	2	19
Empanadas - Chicken w/ Chili con Queso, 2 each	490	33	28	1	17
Enchilada - Beef, 1 each	340	17	27	6	19
Enchilada - Cheese & Onion, 1 each	410	24	27	5	20
Enchilada - Chicken, 1 each	350	23	21	3	11
Fish Taco, 1 each	530	38	33	2	13
Pork Tamale, 1 each	310	17	26	3	12
Soft Taco - Beef, 1 each	340	19	23	2	19
Soft Taco - Chicken, 1 each	250	11	20	1	13
Desserts					
• Border Brownie Sundae w/ Vanilla Ice Cream	1360	78	158	7	17
Chocolate Turtle Empanadas, 4 each	1280	81	131	4	11
Dulce De Leche Cheesecake	1160	72	122	2	15
Kahlua® Ice Cream Pie	850	44	100	5	10
Sizzling Apple Crisp	960	36	157	5	11
Sopapillas	1230	56	136	1	13
• Vanilla Ice Cream, 1 scoop	180	10	19	0	3
Fajita Grill					
Carnitas (roasted pork) Fajitas	830	62	19	6	50
• Chicken Chipotle Fajita Favorites	1160	86	46	8	57
Corn Tortillas, 3 each	230	4	43	5	6
• Grlld Vegetable Fajitas w/ Portobello Mushrooms	390	28	30	7	7
Homemade Flour Tortillas, 3 each	360	11	54	0	8
Lettuce, Sour Cream, Pico de Gallo, Cheese	200	16	5	1	9
Lettuce, Sour Cream, Pico de Gallo, Guacamole	160	13	9	3	2
Monterey Ranch Chicken Fajita Favorites	840	54	17	2	69
Original Mesquite-Grilled Chicken Fajitas	440	18	20	4	48
Original Mesquite-Grilled Shrimp Fajitas	750	63	18	3	28
Original Mesquite-Grilled Steak Fajitas	620	41	18	3	42
Parrilla Butter, 1 oz.	120	13	1	0	0
Smothered Steak Fajitas	860	57	20	0	62
Favoritos					
Brisket Tacos w/ Jalapeño BBQ Sauce, 3 each	1200	56	114	4	54

(• = most healthy • = least healthy) **RESTAURANTS & FAST-FOOD • 249**

RESTAURANTS & FAST-FOOD CHAINS

On the Border Mexican Grill (cont.)

	Cal	Fat	Cbs	Fbr	Prtn
Favoritos (cont.)					
• Corona Extra Dinner	2040	126	136	13	77
Dos XX® Fish Tacos	1590	113	100	5	40
Enchilada Suizas w/ Sauce, 3 each	1110	71	70	12	44
Quesadillas - Double-Stacked Club w/ Dressing	1990	55	89	15	102
Quesadillas - Fajita Chicken	1430	91	59	6	93
Quesadillas - Fajita Chicken & Steak Combo	1450	98	59	6	81
Quesadillas - Fajita Steak	1530	107	59	6	81
Superior Dinner	1350	85	80	13	62
• Tacos - Buffalo Chicken w/ Dressing, 2 each	960	62	61	8	52
Tacos - Carne Asada w/ Dressing, 2 each	1250	83	56	8	70
Tacos - Southwest Chicken w/ Sauce, 3 each	1180	77	63	5	64
Tres Enchilada Dinner - Beef, 3 each	1010	52	80	17	56
Tres Enchilada Dinner - Chicken, 3 each	1040	68	64	10	34
Tres Enchiladas Dinner - Cheese, 3 each	1150	68	79	14	57
Kids Menu					
Border Chicken Strips	570	36	38	2	23
Cheeseburger	500	32	23	1	29
Corn Dog	320	21	11	1	5
Crispy Taco Mexican Dinner - Beef	740	31	77	18	35
Crispy Taco Mexican Dinner - Chicken	740	28	85	17	31
Dessert - Sundae w /Chocolate Syrup	300	13	40	1	4
Dessert - Sundae w/ Strawberry Purée	340	13	52	0	4
Grilled Chicken	130	2	1	0	24
Grilled Chicken Sandwich	630	21	63	2	42
Hamburger	390	23	23	1	22
• Nachos - Bean & Cheese	980	57	71	18	47
Nachos - Cheese	670	47	28	3	31
Side - French Fries	240	13	31	2	3
Side - Mexican Rice	220	6	33	2	3
Side - Salad w/ Chipotle Honey Mustard Dressing	250	22	12	1	1
Side - Salad w/ Ranch Dressing	180	17	5	1	2
• Side - Sautéed Vegetables	70	4	9	3	2
Soft Taco Mexican Dinner - Beef	840	35	91	17	38
Soft Taco Mexican Dinner - Chicken	750	27	89	15	32
Off the Grill					
• Baja Chicken	610	43	50	8	56
Bandera Sirloin	640	43	13	3	43
Carne Asada & Shrimp	1040	74	22	4	69
Pico Chicken & Shrimp	730	51	9	1	65
• Ranchiladas	1360	86	53	9	84
Salad Dressings & Sauces					
Chili Con Carne Sauce, 2 oz.	70	3	6	1	4
Chipotle Honey Mustard Dressing, 2 oz.	310	29	11	0	0
• Chipotle Mayonnaise, 2 oz.	380	42	2	0	0
Fat-free Balsamic Vinaigrette, 2 oz.	50	0	10	0	0
Jalapeño BBQ Sauce, 2 oz.	100	1	20	1	0
Ranch Dressing, 2 oz.	220	23	2	0	0
• Ranchero Sauce, 2 oz.	18	1	3	0	0
Roasted Jalapeño Ranch Dressing, 2 oz.	180	19	2	0	1
Roasted Jalapeño Sauce, 2 oz.	240	26	2	1	0
Salsa Fresca, 2 oz.	20	0	3	1	1
Salsa, 2 oz.	25	1	3	0	0
Smoked Jalapeño Vinaigrette, 2 oz.	231	22	8	0	0

RESTAURANTS & FAST-FOOD CHAINS

On the Border Mexican Grill (cont.)	Cal	Fat	Cbs	Fbr	Prtn
Salad Dressings & Sauces (cont.)					
Sour Cream Sauce, 2 oz.	140	14	2	0	1
Tomatillo Cream Sauce, 2 oz.	120	11	3	0	1
Salads & Soup					
Blackened Chicken Fiesta Salad w/ Dressing	1150	75	54	8	65
Chicken Fiesta Salad w/ Dressing	1140	74	52	7	66
Chicken Tortilla Soup, 1 bowl	350	22	24	5	14
Grande Taco Salad w/ Spicy Chicken	1280	89	74	10	43
Grande Taco Salad w/ Taco Beef	1450	102	78	13	54
Grilled Steak Ensalada w/ Vinaigrette	1120	75	54	8	60
• House Salad	170	10	15	4	6
Sizzling Fajita Salad - Chicken	760	48	23	7	58
Sizzling Fajita Salad - Steak	910	65	24	8	57
Side Items & Extras					
Beans - Black	180	7	19	6	8
Beans - Refried	290	11	36	13	15
Black Bean & Corn Relish, 2 oz.	70	4	6	1	1
• Cheesy Pepper Jack Mashed Potatoes	380	27	26	2	10
Guacamole, 1 scoop	60	5	4	2	1
Mexican Rice	220	6	33	2	3
Pico de Gallo, 1 scoop	20	1	2	1	0
Sautéed Shrimp, 4 each	170	10	1	0	16
Sour Cream, 1 scoop	90	8	3	0	1
Vegetables - Grilled	50	1	8	3	2
Vegetables - Sautéed	70	4	9	3	2

Orange Julius	Cal	Fat	Cbs	Fbr	Prtn
Add a Banana					
1/2 Banana, 3 oz.	60	N/A	13	1	1
1 Banana, 6 oz.	110	1	27	2	1
Beverages					
Bananarilla, 20 oz.	370	9	69	4	4
Cool Cappuccino, 20 oz.	480	13	86	1	15
• Orange Julius®, 20 oz.	270	1	68	1	1
Piña Colada, 20 oz.	410	9	87	4	3
Raspberry Julius, 20 oz.	300	2	76	1	2
Raspberry, 20 oz.	400	10	78	2	4
• Strawberry Banana, 20 oz.	500	9	97	2	4
Strawberry Julius, 20 oz.	280	1	72	1	1
Tripleberry, 20 oz.	460	10	92	3	4
Tropical, 20 oz.	370	9	69	4	4
Fruit Smoothies					
3-Berry Blast, 20 oz.	610	10	144	3	9
Banana Chill, 20 oz.	550	10	134	9	11
Berry Lemon Lively, 20 oz.	450	10	101	1	9
Blackberry Storm, 20 oz.	630	70	129	2	10
Blackberry Toner, 20 oz.	440	10	96	1	9
Blueberrathon, 20 oz.	350	15	89	6	2
Blueberry Burst, 20 oz.	470	5	106	4	7
• Cocoa Latte Swirl, 20 oz.	640	80	122	2	21
Mango Passion, 20 oz.	360	0	80	1	7
Orange Swirl™, 20 oz.	490	90	96	2	4
Peaches & Cream, 20 oz.	500	0	116	4	8
Raspberry Créme, 20 oz.	540	70	107	2	11

(• = most healthy • = least healthy) **RESTAURANTS & FAST-FOOD • 251**

RESTAURANTS & FAST-FOOD CHAINS

Orange Julius (cont.)

	Cal	Fat	Cbs	Fbr	Prtn
Fruit Smoothies (cont.)					
• Raspberry Crush, 20 oz.	330	20	83	3	3
Strawberried Treasure, 20 oz.	550	70	103	2	10
Strawberry Sensation, 20 oz.	430	0	98	2	7
Strawberry Xtreme, 20 oz.	410	5	87	1	8
Tart 'N' Berry™, 20 oz.	450	10	102	5	9
Tropical Tango, 20 oz.	400	25	90	2	2
Tropi-Colada, 20 oz.	560	70	110	3	10
Wild Blue Twist™, 20 oz.	490	5	115	4	7
Nutrition Boost					
• Fiber Plus, 6 g	5	0	4	4	0
Heart Health, 4 g	15	0	3	0	0
• Joint Care, 6 g	20	0	5	0	0

Outback Steakhouse

	Cal	Fat	Cbs	Fbr	Prtn
Add-on Mates					
Grilled Onions	130	N/A	N/A	N/A	N/A
Sauteed Mushrooms	160	N/A	N/A	N/A	N/A
Classics & Pasta					
• Alice Springs Chicken	2000	N/A	N/A	N/A	N/A
• Grilled Pork Chops	1340	N/A	N/A	N/A	N/A
No Rules Pasta	1390	N/A	N/A	N/A	N/A
Fresh Made Sides					
Aussie Chips	350	N/A	N/A	N/A	N/A
Classic Wedge Salad	490	N/A	N/A	N/A	N/A
Dressed Baked Potato	380	N/A	N/A	N/A	N/A
Fresh Steamed Broccoli	130	N/A	N/A	N/A	N/A
• w/o Butter	30	N/A	N/A	N/A	N/A
Fresh Steamed French Green Beans	150	N/A	N/A	N/A	N/A
Fresh Steamed Veggies	160	N/A	N/A	N/A	N/A
House Salad	570	N/A	N/A	N/A	N/A
Roasted Garlic Mashed Potatoes	350	N/A	N/A	N/A	N/A
• Sweet Potato	590	N/A	N/A	N/A	N/A
Walkabout Soup	480	N/A	N/A	N/A	N/A
Whole Grain Wild Rice	190	N/A	N/A	N/A	N/A
Prime Rib & Roasted Sirloin					
Prime Rib, 12 oz.	520	N/A	N/A	N/A	N/A
Prime Rib, 16 oz.	690	N/A	N/A	N/A	N/A
• Prime Rib, 8 oz.	350	N/A	N/A	N/A	N/A
• Slow Roasted Sirloin Medley	1150	N/A	N/A	N/A	N/A
Simply Grilled					
• Baby Back Ribs w/ Chips and Apples	2260	N/A	N/A	N/A	N/A
Baby Back Ribs, 1/2 rack	1520	N/A	N/A	N/A	N/A
Chicken Griller	1400	N/A	N/A	N/A	N/A
Chicken on the Barbie	860	N/A	N/A	N/A	N/A
Filet Griller	1100	N/A	N/A	N/A	N/A
• Rack of Lamb	820	N/A	N/A	N/A	N/A
Salmon Griller	1390	N/A	N/A	N/A	N/A
Scallop Griller	1250	N/A	N/A	N/A	N/A
Shrimp Griller	1880	N/A	N/A	N/A	N/A
Straight from the Sea					
Atlantic Salmon, 7 oz.	1540	N/A	N/A	N/A	N/A
• Atlantic Salmon, 9 oz.	1640	N/A	N/A	N/A	N/A
Boomerang Shrimp	1620	N/A	N/A	N/A	N/A

RESTAURANTS & FAST-FOOD CHAINS

Outback Steakhouse (cont.)

	Cal	Fat	Cbs	Fbr	Prtn
Straight from the Sea (cont.)					
Fresh Tilapia	700	N/A	N/A	N/A	N/A
Lobster Tail, 1 tail	550	N/A	N/A	N/A	N/A
Lobster Tails, 2 tails	670	N/A	N/A	N/A	N/A
Lobster Tails, 3 tails	800	N/A	N/A	N/A	N/A
USDA "Choice" Steaks					
New York Strip, 14 oz.	730	N/A	N/A	N/A	N/A
Outback Special , 12 oz.	860	N/A	N/A	N/A	N/A
Outback Special , 9 oz.	680	N/A	N/A	N/A	N/A
Ribeye, 14 oz.	1210	N/A	N/A	N/A	N/A
The Melbourne, 22 oz.	1410	N/A	N/A	N/A	N/A
Victoria's Center Cut Fillet, 7 oz.	600	N/A	N/A	N/A	N/A
Victoria's Center Cut Fillet, 9 oz.	740	N/A	N/A	N/A	N/A
Victoria's Crowned Fillet w/ Blue Cheese, 7 oz.	830	N/A	N/A	N/A	N/A
Victoria's Crowned Fillet w/ Blue Cheese, 9 oz.	970	N/A	N/A	N/A	N/A
Victoria's Crowned Fillet w/ Horseradish, 7 oz.	820	N/A	N/A	N/A	N/A
Victoria's Crowned Fillet w/ Horseradish, 9 oz.	960	N/A	N/A	N/A	N/A

P.F. Chang's China Bistro

	Cal	Fat	Cbs	Fbr	Prtn
Added Extras					
Chili Bean Sauce	81	1	12	0	3
• Crispy Green Bean Sauce	451	48	5	0	0
Mustard Vinaigrette	66	2	7	0	4
Potsticker Sauce	57	1	0	0	2
Rice Sticks	135	0	33	0	0
• Shrimp Dumpling Sauce	24	0	1	0	3
Special Sauce	55	1	9	0	2
Spicy Plum Sauce	110	0	28	0	0
Sweet and Sour Sauce	57	0	15	0	0
Chicken					
Chang's Spicy Chicken	923	37	88	1	56
Chicken with Black Bean Sauce	678	23	33	1	76
Dali Chicken	1091	52	53	6	91
• Ginger Chicken with Broccoli	656	26	45	7	60
Ginger Chicken with Broccoli - Gluten Free	677	30	43	7	61
Ground Chicken and Eggplant	792	40	73	9	33
• Kung Pao Chicken	1228	79	58	8	74
Mu Shu Chicken	715	38	49	23	47
Orange Peel Chicken	1151	46	127	14	61
Philip's Better Lemon Chicken	1051	42	113	5	58
Sweet and Sour Chicken	764	20	107	3	40
Desserts					
Apple Pie Mini Dessert	170	4	34	1	1
Banana Split Mini Dessert	167	6	28	1	1
Banana Spring Rolls	814	37	130	7	12
Carrot Cake Mini Dessert	295	14	42	1	2
• Coconut-pineapple Ice Cream	111	12	25	0	4
Creamy Strawberry Cheesecake Mini Dessert	239	20	14	1	3
Flourless Chocolate Dome - Gluten Free	572	26	84	8	8
Great Wall Of Chocolate Mini Dessert	336	26	24	2	1
S'mores Mini Dessert	323	12	50	1	3
• The Great Wall Of Chocolate Cake	2237	90	376	13	20
Tiramisu Mini Dessert	202	14	15	0	3
Tres Leche Lemon Dream Mini Dessert	216	8	32	1	4

RESTAURANTS & FAST-FOOD CHAINS

P.F. Chang's China Bistro (cont.)

	Cal	Fat	Cbs	Fbr	Prtn
Meat					
Beef A La Sichuan	1172	64	56	5	86
Chengdu Spiced Lamb	1056	75	34	5	62
Mongolian Beef	1178	73	29	2	96
• Mu Shu Pork	871	50	50	25	57
• Orange Peel Beef	1568	85	115	14	88
Sweet and Sour Pork	1095	46	106	3	61
Wok Charred Beef	941	63	33	8	61
Wok Seared Lamb	1081	80	29	8	62
Noodles, Meins, and Rice					
• Brown Rice - Cup	254	2	53	4	5
Cantonese Chow Fun with Chicken	1045	23	146	5	60
with Beef	1212	38	142	5	69
Chow Mein with Beef	793	26	84	7	54
with Chicken	689	16	84	6	49
with Pork	898	34	83	6	61
with Shrimp	625	13	84	6	41
Chow Mein Combo	912	34	86	6	61
Double Pan-fried Noodles with Beef	1186	56	112	6	53
with Chicken	1072	47	115	7	42
with Pork	1208	60	114	7	50
with Shrimp	1031	46	115	7	37
Dan Dan Noodles	1087	30	145	7	51
Double Pan-fried Noodles Combo	1384	69	118	7	68
Garlic Noodles	612	11	111	6	18
P.F. Chang's Fried Rice with Beef	1228	40	150	5	58
with Chicken	1208	44	151	5	47
with Pork	1360	57	150	5	55
with Shrimp	1154	41	149	4	40
P.F. Chang's Fried Rice Combo	1539	69	154	5	68
Singapore Street Noodles	572	16	81	7	28
Singapore Street Noodles - Gluten Free	566	15	81	4	28
• Tam's Noodles	1678	93	144	6	58
White Rice - Cup	295	1	64	1	6
Seafood					
Cantonese Scallops	408	16	26	4	39
• Cantonese Shrimp	330	12	21	4	33
Chang's Lemon Scallops	952	28	100	3	69
Crispy Honey Shrimp	1061	44	118	2	35
• Hot Fish	1338	71	111	8	60
Kung Pao Scallops	1136	57	66	9	87
Kung Pao Shrimp	977	58	58	9	60
Lemon Pepper Shrimp	701	36	59	5	36
Oolong Marinated Sea Bass	521	12	40	3	64
Orange Peel Shrimp	1010	41	118	14	47
Salt and Pepper Prawns	844	50	55	5	45
Shrimp with Candied Walnuts	1225	80	74	2	60
Sichuan from the Sea Calamari	1078	36	118	4	69
Sichuan from the Sea Scallops	1030	36	98	3	70
Sichuan from the Sea Shrimp	728	37	55	3	44
Wild Alaskan Sockeye Salmon Stmd w/ Ginger	646	36	23	5	60
Sides					
Asian Slaw	585	57	19	5	5
Garlic Snap Peas - Large	205	10	23	7	7

RESTAURANTS & FAST-FOOD CHAINS

P.F. Chang's China Bistro (cont.)

	Cal	Fat	Cbs	Fbr	Prtn
Sides (cont.)					
Garlic Snap Peas - Small	129	7	13	4	4
Shanghai Cucumbers	124	6	8	4	10
Sichuan-style Asparagus - Large	204	6	34	6	11
Sichuan-style Asparagus - Small	97	3	16	3	6
• Spicy Green Beans - Large	602	40	48	13	14
Spicy Green Beans - Small	234	13	23	6	7
Spinach Stir-fried with Garlic - Large	140	6	16	11	12
• Spinach Stir-fried with Garlic - Small	77	3	9	6	7
Soups and Salads					
Bikini Shrimp Salad	192	6	30	4	8
with Watermelon Citrus Vinaigrette Add	240	23	7	0	1
Chang's Chicken Noodle Soup - 1 bowl	512	13	30	2	64
Chang's Wedge	244	19	12	5	8
with Chicken	595	35	12	5	57
with Creamy Wedge Dressing	443	43	8	1	3
Chicken Chopped Salad	401	14	21	5	47
with Our Signature Ginger Dressing	483	48	9	0	1
Egg Drop Soup - 1 bowl	367	14	51	1	7
• Egg Drop Soup - 1 cup	48	2	7	0	1
• Hot and Sour Soup - 1 Bowl	652	18	82	34	37
Hot and Sour Soup - 1 cup	85	2	11	4	5
Wonton Soup - 1 bowl	354	10	44	3	21
Starters					
Chang's Chicken Lettuce Wraps	377	12	35	5	28
Chang's Chicken Lettuce Wraps - Gluten Free	477	12	63	5	31
• Chang's Spare Ribs	1356	89	43	1	93
Chang's Vegetarian Lettuce Wraps	281	4	37	7	25
Crab Wontons	440	26	32	2	19
Crispy Green Beans	507	28	59	8	8
Harvest Spring Rolls	287	15	30	2	6
Northern Style Spare Ribs	720	54	6	0	49
Peking Dumplings - Pan Fried	367	23	21	1	18
Peking Dumplings - Steamed	327	18	21	1	18
Salt And Pepper Calamari	720	11	118	3	33
• Seared Ahi Tuna	210	9	9	1	26
Shrimp Dumplings - Pan Fried	305	13	25	1	21
Shrimp Dumplings - Steamed	265	8	25	1	21
Vegetable Dumplings - Pan Fried	307	11	43	2	9
Vegetable Dumplings - Steamed	267	7	43	2	9
The Grill					
• Asian Marinated New York Strip	1432	86	68	2	92
Citrus Soy Salmon - with Brown Rice	1000	59	42	4	69
Citrus Soy Salmon - with White Rice	1025	58	49	2	70
• Lemongrass Prawns	907	58	65	4	34
Sichuan Chicken Flatbread	1160	80	56	4	52
Traditional Lunch Bowls					
Almond And Cashew Chicken with Brown Rice	909	27	101	9	62
Almond And Cashew Chicken with White Rice,	955	26	112	5	63
Beef with Broccoli with Brown Rice	844	27	87	8	58
Beef with Broccoli with White Rice	890	26	99	5	59
• Buddha's Feast with Brown Rice	541	8	101	11	23
Buddha's Feast with White Rice	587	6	113	7	24
Citrus Soy Salmon with Brown Rice	1047	63	67	6	48

(•= most healthy •= least healthy) **RESTAURANTS & FAST-FOOD • 255**

RESTAURANTS & FAST-FOOD CHAINS

P.F. Chang's China Bistro (cont.)

	Cal	Fat	Cbs	Fbr	Prtn
Traditional Lunch Bowls (cont.)					
• Citrus Soy Salmon with White Rice	1093	62	79	2	49
Crispy Honey Chicken with Brown Rice	943	13	126	6	61
Crispy Honey Chicken with White Rice	989	12	138	2	62
Moo Goo Gai Pan with Brown Rice	545	8	76	7	40
Moo Goo Gai Pan with White Rice	591	6	88	3	41
Pepper Steak with Brown Rice	820	28	82	7	54
Pepper Steak with White Rice	968	39	94	3	55
Shrimp with Lobster Sauce with Brown Rice	686	25	75	6	37
Shrimp with Lobster Sauce with White Rice	732	23	87	2	38
Traditions					
Almond And Cashew Chicken	815	30	63	5	81
Beef with Broccoli	1118	65	38	7	93
Crispy Honey Chicken	867	11	121	3	53
Lo Mein with Beef	1374	80	94	8	67
with Chicken	1198	67	97	8	51
with Pork	1400	54	95	8	63
with Shrimp	1134	64	97	8	43
• Lo Mein Combo	1409	83	98	8	66
Moo Goo Gai Pan	661	34	32	4	54
Pepper Steak	971	48	32	4	95
• Shrimp with Lobster Sauce	480	22	24	1	42
Vegetarian Plates					
• Buddha's Feast - Steamed	137	1	29	10	8
Buddha's Feast - Stir Fried	367	5	66	10	25
Coconut Curry Vegetables	686	46	48	12	30
Stir-fried Eggplant	590	34	64	10	10
• Vegetable Chow Fun	878	8	181	26	22
Vegetarian Ma Po Tofu	537	19	51	6	40

Panda Express

	Cal	Fat	Cbs	Fbr	Prtn
Appetizers					
Chicken Egg Roll, 3 oz.	170	8	17	2	8
• Chicken Potsticker, 6 pieces.	440	25	49	8	11
Cream Cheese Rangoon, 3 pieces	190	8	24	2	5
• Veggie Spring Roll, 2 oz.	80	4	11	2	2
Beef					
Broccoli Beef, 6 oz.	150	7	11	4	11
Mongolian Beef, 6 oz.	180	11	15	2	11
Chicken					
Black Pepper Chicken, 6 oz.	200	12	11	2	13
Kung Pao Chicken, 6 oz.	240	15	12	5	16
Mandarin Chicken, 6 oz.	250	10	8	0	31
• Mushroom Chicken, 6 oz.	130	6	8	3	11
• Orange Chicken, 6 oz.	500	27	42	3	23
Potato Chicken, 6 oz.	200	10	21	2	11
String Bean Chicken Breast, 6 oz.	160	8	10	4	12
Pork					
BBQ Pork, 6 oz.	440	23	15	1	41
Sweet & Sour Pork, 6 oz.	400	23	35	2	13
Rice & Noodles					
Chow Mein, 8 oz.	390	12	59	7	11
• Fried Rice, 8 oz.	450	14	67	6	13
• Steamed Rice, 8 oz.	380	3	81	4	9

RESTAURANTS & FAST-FOOD CHAINS

Panda Express (cont.)

	Cal	Fat	Cbs	Fbr	Prtn
Sauces					
Mandarin Sauce, 2 oz.	70	0	17	0	1
Potsticker Sauce, 2 oz.	35	0	8	0	1
Sweet & Sour Sauce, 2 oz.	80	0	19	0	0
Shrimp					
Crispy Shrimp, 100 g	260	13	26	1	9
Kung Pao Shrimp, 6 oz.	240	14	14	4	16
Tangy Shrimp, 6 oz.	150	5	16	2	9
Soup					
Egg Flower Soup, 12 oz.	88	2	16	0	2
Hot & Sour Soup, 12 oz.	110	4	14	2	5
Veggies					
Eggplant and Tofu, 6 oz.	180	10	20	4	5
Mixed Veggies, 6 oz.	90	7	8	3	2

Panera Bread

	Cal	Fat	Cbs	Fbr	Prtn
Artisan Breads					
Ciabatta, 6 oz.	460	5	98	5	14
Country Demi, 2 oz.	130	0	27	1	5
Country Loaf, 2 oz.	130	0	27	1	5
Country Miche, 2 oz.	120	0	25	1	5
Focaccia, 2 oz.	160	3	29	1	5
French Baguette, 2 oz.	140	0	28	1	5
French Miche, 2 oz.	120	0	25	1	5
Sesame Semolina Demi, 2 oz.	130	1	27	1	5
Sesame Semolina Loaf, 2 oz.	130	1	27	1	4
Sesame Semolina Miche, 2 oz.	130	1	25	1	4
Stone-Milled Rye Loaf, 2 oz.	120	0	25	2	4
Stone-Milled Rye Miche, 2 oz.	120	0	24	2	4
Three Cheese Demi, 2 oz.	140	2	24	1	6
Three Cheese Loaf, 2 oz.	140	2	24	1	6
Three Cheese Miche, 2 oz.	130	2	23	1	6
Three Seed Demi, 2 oz.	140	3	25	2	5
Whole Grain Baguette, 2 oz.	140	1	28	3	6
Whole Grain Loaf, 2 oz.	130	1	26	3	6
Whole Grain Miche, 2 oz.	140	1	27	3	6
Artisan Pastries					
Caramel Apple, 4 oz.	400	19	51	2	7
Cheese, 4 oz.	380	22	38	1	7
Cherry, 5 oz.	420	21	51	1	8
Chocolate Crumb, 4 oz.	470	21	64	3	9
Chocolate, 4 oz.	340	20	37	2	6
Fresh Strawberries & Citrus, 4 oz.	310	16	37	1	6
Pecan Braid, 4 oz.	410	22	48	2	6
Baked Egg Soufflés					
Four Cheese, 6 oz.	470	30	35	2	16
Spinach & Artichoke, 6 oz.	490	32	36	2	18
Spinach & Bacon, 6 oz.	530	34	36	2	19
Turkey Sausage & Potato, 6 oz.	440	27	36	2	14
Brownies					
Caramel Pecan, 4 oz.	470	24	59	2	5
Very Chocolate, 4 oz.	460	22	61	2	5
Cafe Sandwiches - Half Portions					
Chicken Salad on Sesame Semolina	340	12	44	7	15

RESTAURANTS & FAST-FOOD CHAINS

Panera Bread (cont.)

	Cal	Fat	Cbs	Fbr	Prtn
Cafe Sandwiches - Half Portions (cont.)					
Chicken Salad on Whole Grain	290	14	33	6	13
Smoked Ham & Swiss on Rye	340	17	27	2	20
Smoked Ham & Swiss on Stn-Milled Rye	380	16	37	3	22
Smoked Turkey Breast on Country	300	9	39	2	17
• Smoked Turkey Breast on Sourdough	230	8	24	2	15
Tuna Salad on Honey Wheat	350	23	29	2	10
• Tuna Salad on Whole Grain	420	22	43	5	14
Cookies					
Chocolate Chipper, 3 oz.	410	20	55	2	5
Chocolate Duet with Walnuts, 3 oz.	400	22	52	3	6
• Nutty Chocolate Chipper, 3 oz.	430	24	51	3	5
• Nutty Oatmeal Raisin, 3 oz.	340	14	50	3	5
Shortbread, 3 oz.	350	21	36	1	3
Cream Cheese Spreads					
• Plain, 2 oz.	200	19	2	0	4
Reduced Fat Hazelnut, 2 oz.	150	12	6	1	5
Reduced Fat Honey Walnut, 2 oz.	160	11	10	1	5
Reduced Fat Plain, 2 oz.	140	13	2	1	5
Reduced Fat Raspberry, 2 oz.	150	11	8	1	5
Reduced Fat Sun-Dried Tomato Cream, 2 oz.	140	12	4	1	5
• Reduced Fat Veggie, 2 oz.	120	10	3	1	4
Crispani®					
BBQ Chicken, 5 oz.	380	15	42	2	20
Italian Meat Classic, 5 oz.	380	18	38	2	17
Pepperoni, 4 oz.	380	18	38	2	17
Roasted Wild Mushroom, 4 oz.	340	16	38	2	13
• Sausage & Roasted Peppers, 5 oz.	380	18	38	2	15
Three Cheese, 4 oz.	340	15	37	2	15
• Tomato & Fresh Basil, 4 oz.	320	13	37	2	13
Espresso Drinks					
• Caffe Latte, 9 oz.	120	5	12	0	8
Caffe Mocha, 12 oz.	370	15	60	2	11
Cappuccino, 9 oz.	120	5	12	0	8
Caramel Latte, 12 oz.	390	16	53	0	10
• Pumpkin Spice Latte, 13 oz.	410	10	68	0	8
Freshly Baked Bagels					
Asiago Cheese, 5 oz.	350	6	60	2	16
Blueberry, 4 oz.	330	1	69	3	12
• Cinnamon Crunch, 5 oz.	410	8	75	2	11
Cranberry Walnut, 5 oz.	370	5	71	4	13
Dutch Apple & Raisin, 5 oz.	370	3	78	3	10
Everything, 4 oz.	300	2	60	3	12
French Toast, 5 oz.	380	5	73	3	11
Gingerbread, 5 oz.	390	5	77	2	10
• Plain, 4 oz.	290	1	61	3	12
Sesame, 4 oz.	310	4	58	3	12
Whole Grain, 5 oz.	340	3	66	6	13
Frozen Drinks					
Caramel - Grande, 16 oz.	550	23	80	0	5
Mango - Grande, 16 oz.	350	10	60	3	1
• Mocha - Grande, 16 oz.	570	25	88	2	6
• Strawberry Smoothie - Grande, 18 oz.	250	2	53	5	5

RESTAURANTS & FAST-FOOD CHAINS

Panera Bread (cont.)

	Cal	Fat	Cbs	Fbr	Prtn
Hand-Tossed Salads					
Asian Sesame Chicken, half portion	220	11	16	3	16
Caesar, half portion	220	16	13	2	7
• Classic Cafe, half portion	90	5	9	2	1
Fuji Apple Chicken, half portion	290	15	19	3	16
Greek, half portion	260	24	7	3	5
Grilled Chicken Caesar, half portion	280	17	14	2	19
Grilled Salmon, half portion	170	7	16	3	11
Orchard Harvest, half portion	210	12	15	2	5
Hot Drinks					
Chai Tea Latte, 10 oz.	190	4	31	0	7
• Hot Chocolate, 11 oz.	370	15	60	2	11
Hot Panini					
Half Chkn Pomodoro on French, 6 oz.	280	10	25	2	23
Half Chkn Pomodoro on Sesame Semolina, 7 oz.	350	10	43	3	25
• Half Frontega Chicken®, 6 oz.	400	16	40	2	23
Half Portobello & Mozzarella, 6 oz.	330	12	41	2	13
Half Smokehouse Turkey® on Focaccia, 6 oz.	360	12	39	2	23
Half Smokehouse Turkey® on Three Chz, 6 oz.	350	11	37	2	24
Half Turkey Artichoke, 7 oz.	350	11	44	3	20
Iced Drinks					
Iced Green Tea - Grande, 16 oz.	100	0	25	0	0
Iced Chai Tea Latte, 16 oz.	150	4	25	0	6
• Home Style Lemonade - Grande, 16 oz.	90	0	22	0	0
Mini Bundt Cakes					
• Lemon Poppyseed, 5 oz.	460	20	63	0	6
• Pineapple Upside-Down, 6 oz.	520	25	74	2	6
Muffins & Muffies					
Carrot Walnut Muffin, 5 oz.	430	19	61	2	8
• Chocolate Chip Muffie, 3 oz.	240	10	36	2	4
Cranberry Orange Muffin, 5 oz.	400	15	59	1	6
Pumpkin Muffie, 3 oz.	310	7	49	1	4
• Pumpkin Muffin, 6 oz.	590	13	93	1	7
Reduced Fat Wild Blueberry Muffin, 5 oz.	360	10	61	1	6
Wild Blueberry Muffin, 5 oz.	400	16	59	1	6
Panera Kids™					
Deli Sandwich - Roast Beef, 6 oz.	370	13	36	3	27
Deli Sandwich - Smoked Ham, 6 oz.	360	14	35	3	25
Deli Sandwich - Smoked Turkey, 6 oz.	350	12	36	3	25
• Grilled Cheese Sandwich, 4 oz.	290	11	35	3	14
• Peanut Butter & Jelly Sandwich, 5 oz.	420	16	55	5	13
Salad Dressings					
Balsamic Vinaigrette, 2 oz.	130	10	9	0	0
Caesar Dressing, 2 oz.	150	15	3	1	1
Cherry Balsamic Vinaigrette, 2 oz.	130	12	7	0	0
• Fat-Free Raspberry Dressing, 2 oz.	35	0	8	1	1
Fuji Apple Vinaigrette, 2 oz.	150	12	11	0	0
• Greek Dressing, 2 oz.	220	24	0	1	0
Low-Fat Rstd Grlc Meyer Lemon Vinaigrette, 2 oz.	60	2	9	0	0
Reduced-Sugar Asian Sesame Vinaigrette, 2 oz.	90	8	4	1	0
Scones					
• Cinnamon Chip, 5 oz.	530	27	67	2	8
Orange, 5 oz.	430	21	54	1	9
• Tart Cherry, 4 oz.	380	16	58	2	9

RESTAURANTS & FAST-FOOD CHAINS

▶ Panera Bread (cont.)

	Cal	Fat	Cbs	Fbr	Prtn
Scones (cont.)					
Wild Blueberry, 4 oz.	410	15	63	2	6
Signature Sandwiches					
Asiago Roast Beef, half portion	350	16	28	2	24
Bacon Turkey Bravo®, half portion	370	13	42	2	23
Chicken Caesar on Focaccia, half portion	400	16	41	2	22
Chicken Caesar on Three Cheese, half portion	380	15	39	2	22
• Chicken Tomesto on French, half portion	240	7	27	2	17
Chicken Tomesto on Three Cheese, half portion	310	8	40	3	21
Chipotle Chicken on Artisan French, half portion	470	24	39	2	24
Chipotle Chicken on Specialty French, half portion	400	24	25	2	22
• Italian Combo, half portion	530	24	53	3	29
Mediterranean Veggie, half portion	300	6	50	5	11
Sierra Turkey, half portion	420	20	41	2	18
Soups					
Baked Potato, 8 oz.	230	14	21	1	5
Broccoli Cheddar, 8 oz.	230	16	13	1	8
Cream of Chicken & Wild Rice, 8 oz.	200	12	19	1	5
French Onion (with cheese & croutons), 8 oz.	220	10	23	2	9
• French Onion (without cheese & croutons), 8 oz.	80	3	12	2	2
Low-Fat Chicken Noodle, 8 oz.	100	2	15	1	5
Low-Fat Vegetarian Black Bean, 8 oz.	160	1	31	11	9
Low-Fat Vegetarian Garden Vegetable, 8 oz.	90	1	17	2	4
• New England Clam Chowder, 8 oz.	320	28	11	1	6
Parisian Chicken, 9 oz.	170	11	13	2	6
Vegetarian Fiesta Con Queso, 8 oz.	250	16	18	2	8
Specialty Breads					
Asiago Cheese Demi, 2 oz.	150	4	22	1	7
Asiago Cheese Loaf, 2 oz.	150	4	22	1	7
Cinnamon Raisin Loaf, 2 oz.	170	3	32	1	4
Cranberry Walnut Panettone, 2 oz.	210	10	27	1	5
French Baguette, 2 oz.	150	2	30	1	6
French Loaf, 2 oz.	140	2	28	1	6
French Roll, 2 oz.	170	2	34	1	7
Holiday, 2 oz.	150	2	29	1	3
Honey Wheat loaf, 2 oz.	160	3	30	2	5
Sourdough Baguette, 2 oz.	150	0	30	1	6
Sourdough Loaf, 2 oz.	140	0	28	1	5
Sourdough Roll, 3 oz.	190	1	38	2	7
• Sourdough Soup Bowl, 8 oz.	560	2	115	5	22
Sunflower Loaf, 2 oz.	180	6	26	2	6
• Tomato Basil Loaf, 2 oz.	130	1	27	1	5
White Whole Grain Wheat Loaf, 2 oz.	140	2	28	3	5
XL French Loaf, 2 oz.	140	2	28	1	6
Specialty Pastries					
• Bear Claw, 5 oz.	460	27	49	2	10
• Coffee Cake - Cherry Cheese, 2 oz.	210	11	26	1	3
French Croissant, 2 oz.	240	14	25	1	5
Sweet Rolls					
Cinnamon Roll, 6 oz.	610	27	90	5	9
• Cobblestone, 7 oz.	590	12	107	3	6
Pecan Roll, 5 oz.	591	32	73	4	8

RESTAURANTS & FAST-FOOD CHAINS

▶ Papa Gino's

	Cal	Fat	Cbs	Fbr	Prtn
Appetizers & Snacks: Small					
BBQ Chick Tenders, 1/2 portion	259	9	28	1	14
Buff. Chick. Tender, 1/2 portion	199	7	20	1	14
• Cheese Breadsticks, 1/2 portion	535	24	58	2	24
• Chicken Tender, 1/2 portion	190	7	18	1	14
Cinnamon Sticks, 1/2 portion	309	10	50	2	6
French Fries, 1/2 portion	331	19	38	2	4
Marinara Dip Sauce, 1/2 portion	57	1	13	1	3
Mozzarella Sticks, 1/2 portion	347	15	35	1	22
Toasted Ravioli, 1/2 portion	286	15	33	1	7
Appetizers & Snacks: Large					
BBQ Chicken Tender, 1/4 portion	259	9	28	1	14
Buff. Chick. Tender, 1/4 portion	199	7	20	1	14
• Cheese Breadsticks, 1/4 portion	535	24	58	2	24
Cheese Garlic Bread, 1/4 portion	222	5	36	2	7
• Chicken Tender, 1/4 portion	190	7	18	1	14
Cinnamon Stick Icing, 1/4 portion	240	1	57	0	0
French Fries, 1/4 portion	362	22	38	2	4
Mozzarella Sticks, 1/4 portion	347	15	35	1	22
Toasted Ravioli Small, 1/4 portion	286	15	33	1	7
Extras					
Hot Peppers, 1 oz.	0	0	1	0	0
• Mayonnaise, 28 g	213	24	1	0	0
Mushrooms, 1 oz.	7	0	1	0	1
Onions, 0.5 oz.	6	0	1	0	0
Pickles, 1 oz.	0	0	1	0	0
Processed American Cheese, 1 oz.	95	7	3	0	5
Provolone Cheese, 1 oz.	100	8	1	0	7
Sweet Green Pepper, 1 oz.	6	0	1	1	0
Tomato, 60 g	11	0	2	1	1
Kids Meal					
Cheese Slice, 158 g	316	9	44	2	15
Chicken Tender Meal, 219 g	481	26	44	1	20
• Hot Dog Meal, 213 g	511	29	49	2	14
• Penne, 254 g	336	6	61	2	10
Pepperoni Slice, 172 g	388	16	44	2	19
Spaghetti & Meatball, 296 g	456	16	63	2	17
Large Thick Crust Pizza					
BBQ Chicken, 158 g	379	10	53	2	18
Buffalo Chicken, 153 g	350	10	47	2	18
Cheese, 155 g	365	12	47	2	16
Cheeseburger, 178 g	423	16	49	2	20
Chicken Pepper, 190 g	385	12	48	3	21
Fenway, 207 g	414	15	50	3	18
Garlic Chicken, 186 g	398	12	50	3	21
Hawaiian, 182 g	386	11	49	3	20
Meat Combo, 172 g	427	17	47	2	20
• PapaRoni, 169 g	428	18	48	2	19
Pepperoni, 148 g	360	11	49	3	16
• Super Veggie, 204 g	348	10	50	3	14
Works, 189 g	405	15	49	3	18
Large Thin Crust Pizza					
BBQ Chicken, 130 g	273	7	39	1	14
Buffalo Chicken, 125 g	244	7	32	1	14

(• = most healthy • = least healthy)   **RESTAURANTS & FAST-FOOD • 261**

Papa Gino's (cont.)	Cal	Fat	Cbs	Fbr	Prtn
Large Thin Crust Pizza (cont.)					
• Cheese, 110 g	224	6	32	2	10
Chicken Pepper, 163 g	285	10	34	2	16
Garlic Chicken, 159 g	292	11	35	2	16
Meat Combo, 140 g	323	14	33	2	17
• PapaRoni, 138 g	323	15	33	2	16
Pepperoni, 122 g	269	10	32	2	13
Works, 156 g	300	12	34	2	15
Pasta Entrees					
• Broccoli Ravioli, 386 g	445	20	49	4	19
Papa Platter Penne, 641 g	1003	34	136	4	39
Papa Platter Spaghetti, 641 g	1003	34	136	8	39
Pasta Trio Plate, 563 g	916	30	130	5	31
Penne Alfredo Chix, 559 g	1021	42	119	4	46
Penne Alfredo, 417 g	901	37	111	2	29
Penne, 474 g	651	11	118	3	21
Spaghetti & Meatballs, 559 g	893	30	123	7	34
Spaghetti Alfredo Chix Broccoli, 559 g	1021	42	119	7	46
Spaghetti Alfredo, 417 g	901	37	111	5	29
• Spaghetti Chicken Parmesan, 656 g	1080	41	128	7	52
Spaghetti, 474 g	653	11	118	7	21
Pasta Sides					
• Meatballs, 128 g	270	18	9	0	13
Penne Alfredo, 209 g	450	18	55	1	14
Penne, 254 g	336	6	61	2	10
• Spaghetti Alfredo, 209 g	450	18	55	3	14
Spaghetti, 254 g	337	6	61	4	10
Pizza					
Cheese, 1 slice	316	9	44	2	15
Pepperoni, 1 slice	388	16	44	2	19
Salads					
Buffalo Chicken Tender, 325 g	319	15	32	3	17
Caesar, 234 g	191	8	20	5	10
Chicken Bacon Cheddar, 415 g	481	21	26	5	47
Chicken Caesar, 365 g	324	8	16	5	47
Chicken Tender, 308 g	282	10	30	4	19
• Garden, 289 g	176	6	27	5	6
Greek, 335 g	202	11	12	6	13
• Italian Chopped, 357 g	574	50	12	5	22
Single Breadstick, 82 g	215	10	23	1	10
Salads Dressing					
Bleu Cheese, 30 g	150	15	3	0	1
• Caesar, 85 g	397	43	0	0	3
• Fat Free Honey Dijon, 43 g	59	0	13	1	1
Honey Mustard, 30 g	150	14	7	0	0
Olive Oil Vinaigrette, 85 g	170	17	9	0	0
Ranch, 85 g	284	31	3	0	0
Small Thin Crust Pizza					
BBQ Chicken, 105 g	209	4	31	1	10
Buffalo Chicken, 93 g	176	4	24	1	10
• Cheese, 87 g	166	4	25	1	7
Chicken Pepper, 131 g	208	7	25	1	12
Garlic Chicken, 117 g	213	7	27	1	11
• Meat Combo, 113 g	257	11	25	1	14

RESTAURANTS & FAST-FOOD CHAINS

Papa Gino's (cont.)	Cal	Fat	Cbs	Fbr	Prtn
Small Thin Crust Pizza (cont.)					
PapaRoni, 105 g	235	10	25	1	11
Pepperoni, 95 g	203	8	25	1	9
Super Veggie, 144 g	186	5	28	2	8
Works, 127 g	219	8	27	2	11
Subs & Sandwiches: Large					
BLT, 430 g	1025	48	107	6	40
Chicken Cutlet, 358 g	743	18	107	4	39
Chicken Parm, 477 g	1082	44	114	5	59
Italian, 520 g	1243	62	106	6	64
• Meatball Parm, 576 g	1376	63	120	5	67
Meatball, 519 g	1174	54	120	5	52
Seafood Salad, 404 g	949	37	116	5	37
Steak & Cheese, 446 g	1168	53	106	4	63
Steak, 364 g	891	33	99	4	47
Super Steak, 673 g	1235	53	120	7	66
Tuna, 401 g	1086	56	100	5	44
Turkey Club, 487 g	842	21	105	6	56
• Turkey, 333 g	619	2	101	4	47
Vegetarian, 456 g	778	22	113	7	31
Subs & Sandwiches: Panini Sandwiches					
• Basil Chicken, 424 g	1117	62	89	5	52
• Eggplant, 376 g	768	30	101	8	25
Italian Deli, 374 g	950	52	72	3	48
Sausage & Pepper, 431 g	1106	68	76	4	49
Subs & Sandwiches: Small					
BLT, 312 g	683	31	72	4	30
Hot Dog w/ Roll, 128 g	391	25	30	1	12
• Italian, 313 g	905	48	69	3	47
Lobster Roll, 227 g	545	35	31	2	27
Meatball Parm, 327 g	832	36	76	3	41
Meatball, 299 g	731	33	76	3	34
Seafood Salad, 284 g	680	34	69	3	25
Steak & Cheese, 269 g	694	30	68	2	37
Steak, 241 g	600	23	65	2	32
Super Steak, 428 g	741	30	78	5	40
Tuna, 281 g	734	38	67	3	31
Turkey Club, 333 g	600	19	70	3	37
Turkey, 224 g	444	2	72	2	32
Toppings (per large slice)					
Bacon, 13 g	59	4	0	0	4
BBQ Chicken, 99 g	240	9	28	1	11
Black Olives, 11 g	13	1	1	0	0
Broccoli, 20 g	6	0	1	1	1
Buffalo Chicken, 96 g	219	9	24	1	11
Capicola, 6 g	7	0	0	0	1
Cheese, 86 g	208	9	24	1	8
Chicken Pepper, 121 g	247	11	25	2	13
Extra Cheese, 12 g	35	3	0	0	2
Garlic Chicken, 118 g	251	11	25	2	13
Green Pepper, 12 g	2	0	1	0	0
Hamburger, 19 g	59	4	0	0	5
• Meat Combo, 106 g	274	14	25	2	13
Mushrooms, 12 g	3	0	0	0	0

(• = most healthy • = least healthy) **RESTAURANTS & FAST-FOOD • 263**

RESTAURANTS & FAST-FOOD CHAINS

Papa Gino's (cont.)

	Cal	Fat	Cbs	Fbr	Prtn
Toppings (per large Slice) (cont.)					
Naples, 116 g	273	14	25	1	11
Onions, 12 g	5	0	1	0	0
PapaRoni, 105 g	274	14	25	1	12
Pepperoni, 7 g	31	3	0	0	2
Pepperoni, 93 g	238	11	24	1	10
Saus Arrabbiata, 111 g	259	13	25	1	10
Sausage, 21 g	74	7	0	0	3
• Sliced Tomato, 7 g	1	0	0	0	0
Super Veggie, 128 g	222	9	26	2	9
Works, 116 g	258	12	25	2	11

Papa John's Pizza

	Cal	Fat	Cbs	Fbr	Prtn
10" Pizza					
• Cheese Pizza, 91 g	210	8	27	1	9
Pepperoni Pizza, 91 g	220	9	27	1	5
• Sausage Pizza, 95 g	240	11	26	2	9
14" Pizza					
• Cheese Pizza, 132 g	300	11	39	2	13
Pepperoni Pizza, 128 g	310	13	38	2	13
• Sausage Pizza, 134 g	330	15	37	3	13
BBQ Chicken & Bacon					
Original Crust Pizza, 150 g	340	11	44	2	15
• Pan Crust Pizza, 156 g	410	140	44	1	16
• Thin Crust Pizza, 114 g	290	14	29	1	13
Garden Fresh					
Original Crust Pizza, 160 g	280	9	40	2	11
• Pan Crust Pizza, 173 g	360	13	40	2	12
• Thin Crust Pizza, 134 g	210	11	23	2	8
Grilled Chicken Alfredo					
Original Crust Pizza, 132 g	310	12	36	2	15
• Pan Crust Pizza, 138 g	380	16	36	2	15
• Thin Crust Pizza, 96 g	240	13	20	1	12
Hawaiian BBQ Chicken					
Original Crust Pizza, 164 g	340	11	46	2	16
• Pan Crust Pizza, 170 g	420	16	46	1	16
• Thin Crust Pizza, 127 g	290	14	31	1	13
Italian Meats Trio					
Original Crust Pizza, 150 g	340	11	38	2	16
• Pan Crust Pizza, 164 g	440	20	40	2	17
• Thin Crust Pizza, 113 g	280	12	22	2	13
Roma Meats					
Original Crust Pizza, 158 g	340	11	39	3	15
• Pan Crust Pizza, 170 g	430	20	40	2	16
• Thin Crust Pizza, 122 g	280	12	22	2	12
Six Cheese					
Original Crust Pizza, 133 g	320	13	38	2	15
• Pan Crust Pizza, 144 g	400	21	40	1	16
• Thin Crust Pizza, 96 g	250	14	21	1	12
Spicy Italian					
Original Crust Pizza, 147 g	370	11	39	4	15
• Pan Crust Pizza, 159 g	450	15	39	3	16
• Thin Crust Pizza, 110 g	320	14	24	3	12

RESTAURANTS & FAST-FOOD CHAINS

Papa John's Pizza (cont.)

	Cal	Fat	Cbs	Fbr	Prtn
Spinach Alfredo					
Original Crust Pizza, 116 g	280	11	36	2	11
• Pan Crust Pizza, 122 g	360	15	36	1	12
• Thin Crust Pizza, 79 g	220	13	19	1	8
Spinach Alfredo Chicken Tomato					
Original Crust Pizza, 144 g	290	11	37	2	13
• Pan Crust Pizza, 153 g	380	16	37	2	14
• Thin Crust Pizza, 110 g	230	13	21	1	10
The Meats					
Original Crust Pizza, 141 g	350	16	38	2	15
Pan Crust Pizza, 152 g	420	19	38	1	16
• Thin Crust Pizza, 105 g	300	18	23	2	13
The Works					
Original Crust Pizza, 157 g	330	11	39	3	14
• Pan Crust Pizza, 167 g	400	15	39	2	15
• Thin Crust Pizza, 120 g	280	14	24	2	12

Papa Murphy's

	Cal	Fat	Cbs	Fbr	Prtn
Cheesy Bread					
Cheesy Bread, 75 g	220	8	31	8	7
Dessert Pizzas					
Apple, 97 g	245	5	46	22	4
• Cherry, 97 g	235	5	44	18	5
Chocolate Chip Cookies, 57 g	245	11	34	20	3
• Cinnamon Rolls, 111 g	344	10	58	25	6
Cinnamon Wheel, 82 g	250	7	42	17	5
Family Size (16") Original Crust Pizzas					
Barbecue Chicken, 144 g	334	12	36	12	19
• Cheese, 109 g	260	10	29	7	12
Cowboy, 151 g	340	17	31	8	17
Gourmet Chicken Garlic, 137 g	320	14	30	8	18
Gourmet Classic Italian, 146 g	352	18	31	8	17
Gourmet Vegetarian, 144 g	302	13	31	8	14
Hawaiian, 136 g	285	11	33	10	14
Herb Chicken Mediterranean, 128 g	338	15	35	11	17
Murphy's Combination, 158 g	355	18	31	8	17
Papa's All Meat, 141 g	350	17	30	7	18
• Papa's Favorite, 170 g	355	18	31	8	17
Papa-Roni Signature, 125 g	340	17	29	7	16
Pepperoni, 118 g	310	15	29	7	14
Rancher, 140 g	325	15	30	8	17
Specialty of the House, 145 g	310	14	31	8	15
Vegetarian Combo, 160 g	285	12	32	8	13
Veggie Mediterranean, 113 g	320	14	34	11	13
Family Size Calzones					
• Chicken Florentine, 218 g	457	19	46	11	25
Combo, 184 g	434	19	45	11	21
Italian, 209 g	449	20	46	11	22
• Veggie, 197 g	390	16	45	11	18
Family Size Stuffed Pizzas					
5-Meat, 143 g	365	16	38	9	18
• Big Murphy, 157 g	360	16	40	10	17
Chicago-Style, 149 g	365	16	38	10	17
• Chicken and Bacon, 151 g	373	15	38	10	20

(• = most healthy • = least healthy) **RESTAURANTS & FAST-FOOD • 265**

RESTAURANTS & FAST-FOOD CHAINS

Papa Murphy's (cont.)

	Cal	Fat	Cbs	Fbr	Prtn
Large (14") Original Crust Pizzas					
Barbecue Chicken, 134 g	308	11	35	12	17
• Cheese, 98 g	240	10	26	7	11
Cowboy, 137 g	310	16	28	7	15
Gourmet Chicken Garlic, 124 g	291	12	27	7	16
Gourmet Classic Italian, 129 g	315	16	27	7	15
Gourmet Vegetarian, 127 g	273	12	28	7	13
Hawaiian, 124 g	255	10	29	9	13
Herb Chicken Mediterranean, 114 g	300	13	31	10	15
• Murphy's Combination, 141 g	320	16	28	7	16
Papa's All Meat, 125 g	315	16	27	7	17
Papa's Favorite, 153 g	320	16	28	7	16
Pepperoni, 106 g	280	14	26	7	13
Rancher, 125 g	290	14	27	7	15
Specialty of the House, 154 g	290	14	28	7	15
Vegetarian Combo, 145 g	260	11	29	7	12
Veggie Mediterranean, 102 g	285	13	31	10	12
Large (14") Thin Crust deLITE Pizzas					
Barbecue Chicken deLITE, 79 g	181	8	17	4	11
• Cheese deLITE, 58 g	140	7	13	2	8
Cowboy deLITE, 86 g	190	11	13	1	11
Gourmet Chicken Bacon Artichoke deLITE, 78 g	181	9	13	1	12
Gourmet Chicken Garlic deLITE, 76 g	172	9	13	1	11
Gourmet Classic Italian deLITE, 85 g	180	10	13	1	10
Gourmet Vegetarian deLITE, 76 g	161	8	13	1	8
Hawaiian deLITE, 77 g	150	7	15	4	9
Herb Chicken Mediterranean deLITE, 68 g	180	9	16	3	10
Meat deLITE, 76 g	190	11	13	2	11
Murphy's Combination deLITE, 91 g	195	12	14	1	11
Papa's All Meat deLITE, 76 g	187	11	13	1	11
• Papa's Favorite deLITE, 96 g	195	11	14	1	11
Pepperoni deLITE, 64 g	165	9	13	2	9
Rancher deLITE, 77 g	175	9	13	1	10
Specialty of the House deLITE, 82 g	170	9	13	1	10
Vegetarian Combo deLITE, 92 g	150	8	14	1	8
Veggie deLITE, 71 g	152	8	13	1	8
Veggie Mediterranean deLITE, 59 g	165	9	15	3	8
Large Size Calzones					
• Chicken Florentine, 215 g	455	19	45	11	25
Combo, 182 g	440	20	44	11	20
Italian, 196 g	440	20	45	11	21
• Veggie, 186 g	390	16	44	11	18
Large Size Stuffed Pizzas					
5-Meat, 142 g	361	15	37	9	18
• Big Murphy, 152 g	355	15	38	10	17
Chicago-Style, 145 g	356	15	38	9	17
• Chicken and Bacon, 148 g	366	15	38	9	19
Medium (12") Original Crust Pizzas					
Barbecue Chicken, 117 g	273	10	30	10	15
Cheese, 90 g	215	9	24	6	10
Cowboy, 125 g	280	14	25	6	14
Gourmet Chicken Garlic, 112 g	263	12	24	6	15
Gourmet Classic Italian, 125 g	271	13	25	6	14
Gourmet Vegetarian, 113 g	248	11	25	7	11

RESTAURANTS & FAST-FOOD CHAINS

Papa Murphy's (cont.)

	Cal	Fat	Cbs	Fbr	Prtn
Medium (12") Original Crust Pizzas (cont.)					
Hawaiian, 91 g	190	7	22	8	10
Herb Chicken Mediterranean, 103 g	272	12	28	9	14
Murphy's Combination, 131 g	290	15	26	6	14
Papa's All Meat, 113 g	280	14	24	6	15
Papa's Favorite, 138 g	290	15	26	7	14
Pepperoni, 97 g	250	12	24	6	12
Rancher, 114 g	265	12	25	6	14
Specialty of the House, 97 g	210	10	20	5	10
Vegetarian Combo, 133 g	235	10	26	7	11
Veggie Mediterranean, 92 g	255	12	28	9	11
Salads					
Caesar, 120 g	47	2	4	2	4
Chicken Caesar, 163 g	108	3	5	2	15
Club, 189 g	145	9	6	2	12
Garden, 206 g	100	6	8	2	6
Italian, 186 g	136	10	7	2	7
Lasagna, 201 g	255	14	17	4	14

Pei Wei Asian Diner

	Cal	Fat	Cbs	Fbr	Prtn
Dan Dan Noodles					
Chicken, 1/2 portion	390	7	54	3	26
First Tastes					
Crab Wontons, 2 pcs.	190	13	9	0	8
Crispy Potstickers, 2 pcs.	130	7	10	0	6
Edamame, 1/2 portion	156	8	12	5	14
Hot & Sour Soup, 1 bowl	500	28	37	6	24
Hot & Sour Soup, 1 cup	150	9	11	2	7
Minced Chkn w/ Cool Lettuce Wraps, 1/2 portion	250	4	31	3	22
Pei Wei Spring Rolls, 1 roll	90	5	11	1	2
Wonton Soup, 1 bowl	260	5	49	6	12
Wonton Soup, 1 cup	110	2	23	3	5
Fried Rice					
Beef, 1/2 portion	580	21	56	3	35
Chicken, 1/2 portion	470	11	56	3	31
Pork, 1/2 portion	500	16	57	3	28
Scallops, 1/2 portion	410	9	56	3	21
Shrimp, 1/2 portion	420	10	55	3	23
Vegetables & Tofu, 1/2 portion	380	7	60	5	16
Japanese Udon Noodles					
Beef, 1/2 portion	600	26	57	4	32
Chicken, 1/2 portion	490	16	57	4	28
Pork, 1/2 portion	520	21	57	4	25
Scallops, 1/2 portion	450	16	58	4	18
Shrimp, 1/2 portion	460	16	57	4	20
Vegetables & Tofu, 1/2 portion	440	16	63	6	11
Kid's Wei™					
Honey Seared Chicken, 1/2 portion	290	17	19	0	16
Teriyaki Chicken, 1/2 portion	240	5	20	0	23
Lo Mein Noodles					
Beef, 1/2 portion	570	21	61	5	36
Chicken, 1/2 portion	460	11	61	5	31
Pork, 1/2 portion	490	16	62	5	28
Scallops, 1/2 portion	390	8	61	5	21

RESTAURANTS & FAST-FOOD CHAINS

Pei Wei Asian Diner (cont.)

	Cal	Fat	Cbs	Fbr	Prtn
Lo Mein Noodles (cont.)					
Shrimp, 1/2 portion	400	8	60	5	23
Vegetables & Tofu, 1/2 portion	400	8	66	7	16
Pad Thai					
• Beef, 1/2 portion	670	30	63	2	40
Chicken, 1/2 portion	560	20	61	2	35
Pork, 1/2 portion	590	25	62	2	32
Scallops, 1/2	480	16	61	2	25
Shrimp, 1/2 portion	490	17	60	2	27
• Vegetables & Tofu, 1/2 portion	470	17	66	4	18
Rice & Noodles					
Brown Rice, 1/2 portion	170	2	37	3	4
• Egg Noodles, 1/2 portion	210	3	39	2	7
Rice Noodles, 1/2 portion	130	0	32	0	0
• Udon Noodles, 1/2 portion	101	0	20	0	3
White Rice, 1/2 portion	200	0	44	1	4
Salads					
Asian Chopped Chicken Salad, 1/2 portion	280	15	13	2	24
w/o Dressing	200	8	10	2	23
• Pei Wei Spicy Chicken Salad, 1/2 portion	350	16	28	2	22
w/o Dressing	210	3	23	2	22
• Vietnamese Chicken Salad Rolls, 3 rolls	80	4	9	1	3
Sauces & Sides					
Fortune Cookie	30	0	7	0	0
Lettuce Wrap Sauce, 2 oz.	70	5	2	0	4
Lime Vinaigrette, 2 oz.	230	20	13	0	0
• Rice Sticks, 1 cup	130	0	33	0	0
Sesame Ginger Dressing, 2 oz.	170	16	5	0	1
Sweet Chile Sauce, 2 oz.	140	0	34	2	0
Thai Peanut Sauce, 2 oz.	168	11	15	1	5
• Sgntre Dishes: Asian Coconut Curry Beef, 1/2 portion	550	37	20	2	36
Chicken, 1/2 portion	380	19	23	2	30
Pork, 1/2 portion	420	26	24	2	25
Scallops, 1/2 portion	290	16	19	2	18
Shrimp, 1/2 portion	300	17	18	2	21
Vegetables & Tofu, 1/2 portion	220	14	19	2	8
Signature Dishes: Blazing Noodles					
• Beef, 1/2 portion	570	36	23	4	36
Chicken, 1/2 portion	420	22	22	4	30
Pork, 1/2 portion	460	29	23	4	26
Scallops, 1/2 portion	370	21	24	4	18
Shrimp, 1/2 portion	380	22	23	4	21
• Vegetables & Tofu, 1/2 portion	300	17	27	6	10
Signature Dishes: Ginger Broccoli					
• Beef, 1/2 portion	450	22	19	2	37
Chicken, 1/2 portion	300	9	19	2	31
Pork, 1/2 portion	340	16	20	2	26
Scallops, 1/2 portion	220	6	19	2	19
Shrimp, 1/2 portion	230	7	18	2	22
• Vegetables & Tofu, 1/2 portion	170	4	23	4	10
Signature Dishes: Honey Seared					
Chicken, 1/2 portion	420	15	45	1	21
• Pork, 1/2 portion	460	21	46	1	18
• Shrimp, 1/2 portion	370	14	43	0	14

RESTAURANTS & FAST-FOOD CHAINS

Pei Wei Asian Diner (cont.)	Cal	Fat	Cbs	Fbr	Prtn
Signature Dishes: Lemon Pepper					
• Beef, 1/2 portion	550	31	32	2	36
Chicken, 1/2 portion	440	20	34	2	31
Pork, 1/2 portion	480	28	35	2	26
Scallops, 1/2 portion	360	17	35	2	16
Shrimp, 1/2 portion	380	18	34	2	22
Vegetables & Tofu, 1/2 portion	230	10	29	4	10
Signature Dishes: Mandarin Kung Pao					
• Beef, 1/2 portion	610	34	31	3	40
Chicken, 1/2 portion	450	21	28	3	34
Pork, 1/2 portion	500	29	28	3	30
Scallops, 1/2 portion	400	19	32	3	22
Shrimp, 1/2 portion	400	19	28	3	25
Vegetables & Tofu, 1/2 portion	290	15	23	4	13
Signature Dishes: Mongolian					
• Beef, 1/2 portion	420	22	14	1	36
Chicken, 1/2 portion	280	9	14	1	30
Pork, 1/2 portion	320	16	15	1	26
Scallops, 1/2 portion	190	6	13	1	18
Shrimp, 1/2 portion	210	6	12	1	21
Vegetables & Tofu, 1/2 portion	180	6	19	3	10
Signature Dishes: Orange Peel					
• Beef, 1/2 portion	660	31	52	3	42
Chicken, 1/2 portion	520	18	52	3	36
Pork, 1/2 portion	560	25	53	3	31
Scallops, 1/2 portion	440	15	52	3	24
Shrimp, 1/2 portion	460	16	51	3	27
Vegetables & Tofu, 1/2 portion	330	10	46	4	14
Signature Dishes: Pei Wei Spicy					
• Beef, 1/2 portion	480	26	25	2	34
Chicken, 1/2 portion	330	13	25	2	28
Pork, 1/2 portion	380	20	26	2	23
Scallops, 1/2 portion	270	10	27	2	16
Shrimp, 1/2 portion	300	11	29	2	19
• Vegetables & Tofu, 1/2 portion	250	16	21	3	6
Signature Dishes: Spicy Korean					
• Beef, 1/2 portion	490	24	26	3	41
Chicken, 1/2 portion	350	11	26	3	35
Pork, 1/2 portion	390	18	27	3	31
Scallops, 1/2 portion	270	8	25	3	23
Shrimp, 1/2 portion	280	9	24	3	26
Vegetables & Tofu, 1/2 portion	240	9	27	4	15
Signature Dishes: Sweet & Sour					
Chicken, 1/2 portion	440	13	61	2	21
• Pork, 1/2 portion	480	18	61	2	18
• Shrimp, 1/2 portion	390	11	59	2	14
Soba Miso Bowl					
• Beef, 1/2 portion	530	18	53	5	38
Chicken, 1/2 portion	420	8	53	5	34
Pork, 1/2 portion	450	13	53	5	31
• Scallops, 1/2 portion	350	5	52	5	24
Shrimp, 1/2 portion	360	6	51	5	26
Vegetables & Tofu, 1/2 portion	360	7	57	7	19

(• = most healthy • = least healthy) **RESTAURANTS & FAST-FOOD • 269**

RESTAURANTS & FAST-FOOD CHAINS

Pei Wei Asian Diner (cont.)

	Cal	Fat	Cbs	Fbr	Prtn
Teriyaki Bowl with Brown Rice					
• Beef, 1/2 portion	580	17	66	4	33
Chicken, 1/2 portion	460	7	64	4	28
Pork, 1/2 portion	490	13	64	4	25
• Scallops, 1/2 portion	400	5	65	4	18
Shrimp, 1/2 portion	410	5	64	4	20
Vegetables & Tofu, 1/2 portion	410	6	71	7	13
Teriyaki Bowl with White Rice					
• Beef, 1/2 portion	560	16	62	3	32
Chicken, 1/2 portion	440	6	60	3	28
Pork, 1/2 portion	470	11	61	3	24
• Scallops, 1/2 portion	380	4	62	3	18
Shrimp, 1/2 portion	390	5	61	3	20
Vegetables & Tofu, 1/2 portion	390	5	68	5	13

Penn Station

	Cal	Fat	Cbs	Fbr	Prtn
Bread					
Small Bread, 7"	260	0	54	N/A	N/A
Cheeses					
• American, 1 oz.	100	5	1	N/A	N/A
• Provolone, 1 oz.	100	8	1	N/A	N/A
Swiss, 1 oz.	100	8	1	N/A	N/A
Condiments/Toppings					
Honey Mustard, 0.5 oz.	66	6	2	N/A	N/A
• Mayonnaise, 0.5 oz.	101	11	0	N/A	N/A
Olive Oil & Vinegar, 0.5 oz.	96	11	0	N/A	N/A
Oregano, 0.5 tbsp.	16	2	0	N/A	N/A
Parmesan Cheese, 0.5 oz.	25	2	0	N/A	N/A
Pizza Sauce, 1 oz.	18	0	4	N/A	N/A
• Sauerkraut, 4 oz.	16	0	4	N/A	N/A
Meats					
• Artichokes, 1 oz.	8	0	2	N/A	N/A
Bacon, 2 slices	55	4	0	N/A	N/A
Chicken Salad, 1 oz.	66	5	3	N/A	N/A
Chicken, 1 oz.	47	1	0	N/A	N/A
Corned Beef, 1 oz.	73	2	1	N/A	N/A
Ham, 1 oz.	33	1	0	N/A	N/A
• Pepperoni, 1 oz.	140	13	0	N/A	N/A
Salami, 1 oz.	120	11	0	N/A	N/A
Sausage, 1 oz.	90	7	1	N/A	N/A
Steak, 1 oz.	38	2	0	N/A	N/A
Tuna Salad, 1 oz.	60	4	3	N/A	N/A
Turkey (white), 1 oz.	25	0	0	N/A	N/A
Veggies					
• Banana Peppers (Grilled), 0.5 oz.	1	0	0	N/A	N/A
Green Peppers (Grilled), 0.5 oz.	4	0	1	N/A	N/A
Lettuce, 15 oz.	5	0	0	N/A	N/A
Mushrooms (Grilled), 0.5 oz.	3	0	0	N/A	N/A
Pickles, 0.5 oz.	1	0	0	N/A	N/A
Red Onions, 1 oz.	17	0	3	N/A	N/A
Tomato, 1 oz.	5	0	1	N/A	N/A
• Yellow Onions (Grilled), 2 oz.	22	0	5	N/A	N/A

RESTAURANTS & FAST-FOOD CHAINS

Pepe's Mexican	Cal	Fat	Cbs	Fbr	Prtn
Beef Menu					
Beef & Bean Burrito Suizo, 314 g	640	34	55	10	30
Beef & Bean Burrito, 228 g	510	24	52	9	22
Beef & Bean Tostada Suiza, 184 g	440	29	26	4	19
Beef & Bean Tostada, 186 g	380	23	26	5	15
Beef Enchilada Suiza, 124 g	220	11	16	2	13
Beef Flauta - Plain, 57 g	160	9	10	2	8
Beef Flauta with Cheese and Sauce, 80 g	190	12	11	2	10
Beef Taco Crisp, 138 g	210	11	16	3	12
Beef Taco Salad with 4 oz Salsa, 536 g	550	26	52	8	27
Beef Taco Soft Corn, 161 g	250	10	28	4	13
Beef Taco Soft Flour, 146 g	250	11	24	3	13
Refried Beans with Mexican Cheese, 126 g	300	20	22	8	10
Spanish Rice with Ranchera Sauce, 112 g	140	6	21	1	2
Taco Salad w/ 4 oz Salsa - no shell, 475 g	330	19	20	6	22
Burritos					
Beef & Bean Burrito Suizo, 314 g	640	34	55	10	30
Beef & Bean Burrito, 228 g	510	24	52	9	22
Chicken & Bean Burrito Suizo, 314 g	610	31	54	9	30
Chicken & Bean Burrito, 228 g	480	21	51	9	22
Pork & Bean Burrito Suizo, 314 g	600	29	54	10	32
Pork & Bean Burrito, 228 g	470	19	51	9	24
Chicken Menu					
Chicken & Bean Burrito Suizo, 314 g	610	31	54	9	30
Chicken & Bean Burrito, 228 g	480	21	51	9	22
Chicken & Bean Tostada Suiza, 184 g	410	26	25	4	19
Chicken & Bean Tostada, 186 g	360	21	21	6	15
Chicken Enchilada Suiza, 124 g	190	9	15	2	13
Chicken Flauta - Plain, 57 g	190	10	16	2	8
Chicken Flauta with Sauce & Cheese, 80 g	230	13	17	2	11
Chicken Taco Crisp, 138 g	190	9	15	2	12
Chicken Taco Salad with 4 oz Salsa - no shell, 475 g	300	16	19	6	22
Chicken Taco Salad with 4 oz Salsa, 536 g	520	23	51	7	27
Chicken Taco Soft Corn, 161 g	230	8	27	4	13
Chicken Taco Soft Flour, 146 g	230	9	23	2	14
Refried Beans with Mexican Cheese, 126 g	300	20	22	8	10
Spanish Rice with Ranchera Sauce, 112 g	140	6	21	1	2
Flautas					
Beef Flauta - Plain, 57 g	160	9	10	2	8
Beef Flauta with Cheese and Sauce, 80 g	190	12	11	2	10
Chicken Flauta - Plain, 57 g	190	10	16	2	8
Chicken Flauta with Sauce & Cheese, 80 g	230	13	17	2	11
Pork Menu					
Pork & Bean Burrito Suizo, 314 g	600	29	54	10	32
Pork & Bean Burrito, 228 g	470	19	51	9	24
Pork & Bean Tostada Suiza, 184 g	410	25	26	4	20
Pork & Bean Tostada, 186 g	350	20	26	5	16
Pork Enchilada Suiza, 124 g	190	8	15	2	14
Pork Taco Crisp, 135 g	170	6	16	3	13
Pork Taco Salad with 4 oz Salsa - no shell, 475 g	290	13	19	6	24
Pork Taco Salad with 4 oz Salsa, 536 g	500	20	52	8	29
Pork Taco Soft Corn, 160 g	220	6	27	4	14
Pork Taco Soft Flour, 145 g	220	7	24	3	15
Refried Beans with Mexican Cheese, 126 g	300	20	22	8	10

(●= most healthy ●= least healthy)   **RESTAURANTS & FAST-FOOD • 271**

RESTAURANTS & FAST-FOOD CHAINS

Pepe's Mexican (cont.)

	Cal	Fat	Cbs	Fbr	Prtn
Pork Menu (cont.)					
Spanish Rice with Ranchera Sauce, 112 g	140	6	21	1	2
Salads					
Beef Taco Salad with 4 oz Salsa - no shell, 475 g	330	19	20	6	22
• Beef Taco Salad with 4 oz Salsa, 536 g	550	26	52	8	27
Chicken Taco Salad with 4 oz Salsa - no shell, 475 g	300	16	19	6	22
Chicken Taco Salad with 4 oz Salsa, 536 g	520	23	51	7	27
• Pork Taco Salad with 4 oz Salsa - no shell, 475 g	290	13	19	6	24
Pork Taco Salad with 4 oz Salsa, 536 g	500	20	52	8	29
Taco					
Beef Taco Crisp, 138 g	210	11	16	3	12
Beef Taco Soft Corn, 161 g	250	10	28	4	13
• Beef Taco Soft Flour, 146 g	250	11	24	3	13
Chicken Taco Crisp, 138 g	190	9	15	2	12
Chicken Taco Soft Corn, 161 g	230	8	27	4	13
Chicken Taco Soft Flour, 146 g	230	9	23	2	14
• Pork Taco Crisp, 135 g	170	6	16	3	13
Pork Taco Soft Corn, 160 g	220	6	27	4	14
Pork Taco Soft Flour, 145 g	220	7	24	3	15
Tostadas					
• Beef & Bean Tostada Suiza, 184 g	440	29	26	4	19
Beef & Bean Tostada, 186 g	380	23	26	5	15
Chicken & Bean Tostada Suiza, 184 g	410	26	25	4	19
Chicken & Bean Tostada, 186 g	360	21	21	6	15
Pork & Bean Tostada Suiza, 184 g	410	25	26	4	20
• Pork & Bean Tostada, 186 g	350	20	26	5	16

Peter Piper Pizza

	Cal	Fat	Cbs	Fbr	Prtn
Appetizers & Desserts					
Breadsticks, 69 g	250	10	36	0	7
Chicken Strips, 138 g	300	9	26	0	26
Cinnamon Crunch Dessert, 86 g	220	2	49	2	5
• Garlic Cheese Bread, 92 g	310	14	37	2	10
• Wings, 48 g	110	8	0	0	9
Healthier Choices Made Easy					
California Veggie Crust Original, 1 slice	200	6	23	2	12
California Veggie Crust Ultra Thin, 1 slice	130	4	15	1	8
• Cheese Pizza Crust Original, 1 slice	300	6	23	2	12
• Cheese Pizza Crust Ultra Thin, 1 slice	130	4	15	1	8
Chicken Caesar Salad No Dressing	130	4	15	1	8
Cinnamon Crunch Dessert Pie, 1 slice	130	4	15	1	8
Garden Fresh Salad No Dressing	130	4	15	1	8
Mushroom Pizza Crust Original, 1 slice	200	6	23	2	12
Mushroom Pizza Crust Ultra Thin, 1 slice	130	4	15	1	8
Pizza: 14" Large Pizza					
Cheese Hand-tossed, 110 g	290	9	38	2	17
Cheese Original, 111 g	300	9	37	2	18
Cheese Pan, 110 g	290	9	38	2	17
Cheese Thin, 52 g	150	5	14	1	10
Ham & Pineapple Hand-tossed, 115 g	280	7	39	2	15
Ham & Pineapple Original, 116 g	280	7	38	2	17
Ham & Pineapple Pan, 129 g	310	7	46	2	16
• Ham & Pineapple Thin, 55 g	130	4	15	1	9
Pepperoni & Sausage Hand-tossed, 111 g	310	11	38	2	15

RESTAURANTS & FAST-FOOD CHAINS

Peter Piper Pizza (cont.)

	Cal	Fat	Cbs	Fbr	Prtn
Pizza: 14" Large Pizza (cont.)					
Pepperoni & Sausage Original, 112 g	310	11	37	2	17
Pepperoni & Sausage Pan, 125 g	340	11	45	2	16
Pepperoni & Sausage Thin, 53 g	150	7	14	1	9
Pepperoni Hand-tossed, 104 g	290	10	37	2	14
Pepperoni Original, 105 g	300	10	36	2	16
Pepperoni Pan, 118 g	330	10	44	2	15
Pepperoni Thin, 48 g	150	6	13	1	9
Sausage Hand-tossed, 115 g	310	10	39	2	15
Sausage Original, 116 g	310	10	38	2	17
• Sausage Pan, 129 g	340	11	46	3	16
Sausage Thin, 55 g	150	7	14	1	10
Pizza: 14" Large Specialty Pizza					
5 Meat Supreme Hand-tossed, 126 g	350	13	38	2	19
5 Meat Supreme Original, 127 g	350	13	38	2	21
5 Meat Supreme Pan, 140 g	380	13	46	2	20
5 Meat Supreme Thin, 63 g	180	8	14	1	12
California Veggie Hand-tossed, 119 g	270	7	39	2	13
California Veggie Original, 91 g	200	6	23	2	12
California Veggie Pan, 134 g	300	7	47	3	14
• California Veggie Thin, 61 g	130	5	15	1	8
Chicago Classic Hand-tossed, 121 g	300	10	39	2	15
Chicago Classic Original, 121 g	300	10	38	2	17
Chicago Classic Pan, 135 g	340	10	46	3	16
Chicago Classic Thin, 59 g	150	6	15	1	9
NY 3 Chz w/ Pepperoni Hand-tossed, 127 g	380	16	39	2	19
NY 3 Chz w/ Pepperoni Original, 127 g	380	16	38	2	21
• NY 3 Chz w/ Pepperoni Pan, 141 g	410	16	46	2	20
NY 3 Chz w/ Pepperoni Thin, 63 g	200	10	14	1	12
Smoke House Hand-tossed, 129 g	370	15	39	2	21
Smoke House Original, 130 g	370	15	38	2	23
Smoke House Pan, 143 g	400	15	46	2	22
Smoke House Thin, 65 g	200	9	15	1	13
The Werax Hand-tossed, 139 g	310	11	39	2	16
The Werax Original, 140 g	320	11	38	2	17
The Werax Pan, 153 g	350	11	46	2	16
The Werax Thin, 71 g	160	7	14	1	10
Pizza: 16" Extra Large Pizza					
Cheese Hand-tossed, 98 g	260	8	33	1	15
Cheese Original, 98 g	260	8	32	1	17
Cheese Pan, 107 g	290	8	38	2	16
Cheese Thin, 51 g	140	5	13	1	10
Ham & Pineapple Hand-tossed, 103 g	250	6	35	1	13
Ham & Pineapple Original, 103 g	250	6	33	1	14
Ham & Pineapple Pan, 112 g	270	6	39	2	14
• Ham & Pineapple Thin, 55 g	130	4	14	1	9
Pepperoni & Sausage Hand-tossed, 99 g	280	10	33	2	14
Pepperoni & Sausage Original, 99 g	280	10	32	2	15
Pepperoni & Sausage Pan, 109 g	300	10	38	2	14
Pepperoni & Sausage Thin, 52 g	150	7	13	1	9
Pepperoni Hand-tossed, 92 g	260	8	33	1	13
Pepperoni Original, 92 g	260	8	32	1	14
Pepperoni Pan, 101 g	280	9	37	2	13
Pepperoni Thin, 47 g	140	6	13	1	9

(• = most healthy • = least healthy) **RESTAURANTS & FAST-FOOD • 273**

RESTAURANTS & FAST-FOOD CHAINS

Peter Piper Pizza (cont.)

	Cal	Fat	Cbs	Fbr	Prtn
Pizza: 16" Extra Large Pizza (cont.)					
Sausage Hand-tossed, 104 g	280	10	34	2	14
Sausage Original, 104 g	280	10	33	2	16
• Sausage Pan, 113 g	300	10	39	2	15
Sausage Thin, 56 g	150	7	14	1	10
Pizza: 16" Extra Large Specialty Pizza					
5 Meat Supreme Hand-tossed, 115 g	320	13	34	2	18
5 Meat Supreme Original, 115 g	320	13	33	2	20
5 Meat Supreme Pan, 125 g	340	13	39	2	19
5 Meat Supreme Thin, 64 g	190	9	14	1	13
California Veggie Hand-tossed, 106 g	240	6	34	2	12
California Veggie Original, 106 g	240	6	33	2	13
California Veggie Pan, 115 g	260	6	39	2	12
• California Veggie Thin, 57 g	130	4	14	1	8
Chicago Classic Hand-tossed, 111 g	270	9	34	2	14
Chicago Classic Original, 111 g	270	9	33	2	15
Chicago Classic Pan, 120 g	290	9	39	2	14
Chicago Classic Thin, 61 g	150	6	14	1	9
New York 3 Cheese with Pepperoni Hand-tossed, 113 g	340	14	34	2	17
New York 3 Cheese with Pepperoni Original, 112 g	340	14	32	1	19
• New York 3 Cheese with Pepperoni Pan, 122 g	360	15	39	2	18
New York 3 Cheese with Pepperoni Thin, 62 g	200	10	14	1	12
Smoke House Hand-tossed, 116 g	340	13	34	2	19
Smoke House Original, 116 g	340	13	33	2	21
Smoke House Pan, 126 g	360	14	39	2	20
Smoke House Thin, 65 g	200	10	14	1	14
The Werax Hand-tossed, 128 g	280	10	34	2	14
The Werax Original, 128 g	290	10	33	2	16
The Werax Pan, 137 g	310	10	39	2	15
The Werax Thin, 74 g	160	7	14	1	10
Salads					
Chicken Caesar, 229 g	200	8	10	4	21
• Family, 371 g	290	16	14	2	24
Garden, 250 g	50	0	10	2	3
Italian Chef, 114 g	20	0	4	0	1
• Side, 145 g	20	0	4	1	2

Petro's

	Cal	Fat	Cbs	Fbr	Prtn
Chili: Large					
• Chicken	375	6	58	N/A	24
Original	504	19	57	N/A	28
• Veggie	525	15	79	N/A	19
Chili: Medium					
• Chicken	275	4	43	N/A	18
Original	370	14	42	N/A	21
• Veggie	385	11	58	N/A	14
Chili: Small					
• Chicken	175	3	27	N/A	11
Original	235	9	26	N/A	13
• Veggie	245	7	37	N/A	9
Large Petro®					
• Chicken	969	52	88	5	39
Original	1073	60	87	5	42
• Veggie	1089	60	105	5	35

RESTAURANTS & FAST-FOOD CHAINS

Petro's (cont.)

	Cal	Fat	Cbs	Fbr	Prtn
Lite Pasta Petro®					
Large	678	5	108	9	52
Medium	494	4	80	7	33
Small	333	2	53	5	25
Lite Petro®					
Large	787	24	99	4	42
Medium	532	16	66	3	30
Small	382	12	48	2	21
Medium Petro®					
Chicken	665	36	59	3	27
Original	734	43	58	3	29
Veggie	745	41	70	3	24
Miscellaneous: Baked Potatoes					
#1 Lite	363	0	74	7	18
#2 Butter Sour Cream	482	18	74	8	8
#3 Loaded	679	33	78	9	21
#4 Loaded w/ Chili	780	37	90	9	26
#5 Broccoli 3 Cheese	657	30	77	9	21
Miscellaneous: Hot Dogs					
Chili	315	17	28	2	11
Chili/cheese	347	19	29	2	14
Loaded	352	19	30	2	14
Plain	266	14	22	0	9
Slaw	352	16	23	0	9
Pasta Petro®					
Large	848	37	91	9	40
Medium	627	27	68	10	30
Small	406	17	46	6	20
Pee Wee Petro®					
Chicken	259	14	23	1	11
Original	284	16	22	1	12
Veggie	289	16	27	1	10
Salads: Garden Salads					
Large	86	1	16	7	7
Small	43	1	8	4	3
Salads: Petro Salads					
Grilled Chicken	742	41	42	8	54
Original	570	36	42	2	25
Small Petro®					
Chicken	464	24	43	2	19
Original	516	30	43	2	21
Veggie	524	28	52	2	17

Philly Connection

	Cal	Fat	Cbs	Fbr	Prtn
Original Cheesesteak Sandwich					
Regular, 10"	623	15	73	3	48
Small, 7"	455	11	55	2	35

Piccadilly

	Cal	Fat	Cbs	Fbr	Prtn
Low Carb Items					
Au Jus, 3 fl.oz.	6	0	1	0	0
Beans, Green, Fresh, 5 oz.	136	11	8	4	3
Beef, Chopped Steak, Fried Jumbo, 8 oz.	737	59	11	0	34
Beef, Chopped Steak, Fried Regular, 5 oz.	414	33	6	0	19

(• = most healthy • = least healthy) **RESTAURANTS & FAST-FOOD • 275**

RESTAURANTS & FAST-FOOD CHAINS

▶ Piccadilly (cont.)

	Cal	Fat	Cbs	Fbr	Prtn
Low Carb Items (cont.)					
Beef, Roast Leg (Small), 4 oz.	352	22	2	1	35
Beef, Steak, Filet Mignon, 6 oz.	341	20	1	0	36
Beef, Steak, New Your Strip, 10 oz.	876	71	1	0	55
Beef, Steak, Ribeye or Sirloin Strip, 7 oz.	673	58	1	0	35
Beef, Steak, Ribeye, 10 oz.	1042	91	2	1	50
• Beef, Steak, Ribeye, 14 oz.	1353	116	2	1	70
Broccoli w/Cheese Sauce, full portion	106	7	9	3	3
Broccoli, Fresh Florets, 4 oz.	90	7	5	3	3
Brussel Sprouts, Buttered, full portion	91	6	8	4	3
Cabbage, Bacon Seasoned, Steamed, full portion	106	8	6	2	2
Cabbage, Buttered, Steamed, full portion	68	5	6	2	1
Cauliflower, Buttered, full portion	89	6	8	4	3
Cheese Sauce, 2 fl.oz.	35	1	5	0	1
Chicken Breast, Mesquite Smoke	212	8	1	1	34
Chicken Breast, Mesquite w BBQ sauce	240	9	6	0	35
Chicken, Baked (Quarters)	849	61	6	1	64
Chicken, Baked Cajun, Boneless Breast	431	27	9	1	35
Chicken, Baked Italian, Boneless Breast	548	41	8	1	35
Chicken, Barbecued (Quarters)	796	53	12	1	64
Chicken, Rotisserie- Herb Style (Dark), 1 quarter	827	65	12	1	48
Chicken, Rotisserie- Herb Style (Half), 1 half	1179	75	4	1	123
Chicken, Rotisserie- Herb Style (White), 1 quarter	521	31	2	1	65
Chicken, SW Chicken Breast, full portion	522	35	9	1	45
Cottage Cheese, Creamed, 4 oz.	117	5	3	0	14
Cucumbers and Sour Cream, 5 oz.	86	6	6	1	2
Fish, Basa, Blackened	408	32	2	1	26
Fish, Basa, Cajun Baked	263	15	4	1	27
Fish, Basa, Stuffed	438	30	9	1	32
Fish, Catfish Filet, Blackened	523	43	2	1	29
Fish, Catfish Filet, Stuffed	552	40	9	1	35
Fish, Catfish, Cajun Baked, full portion	404	28	6	1	30
Fish, Grouper Filet, Baked, 6 oz.	305	9	8	1	46
Fish, Tilapia, Cajun Baked, full portion	267	19	7	2	18
Fish, Trout Filets, Baked, full portion	464	19	10	1	59
Fish, Trout, Almondine, Baked, full portion	490	22	11	1	60
Gelatin, Plain Sugar- Free, full portion	58	0	1	0	10
Greens, Collard, Mustard, Turnip, 3 oz.	135	10	3	2	4
Greens, Turnip w/Diced Turnips, 3 oz.	150	12	4	2	4
Gumbo, Chicken (no rice), 10 oz.	98	2	11	1	8
Gumbo, Chicken and Sausage (no rice), 10 oz.	224	15	10	1	12
Okra, Creole, full portion	79	4	9	3	2
Peas, Sugar Snap, Mixed, 5 oz.	102	5	10	3	3
Pork Loin, Bone In, Roast, 5 oz.	373	13	10	1	49
Salad Dressing, Blue Cheese, 2 tbsp	160	18	1	0	1
Salad Dressing, French, 2 tbsp	130	13	5	0	0
Salad Dressing, Italian, 2 tbsp	160	17	1	0	0
Salad Dressing, Ranch, 2 tbsp	150	17	1	0	1
Salad Dressing, Ranch, Fat Free, 2 tbsp	36	0	7	1	1
Salad Dressing, Thousand Island, 2 tbsp	170	18	2	0	0
Salad, Asparagus and Tomato, full portion	88	5	10	2	2
Salad, Caesar, 3 oz.	143	11	7	1	5
Salad, Cauliflower, Fresh, 4 oz.	117	8	9	2	4
Salad, Chef's (Small), 6 oz.	143	9	4	1	13

RESTAURANTS & FAST-FOOD CHAINS

Piccadilly (cont.)

	Cal	Fat	Cbs	Fbr	Prtn
Low Carb Items (cont.)					
Salad, Coleslaw, Italian, 4 oz.	163	16	5	2	1
Salad, Coleslaw, Kosher Style, 4 oz.	143	13	7	2	1
Salad, Combination, 4 oz.	73	5	5	1	2
Salad, Cucumber and Celery, 4 oz.	74	4	9	1	1
Salad, Cucumber and Tomato, 4 oz.	41	0	10	1	1
Salad, Cucumber Mix, 6 oz.	61	4	7	2	1
Salad, Louisianne Bowl, full portion	44	3	2	1	4
Salad, Mexican, 4 oz.	58	3	8	1	1
Salad, Piccadilly Bowl, full portion	27	0	6	2	1
Salad, Spring Salad Bowl (Small), 3 oz.	15	0	3	1	1
Salad, Tomato, Cucumber and Onion, 4 oz.	44	0	10	2	1
Salad, Veggie Combination w/Cherry Tom, full portion	68	4	9	2	1
Spinach, Buttered, or Bacon Seasoned, 4 oz.	80	6	3	3	3
Turkey Breast, Carved, 6 oz.	267	10	5	0	37
Vegetables, Mixed, 4 oz.	137	7	17	4	4
Popular Items					
Beans, Green, Fresh, 5 oz.	136	11	8	4	3
Beef, Roast, 6 oz.	481	30	3	1	48
Blueberry Pie, Sugar-Free, 1 slice	314	17	42	3	5
Broccoli, Fresh Florets, 4 oz.	90	7	5	3	3
Cherry Pie, Sugar-Free, 1 slice	334	17	45	1	5
Chicken, Grilled Breast, 6 oz.	478	26	23	1	36
• Chocolate Almond Pie, Sugar Free, 1 slice	612	44	49	2	5
Corn, Fresh, 4 oz.	125	6	18	1	3
Fish, Tilapia, Baked, full portion	210	11	10	1	17
Okra, Fried, 3 oz.	242	13	26	4	4
Pork Loin, Marinated Boneless, 6 oz.	365	24	1	0	34
Rolls, White, Parker House, 1 each	147	5	22	1	3
Rolls, Whole Wheat, 1 each	231	8	37	5	6
Salad Dressing, Ranch, Fat-Free, 2 tbsp.	36	0	7	1	1
Salad, Piccadilly Fruit, 6 oz.	78	0	20	3	1
Salad, Shrimp Remoulade, 12 oz.	516	28	33	5	31
• Salad, Spring Bowl, 3 oz.	15	0	3	1	1
Shrimp, Fried, full portion	462	19	34	2	36

Pizza Hut

	Cal	Fat	Cbs	Fbr	Prtn
Appetizers					
Breadsticks, 1 bread	150	6	20	1	4
Cheese Breadsticks, 1 bread	200	10	21	1	7
Hot Wings, 2 pieces	120	7	1	0	11
Mild Wings, 2 pieces	110	7	2	0	11
• Wing Blue Cheese Dipping Sauce, 2 oz.	220	23	3	0	1
Wing Ranch Dipping Sauce, 2 oz.	220	23	3	0	1
Desserts					
Apple Dessert Pizza, 101 g	260	5	52	1	4
Cherry Dessert Pizza, 101 g	260	5	47	1	4
• Cinnamon Sticks, 55 g	170	5	27	1	4
White Icing Dipping Cup, 2 oz.	190	0	47	0	0
Dressings & Dipping Sauces					
• Breadstick Dipping Sauce, 3 oz.	40	0	8	2	1
French Dressing, 30 g	150	13	9	0	0
Italian Dressing, 30 g	140	15	2	0	0
Lite Italian Dressing, 30 g	70	5	5	0	0

RESTAURANTS & FAST-FOOD CHAINS

Pizza Hut (cont.)	Cal	Fat	Cbs	Fbr	Prtn
Dressings & Dipping Sauces (cont.)					
Lite Ranch Dressing, 30 g	60	6	1	0	0
Ranch Dressing, 30 g	100	10	2	0	1
Thousand Island Dressing, 30 g	120	11	5	0	0
Pizza: 12" Medium Hand-Tossed Style Pizzas					
Cheese Only, 98 g	230	10	25	1	12
Italian Sausage & Red Onion, 114 g	260	12	26	1	12
• Meat Lover's, 129 g	340	19	25	1	17
Pepperoni & Mushroom, 104 g	230	9	25	1	11
Pepperoni, 96 g	240	11	24	1	12
Quartered Ham & Pineapple, 104 g	220	8	26	1	10
Supreme, 122 g	270	13	26	2	13
• Veggie Lover's®, 115 g	210	8	26	2	10
Pizza: 12" Medium Pan Pizzas					
Cheese Only, 104 g	270	13	27	1	11
Italian Sausage & Red Onion, 119 g	300	15	28	1	12
• Meat Lover's®, 135 g	370	22	28	2	17
Pepperoni & Mushroom, 109 g	260	13	27	1	11
Pepperoni, 102 g	280	14	27	1	12
Quartered Ham & Pineapple, 109 g	250	11	28	1	10
Supreme, 127 g	310	16	28	2	13
• Veggie Lover's®, 119 g	250	11	28	2	10
Pizza: 12" Medium Thin 'N Crispy Pizzas					
Cheese Only, 79 g	200	8	21	1	10
Italian Sausage & Red Onion, 97 g	230	11	23	1	10
• Meat Lover's®, 111 g	310	18	22	1	15
Pepperoni & Mushroom, 87 g	190	8	21	1	9
Pepperoni, 77 g	210	10	21	1	10
• Quartered Ham & Pineapple, 87 g	180	6	23	1	9
Supreme, 106 g	230	11	22	1	11
Veggie Lover's®, 101 g	180	7	23	1	8
Pizza: 14" Large Hand-Tossed Style Pizzas					
Cheese Only, 142 g	340	14	36	2	17
Italian Sausage & Red Onion, 163 g	370	17	38	2	17
• Meat Lover's®, 187 g	490	27	37	2	24
Pepperoni & Mushroom, 149 g	330	14	36	2	16
Pepperoni, 140 g	360	16	35	2	17
• Quartered Ham & Pineapple, 150 g	310	11	38	2	15
Supreme, 174 g	390	18	37	2	19
Veggie Lover's®, 163 g	310	12	37	2	14
Pizza: 14" Large Pan Pizza					
Cheese Only, 146 g	390	19	38	2	16
Italian Sausage & Red Onion, 165 g	420	22	39	2	17
• Meat Lover's®, 190 g	530	31	39	2	23
Pepperoni & Mushroom, 151 g	380	18	37	2	15
Pepperoni, 143 g	400	21	37	2	16
Quartered Ham & Pineapple, 152 g	360	16	39	2	15
Supreme, 176 g	440	23	39	2	18
• Veggie Lover's®, 163 g	350	16	39	2	14
Pizza: 14" Large Stuffed Crust Pizzas					
Cheese Only, 150 g	360	16	37	2	18
Italian Sausage & Red Onion, 174 g	410	20	39	2	19
• Meat Lover's®, 199 g	520	29	38	2	26
Pepperoni & Mushroom, 160 g	360	16	37	2	18

RESTAURANTS & FAST-FOOD CHAINS

Pizza Hut (cont.)	Cal	Fat	Cbs	Fbr	Prtn
Pizza: 14" Large Stuffed Crust Pizzas (cont.)					
Pepperoni, 152 g	390	19	37	2	19
Quartered Ham & Pineapple, 161 g	350	14	39	2	17
Supreme, 185 g	420	21	39	2	21
• Veggie Lover's®, 173 g	340	14	38	2	16
Pizza: 14" Large Thin N' Crispy Pizza					
Cheese Only, 111 g	280	12	30	1	14
Italian Sausage & Red Onion, 136 g	320	15	32	2	14
• Meat Lover's®, 157 g	430	25	31	2	21
Pepperoni & Mushroom, 122 g	270	12	30	1	13
Pepperoni, 109 g	300	14	29	1	14
Quartered Ham & Pineapple, 123 g	260	9	32	1	12
Supreme, 148 g	330	16	31	2	16
Veggie Lover's®, 141 g	260	10	31	2	12
Pizza: 6" Personal Pan Pizzas					
Cheese Only, 249 g	620	26	69	3	28
Italian Sausage & Red Onion, 286 g	690	33	71	4	29
• Meat Lover's®, 333 g	890	49	70	4	41
Pepperoni & Mushroom, 256 g	600	25	68	3	26
Pepperoni, 245 g	640	29	67	3	28
Quartered Ham & Pineapple, 258 g	570	21	70	3	25
Supreme, 303 g	710	34	70	4	32
• Veggie Lover's®, 275 g	560	22	70	4	24
Pizza: XL Full House Pizza™					
Cheese Only, 114 g	280	12	30	2	12
Italian Sausage & Red Onion, 130 g	300	14	32	2	12
• Meat Lover's®, 143 g	370	20	31	2	17
Pepperoni & Mushroom, 121 g	270	11	30	2	11
Pepperoni, 111 g	280	13	30	2	12
Quartered Ham & Pineapple, 121 g	260	10	32	2	11
Supreme, 139 g	310	14	31	2	13
Veggie Lover's®, 135 g	260	10	31	2	10

Pizza Pizza	Cal	Fat	Cbs	Fbr	Prtn
Classic Pizza					
Beacon Double Cheeseburger, 97 g	220	7	29	1	11
Big Bacon Bonanza, 93 g	220	7	29	1	10
Canadian Eh!, 112 g	230	7	30	2	11
Cheese, 89 g	200	5	29	1	9
Classic Super, 110 g	210	6	30	2	10
• Deep Dish Pepperoni, 129 g	330	11	45	2	14
Garden Veggie, 111 g	190	5	30	2	8
New York Pepperoni, 92 g	230	8	29	2	10
Pepperoni & Mushroom, 105 g	210	6	30	2	10
Pepperoni, 93 g	210	6	29	1	10
Silican, 108 g	240	9	30	1	10
Spicy BBQ Chicken, 104 g	200	5	30	2	10
Tropical Hawaiian, 100 g	220	7	30	1	10
Signature Pizza					
Bacon Chicken Mushroom Melt, 112 g	270	12	29	1	12
Chicken Bruschetta Parm, 94 g	180	6	22	1	10
Chicken Mango, 115 g	220	7	30	3	11
Garden Riviera, 107 g	220	6	31	2	9
• Meat Supreme, 120 g	290	13	30	1	14

(•= most healthy •= least healthy) **RESTAURANTS & FAST-FOOD • 279**

RESTAURANTS & FAST-FOOD CHAINS

Pizza Pizza (cont.)

	Cal	Fat	Cbs	Fbr	Prtn
Signature Pizza (cont.)					
Mediterranean Vegetarian, 125 g	210	6	31	2	9
Napa Valley, 86 g	200	8	22	1	10
Pesto Amore, 76 g	170	7	19	2	8
Philly Cheese Steak, 116 g	230	6	31	2	12
• Sweet Chili Chicken, 91 g	170	5	26	2	9
Trio Pomodoro, 91 g	180	6	22	1	8

Planet Smoothie

	Cal	Fat	Cbs	Fbr	Prtn
Smoothies					
2 Piece Bikini-Chocolate™, 22 oz.	321	1	80	4	5
2 Piece Bikini-Strawberry™, 22 oz.	286	1	72	4	4
Acai (Ah-SIGH-ee), 22 oz.	510	6	118	11	3
Berry Bada-Bing™, 22 oz.	362	0	88	5	9
Big Bang™, 22 oz.	347	1	80	5	14
Billy Bob Banana™, 22 oz.	312	1	78	5	4
• Captain Kid (12 oz)™, 22 oz.	194	2	47	2	1
Chocolate Chimp™, 22 oz.	400	1	93	4	15
Chocolate Elvis™, 22 oz.	522	9	109	5	13
Frozen Goat™, 22 oz.	358	1	85	2	8
Grape Ape™, 22 oz.	304	1	78	2	1
Hangover Over™, 22 oz.	312	1	78	4	6
Leapin' Lizard™, 22 oz.	209	0	55	3	1
Lunar Lemonade Raspberry™, 22 oz.	375	1	97	4	2
Lunar Lemonade™, 22 oz.	378	1	98	4	2
Mediterranean Monster™, 22 oz.	310	1	80	4	2
Merlin's Pineapple LB™, 22 oz.	413	2	57	2	46
Merlin's Pineapple Myoplex™, 22 oz.	392	2	53	2	43
Merlin's Strawberry LB™, 22 oz.	484	2	78	4	46
Merlin's Strawberry Myoplex™, 22 oz.	463	2	74	4	43
Mr. Mongo-Chocolate™, 22 oz.	516	1	117	4	21
Mr. Mongo-Strawberry, 22 oz.	421	1	92	4	19
• PBJ™, 22 oz.	560	17	97	6	15
Rasmanian Devil™, 22 oz.	265	1	66	6	3
Road Runner™, 22 oz.	279	1	72	6	2
Screamsicle™, 22 oz.	365	2	86	3	6
Shag-a-delic™, 22 oz.	430	1	104	5	7
Spazz™, 22 oz.	266	1	68	4	3
The Last Mango™, 22 oz.	354	3	83	4	3
Thelma & Louise™, 22 oz.	226	0	59	3	1
Twig & Berries™, 22 oz.	297	1	74	4	6
Vinnie del Rocco™, 22 oz.	385	4	92	6	3
Werewolf™, 22 oz.	261	1	67	4	3
Yo' Adriane™, 22 oz.	263	0	65	3	6
Zeus Juice™, 22 oz.	248	1	65	4	1

Pollo Tropical

	Cal	Fat	Cbs	Fbr	Prtn
Chicken					
• 1/4 Chicken dark meat w/o skin, 3 oz.	191	10	0	0	25
1/4 Chicken dark meat, 4 oz.	291	18	0	0	32
1/4 Chicken white meat w/o skin, 4 oz.	204	6	0	0	36
• 1/4 Chicken white meat, 6 oz.	323	16	0	0	43
Boneless Chicken Breast, 6 oz.	241	3	0	0	52

▶ Pollo Tropical (cont.)

	Cal	Fat	Cbs	Fbr	Prtn
Condiments					
BBQ Sauce, 2 oz.	83	0	20	0	0
Caesar Dressing, 1 oz.	161	17	1	0	2
• Extra dressing is 1.75 oz, 2 oz.	281	30	2	0	3
Guacamole Sauce, 2 oz.	75	6	3	3	0
Guava BBQ Sauce, 2 oz.	83	0	22	0	0
Mojo Sauce, 1 oz.	97	9	3	0	0
Mustard Curry Sauce, 2 oz.	265	30	0	0	0
• Salsa, 2 oz.	8	0	2	0	0
Desserts					
Flan, 5 oz.	390	13	59	1	9
• Key Lime, 4 oz.	210	9	25	0	8
• Tres Leches (Caribbean Cream Cake), 5 oz.	410	9	76	0	9
Ribs					
¼ Rack Ribs, 2 oz.	200	15	1	0	14
½ Rack Ribs, 4 oz.	400	31	2	0	28
Roast Pork					
Roast Pork, 6 oz.	392	23	0	0	48
Salads					
Chicken Caesar Salad, 14,45 oz.	669	41	3	58	
Sandwiches					
• Chicken Caesar Sandwich, 13 oz.	881	34	71	5	70
Grilled Chicken Sandwich, 15 oz.	827	24	84	6	65
• Roast Pork Sandwich, 12 oz.	773	26	83	5	53
Shrimp					
Shrimp Skewer (One Skewer), 108 oz.	1	1	0	0	24
Sides					
• Balsamic Tomato, Combo Side, 4 oz.	88	1	7	1	1
Balsamic Tomato, Small Side, 8 oz.	176	2	14	2	2
Black Beans, Combo Side, 4 oz.	90	3	18	7	6
Black Beans, Small Side, 9 oz.	203	6	41	16	14
Black Beans/White Rice Combo side, 9 oz.	294	6	58	8	9
• Black Beans/White Rice Value side, 13 oz.	458	9	90	11	14
Boiled Yuca Combo Side, 8 oz.	188	0	51	4	0
Boiled Yuca Small Side, 10 oz.	251	0	68	5	0
Caesar Salad, Combo Side, 3 oz.	130	11	4	1	3
Caesar Salad, Small Side, 4 oz.	207	18	6	1	4
Caribbean Chicken Soup, Large Bowl, 16 oz.	237	3	40	5	17
Caribbean Chicken Soup, Small Bowl, 8 oz.	121	2	21	3	9
Corn, Combo Side, 4 oz.	121	4	19	5	3
Corn, Small Side, 8 oz.	225	8	37	10	6
French Fries, Combo Side, 4 oz.	311	15	40	4	4
French Fries, Small Side, 4 oz.	311	15	40	4	4
Tropical Shrimp Soup, Large Bowl, 16 oz.	280	5	38	0	20
Tropical Shrimp Soup, Small Bowl, 8 oz.	134	3	18	0	10
White Rice, Combo Side, 5 oz.	203	3	40	1	3
White Rice, Small Side, 8 oz.	339	6	66	2	6
Yellow Rice w/Veg, Combo Side, 5 oz.	163	3	31	1	4
Yellow Rice w/Veg, Small Side, 8 oz.	245	4	47	2	6
Steaks					
Beef skewers / Two Per Serving, 4 oz.	289	19	4	0	26
• Beef skewers, 1 oz.	77	5	1	0	7
• Steak & Chicken (dark meat), 6 oz.	437	28	2	0	46
Steak & Shrimp, 255 oz.	330	11	2	0	37

(• = most healthy • = least healthy)

RESTAURANTS & FAST-FOOD CHAINS

Pollo Tropical (cont.)

	Cal	Fat	Cbs	Fbr	Prtn
Tropical Favorites					
Bananas Tropical®, 7 oz.	437	11	89	9	4
Yucatan Fries®, 6 oz.	497	24	69	3	2
Tropichops®					
• Chkn w/ Yellow Rice & Veggies, 10 oz.	341	5	50	2	23
Chkn w/ Yellow Rice & Veggies, 23 oz.	864	21	93	4	74
Grilled Chicken Deluxe, 13 oz.	409	6	52	3	37
Grilled Chicken Deluxe, 25 oz.	753	11	91	5	72
Pork w/ White Rice & Black Beans, 20 oz.	714	23	97	12	38
• Pork w/ White Rice & Black Beans, 31 oz.	1273	50	147	18	71
Pork w/ Yellow Rice & Vegetables, 12 oz.	480	21	91	5	35
Pork w/ Yellow Rice & Vegetables, 30 oz.	1020	43	96	6	62
Ropa Vieja (shredded beef), 19 oz.	618	17	98	13	28
Ropa Vieja (shredded beef), 33 oz.	1160	41	161	20	51
Shrimp Creole TropiChop MAX, 26 oz.	1002	29	129	7	54
Shrimp Creole TropiChop, 14 oz.	506	11	75	3	27
Vegetarian TropiChop Max®, 31 oz.	950	21	177	26	26
Vegetarian TropiChop®, 19 oz.	580	13	109	16	17
Wraps					
Chx Caesar Wrap, 13 oz.	901	48	64	4	49
• Chx Classic Wrap, 13 oz.	694	26	68	5	43
Curry Chx Wrap, 14 oz.	930	43	94	6	40
• Steak Wrap, 15 oz.	993	48	106	6	32

Popeye's Chicken and Biscuits

	Cal	Fat	Cbs	Fbr	Prtn
Cajun Wings					
Cajun Wing segments, 244 g	595	43	19	0	34
Louisiana Legends					
• Chicken & Sausage Jambalaya, 453 g	660	33	60	3	30
• Chicken Etouffee, 453 g	480	30	18	6	36
Crawfish Etouffee, 453 g	540	15	75	6	21
Smothered Chicken, 453 g	630	24	72	3	30
Mild Chicken					
• Breast, 179 g	350	20	8	0	33
• Leg, 63 g	110	7	3	0	11
Strips, 116 g	250	10	16	1	22
Thigh, 111 g	280	20	7	0	16
Wing, 59 g	150	10	5	0	9
Mild Chicken (Skinless and Breading Removed)					
Breast, 123 g	120	2	0	0	24
Leg, 52 g	50	2	0	0	9
• Strips, 94 g	130	3	3	0	25
Thigh, 72 g	80	4	0	0	11
• Wing, 42 g	40	2	0	1	7
Sandwiches					
Deluxe w/ Mayo, 265 g	630	31	53	3	35
Deluxe w/o Mayo, 237 g	480	15	54	3	33
Seafood					
Popcorn Shrimp, 85 g	280	16	22	1	12
Sides					
Biscuits, 60 g	240	13	26	1	4
Cajun Rice, 117 g	170	6	22	2	8
Chicken Etouffee, 151 g	160	10	6	2	12
Cinnamon Apple Turnover, 86 g	250	12	34	2	3

RESTAURANTS & FAST-FOOD CHAINS

Popeye's Chicken and Biscuits (cont.)	Cal	Fat	Cbs	Fbr	Prtn
Sides (cont.)					
Coleslaw, 138 g	260	23	14	9	1
Corn on the Cob, 284 g	190	2	37	4	6
Crawfish Etouffee, 151 g	180	5	25	2	7
French Fries, 88 g	310	17	35	3	4
• Green Beans, 100 g	70	1	14	2	2
Jambalaya, 151 g	220	11	20	1	10
Mashed Potatoes w/ Gravy, 142 g	130	4	18	2	3
Mashed Potatoes w/o Gravy, 113 g	100	3	17	1	1
• Red Beans & Rice, 174 g	320	19	31	17	10
Smothered Chicken, 151 g	210	8	24	1	10
Spicy Chicken					
• Breast, 179 g	360	22	8	1	31
Leg, 63 g	100	5	3	0	9
Strips, 116 g	270	11	21	1	22
Thigh, 111 g	300	24	7	0	15
Wing, 59 g	140	9	5	0	9
Spicy Chicken (Skinless and Breading Removed)					
Breast, 123 g	120	2	1	1	25
Leg, 52 g	50	2	0	0	9
• Strips, 94 g	150	4	5	0	23
Thigh, 72 g	80	3	2	0	12
• Wing, 42 g	40	2	0	1	6

Port of Subs	Cal	Fat	Cbs	Fbr	Prtn
Brownies					
Brownies, 5 oz.	300	10	48	1	4
Cold Submarine Sandwiches					
Bacon Lettuce & Tomato, 8 oz.	519	30	43	3	20
• Ham American, 10 oz.	382	20	45	3	29
• Ham Salami Capicolla Pepperoni Provolone, 10 oz.	532	26	45	3	28
Ham Salami Provolone, 9 oz.	469	21	45	3	24
Ham Turkey Provolone, 10 oz.	434	15	46	3	26
Peppered Pastrami Swiss, 9 oz.	439	17	44	3	21
Peppered Pastrami Turkey Swiss, 8 oz.	511	26	44	3	23
Roast Beef Provolone, 10 oz.	421	14	43	3	27
Roast Beef Turkey Provolone, 10 oz.	421	14	45	3	26
Roasted Chicken Breast Provolone, 10 oz.	410	13	45	3	28
Salami Pepperoni Provolone, 8 oz.	511	27	45	3	26
Salami Provolone, 8 oz.	479	25	45	3	23
Salami Turkey Provolone, 9 oz.	465	20	46	3	23
Smoked Ham Swiss, 10 oz.	447	17	45	3	23
Smoked Ham Turkey Cheddar, 10 oz.	431	15	47	3	25
Tuna (w/o cheese), 9 oz.	422	18	45	3	19
Turkey Provolone, 11 oz.	421	14	47	3	25
Fresh Salads					
Caesar Salad, 6 oz.	333	30	7	2	3
Chef Salad, 11 oz.	388	25	13	2	26
• Garden Salad, 8 oz.	93	5	10	2	2
Grilled Chicken Caesar Salad, 13 oz.	541	34	15	5	37
Grilled Chicken Salad, 13 oz.	300	10	16	3	36
Macaroni Salad, 8 oz.	440	30	36	3	7
Potato Salad, 8 oz.	360	26	54	6	4
Tuna Salad, 11 oz.	311	23	12	2	16

(•= most healthy •= least healthy) **RESTAURANTS & FAST-FOOD • 283**

RESTAURANTS & FAST-FOOD CHAINS

Port of Subs (cont.)

	Cal	Fat	Cbs	Fbr	Prtn
Hot Sandwiches					
• Grilled Chicken, 9 oz.	563	11	68	3	43
• Hot Pastrami, 9 oz.	758	17	62	3	42
Meatball, 9 oz.	653	25	76	4	29
Kid's Meal Sandwich					
Ham, 3 oz.	200	3	4	1	10
• Salami, 3 oz.	254	9	4	1	9
• Turkey, 3 oz.	190	3	4	1	8
Sandwiches					
• Ham Turkey, 10 oz.	328	5	46	3	22
Peppered Pastrami, 8 oz.	293	4	44	3	16
Roast Beef Turkey, 9 oz.	315	4	45	3	22
Roast Beef, 9 oz.	315	4	43	3	23
Roasted Chicken Breast, 9 oz.	304	3	44	3	24
Smoked Ham Turkey, 10 oz.	320	5	46	3	21
Smoked Ham, 8 oz.	301	4	44	3	18
Turkey, 10 oz.	315	4	47	3	21
• Vegetarian (w/o cheese), 7 oz.	238	2	44	4	7
Soup - Medium					
Boston Clam Chowder, 6 oz.	105	4	13	1	4
• Broccoli Cheese, 6 oz.	120	6	13	2	5
• Minestrone, 6 oz.	53	1	8	2	2
Roasted Chicken Noodle, 6 oz.	83	2	9	1	7
Wraps					
Chicken Caesar, 11 oz.	762	35	63	3	42
• Hot Grilled Chkn Smokey Cheddar, 11 oz.	661	23	63	3	47
Tortilla Only, 4 oz.	330	8	55	2	7
• Turkey & Bacon Ranch, 12 oz.	785	44	190	2	33

Pret a Manger

	Cal	Fat	Cbs	Fbr	Prtn
Bagels					
Cinnamon Bagel, 113 g	300	0	64	2	12
with Cream Cheese, 142 g	390	9	65	2	14
• Plain Bagel, 113 g	300	0	0	0	12
• with Cream Cheese, 160 g	460	16	65	0	15
Sesame Bagel, 113 g	300	8	64	0	12
with Cream Cheese, 142 g	390	17	65	0	14
Baguettes					
All Natural Smoked Ham & Swiss, 625 g	620	16	66	3	35
Bell & Evans Chicken & Mozzarella, 344 g	580	19	72	4	32
Cream Chz, Tomato & Basil Brkfst, 176 g	390	19	45	2	12
Just Made French Brie & Basil, 280 g	560	23	66	3	24
Organic Egg & Bacon Brkfst, 146 g	410	18	42	2	17
Organic Egg & Tomato Brkfst, 153 g	340	12	43	2	13
Pret's Classic Tuna Salad, 295 g	580	20	67	3	31
• Slow-Roast Beef, Arugula & Parmegiano, 245 g	670	13	65	3	41
Chips & Popcorn					
Cracked Pepper Potato Chips, 1 oz.	150	9	16	2	2
Lightly Salted Potato Chips, 1 oz.	150	9	15	2	2
• New York Cheddar Potato Chips, 28 g	180	9	15	1	2
• Pret's Organic Popcorn, 32 g	131	6	19	1	3
Salt & Vinegar Potato Chips, 1 oz.	150	9	16	1	2
Spicy Thai Potato Chips., 28 g	150	9	15	1	2
Yogurt & Green Onion Potato Chips, 28 g	150	9	15	1	2

RESTAURANTS & FAST-FOOD CHAINS

◗ Pret a Manger (cont.)

	Cal	Fat	Cbs	Fbr	Prtn
Cookies, Cakes & Treats					
Banana Cake, 128 g	420	24	48	1	4
Carrot Cake, 128 g	460	29	47	1	5
Chocolate Brownie, 96 g	390	20	51	3	3
Chocolate Cake, 128 g	470	19	71	2	6
Chocolate Chunk Cookie, 71 g	310	16	43	2	3
Fruit & Oat Slice, 96 g	410	18	55	5	7
Harvest Cookie, 43 g	180	8	24	2	3
Love Bar, 105 g	460	25	54	4	8
• Mini Brownie, 45 g	180	9	24	1	1
• Pecan Pie, 128 g	510	27	63	2	6
Raspberry Bar, 104 g	420	20	60	0	4
Croissants					
• Almond Croissant, 74 g	265	15	27	1	5
Pain au Chocolate, 62 g	221	12	24	1	4
• Plain Croissant, 34 g	130	7	13	1	2
Juices & Smoothies					
• Blueberry Pomegranate Smoothie, 240ml.	160	2	29	0	7
Carrot Juice, 236 ml.	72	0	15	3	2
Cranberry Apple Cider, 80 oz.	60	0	14	0	0
• Iced Tea & Lemonade, 8 oz.	40	0	12	2	1
Lemonade, 8 oz.	130	0	30	0	0
Mango Smoothie, 8 oz.	130	0	33	4	1
Organic Grapefruit Juice, 8 oz.	100	0	23	0	1
Organic Orange Juice, 8 oz.	110	0	27	0	1
Raspberry Smoothie, 8 oz.	120	0	28	2	1
Muffins					
Banana Nut Muffin, 55 g	170	7	25	1	3
Blueberry Muffin, 55 g	150	4	26	1	3
Carrot & Zucchini Muffin, 55 g	190	10	24	2	3
• Hot Oatmeal, 149 g	530	10	99	9	11
Lemon Poppyseed Muffin, 55 g	180	8	24	1	4
• Raisin Bran Muffin, 55 g	120	3	3	3	3
Pret Yogurt Pots - Low Fat					
Blueberry & Granola PretPot, 283 g	350	16	43	4	11
• Honey & Banana PretPot, 337 g	530	18	84	5	13
Honey & Granola PretPot, 203 g	330	14	47	3	9
• Strawberry & Rhubarb PretPot, 197 g	170	6	28	0	6
Yoga Bunny PretPot, 187 g	240	12	28	3	8
Salad Dressing					
Balsamic Dressing Cup, 1 oz.	110	9	5	0	0
• Caesar Dressing Cup, 1 oz.	160	17	3	0	1
Honey Dijon Dressing Cup, 1 oz.	70	6	3	0	0
• Toasted Sesame Dressing Cup, 1 oz.	60	4	7	1	1
Salads					
• All Natural Cobb & Greens, 287 g	460	25	33	5	27
Bell & Evans Grilled Chicken Caesar, 338 g	390	15	24	4	25
• Pret's Salmon Sushi, 293 g	350	15	37	6	17
Pret's Tuna Sushi, 315 g	430	20	36	3	27
Chicken & Avocado Salad, 349 g	420	29	38	12	22
Sandwiches					
Bell & Evans Chicken and Bacon, 267 g	520	15	59	9	27
Bell & Evans Chicken Avocado, 257 g	580	23	62	14	23
• Bell & Evans Chicken Coronation, 303 g	320	27	78	11	28

RESTAURANTS & FAST-FOOD CHAINS

❯ Pret a Manger (cont.)

	Cal	Fat	Cbs	Fbr	Prtn
Sandwiches (cont.)					
Holiday Lunch, 288 g	490	13	70	5	21
Avocado Grana Padana Parmegiano, 293 g	560	27	59	14	12
Bacon, Lettuce & Tomato, 232 g	550	21	51	7	20
Murray's Natural Turkey Club, 341 g	530	21	59	13	27
• Organic Egg Salad, Spinach & Parmegiano, 301 g	580	27	54	8	18
Pret's Classic Tuna Salad, 282 g	430	19	43	5	27
Soups					
Angus Steak Chilli Medium, 12 oz.	345	14	29	6	27
Beef Stew Medium, 12 oz.	285	7	26	5	9
Broccoli & Cheddar Medium, 1 2 oz.	360	29	14	3	14
Butternut Squash Medium, 12 oz.	270	11	27	5	6
• Chicken Corn Chowder Medium, 12 oz.	375	24	27	3	12
Chicken Fajita Medium, 12 oz.	345	18	26	6	20
Chicken Noodle Medium, 12 oz.	180	3	21	3	17
Chicken Pot Pie Medium, 12 oz.	345	17	18	1	42
Italian Wedding w/ Meatball, 12 oz.	210	5	27	1	14
Leek and Potato Medium, 12 oz.	195	11	21	3	5
Loaded Potato Medium, 12 oz.	315	21	14	3	18
Mediterranean Eggplant & Zucchini, 12 oz.	120	8	9	3	5
Moroccan Lentil Medium, 12 oz.	345	17	36	5	12
Roasted Vegetable Medium, 12 oz.	225	14	21	3	3
Shrimp & Roast Corn Medium, 12	285	17	21	3	15
Thai Chicken with Curry Medium, 12 oz.	240	9	29	3	14
Tomato and Garden Vegetable, 12 oz.	150	4	21	6	8
• Tomato Basil Medium, 12 oz.	120	5	12	5	8
White Bean & Escarole Medium, 12 oz.	330	11	42	8	17
White Chicken Cilantro Medium, 12 oz.	375	14	35	6	30
Zesty Green Pea w/ Mint, 12 oz.	360	7	57	21	20
The Ridiculous No Bread Sandwich					
• No Bread Crayfish & Avocado, 228 g	200	14	11	7	12
No Bread Grilled Chicken Provencal, 318 g	240	16	20	4	17
No Bread Mezze, 238 g	410	17	51	8	14
• No Bread More Than Mozzarella, 376 g	420	35	16	8	17
• No Bread Rock Shrimp Cocktail, 312 g	310	21	14	7	19
Wraps					
• Bell & Evans Chicken Jalepeño Hot Wrap, 374 g	550	24	57	8	41
• Marguerita Pizza Hot Wrap, 303 g	820	43	55	6	27
Natural Reuben Hot Wrap, 230 g	600	34	41	5	32

❯ Pretzel Time

	Cal	Fat	Cbs	Fbr	Prtn
Bites					
Bites Cinnamon Sugar, 165 g	520	12	95	3	9
Bites Large, 165 g	510	13	88	3	10
• Bites Medium, 210 g	640	16	112	4	13
Bites Small, 150 g	450	11	80	3	9
• PT Pretzel Dog, 167 g	440	27	34	1	15
Breezers					
Coffee, 20 fl.oz.	640	21	107	0	6
• Mochas, 20 fl.oz.	620	20	106	0	6
Peach, 20 fl.oz.	650	20	117	0	6
Raspberry, 20 fl.oz.	650	20	117	0	6
Strawberry Banana, 20 fl.oz.	650	20	115	0	6

RESTAURANTS & FAST-FOOD CHAINS

Pretzel Time (cont.)	Cal	Fat	Cbs	Fbr	Prtn
Pretzels					
• Caramel Nut, 129 g	390	7	74	2	7
Cinnamon Sugar, 122 g	370	8	68	2	7
Garlic, 118 g	350	7	64	2	7
Original, 114 g	340	7	61	2	7
Parmesan, 119 g	360	9	61	2	9
Plain, 108 g	290	2	61	2	7
• Ranch, 117 g	240	7	63	2	7
Sauces					
Caramel, 2 oz.	140	0	35	0	1
Cheddar Cheese, 2 oz.	70	5	6	0	1
Cream Cheese Icing, 2 oz.	180	9	22	0	1
• Cream Cheese, 2 oz.	200	20	4	0	2
Ketchup, 18 g	20	0	4	0	0
• Mustard, 10 g	5	0	1	0	0
Nacho Cheese, 2 oz.	80	5	7	0	1
Pizza Cheese, 2 oz.	30	1	6	2	1

Pretzelmaker	Cal	Fat	Cbs	Fbr	Prtn
Bites					
Bites Cinnamon Sugar, 165 g	520	12	95	3	9
Bites Large, 165 g	510	13	88	3	10
• Bites Medium, 210 g	640	16	112	4	13
• Bites Small, 150 g	450	11	80	3	9
Breezers					
Coffee, 20 fl.oz.	640	21	107	0	6
• Mochas, 20 fl.oz.	620	20	106	0	6
• Peach, 20 fl.oz.	650	20	117	0	6
Raspberry, 20 fl.oz.	650	20	117	0	6
Strawberry Banana, 20 fl.oz.	650	20	115	0	6
Pretzels					
Caramel Nut, 129 g	390	7	74	2	7
Cinnamon Sugar, 122 g	370	8	68	2	7
Garlic, 118 g	350	7	64	2	7
Original, 114 g	340	7	61	2	7
Parmesan, 119 g	360	9	61	2	9
Plain, 108 g	290	2	61	2	7
• PT Pretzel Dog, 167 g	440	27	34	1	15
• Ranch, 117 g	240	7	63	2	7
Sauces					
Caramel, 2 oz.	140	0	35	0	1
Cheddar Cheese, 2 oz.	70	5	6	0	1
Cream Cheese Icing, 2 oz.	180	9	22	0	1
• Cream Cheese, 2 oz.	200	20	4	0	2
Ketchup, 18 g	20	0	4	0	0
• Mustard, 10 g	5	0	1	0	0
Nacho Cheese, 2 oz.	80	5	7	0	1
Pizza Cheese, 2 oz.	30	1	6	2	1

Qdoba Mexican Grill	Cal	Fat	Cbs	Fbr	Prtn
Burritos					
• Fajita Ranchera Naked Burrito	530	23	35	18	45
• Grilled Vegetable Burrito	790	18	130	25	26
Naked Steak Burrito	610	18	69	17	42

(• = most healthy • = least healthy) **RESTAURANTS & FAST-FOOD • 287**

RESTAURANTS & FAST-FOOD CHAINS

Qdoba Mexican Grill (cont.)

	Cal	Fat	Cbs	Fbr	Prtn
Specialties					
Chicken Mexican Gumbo, 1 bowl	710	23	81	17	45
Tortilla Soup, 1 bowl	150	7	15	2	6
Tacos & Salad					
• 2 Grilled Vegetable Soft Tacos	340	16	40	8	14
• Grilled Veggie Naked Taco Salad	240	8	33	11	10
Naked Chicken Taco Salad	310	10	25	8	30

Quizno's Sub

	Cal	Fat	Cbs	Fbr	Prtn
Meals					
Small Traditional on wheat	490	N/A	N/A	N/A	N/A
Small Turkey Ranch & Swiss on wheat	470	N/A	N/A	N/A	N/A
Salads					
• Black & Bleu	380	N/A	N/A	N/A	N/A
Classic Cobb	400	N/A	N/A	N/A	N/A
• Raspberry Chipotle Salad	500	N/A	N/A	N/A	N/A
Sammies					
Alpine Chicken	310	N/A	N/A	N/A	N/A
Bistro Steak Melt	320	N/A	N/A	N/A	N/A
• Italiano	325	N/A	N/A	N/A	N/A
• Sonoma Turkey	300	N/A	N/A	N/A	N/A
Sides					
Cup of Chili	140	N/A	N/A	N/A	N/A
• Side Salad w/ Fat Free Blsmc Vinaigrette	130	N/A	N/A	N/A	N/A
• Side Salad with Raspberry Chipotle	220	N/A	N/A	N/A	N/A
Side Salad w/ Reduced Fat Bttrmlk Ranch	130	N/A	N/A	N/A	N/A
Subs					
• Baja Chicken, 6"	500	N/A	N/A	N/A	N/A
Black Angus Steak, 6"	480	N/A	N/A	N/A	N/A
• Honey Bourbon Chicken, 6"	320	N/A	N/A	N/A	N/A
Steakhouse Beef Dip, 6"	430	N/A	N/A	N/A	N/A
The Traditional, 6"	360	N/A	N/A	N/A	N/A
Turkey Bacon Guacamole, 6"	440	N/A	N/A	N/A	N/A
Turkey Ranch & Swiss, 6"	340	N/A	N/A	N/A	N/A
Tuscan Turkey, 6"	400	N/A	N/A	N/A	N/A

Ranch 1

	Cal	Fat	Cbs	Fbr	Prtn
Salads					
• Chicken on Gourmet Greens Salad, 15 oz.	350	11	31	5	32
Gourmet Greens Salad, 12 oz.	220	7	31	5	10
• Zesty Caesar Salad, 7 oz.	180	3	31	4	8
Zesty Chicken Caesar Salad, 9 oz.	290	6	31	4	26
Side Kicks					
• Fruit Cup, 8 oz.	90	1	18	2	3
• Ranch Fries (Large), 6 oz.	420	17	62	7	6
Ranch Fries (Regular), 5 oz.	350	14	51	5	5
Signature Sandwiches					
American Rancher, 9 oz.	390	10	51	3	25
• Club Sandwich, 9 oz.	470	16	53	3	29
Grilled Chicken Philly Sandwich, 9 oz.	450	14	53	3	28
• Ranch Classic, 9 oz.	370	5	53	3	26
Spicy Grilled Chicken Sandwich, 9 oz.	420	11	58	3	23
Specialities					
Baked Potato with Broccoli, 18 oz.	510	1	117	12	12

RESTAURANTS & FAST-FOOD CHAINS

Ranch 1 (cont.)

Specialities (cont.)	Cal	Fat	Cbs	Fbr	Prtn
• Baked Potato with Cheese, 19 oz.	790	25	118	11	23
Baked Potato with Chicken, 14 oz.	610	4	114	11	30
Chicken Tenders (all white meat), 7 oz.	370	15	7	0	52
Grilled Chicken & Vegetable Platter, 25 oz.	790	7	129	16	54
• Grilled Chicken Fajita, 7 oz.	330	16	25	4	22
Grilled Chicken Hot Pasta, 19 oz.	590	10	86	6	37

Red Robin

Chicken Burgers	Cal	Fat	Cbs	Fbr	Prtn
Blackened Chicken Burger, 345 g	791	48	50	2	45
• California Chicken Burger, 406 g	982	62	50	3	54
Crispy Chicken Burger, 368 g	929	56	71	4	37
Jamaican Jerk'd, 361 g	678	34	53	2	42
Teriyaki Chicken Burger, 435 g	900	47	65	3	56
Whiskey River BBQ Chicken Burger, 398 g	954	51	72	4	49

Classic Gourmet Burgers					
5 Alarm Burger, 372 g	907	58	50	3	47
• A.1. Peppercorn Burger, 378 g	1440	97	94	3	54
Blackened Bayou Burger, 364 g	858	57	44	2	43
Bleu Ribbon Burger, 393 g	1062	63	71	3	47
Guacamole Bacon Burger, 407 g	1151	76	52	3	63
Monster Burger, 485 g	1151	69	57	3	75
Red Robin Bacon Cheeseburger, 344 g	1030	70	47	3	52
• Red Robin Gourmet Cheeseburger	850	49	57	3	46
Royal Red Robin Burger, 408 g	1178	82	48	3	60
Santa Fe Burger, 384 g	1036	63	63	5	47
Sauteed Shroom Burger, 440 g	971	60	52	4	60
Sicilian Burger, 435 g	1070	66	46	2	68
The Banzai Burger, 421 g	1054	63	69	3	49
Whiskey River BBQ Burger, 402 g	1129	69	72	4	50

Desserts					
• Birthday Sundae, 138 g	312	17	49	2	6
Hot Apple Crisp, 497 g	784	13	165	12	8
Hot Fudge Sundae, 277 g	673	37	119	5	12
Kid's Sundae, 141 g	324	18	52	2	6
• Mountain High Mudd Pie, 441 g	1390	69	205	10	21

Entrees					
Arctic Code Fish & Chips, 446 g	991	60	76	8	36
Carnitas Fajitas, 676 g	1159	63	81	6	61
Chicken Fajitas, 634 g	1051	49	80	6	66
• Chicken Parmigiano Pasta, 968 g	1542	73	152	9	72
Clucks & Fries Buffalo Style, 545 g	1486	106	91	7	45
Clucks & Fries, 419 g	1261	80	90	6	43
• Ensenada Chicken Platter, 563 g	590	30	14	4	64
Jumbo Shrimp & Slaw Platter, 712 g	1235	58	120	10	42
Red's Rice Bowl, 839 g	1008	29	142	5	43
Shrimp & Cod Duo, 749 g	1407	83	107	9	40
Southwest Chicken Pasta, 875 g	1539	89	121	7	60

Insanely Delicious Burgers					
Bruschetta Chicken Burger, 375 g	876	54	54	4	46
Chili Chili Cheeseburger, 405 g	979	57	58	6	58
Honky Tonk BBQ Pork Burger, 389 g	679	24	78	5	41
• Prime Rib Dip, 675 g	988	56	57	3	78

(• = most healthy) (• = least healthy) **RESTAURANTS & FAST-FOOD • 289**

RESTAURANTS & FAST-FOOD CHAINS

Red Robin (cont.)

	Cal	Fat	Cbs	Fbr	Prtn
Kid's Menu: Kids					
Carnival Corn Dog, 197 g	490	20	62	4	14
• Cheesey Mac 'n Cheesey, 435 g	481	22	57	4	14
Chick-Chick-Chicken Fingers, 180 g	481	24	44	3	22
• Chick-n-Cheese Quesadilla, 306 g	763	35	60	4	46
Grilled Cheesewich, 242 g	635	38	56	4	18
Grilled Chick-N-Parmesan Noodles, 272 g	518	28	44	0	24
Red Robin Burger, 206 g	541	24	52	4	24
Red Robinetti Spaghetti, 522 g	614	15	95	2	21
Red's Pizzeria Pizza, 263 g	561	26	54	2	31
Lighten Up Burgers					
Crispy Fish Burger, 289 g	565	27	58	3	24
• Grilled Salmon Burger, 359 g	745	38	52	2	36
Grilled Turkey Burger, 273 g	704	43	51	3	30
• Lettuce-Wrapped Protein Burger, 387 g	439	27	10	3	36
The Garden Burger, 296 g	517	18	63	10	23
Salads					
Apple Harvest Chicken Salad, 512 g	603	34	39	8	33
Asian Chicken Salad, 610 g	488	6	70	7	39
Cobb Salad, 712 g	832	50	45	12	57
• Crispy Chicken Tender Salad, 671 g	1326	87	84	7	54
Fajita Fiesta Pollo Salad, 756 g	1238	85	67	12	52
Mighty Caesar Salad, 436 g	784	51	60	9	15
Mighty Caesar-Blackened Chicken, 563 g	980	61	61	9	42
Mighty Caesar-Grilled Chicken, 557 g	980	61	61	9	42
Mighty Caesar-Salmon, 577 g	960	57	60	9	42
Side Caesar Salad, 281 g	611	31	65	7	14
• Side Dinner Salad, 212 g	217	13	15	4	10
Sandwiches					
BLTA Croissant, 673 g	1077	66	114	14	41
Shareable Starters					
Cheeseburger Con Queso, 456 g	1303	85	75	6	60
Chili Chili Nachos w/ Chicken, 634 g	1379	89	67	14	75
Chili Chili Nachos, 513 g	1183	80	66	14	48
Creamy Artichoke & Spanish Dip, 520 g	1201	73	101	17	39
Fresh-Fried Cheese Sticks, 415 g	1181	70	86	5	52
• Guacamole, Salsa & Chips, 344 g	800	47	88	15	10
Just-in-quesadilla, 574 g	1073	55	72	8	60
RR's Buzzard Wings, 427 g	1023	81	4	3	74
• Towering Onion Rings, 541 g	1837	124	160	10	18
Soups					
• Chicken Tortilla Soup, 1 cup	173	9	11	2	10
• Clamdigger's Clam Chowder, 1 cup	346	20	26	1	13
French Onion Soup Cup, 1 cup	280	11	27	3	11
Red's Homemade Chili, 1 cup	302	19	16	4	20
Wraps					
Caesar's Chicken Wrap, 677 g	1244	60	122	10	46
Whiskey River BBQ Chicken Wrap, 740 g	1526	81	138	11	58

Red Lobster

	Cal	Fat	Cbs	Fbr	Prtn
Appetizers					
Buffalo Chicken Wings	680	N/A	N/A	N/A	N/A
Chicken Breast Strips	690	N/A	N/A	N/A	N/A
Chilled Jumbo Shrimp Cocktail	121	N/A	N/A	N/A	N/A

RESTAURANTS & FAST-FOOD CHAINS

Red Lobster (cont.)	Cal	Fat	Cbs	Fbr	Prtn
Appetizers (cont.)					
Crispy Calamari and Vegetables	1520	N/A	N/A	N/A	N/A
Hand-Shucked Oysters on the Half Shell, 6 pcs.	50	N/A	N/A	N/A	N/A
Lobster Pizza	720	N/A	N/A	N/A	N/A
Lobster, Artichoke and Seafood Dip	1080	N/A	N/A	N/A	N/A
Lobster, Crab & Seafood-Stuffed Mshrms	380	N/A	N/A	N/A	N/A
Mozzarella Cheesesticks	680	N/A	N/A	N/A	N/A
New England Seafood Sampler	890	N/A	N/A	N/A	N/A
Pan-Seared Crab Cakes	360	N/A	N/A	N/A	N/A
Parrot Bay Jumbo Coconut Shrimp	588	N/A	N/A	N/A	N/A
Southwestern Lobster Rolls	780	N/A	N/A	N/A	N/A
Steamed Clams	430	N/A	N/A	N/A	N/A
Ultimate Fondue	1490	N/A	N/A	N/A	N/A
Condiments and Sauces					
Add Petite Shrimp to your Salad	15	N/A	N/A	N/A	N/A
Baked Potato	190	N/A	N/A	N/A	N/A
add Butter	90	N/A	N/A	N/A	N/A
add Sour Cream	30	N/A	N/A	N/A	N/A
Caesar Salad	270	N/A	N/A	N/A	N/A
Cheddar Bay Biscuit, 1 biscuit	150	N/A	N/A	N/A	N/A
Coleslaw	200	N/A	N/A	N/A	N/A
• Creamy Lobster Topped Baked Potato	370	N/A	N/A	N/A	N/A
Creamy Lobster Topped Mashed Potatoes	360	N/A	N/A	N/A	N/A
Fresh Asparagus	60	N/A	N/A	N/A	N/A
Fresh Broccoli	45	N/A	N/A	N/A	N/A
Fries	330	N/A	N/A	N/A	N/A
Garden Salad	90	N/A	N/A	N/A	N/A
Home-Style Mashed Potatoes	180	N/A	N/A	N/A	N/A
• Lemon Wedge	5	N/A	N/A	N/A	N/A
Wild Rice Pilaf	180	N/A	N/A	N/A	N/A
Create Your Own Appetizer Combo					
Chicken Breast Strips	414	N/A	N/A	N/A	N/A
Clam Strips	370	N/A	N/A	N/A	N/A
• Crispy Calamari and Vegetables	775	N/A	N/A	N/A	N/A
Mozzarella Cheesesticks	340	N/A	N/A	N/A	N/A
• Stuffed Mushrooms	220	N/A	N/A	N/A	N/A
Create Your Own Feast					
Crab Linguini Alfredo	560	N/A	N/A	N/A	N/A
Garlic Shrimp Scampi	195	N/A	N/A	N/A	N/A
Garlic-Grilled Jumbo Shrimp	105	N/A	N/A	N/A	N/A
Grilled Salmon	210	N/A	N/A	N/A	N/A
Grilled Sirloin Steak	250	N/A	N/A	N/A	N/A
• Parrot Bay Jumbo Coconut Shrimp	784	N/A	N/A	N/A	N/A
Seafood-Stuffed Flounder	160	N/A	N/A	N/A	N/A
Shrimp Linguini Alfredo	550	N/A	N/A	N/A	N/A
• Steamed Snow Crab Legs	80	N/A	N/A	N/A	N/A
Walt's Favorite Shrimp	466	N/A	N/A	N/A	N/A
Dipping Sauces					
100% Melted Butter, 1 oz.	230	N/A	N/A	N/A	N/A
Cocktail Sauce, 1 oz.	50	N/A	N/A	N/A	N/A
• Honey Mustard Dipping Sauce, 1 oz.	240	N/A	N/A	N/A	N/A
Horseradish, 1 oz.	20	N/A	N/A	N/A	N/A
Ketchup, 1 oz.	30	N/A	N/A	N/A	N/A
Marinara Sauce, 1 oz.	30	N/A	N/A	N/A	N/A

RESTAURANTS & FAST-FOOD CHAINS

Red Lobster (cont.)

	Cal	Fat	Cbs	Fbr	Prtn
Dipping Sauces (cont.)					
• Pico de Gallo, 1 oz.	10	N/A	N/A	N/A	N/A
Piña Colada Sauce, 1 oz.	120	N/A	N/A	N/A	N/A
Remoulade, 2 oz.	150	N/A	N/A	N/A	N/A
Sweet and Spicy Glaze, 1 oz.	90	N/A	N/A	N/A	N/A
Tartar Sauce, 1 oz.	130	N/A	N/A	N/A	N/A
Dressings					
Balsamic Vinaigrette, 1 oz.	60	N/A	N/A	N/A	N/A
Blue Cheese, 1 oz.	170	N/A	N/A	N/A	N/A
• Caesar, 1 oz.	200	N/A	N/A	N/A	N/A
French, 1 oz.	120	N/A	N/A	N/A	N/A
Honey Mustard Dressing, 1 oz.	100	N/A	N/A	N/A	N/A
• Ranch (Fat-Free), 1 oz.	40	N/A	N/A	N/A	N/A
Ranch, 1 oz.	110	N/A	N/A	N/A	N/A
Thousand Island, 1 oz.	130	N/A	N/A	N/A	N/A
Lobster & Crab					
Chef's Signature Lobster & Shrimp Pasta	1020	N/A	N/A	N/A	N/A
• Crab Linguini Alfredo	1120	N/A	N/A	N/A	N/A
• Live Maine Lobster, 1 1/4 lb	45	N/A	N/A	N/A	N/A
Lobster & Seafood Mixed Grill	630	N/A	N/A	N/A	N/A
North Pacific King Crab Legs	390	N/A	N/A	N/A	N/A
Rock Lobster Tail	90	N/A	N/A	N/A	N/A
Snow Crab Legs, 1 lb	160	N/A	N/A	N/A	N/A
Other					
Steamed King Crab Legs, 1/2 lb	130	N/A	N/A	N/A	N/A
Steamed Snow Crab Legs, 1/2 lb	80	N/A	N/A	N/A	N/A
Shrimp					
Crunchy Popcorn Shrimp	560	N/A	N/A	N/A	N/A
• Garlic-Grilled Jumbo Shrimp	245	N/A	N/A	N/A	N/A
Maui Luau Shrimp and Salmon	790	N/A	N/A	N/A	N/A
• Parrot Bay Jumbo Coconut Shrimp	980	N/A	N/A	N/A	N/A
Shrimp Linguini Alfredo	550	N/A	N/A	N/A	N/A
Spicy Asian-Garlic Jumbo Shrimp	245	N/A	N/A	N/A	N/A
Tequila-Lime Jumbo Shrimp	360	N/A	N/A	N/A	N/A
Walt's Favorite Shrimp	700	N/A	N/A	N/A	N/A
Shrimp Your Way					
• Coconut Shrimp Bites	290	N/A	N/A	N/A	N/A
Fried Shrimp	190	N/A	N/A	N/A	N/A
Popcorn Shrimp	180	N/A	N/A	N/A	N/A
• Scampi	130	N/A	N/A	N/A	N/A
Signature Combinations					
• Admiral's Feast	1506	N/A	N/A	N/A	N/A
Seaside Shrimp Trio	1030	N/A	N/A	N/A	N/A
• Ultimate Feast	638	N/A	N/A	N/A	N/A
Soups & Salads					
• Apple-Walnut Chicken Salad	900	N/A	N/A	N/A	N/A
• Manhattan Clam Chowder, 1 cup	80	N/A	N/A	N/A	N/A
New England Clam Chowder, 1 cup	240	N/A	N/A	N/A	N/A
Seafood Caesar Salad	680	N/A	N/A	N/A	N/A
Specialty Drinks					
• Sail Away Smoothie - Banana Bay Choco	460	N/A	N/A	N/A	N/A
Sail Away Smoothie - Strawberry Banana	340	N/A	N/A	N/A	N/A
Sail Away Smoothie - Sunset Strawberry	250	N/A	N/A	N/A	N/A
• Tropical Freezes - Orange or Pineapple	250	N/A	N/A	N/A	N/A

RESTAURANTS & FAST-FOOD CHAINS

Red Lobster (cont.)

	Cal	Fat	Cbs	Fbr	Prtn
Steak & Chicken					
Aztec Chicken	755	N/A	N/A	N/A	N/A
Cajun Chicken Linguini Alfredo	1260	N/A	N/A	N/A	N/A
Grilled Center-Cut New York Strip	480	N/A	N/A	N/A	N/A
Grilled Chicken Breast	610	N/A	N/A	N/A	N/A
Honey BBQ Shrimp and Chicken	710	N/A	N/A	N/A	N/A
New York Steak and Rock Lobster Tail	570	N/A	N/A	N/A	N/A
New York Strip Steak and Shrimp	946	N/A	N/A	N/A	N/A
Sirloin Steak and Rock Lobster Tail	340	N/A	N/A	N/A	N/A
Sirloin Steak and Shrimp	716	N/A	N/A	N/A	N/A
Steak Lobster-and-Shrimp Oscar	990	N/A	N/A	N/A	N/A
Traditional Favorites					
Broiled Seafood Platter	280	N/A	N/A	N/A	N/A
Classic Fried Seafood Platter	1090	N/A	N/A	N/A	N/A
Farm-Raised Catfish - Blackened	380	N/A	N/A	N/A	N/A
Farm-Raised Catfish - Golden-Fried	440	N/A	N/A	N/A	N/A
Golden-Fried Flounder	440	N/A	N/A	N/A	N/A
Oven-Broiled Flounder	280	N/A	N/A	N/A	N/A
Seafood-Stuffed Flounder	320	N/A	N/A	N/A	N/A

Rita's

	Cal	Fat	Cbs	Fbr	Prtn
Ice					
Cream Ice Regular, 12 oz.	312	4	70	1	1
Custard Regular, 7 oz.	385	21	43	1	7
Gelati w/ Choc. Cust. Regular, 10 oz.	351	11	60	1	4
Gelati w/ Van. Cust. Regular, 10 oz.	366	13	59	0	4
Ice Regular, 12 oz.	263	0	69	0	0
Misto w/ Choc. Cust. Regular, 15 oz.	409	7	90	1	3
Misto w/ Van. Cust. Regular, 15 oz.	420	7	90	0	3
Made with Cream Ice					
Gelati w/ Choc. Cust. Regular, 10 oz.	368	13	60	1	5
Gelati w/ Van. Cust. Regular, 10 oz.	392	15	61	0	5
Misto w/ Choc. Cust. Regular, 15 oz.	463	11	90	1	3
Misto w/ Van. Cust. Regular, 15 oz.	473	12	90	0	3

Robeks

	Cal	Fat	Cbs	Fbr	Prtn
Bowls					
Açai Energy Bowl™, 12 oz.	267	3	55	6	3
Super Açai Bowl™, 12 oz.	314	6	61	7	4
Frozen Yogurt					
Average, 12 oz.	250	0	58	1	10
Shakes & Freezes					
800 lb. Gorilla™, 12 oz.	375	9	50	2	26
Bananasplit Shake, 12 oz.	302	0	69	2	11
Lemon Freeze, 12 oz.	279	2	60	0	2
Orange Freeze, 12 oz.	242	0	56	1	9
P-Nut Power Shake, 12 oz.	422	18	52	4	17
Smoothies					
Açai Energizer™, 12 oz.	167	1	36	2	2
Awesome Açai™, 12 oz.	183	1	42	2	3
Banzai Blueberry™, 12 oz.	175	1	38	3	3
Berry Brilliance®, 12 oz.	194	1	45	2	3
Big Wednesday®, 12 oz.	172	1	40	1	1
Cardio Cooler™, 12 oz.	215	1	44	3	9

(• = most healthy • = least healthy) **RESTAURANTS & FAST-FOOD • 293**

RESTAURANTS & FAST-FOOD CHAINS

Robeks (cont.)

	Cal	Fat	Cbs	Fbr	Prtn
Smoothies (cont.)					
Citrus Stinger™, 12 oz.	194	1	40	2	5
Cranberry Quest™, 12 oz.	173	0	40	1	2
Dr. Robeks®, 12 oz.	181	1	40	3	3
Green Tea Sensation™, 12 oz.	222	1	42	1	6
Guava Lava™, 12 oz.	180	1	42	2	2
Hummingbird®, 12 oz.	185	1	44	1	2
Innite Orange®, 12 oz.	181	0	42	3	4
Mahalo Mango®, 12 oz.	174	1	42	1	2
• Malibu Peach™, 12 oz.	153	0	36	1	3
Outrageous Raspberry, 12 oz.	174	1	39	2	2
Passionfruit Cove®, 12 oz.	168	1	38	1	2
Pina Koolada™, 12 oz.	261	8	46	3	3
Polar Pineapple™, 12 oz.	164	1	38	1	1
Pomegranate Passion™, 12 oz.	196	0	48	1	4
Pomegranate Power™, 12 oz.	211	0	50	1	3
• Pro Arobek®, 12 oz.	265	1	54	3	15
Raspberry Romance®, 12 oz.	172	0	42	2	4
Robeks MuscleMax™, 12 oz.	202	1	38	2	11
Robeks Rejuvenator™, 12 oz.	193	1	43	2	5
South Pacific Squeeze®, 12 oz.	188	1	42	3	2
Strawnana Berry™, 12 oz.	179	0	44	2	3
Venice Burner®, 12 oz.	231	1	46	4	9
Zen Berry®, 12 oz.	190	1	45	5	3

Rockfish Seafood Grill

	Cal	Fat	Cbs	Fbr	Prtn
Be The Chef: Choose A Fish					
Ahi Tuna	248	N/A	N/A	N/A	N/A
Alaskan Flounder	255	N/A	N/A	N/A	N/A
• Chicken	188	N/A	N/A	N/A	N/A
North Atlantic Salmon	356	N/A	N/A	N/A	N/A
Shrimp	325	N/A	N/A	N/A	N/A
Tilapia	341	N/A	N/A	N/A	N/A
Trophy Rainbow Trout	355	N/A	N/A	N/A	N/A
• U.S. Farm- Raised Catfish	488	N/A	N/A	N/A	N/A
Be The Chef: Choose A Prep Style					
Blackened	17	N/A	N/A	N/A	N/A
Be The Chef: Choose A Sauce					
Ancho Cream	102	N/A	N/A	N/A	N/A
• Lemon-Butter	244	N/A	N/A	N/A	N/A
Maple Glaze	106	N/A	N/A	N/A	N/A
Pontchartrain	115	N/A	N/A	N/A	N/A
Roasted Red Pepper	34	N/A	N/A	N/A	N/A
• Tomatillo Salsa	18	N/A	N/A	N/A	N/A
Be The Chef: Choose A Side					
Mixed Veggies	17	N/A	N/A	N/A	N/A
• New Potatoes	152	N/A	N/A	N/A	N/A
• Steamed Spinach	17	N/A	N/A	N/A	N/A
Wild Rice	100	N/A	N/A	N/A	N/A
Salads					
Pacific Cove Crab Salad	423	18	33	N/A	29
Roaring River Salmon Salad	462	19	30	N/A	43
Seared Ahi Tuna Salad	335	14	10	N/A	42
• Small Southwest Caesar Salad	251	34	17	N/A	2

RESTAURANTS & FAST-FOOD CHAINS

Rockfish Seafood Grill (cont.)

	Cal	Fat	Cbs	Fbr	Prtn
Stream					
Ahi Tuna Ciabatta	516	17	41	N/A	46
Baked & Stuffed Shrimp	493	34	19	N/A	23
• Louisiana Gumbo	445	16	54	N/A	15
• Santa Fe Fish Tacos	564	18	101	N/A	46
Tilapia In The Bag	501	18	31	N/A	61
Tilapia Pontchartrain	493	24	9	N/A	61

Rocky Rococo

	Cal	Fat	Cbs	Fbr	Prtn
Bread					
Breadsticks w/ Jalapeño Chz Sauce, 8 oz.	531	18	72	2	17
Breadsticks with Marinara Sauce, 8 oz.	420	7	72	3	18
• Wheat muffin, 1 muffin	200	4	38	5	5
Pasta					
Can't Decide, 14 oz.	464	9	77	4	17
Fettuccine with Alfredo Sauce, 14 oz.	459	14	66	3	16
Light Fettuccine with Alfredo Sauce, 7 oz.	229	7	33	1	8
Light Spaghetti with Meat Sauce, 7 oz.	250	3	44	3	10
Light Spaghetti with Meatballs, 8 oz.	314	8	45	3	15
Light Spaghetti with Tomato Sauce, 7 oz.	235	2	44	3	9
Spaghetti with Meat Sauce, 14 oz.	499	7	87	6	19
Spaghetti with Meatballs, 15 oz.	628	16	89	6	29
Spaghetti with Tomato Sauce, 14 oz.	470	4	87	6	18
Pizza					
Cheese, 1 slice	380	9	54	1	18
Garden, 1 slice	391	10	56	1	19
Pepperoni, 1 slice	427	13	54	1	20
Sausage Mushroom, 1 slice	499	19	55	1	24
Sausage, 1 slice	495	19	54	1	23

Roly Poly

	Cal	Fat	Cbs	Fbr	Prtn
Egg Items					
All American Egg Roly on Low-carb	441	26	24	16	32
All American Egg Roly on Wheat	458	26	27	3	31
• All American Egg Roly on White	468	26	29	1	30
Christo Melt on Low-carb	313	15	24	16	22
Christo Melt on Wheat	330	16	27	4	21
Christo Melt on White	340	16	30	2	21
Steak and Eggs on Low-carb	319	15	26	16	20
Steak and Eggs on Wheat	336	16	29	4	19
Steak and Eggs on White	346	16	31	2	19
Veggie Scramble Egg Roly on Low-carb	296	15	26	17	15
Veggie Scramble Egg Roly on Wheat	314	16	29	4	14
Veggie Scramble Egg Roly on White	324	16	32	3	14
Western Egg Roly on Low-carb	310	17	26	17	16
Western Egg Roly on Wheat	328	17	29	4	15
Western Egg Roly on White	338	18	32	2	14
Kids Items					
Kids Cheese Dog on Low-carb	246	14	22	16	11
Kids Cheese Dog on Wheat	264	14	25	3	10
Kids Cheese Dog on White	274	15	28	1	10
• Kids Chicken Melt on Low-carb	193	7	22	16	12
Kids Chicken Melt on Wheat	210	7	25	3	10
Kids Chicken Melt on White	220	8	28	1	10

(•= most healthy •= least healthy) **RESTAURANTS & FAST-FOOD • 295**

RESTAURANTS & FAST-FOOD CHAINS

Roly Poly (cont.)

	Cal	Fat	Cbs	Fbr	Prtn
Kids Items (cont.)					
Kids Grilled Cheese on Low-carb	200	10	22	16	10
Kids Grilled Cheese on Wheat	218	10	24	3	8
Kids Grilled Cheese on White	228	10	27	1	8
Kids Meat and Cheese on Low-carb	193	7	22	16	12
Kids Meat and Cheese on Wheat	210	7	25	3	10
Kids Meat and Cheese on White	220	8	28	1	10
Kids Peanut Butter and Jelly on Low-carb	255	11	34	16	8
Kids Peanut Butter and Jelly on Wheat	272	11	36	4	8
• Kids Peanut Butter and Jelly on White	282	11	39	2	8
Salad					
Alpine Chef	412	24	14	4	38
• Chipotle Caesar	599	31	23	4	51
Cobb Salad	566	34	12	4	47
• Greek Salad	242	16	17	4	9
Las Olas Salad	349	14	12	3	36
Spa Salad	255	15	26	7	9
Walnut Spinach	515	43	15	7	24
Sandwich: Black Forest Ham & Roast Pork					
BarBQ Pork Melt Wheat	302	10	26	3	22
BarBQ Pork Melt White	315	10	27	1	22
Italian Classic Wheat	328	12	28	4	18
Italian Classic White	341	12	29	2	18
• Key West Cuban Mix Wheat	297	9	28	4	27
Key West Cuban Mix White	310	9	28	2	27
Peachtree Melt Wheat	327	11	28	3	16
Peachtree Melt White	340	11	29	1	16
Porky's Nightmare Wheat	312	12	26	4	21
Porky's Nightmare White	325	12	28	2	21
• Southside Club Wheat	364	18	29	4	22
Southside Club White	374	19	32	3	22
Sandwich: Chicken					
Basil Cashew Chicken Wheat	288	11	27	3	15
Basil Cashew Chicken White	301	11	28	3	14
Buffalo Chicken Melt Wheat	355	11	33	4	26
Buffalo Chicken Melt White	365	12	35	2	25
Buffalo Slim Wheat	279	6	26	4	14
Catalina Chicken Salad Wheat	305	12	27	5	17
Catalina Chicken Salad White	318	13	28	3	17
Chicken Caesar Wheat	312	12	28	6	15
Chicken Caesar White	325	12	30	4	14
Chicken Cordonbleu Wheat	303	11	27	4	23
Chicken Cordonbleu White	319	11	28	2	23
Chicken Fajita Wheat	279	8	27	4	22
Chicken Fajita White	292	8	28	2	22
• Chicken Popper Wheat	246	7	29	4	19
Chicken Popper White	259	7	30	2	19
Cobb Salad Wheat	318	14	28	5	11
Cobb Salad White	331	14	29	3	11
Delhi Chicken Wheat	319	12	32	5	18
Delhi Chicken White	332	13	33	3	17
Hickory Chicken Wheat	336	11	27	4	23
Hickory Chicken White	349	11	29	2	23
Oriental Chicken Wheat	262	6	31	5	19

RESTAURANTS & FAST-FOOD CHAINS

Roly Poly (cont.)	Cal	Fat	Cbs	Fbr	Prtn
Sandwich: Chicken (cont.)					
Oriental Chicken White	275	6	32	3	19
Pesto Chicken Wheat	410	18	31	4	27
Pesto Chicken White	420	18	34	2	27
Santa Fe Chicken Wheat	272	8	27	4	21
Santa Fe Chicken White	285	8	28	2	21
Sandwich: Sliced Steak & Roast Beef					
Chipotle Cheesesteak Wheat	363	17	29	4	24
Chipotle Cheesesteak White	373	17	32	2	24
Pepper Steak Wheat	237	9	26	4	17
Pepper Steak White	250	9	28	2	17
Philly Melt Wheat	257	7	26	3	18
Philly Melt White	270	7	27	1	18
Ranch Roast Wheat	316	14	28	5	19
Ranch Roast White	329	14	29	3	19
Russian Beef Wheat	282	11	26	4	17
Russian Beef White	295	11	28	2	17
Santa Fe Steak Wheat	279	8	27	4	21
Santa Fe Steak White	292	8	28	2	21
Steak Fajita Wheat	283	8	27	4	22
Steak Fajita White	296	8	28	2	22
Sandwich: Tuna Salad					
• Popeye's Tuna Wheat	309	5	30	4	18
Texas Tuna Melt Wheat	309	13	26	4	17
Texas Tuna Melt White	322	14	27	2	17
Thai Hot Tuna Wheat	327	13	27	5	16
• Thai Hot Tuna White	340	13	28	3	15
Tuna Luau Wheat	323	15	29	4	17
Tuna Luau White	336	15	30	2	17
Sandwich: Turkey & Smoked Turkey					
California Turkey Wheat	319	14	34	5	21
California Turkey White	332	14	35	3	20
Cider House Melt Wheat	252	5	284	5	19
Greek Turkey Wheat	256	5	30	5	17
Hickory Christo Wheat	302	10	28	5	19
Hickory Christo White	315	10	29	3	19
Hot Honey Wheat	291	9	28	6	21
Hot Honey White	304	9	30	4	20
Italian Turkey Wheat	320	12	31	6	20
Italian Turkey White	333	12	32	4	20
Pesto Turkey Club Wheat	382	20	31	5	22
• Pesto Turkey Club White	392	20	34	3	22
Smokehouse Turkey Wheat	319	11	28	5	19
Smokehouse Turkey White	332	11	29	3	19
Thanksgiving Wheat	276	8	30	3	17
Thanksgiving White	289	8	32	1	17
Turkey Applejack Wheat	311	13	27	4	19
Turkey Applejack White	324	13	28	2	19
Tuscan Turkey Wheat	228	4	31	5	17
• Tuscan Turkey White	241	4	32	3	16
Wild Turkey Wheat	275	12	29	6	18
Wild Turkey White	288	12	30	4	18
Sandwich: Veggie & Cheese					
California Hummer Wheat	305	14	29	6	9

(• = most healthy • = least healthy)

RESTAURANTS & FAST-FOOD CHAINS

Roly Poly (cont.)

	Cal	Fat	Cbs	Fbr	Prtn
Sandwich: Veggie & Cheese (cont.)					
California Hummer White	318	14	31	4	9
French Twist Wheat	264	11	28	5	9
French Twist White	277	11	29	3	9
Italian Veggie Wheat	246	9	29	6	9
Italian Veggie White	259	9	30	4	9
Monster Veggie Wheat	275	10	29	7	9
Monster Veggie White	288	10	31	5	9
Nut & Honey Wheat	360	18	35	8	11
• Nut & Honey White	373	19	37	6	11
Spinach Stuffer Wheat	229	8	31	5	10
Spinach Stuffer White	242	9	32	3	9
• Ultimate Veggie Wheat	196	4	31	7	6
Ultimate Veggie White	209	4	32	5	6
Veggie Fajita Wheat	229	8	28	6	9
Veggie Fajita White	242	9	30	4	8
Sandwiches Special					
Alpine Chicken Melt on Wheat	456	18	33	6	36
Alpine Chicken Melt on White	466	18	36	5	36
BBQ Veggie Ranchero on Wheat	321	5	31	5	15
Buffalo Chicken Melt on Low-carb	338	11	30	17	27
Buffalo Chicken Melt on Wheat	355	11	33	4	26
Buffalo Chicken Melt on White	365	12	35	2	25
Cajun Chicken Melt on Low-carb	378	15	28	17	31
Cajun Chicken Melt on Wheat	395	16	30	4	29
Cajun Chicken Melt on White	405	16	33	3	29
Cajun Club on Low-carb	343	16	30	18	23
Cajun Club on Wheat	361	17	33	5	21
Cajun Club on White	371	17	35	3	21
Caribbean Mix on Low-carb	454	19	42	20	29
Caribbean Mix on Wheat	472	20	44	8	28
Caribbean Mix on White	418	20	31	2	28
Carnita Chicken on Low-carb	373	13	32	18	30
Carnita Chicken on Wheat	391	13	35	6	29
Carnita Chicken on White	401	14	37	4	29
Carnita Steak on Low-carb	364	15	32	18	27
Carnita Steak on Wheat	382	15	34	6	26
Carnita Steak on White	392	16	37	4	26
Carolina Shrimp Melt on Low-carb	258	11	25	16	18
Carolina Shrimp Melt on Wheat	276	11	27	4	17
Carolina Shrimp Melt on White	286	12	30	2	16
Cherry Pecan Chicken Club on Low-carb	593	34	41	20	33
Cherry Pecan Chicken Club on Wheat	640	37	44	7	32
• Cherry Pecan Chicken Club on White	650	38	47	5	31
Chicken Bruschetta on Low-carb	339	11	30	18	29
Chicken Bruschetta on Wheat	357	11	33	6	28
Chicken Bruschetta on White	367	11	35	4	27
Chicken Pizza on Low-carb	392	16	29	17	32
Chicken Pizza on Wheat	409	16	31	4	30
Chicken Pizza on White	419	17	34	2	30
Chipotle Cheesesteak on Low-carb	346	16	26	16	25
Chipotle Cheesesteak on Wheat	363	17	29	4	24
Chipotle Cheesesteak on White	373	17	32	2	24
Chipotle Chicken on Low-carb	405	18	27	17	31

RESTAURANTS & FAST-FOOD CHAINS

Roly Poly (cont.)

	Cal	Fat	Cbs	Fbr	Prtn
Sandwiches Special (cont.)					
Chipotle Chicken on Wheat	423	18	30	4	30
Chipotle Chicken on White	433	19	33	2	30
Coney Island Melt on Low-carb	442	29	26	17	21
Coney Island Melt on Wheat	460	29	29	4	20
Coney Island Melt on White	470	30	31	3	20
Creole Chicken on Low-carb	231	5	27	17	20
• Creole Chicken on Wheat	218	5	25	5	11
Creole Chicken on Wheat	248	5	30	4	19
Creole Chicken on White	258	6	33	3	19
Extreme Veggie on Wheat	263	11	35	6	8
Extreme Veggie on White	273	12	38	5	8
Ginger Shrimp on Wheat	282	5	26	4	9
Grand Central on Low-carb	380	20	33	18	21
Grand Central on Wheat	398	20	36	5	20
Grand Central on White	408	20	38	3	20
Guilt Free Cobbler on Wheat	307	4	32	3	21
Harvest Melt on Wheat	223	4	30	7	11
Hawaiian Chicken on Wheat	284	6	29	3	17
Holiday Meltdown on Low-carb	384	19	30	17	25
Holiday Meltdown on Wheat	402	19	33	4	24
Holiday Meltdown on White	412	20	36	2	24
Huevos Rancheros on Low-carb	331	17	30	18	17
Huevos Rancheros on Wheat	349	17	33	5	16
Huevos Rancheros on White	359	18	35	4	16
Indian Chicken on Wheat	299	6	29	5	13
Longhorn Melt on Low-carb	402	20	27	17	29
Longhorn Melt on Wheat	419	21	30	4	28
Longhorn Melt on White	429	21	32	2	28
Mandarin Tuna on Low-carb	249	5	32	17	23
Mandarin Tuna on Wheat	266	5	34	4	22
Mandarin Tuna on White	276	6	37	2	22
Monster Fajita on Low-carb	373	17	29	18	27
Monster Fajita on Wheat	391	17	31	5	26
Monster Fajita on White	401	17	34	3	26
Monterey Chicken on Low-carb	419	18	32	18	31
Monterey Chicken on Wheat	437	18	35	5	30
Monterey Chicken on White	447	19	37	4	30
Moroccan Tofu on Low-carb	229	10	28	18	11
Moroccan Tofu on Wheat	246	10	31	5	10
Moroccan Tofu on White	256	10	33	3	10
Nantucket Lobster on Low-carb	310	16	31	17	13
Nantucket Lobster on Wheat	328	17	34	5	12
Nantucket Lobster on White	338	17	36	3	12
New Orleans Melt on Low-carb	276	11	26	17	19
New Orleans Melt on Wheat	293	11	29	4	18
New Orleans Melt on White	303	11	32	3	17
New Yorker on Low-carb	290	12	28	17	21
New Yorker on Wheat	308	12	31	4	20
New Yorker on White	318	13	33	3	20
Orange County Smoked Turkey on Lowcarb	493	30	31	20	29
Orange County Smoked Turkey on Wheat	511	30	34	7	28
Orange County Smoked Turkey on White	521	31	37	5	27
Palm Beach Tuna on Low-carb	293	11	30	17	24

(•= most healthy •= least healthy) **RESTAURANTS & FAST-FOOD • 299**

Roly Poly (cont.)

	Cal	Fat	Cbs	Fbr	Prtn
Sandwiches Special (cont.)					
Palm Beach Tuna on Wheat	311	11	33	5	23
Palm Beach Tuna on White	321	12	35	3	22
Peking Chicken on Wheat	230	6	28	5	9
Pesto Chicken on Low-carb	392	18	28	16	28
Pesto Chicken on Wheat	410	18	31	4	27
Pesto Chicken on White	420	18	34	2	27
Pesto Club on Low-carb	349	17	30	18	22
Pesto Club on Wheat	366	17	33	5	22
Pesto Club on White	376	17	36	4	22
Popeye's Tuna on Low- Carb	237	5	30	17	23
Popeye's Tuna on Wheat	254	5	33	5	22
Popeye's Tuna on White	264	6	35	3	22
Ranchero Chicken on Low-carb	364	12	32	18	28
Ranchero Chicken on Wheat	382	13	35	5	27
Ranchero Chicken on White	392	13	38	4	27
Ranchero Steak on Low-carb	356	14	32	18	25
Ranchero Steak on Wheat	373	15	35	5	24
Ranchero Steak on White	383	15	37	4	24
Roly Poly Pounder on Low-carb	425	20	30	17	32
Roly Poly Pounder on Wheat	443	20	33	5	31
Roly Poly Pounder on White	453	21	36	3	31
Roly Polynesian on Low-carb	372	16	29	16	28
Roly Polynesian on Wheat	390	17	31	4	27
Roly Polynesian on White	400	17	34	2	27
Roly Reuben on Low-carb	350	20	23	17	20
Roly Reuben on Wheat	367	20	26	4	19
Roly Reuben on White	377	21	29	2	19
Roma Chicken on Low-carb	340	10	30	19	29
Roma Chicken on Wheat	358	11	33	6	28
Roma Chicken on White	368	11	36	5	28
Shrimp Club on Low-carb	319	18	26	18	17
Shrimp Club on Wheat	336	18	28	5	16
Shrimp Club on White	346	19	31	4	16
Steak & Bearnaise on Low-carb	345	16	25	16	24
Steak & Bearnaise on Wheat	363	17	28	3	23
Steak & Bearnaise on White	373	17	31	2	23
Teriyaki Tuna on Low-carb	399	22	29	18	29
Teriyaki Tuna on Wheat	417	22	31	5	28
Teriyaki Tuna on White	427	22	34	3	27
Thai Peanut Chicken on Low-carb	378	15	27	17	31
Thai Peanut Chicken on Wheat	395	16	30	4	30
Thai Peanut Chicken on White	405	16	33	3	30
Thai Peanut Tofu on Low-carb	218	9	28	18	11
Thai Peanut Tofu on Wheat	236	9	31	5	10
Thai Peanut Tofu on White	246	9	34	3	10
Tofu Tahini on Low- Carb	220	9	28	18	11
Tofu Tahini on Wheat	238	9	30	5	10
Tofu Tahini on White	248	10	33	3	10
Tuna Club on Low-carb	385	21	26	17	29
Tuna Club on Wheat	403	21	29	4	28
Tuna Club on White	413	22	32	3	28
Turkey Saga on Low-carb	329	17	29	18	20
Turkey Saga on Wheat	348	17	32	5	19

RESTAURANTS & FAST-FOOD CHAINS

Roly Poly (cont.)

	Cal	Fat	Cbs	Fbr	Prtn
Sandwiches Special (cont.)					
Turkey Saga on White	357	17	35	3	19
Westport Club on Wheat	382	19	32	5	24
Westport Club on White	392	19	35	3	24
Soup: Classic Soups					
Baja Chicken Enchilada	210	14	12	2	10
Broccoli Cheddar	160	11	10	1	6
Clam Chowder	150	5	12	1	4
Classic Chili	160	5	18	6	9
Harvest Mushroom Bisque	90	5	11	1	3
Loaded Baked Potato	170	11	15	1	4
Mexican Style Chicken Tortilla	130	3	18	3	8
• Old Fashioned Chicken Noodle	70	2	11	1	4
Roasted Garlic Tomato	160	11	12	1	3
Seafood Bisque	217	14	12	1	8
Soup: Classic Vegetarian Soups					
Corn & Green Chile Bisque	130	7	14	1	3
• Garden Vegetable	60	0	12	2	3
Spring Asparagus	130	9	10	1	4
Sweet Items					
Apple Strudel	393	19	51	3	9
Chocolate Cheesecake	456	24	58	4	8
• Fruit Melt	289	14	36	1	6
Peach Granola	456	24	58	4	8
• Rock N Roll Sweet Roly	456	24	58	4	8

Round Table Pizza

	Cal	Fat	Cbs	Fbr	Prtn
Appetizers and Sandwiches					
Buffalo Wings, 12 wings	860	62	10	0	67
Buffalo Wings, 6 wings	420	28	2	0	38
Chicken Club, 353 g	760	34	67	3	46
Garlic Bread w/ Cheese, 189 g	630	33	59	2	21
Garlic Bread, 132 g	470	21	59	2	11
Garlic Parmesan Twists, 3 pcs.	500	14	73	3	17
• Garlic Parmesan Twists, 6 pcs.	1010	29	146	6	34
Ham Club, 375 g	810	37	76	3	36
Honey BBQ Wings, 12 wings	930	55	27	0	71
• Honey BBQ Wings, 6 wings	390	25	8	0	35
RT Pizza Sandwich, 271 g	690	34	65	4	30
RT Veggie Sandwich, 306 g	680	29	79	5	23
Turkey Club, 375 g	800	37	75	3	39
Turkey Sante Fe, 369 g	850	44	74	4	37
Large Cheese					
Original Crust, 1 slice	210	8	25	1	11
• Pan Crust, 1 slice	290	10	38	2	13
• Skinny Crust, 1 slice	180	8	18	1	10
Large Chicken & Garlic Gourmet™					
Original Crust, 1 slice	230	9	25	1	13
• Pan Crust, 1 slice	320	11	39	2	16
• Skinny Crust, 1 slice	200	9	19	1	12
Large Chicken Smokehouse					
Original Crust, 1 slice	250	10	26	1	14
• Pan Crust, 1 slice	360	15	40	2	16
• Skinny Crust, 1 slice	220	10	20	1	13

(•= most healthy •= least healthy) **RESTAURANTS & FAST-FOOD • 301**

RESTAURANTS & FAST-FOOD CHAINS

Round Table Pizza (cont.)	Cal	Fat	Cbs	Fbr	Prtn
Large Gourmet Veggie™					
Original Crust, 1 slice	220	9	26	2	10
• Pan Crust, 1 slice	310	10	40	2	13
• Skinny Crust, 1 slice	190	8	20	1	9
Large Guinevere's Garden Delight®					
Original Crust, 1 slice	210	7	26	2	10
• Pan Crust, 1 slice	290	9	39	2	13
• Skinny Crust, 1 slice	170	7	20	2	9
Large Hawaiian					
Original Crust, 1 slice	210	7	26	1	11
• Pan Crust, 1 slice	290	9	39	2	14
• Skinny Crust, 1 slice	180	7	20	1	10
Large Italian Garlic Supreme™					
Original Crust, 1 slice	270	14	25	1	12
• Pan Crust, 1 slice	360	16	39	2	15
• Skinny Crust, 1 slice	240	14	18	1	11
Large King Arthur's Supreme®					
Original Crust, 1 slice	270	14	26	2	12
• Pan Crust, 1 slice	340	14	39	2	15
• Skinny Crust, 1 slice	240	14	19	1	11
Large Maui Zaui™ (Polynesian Sauce)					
Original Crust, 1 slice	250	9	28	1	12
• Pan Crust, 1 slice	330	11	42	2	15
• Skinny Crust, 1 slice	210	9	21	1	11
Large Maui Zaui™ (Zesty Red Sauce)					
Original Crust, 1 slice	240	9	27	1	12
• Pan Crust, 1 slice	320	11	40	2	16
• Skinny Crust, 1 slice	210	9	20	1	12
Large Montague's All Meat Marvel®					
Original Crust, 1 slice	300	17	25	1	13
• Pan Crust, 1 slice	350	16	38	2	15
• Skinny Crust, 1 slice	260	16	18	1	12
Large Pepperoni					
Original Crust, 1 slice	240	11	24	1	11
• Pan Crust, 1 slice	320	12	38	2	14
• Skinny Crust, 1 slice	210	11	18	1	10
Large Smokehouse Combo					
Original Crust, 1 slice	270	13	26	1	13
• Pan Crust, 1 slice	360	15	40	2	16
• Skinny Crust, 1 slice	240	13	20	1	12
Large Ulti-Meat					
Original Crust, 1 slice	290	15	24	1	13
• Pan Crust, 1 slice	370	17	37	2	16
• Skinny Crust, 1 slice	260	15	18	1	13
Large Wombo Combo					
Original Crust, 1 slice	270	12	26	2	13
• Pan Crust, 1 slice	350	14	39	2	16
• Skinny Crust, 1 slice	230	12	19	1	12
Salads					
• Caesar Salad Small, 128 g	140	7	11	2	6
Garden Salad Small, 177 g	100	4	14	2	2
• Side of Chicken, 57 g	70	1	1	0	14

RESTAURANTS & FAST-FOOD CHAINS

Rubio's

	Cal	Fat	Cbs	Fbr	Prtn
Burritos					
Baja Grill Burrito Carnitas, 379 g	660	32	57	6	36
Baja Grill Burrito Chicken, 379 g	650	28	58	6	44
Baja Grill Burrito Steak, 379 g	650	29	57	6	43
Bean & Cheese Burrito, 371 g	810	37	87	5	32
Big Burrito Especial Carnitas, 522 g	940	42	107	6	36
Big Burrito Especial Chicken, 522 g	940	38	107	6	44
Big Burrito Especial Steak, 522 g	940	39	106	6	43
Fish Burrito, 379 g	770	45	76	7	19
Grilled Mesquite Shrimp Burrito, 368 g	780	40	72	4	30
Mahi Mahi Burrito, 369 g	720	39	55	5	40
Make it a Wet Burrito, 132 g	120	8	9	1	4
Classic Taco Plates					
Original #1 (2 Fish Tacos), 429 g	900	42	110	7	20
Pesky (2 Especial Fish Tacos), 485 g	1040	53	113	9	27
Two Carnitas Tacos, 429 g	780	29	100	8	31
Two Chicken Tacos, 457 g	930	42	101	8	37
• Two Steak Tacos, 429 g	780	27	100	8	36
Enchilada & Fish Taco					
• Carnitas Enchilada & Fish Taco, 594 g	1170	53	128	10	45
• Cheese Enchilada & Fish Taco, 559 g	1120	51	127	10	39
Chicken Enchilada & Fish Taco, 594 g	1170	51	128	10	48
Enchilada Plates					
• Carnitas, 626 g	1240	58	124	9	58
• Cheese, 555 g	1140	53	122	9	46
Chicken, 626 g	1240	54	124	9	65
HealthMex®					
Chicken Burrito, 359 g	550	16	70	6	34
Chicken Salad, 471 g	270	3	36	5	26
Chicken Taco, 132 g	150	2	21	1	12
• Mahi Mahi Burrito, 374 g	560	16	69	6	38
Mahi Mahi Salad, 484 g	270	3	35	7	28
Mahi Mahi Taco, 139 g	150	2	21	1	12
Kid's Meals					
Add Black Beans, 103 g	100	2	14	2	6
Add Chips, 43 g	210	11	28	3	3
Add Mini Churro, 23 g	80	4	11	0	1
Add Pinto Beans, 103 g	110	3	19	7	3
Add Rice, 57 g	80	0	17	1	1
• Bean & Cheese Burrito, 258 g	570	21	71	9	21
Cheese Quesadilla, 116 g	360	18	32	1	17
Chicken Bites, 5 pcs.	230	8	19	1	19
• Chicken Taquitos, 2 pcs.	210	9	18	2	13
World Famous Fish Taco, 115 g	300	16	26	2	10
Quesadillas, Etc.					
Cheese Quesadilla, 338 g	890	59	55	5	35
Chicken Quesadilla, 423 g	1000	61	57	5	58
• Chicken Taquitos (3), 186 g	380	21	35	5	18
Nachos Grande Chicken, 536 g	1450	83	117	5	62
• Nachos Grande Steak, 536 g	1450	84	116	5	61
Nachos Grande, 451 g	1330	81	115	5	39
Shrimp Quesadilla, 446 g	1000	63	56	5	51
Steak Quesadilla, 423 g	1000	62	56	5	57

RESTAURANTS & FAST-FOOD CHAINS

Rubio's (cont.)

	Cal	Fat	Cbs	Fbr	Prtn
Salads & Bowls					
Baja Caesar Salad, 439 g	520	40	15	4	31
Chipotle Ranch Salad Chicken, 489 g	530	35	27	7	30
Chopped Salad Chicken, 512 g	600	35	37	8	36
• Fiesta Salad Chicken, 431 g	500	35	14	6	35
• Grande Bowl Chicken, 520 g	780	43	56	9	41
Sides					
Black Beans, large, 347 g	400	3	68	9	23
Black Beans, small, 96 g	110	1	19	3	7
Brownie, 85 g	430	22	57	2	6
Chips, large, 113 g	580	29	74	9	7
Chips, small, 43 g	220	11	28	3	3
Churro, 45 g	170	8	22	0	2
• Guacamole & Chips, 265 g	790	49	85	16	10
Make It A Combo (small beans & chips), 139 g	350	13	53	N/A	4
Pinto Beans, large, 347 g	460	4	90	5	14
Pinto Beans, small, 96 g	130	2	25	1	4
Rice, large, 227 g	390	21	48	2	4
• Rice, small, 57 g	100	5	12	0	1
Street Tacos					
Carnitas, 69 g	110	4	9	1	8
Chicken, 69 g	110	3	9	1	11
Steak, 69 g	110	3	9	1	10
Tacos					
Carnitas Taco, 136 g	210	9	21	1	12
Chicken Taco, 151 g	280	15	22	1	15
• Especial Fish Taco, 170 g	350	22	28	2	11
Mahi Mahi Taco, 158 g	280	15	22	2	15
Shrimp Taco, 149 g	290	16	23	2	13
• Steak Taco, 136 g	210	8	21	1	15
World Famous Fish Taco, 142 g	290	16	27	1	8

Ruby Tuesday

	Cal	Fat	Cbs	Fbr	Prtn
Appetizers					
• Asian Dumplings, 1/4 portion	110	5	11	1	N/A
Chicken Quesadilla, 1/4 portion	228	14	12	1	N/A
• Classic Sampler, 1/4 portion	338	19	25	2	N/A
Fire Wings, 1/4 portion	219	16	2	1	N/A
Fresh Avocado Quesadilla, 1/4 portion	172	13	12	1	N/A
Fresh Guacamole Dip, 1/4 portion	288	18	24	7	N/A
Grand Sampler, 1/4 portion	324	19	17	2	N/A
Jumbo Lump Crab Cake, 1/4 portion	111	8	3	1	N/A
Queso Dip & Chips, 1/4 portion	308	19	25	2	N/A
Southwestern Spring Rolls, 1/4 portion	176	10	14	1	N/A
Spinach Artichoke Dip, 1/4 portion	332	20	27	3	N/A
Thai Phoon Shrimp, 1/4 portion	194	13	11	1	N/A
Wisconsin Cheddar Fries, 1/4 portion	302	17	25	2	N/A
Chicken					
Bistro Barbecue Chicken	618	29	13	0	N/A
• Chicken & Broccoli Pasta	1713	95	105	13	N/A
Chicken Bella	626	36	11	3	N/A
• Chicken Fresco	464	23	6	1	N/A
Chicken Oscar	469	22	3	1	N/A
Gourmet Chicken Pot Pie	1411	111	37	5	N/A

Ruby Tuesday (cont.)	Cal	Fat	Cbs	Fbr	Prtn
Chicken (cont.)					
Parmesan Chicken Pasta	1654	96	115	11	N/A
Desserts					
Blondie	677	31	91	2	N/A
Chocolate Chip Cookie	320	15	40	2	N/A
Chocolate Tall cake	605	21	93	1	N/A
Double Chocolate Cake	979	48	118	6	N/A
Gourmet Cookie & Ice Cream	800	37	103	2	N/A
Strawberry Cream Puff	840	40	100	3	N/A
White Chocolate Macadamia Nut Cookie	340	20	38	1	N/A
Fresh Combinations					
Broccoli & Cheese Soup	443	34	20	1	N/A
Chicken & Broccoli Quiche	735	58	23	1	N/A
Gourmet Chicken Pot Pie	985	80	29	3	N/A
Ruby Minis, 2 pcs.	655	45	36	1	N/A
Turkey Minis, 2 pcs.	517	33	32	1	N/A
White Bean Chicken Chili	223	7	18	7	N/A
Handcrafted Burgers					
Alpine Swiss Burger	1374	98	60	6	N/A
Avocado Chicken Burger	864	51	47	5	N/A
Avocado Turkey Burger	1034	63	49	7	N/A
Bacon Cheeseburger	1193	85	48	4	N/A
Bella Turkey Burger	1145	71	56	6	N/A
Bison Bacon Cheeseburger	1072	71	48	5	N/A
Bison Burger	892	57	48	5	N/A
Blue Cheese Burger	1280	93	48	4	N/A
Buffalo Chicken Burger	1041	71	62	5	N/A
Chicken BLT Burger	981	63	59	5	N/A
Classic Cheeseburger	1103	78	48	4	N/A
Hickory Chicken Burger	863	47	59	3	N/A
Ruby's Classic Burger	1013	71	48	4	N/A
Smokehouse Burger	1392	96	71	6	N/A
Turkey Burger	812	45	49	4	N/A
Veggie Burger	953	52	60	15	N/A
Kids' Meals					
Chicken Breast & broccoli	276	12	5	3	N/A
Chicken Tenders & fries	714	31	74	7	N/A
Chop Steak & mashed potatoes	517	37	21	3	N/A
Fried Shrimp & fries	571	21	71	6	N/A
Grilled Cheese & fries	929	50	88	7	N/A
Macaroni & Cheese	595	33	54	0	N/A
Mini Cheeseburgers & fries	907	49	82	5	N/A
Pasta with Marinara	314	4	53	7	N/A
Turkey Minis & fries	893	47	82	6	N/A
Premium Burgers					
Jumbo Lump Crab Burger	755	45	57	6	N/A
Triple Prime Burger	883	56	50	3	N/A
Triple Prime Cheddar Burger	1063	70	50	3	N/A
Ribs: Premium Baby Back Ribs					
Classic BBQ , Full Rack	986	65	29	0	N/A
Classic BBQ , Half Rack	493	32	14	0	N/A
Memphis Dry Rub , Full Rack	1070	79	7	0	N/A
Memphis Dry Rub , Half Rack	535	40	3	0	N/A

RESTAURANTS & FAST-FOOD CHAINS

Ruby Tuesday (cont.)

	Cal	Fat	Cbs	Fbr	Prtn
Ruby Minis					
Ruby Minis, 4 pcs.	1310	90	72	2	N/A
Salads					
Carolina Chicken Salad	1022	72	38	7	N/A
Club House Salad	896	60	30	8	N/A
Seafood					
Asian Glazed Salmon	424	27	7	0	N/A
• Creole Catch	312	16	0	0	N/A
Lemon Grilled Salmon	458	32	1	0	N/A
Louisiana Fried Shrimp	423	17	38	2	N/A
New Orleans Seafood	495	31	2	0	N/A
• Parmesan Shrimp Pasta	1221	64	98	10	N/A
Side Items					
Baked Potato (w/ butter & sour cream)	459	19	51	11	N/A
• Baked Potato (w/ cheese & bacon)	614	32	52	11	N/A
Brown Rice Pilaf (w/ cheese & tomatoes)	221	6	33	2	N/A
Creamy Mashed Cauliflower	153	10	9	5	N/A
Fresh Hot Fries	359	13	52	5	N/A
Fresh Steamed Broccoli	129	8	5	3	N/A
• Premium Baby Green Beans	85	5	5	3	N/A
Sautéed Baby Portabella Mushrooms	173	14	7	2	N/A
Toast	160	9	16	1	N/A
Tomato & Mozzarella Salad	112	7	6	1	N/A
Tossed Caesar Salad	174	15	5	2	N/A
White Cheddar Mashed Potatoes	274	16	21	3	N/A
Steaks					
• Peppercorn Mushroom Sirloin, 9 oz.	604	36	14	2	N/A
• Petite Sirloin, 7 oz.	206	5	2	0	N/A
Premium Aged Prime Sirloin, 12 oz.	544	30	0	0	N/A
Rib Eye, 9 oz.	591	35	5	1	N/A
Top Sirloin, 9 oz	256	6	2	0	N/A

Runza

	Cal	Fat	Cbs	Fbr	Prtn
Chicken Sandwiches					
• BBQ Chicken - Crispy, 196 g	517	19	56	4	30
BBQ Chicken - Grilled, 192 g	392	9	46	4	31
Smothered Chicken - Crispy, 213 g	497	19	52	5	30
• Smothered Chicken - Grilled, 207 g	381	10	41	3	31
Special Deluxe Chicken - Crispy, 201 g	483	19	51	4	27
Special Deluxe Chicken - Grilled, 207 g	382	12	40	3	29
Desserts					
Blue Raspberry Runza® Slushie™ - medium, 519 g	302	0	76	0	0
Cake Cone w/ Choco Ice Cream, 146 g	250	7	38	0	5
Cake Cone w/ Swirl Ice Cream, 146 g	250	7	38	0	5
Cake Cone w/ Vanilla Ice Cream, 146 g	250	7	38	0	5
Cherry Runza® Slushie™ - medium, 519 g	302	0	76	0	0
Choco Ice Cream Dish - medium, 140 g	230	7	33	0	5
Chocolate Shake - regular, 341 g	511	16	80	0	11
Chocolate Sundae, 168 g	300	7	51	0	5
Cookie Dough Sundae, 176 g	360	11	57	0	6
Crushed Butterfinger® Topping - regular, 41 g	179	7	29	0	2
Crushed Oreo® Topping - regular, 29 g	140	6	20	1	1
Grape Runza® Slushie™ - medium, 519 g	313	0	78	0	0
• Kid-size Cake Cone w/ Vanilla Ice Cream, 59 g	110	3	16	0	2

Runza (cont.)

	Cal	Fat	Cbs	Fbr	Prtn
Desserts (cont.)					
Mini M&M's® Topping - regular, 61 g	301	14	42	1	3
• Oreo® Cappuccino Shake - regular, 343 g	606	24	85	0	12
Pepsi® Runza® Slushie™ - medium, 519 g	224	0	60	0	0
Reeses® Mini Topping - regular, 58 g	297	15	34	1	7
Snickers® Topping - regular, 38 g	181	9	22	1	3
Strawberry Shake - regular, 314 g	471	16	72	0	10
Strawberry Sundae, 210 g	340	7	60	1	5
Swirl Ice Cream Dish - medium, 140 g	230	7	33	0	5
Turtle Sundae, 170 g	330	12	48	0	6
Vanilla Ice Cream Dish - medium, 140 g	230	7	33	0	5
Vanilla Shake - regular, 327 g	465	16	69	0	11
Waffle Cone w/ Choco Ice Cream, 146 g	270	7	42	1	5
Waffle Cone w/ Swirl Ice Cream, 146 g	270	7	42	1	5
Waffle Cone w/ Vanilla Ice Cream, 146 g	270	7	42	1	5
Dressings & Sauces					
Asian Sesame Ginger, 68 g	300	26	14	0	0
BBQ Sauce, 73 g	113	1	28	0	0
• Caesar, 71 g	408	45	3	0	3
Dorothy Lynch, 70 g	264	14	29	0	0
Honey Mustard, 49 g	238	22	10	0	0
Jalapeño Ranch, 65 g	276	28	2	0	2
Lite Italian, 70 g	84	5	10	0	0
Poppyseed, 74 g	390	36	18	0	0
Ranch, 67 g	299	32	5	0	0
• Raspberry Vinaigrette, 58 g	25	0	6	0	0
Reduced Calorie Ranch, 70 g	168	11	17	0	0
Fries & Onion Rings					
• French Fries - large, 196 g	625	35	70	8	7
French Fries - medium, 129 g	412	23	46	5	4
French Fries - small, 87 g	278	15	31	3	3
Frings®, 180 g	538	28	64	4	7
• Onion Ring Dip, 59 g	89	6	4	1	0
Onion Rings - large, 184 g	591	32	66	4	9
Onion Rings - medium, 115 g	369	20	41	2	5
Kids Meals (includes small fry, no drink)					
Kids Runza® Sandwich, 195 g	527	24	64	5	14
• Mini Corn Dogs (5), 79 g	276	17	25	1	6
• Mini Corn Dogs (10), 166 g	554	32	56	4	9
Polish Dog, 138 g	424	26	30	4	16
Legendary Hamburgers					
• 1/2 lb. Double Chzburger (The Runza® Way), 295 g	639	32	37	3	50
1/4 lb. Bacon Cheeseburger, 193 g	514	29	36	3	28
1/4 lb. Chzburger (The Runza® Way), 207 g	429	21	32	3	28
1/4 lb. French Onion Burger, 236 g	550	34	28	2	29
1/4 lb. Legend Supreme, 203 g	767	37	62	7	46
1/4 lb. Swiss Chz Mushroom, 174 g	448	25	36	3	21
Other Sandwiches/Variety					
Chicken Strips, 167 g	464	25	42	3	16
• Chicken Strips, 2 pcs.	186	10	11	0	13
Fish Sandwich, 178 g	492	24	50	2	19
Junior Cheeseburger, 133 g	327	17	28	3	17
Junior Chzburger (The Runza® Way), 149 g	306	14	30	3	16
Junior Swiss Mushroom Burger, 149 g	381	21	26	0	23

(• = most healthy • = least healthy) **RESTAURANTS & FAST-FOOD • 307**

RESTAURANTS & FAST-FOOD CHAINS

Runza (cont.)

	Cal	Fat	Cbs	Fbr	Prtn
Other Sandwiches/Variety (cont.)					
• Small Hamburger (plain), 168 g	497	24	55	5	16
Other					
American Cheese, 19 g	58	4	1	0	4
• Bacon, 20 g	122	11	0	0	5
Mayo, 9 g	35	3	1	0	0
• Mushrooms, 38 g	7	0	1	1	1
Swiss Cheese, 19 g	70	5	0	0	4
The Runza® Way, 68 g	25	0	5	1	1
OvenStuff'd® Sandwiches					
Cheese, 234 g	555	21	66	4	26
• Original, 215 g	497	17	65	4	22
• Swiss Cheese Mushroom, 275 g	589	25	68	8	23
Salads (w/o Dressing)					
Chicken Caesar w/ Croutons, 350 g	300	13	14	4	32
Shanghai Chicken, 370 g	300	7	32	7	28
• Side Salad, 129 g	28	1	4	2	2
Southwest Chicken w/ Salsa, 317 g	440	23	35	6	22
• Sweet Berry Chicken, 422 g	630	31	50	10	37
Tossed Salad w/ Crispy Chicken, 360 g	437	27	29	5	19
Tossed Salad w/ Croutons, 302 g	290	15	25	6	13
Tossed Salad w/ Grilled Chicken, 336 g	276	13	13	4	26
Soups					
Boston Clam Chowder - Bowl, 276 g	321	23	33	1	6
Boston Clam Chowder - Cup, 180 g	209	15	22	1	4
Broccoli Cheese - Bowl, 310 g	361	27	35	1	8
Broccoli Cheese - Cup, 209 g	243	18	23	1	5
Cauliflower Cheese - Bowl, 287 g	334	26	32	1	4
Cauliflower Cheese - Cup, 162 g	189	15	18	1	2
Chicken Noodle - Bowl, 305 g	171	5	21	1	11
Chicken Noodle - Cup, 191 g	107	3	13	1	7
Homemade Chili - Bowl, 334 g	309	10	26	10	29
Homemade Chili - Cup, 218 g	202	6	17	6	19
Potato w/ Bacon - Bowl, 296 g	306	20	40	3	3
Potato w/ Bacon - Cup, 180 g	186	12	24	2	2
Vegetable Beef - Bowl, 270 g	105	3	13	2	6
• Vegetable Beef - Cup, 191 g	74	2	9	2	4
Vegetable Cheese - Bowl, 296 g	332	22	28	3	6
Vegetable Cheese - Cup, 209 g	234	15	20	2	5
• Wisconsin Cheese - Bowl, 299 g	425	35	36	1	5
Wisconsin Cheese - Cup, 194 g	276	23	23	1	3

Sammy's Woodfired Pizza

	Cal	Fat	Cbs	Fbr	Prtn
Chinese Chicken Salad	450	12	47	8	40
Chopped Chicken Salad	425	11	30	6	52
• Fresh Tomato Basil Soup	110	5	10	3	7
Oak Roasted Salmon on Ponzu Salad	470	19	21	5	50
Roast Chicken Pesto Wrap	480	20	22	5	52
• Tomato Angel Hair Pasta	700	18	115	9	24

Samurai Sam's Teriyaki Grill

	Cal	Fat	Cbs	Fbr	Prtn
Other Bowls - Regular					
• Low Carb Bowl, 326 g	230	4	16	5	33
Spicy Beef 'n Broccoli Bowl - Brown Rice, 475 g	580	14	85	7	26

RESTAURANTS & FAST-FOOD CHAINS

Samurai Sam's Teriyaki Grill (cont.)	Cal	Fat	Cbs	Fbr	Prtn
Other Bowls - Regular (cont.)					
Spicy Beef 'n Broccoli Bowl, 475 g	620	13	97	3	26
Sumo Bowl - Brown Rice, 808 g	1022	23	111	9	81
Sumo Bowl - White Rice, 808 g	1083	21	128	3	81
Sides, Salads & Kids Meals					
Asian Noodle Soup, 208 g	89	2	14	1	5
Chinese Ginger Dressing, 28 g	85	5	9	0	0
Chinese Salad Dressing, 100 g	230	7	44	0	0
Crab Rangoon, 3 pcs.	210	12	20	1	7
Grilled Chicken Egg Roll, 85 g	150	7	17	1	7
Kid's Bowl, White Chicken - Brown Rice, 198 g	262	3	37	2	20
Kid's Bowl, White Chicken - White Rice, 198 g	282	2	43	0	20
Oriental Chicken Salad, 283 g	220	4	9	3	36
Oriental Dressing, 28 g	70	2	12	0	0
Sesame Garden Toss Salad, 475 g	490	13	57	6	41
• Side Salad, 57 g	10	0	2	1	1
Teriyaki Sauce (on the side), 28 g	40	0	9	0	1
Sweet & Sour Bowls - Regular					
Dark Chicken - Brown Rice, 665 g	570	12	84	9	32
• Dark Chicken, 665 g	610	10	96	6	32
White Chicken - Brown Rice, 665 g	540	6	85	9	37
White Chicken, 665 g	580	5	96	6	37
Teriyaki Bowls - Regular					
Dark Chicken - Brown Rice, 411 g	500	11	68	5	31
Dark Chicken - Reg, 411 g	540	10	79	2	31
Dark Chicken & Shrimp - Brown Rice, 404 g	451	7	67	5	29
Dark Chicken & Shrimp, 404 g	492	6	78	2	29
Dark Chicken & Steak , 411 g	540	9	83	2	27
Dark Chkn & Steak - Brown Rice, 411 g	490	10	71	5	27
Salmon - Brown Rice, 588 g	582	5	104	8	33
Salmon, 588 g	643	3	121	3	33
Shrimp - Brown Rice, 411 g	407	3	65	5	28
Steak - Brown Rice, 411 g	490	9	74	5	23
Steak & Shrimp Bowl - Brown Rice, 404 g	442	6	66	5	25
Steak & Shrimp Bowl, 404 g	483	5	77	2	26
Steak , 411 g	530	8	86	2	23
• Teriyaki Bowl White Chicken - Lrg, 581 g	740	6	114	2	52
• Veggie - Brown Rice, 369 g	323	2	69	7	8
Veggie, 369 g	363	1	81	3	8
White Chicken - Brown Rice, 411 g	470	5	68	5	36
White Chicken - Reg, 411 g	520	4	79	2	37
White Chicken & Shrimp - Brown, 404 g	437	4	67	5	32
White Chicken & Shrimp, 404 g	478	3	78	2	32
White Chicken & Steak, 411 g	520	6	83	2	30
White Chkn & Steak - Brown Rice, 411 g	480	7	71	5	30
Wraps					
Dark Chicken - Brown Rice, 391 g	650	17	90	9	34
Dark Chicken & Steak - Brown Rice, 391 g	630	14	93	9	33
Dark Chicken & Steak, 391 g	650	13	98	8	33
• Dark Chicken, 391 g	670	16	95	8	34
Steak - Brown Rice, 391 g	630	15	95	9	27
Steak, 391 g	650	14	101	8	27
• Veggie - Brown Rice, 320 g	490	9	89	10	13
Veggie, 320 g	510	8	94	8	14

RESTAURANTS & FAST-FOOD CHAINS

Samurai Sam's Teriyaki Grill (cont.)

	Cal	Fat	Cbs	Fbr	Prtn
Wraps (cont.)					
White Chicken - Brown Rice, 391 g	620	12	90	9	39
White Chicken & Steak - Brn Rice, 391 g	628	13	89	9	33
White Chicken & Steak, 391 g	649	13	95	8	33
White Chicken, 391 g	640	11	96	8	39
Yakisoba Bowls					
Dark Chicken & Steak, 570 g	825	22	113	6	54
• Dark Chicken, 570 g	842	24	114	6	60
Steak, 570 g	809	20	112	6	48
• Veggie, 400 g	509	8	110	6	19
White Chicken & Steak, 570 g	801	17	113	6	59
White Chicken, 570 g	794	14	114	6	70
Yakisoba Bowl - Shrimp, 570 g	677	10	110	6	55

Schlotzsky's

	Cal	Fat	Cbs	Fbr	Prtn
Buns / Tortilla					
Dark Rye, Medium	330	2	68	3	11
• Dark Rye, Small	230	1	47	2	7
Flour Tortilla	300	9	47	1	8
• Jalapeño Cheese, Medium	340	4	63	2	12
Jalapeño Cheese, Small	230	3	44	2	8
Sourdough, Medium	330	2	67	2	11
Sourdough, Small	230	2	46	2	7
Wheat, Medium	340	3	67	4	12
Wheat, Small	230	2	46	3	8
Chips					
Barbecue, 2 oz. bag	220	12	25	1	3
Cracked Pepper, 2 oz. bag	220	12	25	1	3
Jalapeño, 2 oz. bag	220	12	25	1	3
Regular (Plain), 2 oz. bag	220	12	25	1	3
Salt & Vinegar, 2 oz. bag	220	12	25	1	3
Sour Cream & Onion, 2 oz. bag	220	12	25	1	3
Desserts					
Brownie	415	24	47	2	6
• Carrot Cake	717	42	80	3	7
Cheesecake	350	23	30	1	6
Cookie, Chocolate Chip	162	7	24	1	2
Cookie, Fudge Chocolate Chip	164	8	22	1	2
• Cookie, Oatmeal Raisin	148	5	24	1	2
Cookie, Sugar	154	7	22	0	2
Cookie, White Chocolate Macadamia	170	8	22	0	2
Drinks					
Lemonade Medium, 20 oz.	243	0	45	0	0
Raspberry Lemonade Medium, 20 oz.	243	0	45	0	0
Gourmet Pizzas					
• Baby Spinach Salad	471	8	83	4	18
Bacon Tomato & Portobello	614	22	76	4	29
BBQ Chicken & Jalapeño	684	16	98	3	57
Combination Special	639	25	76	4	27
Double Cheese	597	21	74	3	27
Fresh Tomato & Pesto	556	19	73	3	25
Grilled Chicken & Pesto	652	22	74	4	59
Mediterranean	560	20	74	4	21
Pepperoni & Double Cheese	686	30	74	3	31

Schlotzsky's (cont.)	Cal	Fat	Cbs	Fbr	Prtn
Gourmet Pizzas (cont.)					
Smoked Turkey & Jalapeño	642	19	78	4	39
• Thai Chicken	693	22	85	4	58
Vegetarian Special	540	17	74	4	22
Kid's Meals					
Cheese Pizza	479	13	73	3	18
Cheese Sandwich	397	15	48	2	17
Ham & Cheese Sandwich	427	16	49	2	21
• Pepperoni Pizza	523	17	73	3	20
Turkey Sandwich	298	5	49	2	15
Oven-Toasted Sandwiches					
• Albuquerque Turkey, Medium	964	40	80	6	52
Albuquerque Turkey, Small	687	36	56	4	36
Angus Beef & Provolone, Medium	757	29	80	4	41
Angus Beef & Provolone, Small	503	19	56	3	27
Angus Corned Beef Reuben, Medium	918	41	78	5	59
• Angus Corned Beef Reuben, Small	331	28	54	3	40
Angus Corned Beef, Medium	582	13	77	6	40
Angus Corned Beef, Small	395	9	53	4	27
Angus Pastrami & Swiss, Medium	905	36	82	6	64
Angus Pastrami & Swiss, Small	611	24	56	4	43
Angus Pastrami Reuben, Medium	918	40	78	5	61
Angus Pastrami Reuben, Small	629	27	54	3	41
Angus Roast Beef & Cheese, Medium	783	33	73	4	47
Angus Roast Beef & Cheese, Small	538	22	50	3	33
BLT, Medium	543	18	74	4	22
BLT, Small	364	12	50	2	14
Cheese The Original®-Style, Medium	790	38	74	4	39
Cheese The Original®-Style, Small	566	28	51	3	28
Chicken & Pesto, Medium	564	14	72	4	40
Chicken & Pesto, Small	387	10	50	3	27
Chicken Breast, Medium	509	6	77	5	38
Chicken Breast, Small	345	4	52	3	26
Chipotle Chicken, Medium	540	12	72	4	38
Chipotle Chicken, Small	379	10	47	3	27
Chipotle Grilled Chicken, Medium	578	13	76	4	80
Chipotle Grilled Chicken, Small	405	10	50	3	56
Deluxe The Original®-Style, Medium	954	46	78	4	55
Deluxe The Original®-Style, Small	742	38	55	3	43
Dijon Chicken, Medium	576	11	79	8	44
Dijon Chicken, Small	391	7	54	5	30
Dijon Grilled Chicken, Medium	614	12	83	9	86
Dijon Grilled Chicken, Small	417	8	57	6	58
Fresh Veggie, Medium	483	12	77	6	18
Fresh Veggie, Small	355	10	52	4	14
Grilled Chicken & Pesto, Medium	603	15	76	5	82
Grilled Chicken & Pesto, Small	413	10	52	3	56
Grilled Chicken Breast, Medium	545	7	80	5	80
Grilled Chicken Breast, Small	372	5	55	3	55
Ham & Cheese The Original®-Style, Med.	731	27	78	4	44
Ham & Cheese The Original®-Style, Small	512	19	54	3	31
Homestyle Tuna, Medium	596	20	73	5	30
Homestyle Tuna, Small	410	14	51	4	21
Mediterranean Tuna, Medium	536	11	76	6	31

RESTAURANTS & FAST-FOOD CHAINS

Schlotzsky's (cont.)

	Cal	Fat	Cbs	Fbr	Prtn
Oven-Toasted Sandwiches (cont.)					
Mediterranean Tuna, Small	363	8	52	4	21
Santa Fe Chicken, Medium	619	15	76	5	45
Santa Fe Chicken, Small	425	10	53	4	31
Santa Fe Grilled Chicken, Medium	657	16	80	6	87
Santa Fe Grilled Chicken, Small	452	11	55	3	59
Smoked Turkey Breast, Medium	500	7	76	4	33
Smoked Turkey Breast, Small	345	5	53	2	23
Smoked Turkey Reuben, Medium	889	37	83	5	56
Smoked Turkey Reuben, Small	609	25	58	3	38
Texas Schlotzsky's™, Medium	756	31	73	4	44
Texas Schlotzsky's™, Small	540	23	51	2	32
The Original®, Medium	770	34	76	4	31
The Original®, Small	563	27	52	3	28
Turkey & Guacamole, Medium	552	12	80	6	34
Turkey & Guacamole, Small	364	7	54	4	22
Turkey Bacon Club, Medium	770	29	76	5	52
Turkey Bacon Club, Small	562	23	53	4	36
Turkey The Original®-Style, Medium	815	33	78	4	51
Turkey The Original®-Style, Small	596	26	54	3	37
Panini					
Classic Swiss & Tomato	624	26	63	1	33
Grilled Chicken Romano	539	15	61	1	57
• Mozzarella & Portobello	485	15	63	2	24
• Panini Italiano	736	32	67	2	43
Smoked Ham Crostini	644	23	67	2	39
Smoked Turkey & Guacamole	579	21	67	4	30
Salads					
Baby Spinach & Feta	197	15	10	4	10
Caesar	103	5	10	3	6
Chicken Salad	292	15	12	3	61
Fruit	100	0	25	2	1
Garden	51	1	12	4	3
Greek	137	8	13	4	7
Grilled Chicken Caesar	221	8	12	3	53
Ham & Turkey Chef	249	13	14	4	23
Pasta Salad	68	3	12	1	0
Potato Salad	242	13	29	3	3
• Side Salad	26	1	7	2	1
• Turkey Chef	293	15	15	4	30
Soups					
Boston Clam Chowder, 1 bowl	323	17	34	2	9
Boston Clam Chowder, 1 cup	217	11	23	1	6
Broccoli Cheese Soup, 1 bowl	303	20	20	1	7
Broccoli Cheese Soup, 1 cup	187	12	13	1	4
Chicken Tortilla Soup, 1 bowl	225	9	20	1	15
Chicken Tortilla Soup, 1 cup	150	6	13	1	10
Hearty Vegetable Beef Soup, 1 bowl	165	8	18	3	9
Hearty Vegetable Beef Soup, 1 cup	109	5	12	2	6
Old Fshnd Chicken Noodle Soup, 1 bowl	135	2	17	1	11
Old Fshnd Chicken Noodle Soup, 1 cup	90	2	11	1	7
Potato w/ Bacon, 1 bowl	271	13	38	3	4
Potato w/ Bacon, 1 cup	182	9	26	2	3
Timberline Chili, 1 bowl	345	12	39	12	23

RESTAURANTS & FAST-FOOD CHAINS

Schlotzsky's (cont.)

	Cal	Fat	Cbs	Fbr	Prtn
Soups (cont.)					
Timberline Chili, 1 cup	227	8	26	8	15
Vegetarian Vegetable Soup, 1 bowl	122	1	27	6	3
Vegetarian Vegetable Soup, 1 cup	85	1	19	4	2
Wisconsin Cheese Soup, 1 bowl	460	33	36	2	8
Wisconsin Cheese Soup, 1 cup	306	22	24	1	6
Wraps					
Asian Chicken	505	11	79	5	44
Parmesan Chicken Caesar	630	33	56	5	54
Wraps ~ Following Selections Vary by Restaurant					
Feta & Portobello	618	39	55	4	14
Grilled Chicken & Guacamole	667	36	58	7	50
Homestyle Tuna	480	20	55	4	21
Mediterranean Tuna	440	14	57	5	21

Sheetz

	Cal	Fat	Cbs	Fbr	Prtn
Bakery Cookies					
Chocolate Chunk Cookie, 1 cookie	209	11	27	0	2
Chocolate No-Bake, 1 cookie	180	8	24	1	4
Oatmeal Raisin Cookie, 1 cookie	194	7	29	1	4
Peanut Butter Cookie, 1 cookie	229	14	22	1	4
Peanut Butter No-Bake, 1 cookie	180	8	24	1	3
Pink Iced Cookie, 1 cookie	180	7	29	0	2
Raisin Filled Cookie, 1 cookie	220	8	35	0	2
Coffeez®					
Breakfast Blend, 16 g	10	0	2	0	0
Colombian, 16 g	10	0	2	0	0
House Blend, 16 g	10	0	2	0	0
Pumpkin Spice, 16 g	10	0	2	0	0
Serious Dark Roast, 16 g	10	0	2	0	0
Vanilla Nut Cream, 16 g	10	0	2	0	0
Winter Wonderland, 16 g	10	0	2	0	0
Coffeez® Creamer					
Amaretto Creamer, 1 g	40	2	7	0	0
Cinnamon Hazelnut Creamer, 1 g	40	2	7	0	0
French Vanilla Creamer, 1 g	45	2	6	0	0
Half & Half Creamer, 1 g	15	1	0	0	0
Mocha Creamer, 1 g	40	2	6	0	0
Cupo'ccino® / Hot Chocolate					
Almond Amaretto Cupo'ccino, 16 g	276	8	52	0	2
Blueberry Crumb Cupo'ccino, 16 g	280	8	52	0	0
Creme Burlee Cupo'ccino, 16 g	280	8	50	0	2
Fat Free French Vanilla Cupo'ccino, 16 g	140	0	34	0	2
French Vanilla Cupo'ccino, 16 g	284	10	50	0	2
Harvest Spice Cupo'ccino, 16 g	278	10	48	0	2
Hot Chocolate, 16 g	248	4	52	2	4
Mocha Canela, 16 g	240	4	52	2	4
PB Marshmallow Parfait, 16 g	260	7	52	0	0
Sugar Free Caramel Pecan, 16 g	224	7	40	0	2
Vanilla Chai Cupo'ccino, 16 g	277	8	51	1	3
Other Goodies					
Apple Turnover, 1 piece	340	6	33	1	3
Blueberry Muffin, 1 piece	377	2	53	2	7
Blueberry Pie, 1 piece	440	11	57	1	4

RESTAURANTS & FAST-FOOD CHAINS

Sheetz (cont.)

	Cal	Fat	Cbs	Fbr	Prtn
Other Goodies (cont.)					
Carrot Muffin, 1 piece	415	3	58	3	7
Cherry Pie, 1 piece	460	11	61	0	4
Cherry Turnover, 1 piece	341	6	34	1	4
Chocolate Chunk Brownie, 1 piece	350	10	41	2	4
• Cinnamon Coffee Cake, 1 piece	550	6	68	1	7
Cinnamon Roll, 1 piece	240	3	32	1	5
• Double Dutch Brownie, 1 piece	180	2	28	1	2
Eclair Pie, 1 piece	550	16	63	0	4
Espresso Brownie, 1 piece	430	16	48	3	5
Glazed Honey Bun, 1 piece	246	2	35	1	5
Golden Honey Bun, 1 piece	334	3	41	1	8
Honey Pecan Bar, 1 piece	420	12	31	2	3
Peach Pie, 1 piece	430	11	54	1	4
Peanut Butter Gobbz, 1 piece	550	7	58	0	4
Rasp White Chocolate Scone, 1 piece	411	6	54	1	5
Sweet Dough Swirls, 1 piece	310	3	48	2	7

Shoney's

	Cal	Fat	Cbs	Fbr	Prtn
Blue Plate Specials					
Baked Whitefish	507	8	58	0	48
Bread Service - 2 sl. w/ Oleo	263	7	43	0	7
Cajun Whitefish	480	10	56	0	40
Corn	173	9	23	1	2
Cranberry Sauce, 2 oz.	64	0	17	1	0
Grandma's Meatloaf - w/ Glaze	1092	47	93	1	72
Grandma's Meatloaf - w/ Gravy	1089	49	87	1	72
Green Beans	124	6	14	7	2
Grilled Liver 'n' Onions	711	22	79	2	49
Ham Steak Dinner	667	26	60	0	48
Macaroni & Cheese	241	14	18	1	10
• Mashed Potatoes w/ Gravy	223	10	30	1	4
• Original Country Fried Steak	1151	62	103	1	47
Roast Beef Platter	880	30	96	5	59
Breakfast					
Apple Cinnamon Jelly, 1 packet	35	0	9	0	0
Bacon, 3 strips	120	11	0	0	6
• Biscuits & Gravy	683	32	88	2	11
Biscuits, each	309	14	41	1	5
Creamer, Half & Half, 15 g	20	2	1	0	0
Grape Jelly, 1 packet	35	0	9	0	0
• Grits, 4 oz.	105	6	11	0	1
Hashbrowns, 4 oz.	238	15	25	0	3
Margarine, 1 packet	36	4	0	0	0
Sausage Patties, 1 pc.	209	18	1	0	11
Sourdough Toast w/ oleo, 2 slices	206	5	50	1	9
Strawberry Jam, 1 packet	35	0	9	0	0
Wheat Toast w/ oleo, 2 slices	188	9	24	4	5
White Toast w/ oleo, 2 slices	202	9	26	1	4
Breakfast Bar					
Bacon, 3 strips	120	11	0	0	6
Biscuits, each	309	14	41	1	5
Breakfast Bar Gravy, 2 oz.	54	4	5	0	0
Breakfast Potato Casserole, 4 oz.	43	4	1	0	2

RESTAURANTS & FAST-FOOD CHAINS

Shoney's (cont.)

	Cal	Fat	Cbs	Fbr	Prtn
Breakfast Bar (cont.)					
Cake, Apple Spice, 1 piece	120	13	13	0	1
Cake, Banana Bash, 1 piece	130	9	13	0	2
Cake, Brunch Berry, 1 piece	120	13	41	1	4
Cake, Buttercreme, 1 piece	130	8	15	0	1
Cake, Double Chocolate, 1 piece	130	8	15	1	1
Cake, Luscious Lemon, 1 piece	130	7	15	0	1
Cake, Orange Cranberry, 1 piece	120	0	19	0	1
Cake, Shortcake, 1 piece	50	0	11	0	1
Cheese Sauce, 1 tbsp.	59	3	7	0	0
Cheese, Cheddar, Fancy, 1 tbsp.	27	2	1	0	2
Chicken Wings, Mild, 1 piece	64	3	3	0	5
Cottage Cheese, 1 tbsp.	15	0	1	0	2
Donuts, Powdered, 1 piece	175	9	23	0	0
Eggs, Breakfast Bar, 1/2 cup	120	7	3	0	11
French Toast Sticks, 4 pieces	380	16	53	2	7
Grits, 4 oz.	105	6	11	0	1
Ham, Diced, 1 tbsp.	16	1	0	0	2
Hashbrowns, 4 oz.	238	15	25	0	3
Honey, 1 packet	45	0	11	0	0
Jelly, Apple/Cinnamon, 1 packet	35	0	9	0	0
Jelly, Grape, 1 packet	35	0	9	0	0
Jelly, Strawberry Jam, 1 packet	35	0	9	0	0
Margarine, Parkay, 1 tbsp.	101	11	0	0	0
Milk, White, 1/2 cup	74	4	6	0	4
Oleo, Country Crock Individuals	36	4	0	0	0
Omelet Topping, 1 oz.	22	1	2	0	0
Pancakes, each	318	7	56	0	7
Peppers, Jalapeño, Sliced, 1 tbsp.	2	0	0	0	0
Sauce, Hot Louisiana, 1 tsp	0	0	0	0	0
Sauce, Salsa, 1 tbsp	5	0	1	0	0
Sausage Patty, 1 piece	209	18	1	0	11
Smoked Sausage, 1 piece	180	16	3	0	7
Strawberry Banana Topping, 4 oz.	84	0	20	2	1
Syrup, Pancake & Waffle, 2 tbsp	80	0	21	0	0
Topping, Apple Crisp, 1/4 cup	87	0	22	0	0
Topping, Apple, 1/4 cup	96	0	24	0	0
Topping, Peach, 1/4 cup	54	0	13	1	0
Topping, Strawberry, 1/4 cup	158	0	41	0	0
Tortillas, Flour, 1 piece	133	3	21	1	4
Whipped Topping, 1 scoop	9	1	1	0	0
Breakfast Menu Selections					
All Star Breakfast (Add Options)	190	15	1	0	13
Big Eater Steak Breakfast (Add Options)	629	41	1	0	60
C/F Steak Breakfast	994	66	49	1	50
Deluxe Pancake Platter	1609	32	299	0	29
Half Stack Pancake Platter	932	14	187	0	15
Sausage/Biscuit, 1 pc.	539	34	42	1	16
Sunrise Breakfast	973	60	88	2	22
Burgers					
A-A Bacon Cheeseburger	891	49	44	3	66
All-American Burger	688	32	44	2	54
Famous Patty Melt	946	60	40	5	59
Half-O-Pound Burger	1351	53	130	1	89

(• = most healthy • = least healthy)

RESTAURANTS & FAST-FOOD CHAINS

Shoney's (cont.)

	Cal	Fat	Cbs	Fbr	Prtn
Burgers (cont.)					
Mushroom Swiss Burger	969	58	49	4	64
Chicken					
Charbroiled Blackened Chicken	831	26	100	1	47
• Charbroiled Chicken Breast	797	23	99	1	47
• Chicken Stir-Fry	1200	35	172	5	48
Fried Chicken Tenderloins	1157	61	121	6	30
Monterey Chicken	909	40	84	3	53
Smothered Chicken	891	34	90	2	56
Condiments/Add-Ons/Sides					
American Cheese, 1 slice	107	9	1	0	6
Bacon, 1 slice	40	4	0	0	2
BBQ Sauce, per 2 oz.	71	1	11	0	0
Catsup, 1 oz.	30	0	8	0	0
French Fries, 4 oz.	213	11	25	3	3
Grilled Onions, 2 oz.	67	6	4	1	1
Mayonnaise, 1 oz.	203	23	1	0	0
Monterey Jack Cheese, 1 slice	159	13	0	0	10
• Mustard, 1 oz.	21	1	2	1	1
• Onion Rings, 7 rings	500	15	83	4	12
Sauteed Mushrooms, 3 oz.	107	10	5	1	2
Secret Sauce, 1 2 oz.	168	16	4	N/A	0
Secret Sauce, per 2 oz.	168	16	4	N/A	0
Sweet & Sour Sauce, per, 2 oz.	67	0	17	0	0
Swiss Cheese, 1 slice	160	12	1	0	12
Desserts					
Apple Nutrasweet Pie	454	18	64	3	4
Apple Pie a la Mode	1203	53	174	9	12
Caramel Sundae	621	27	83	0	10
Cheesecake, 1 slice	364	26	23	0	5
Cherry Nutrasweet Pie	467	18	66	4	6
Chocolate Milk Shake	1082	51	141	4	25
Hot Fudge Sundae	599	30	75	0	10
• Original Strawberry Pie	332	17	45	2	2
Peach Nutrasweet Pie	479	21	68	4	4
Strawberry Milk Shake	1115	50	151	1	23
Strawberry Sundae	609	27	85	1	9
Ultimate Hot Fudge Cake	875	37	126	3	14
Vanilla Milk Shake	1076	50	140	0	23
Walnut Brownie a la Mode	576	34	61	0	10

Silver Mine Subs

	Cal	Fat	Cbs	Fbr	Prtn
8" Cold Sub Sandwiches (on white bread)					
California Gulch, 363 g	736	36	66	2	36
Caribou - medium, 350 g	704	34	59	2	40
Comstock, 352 g	657	28	55	1	41
• Dodge City, 362 g	1011	69	57	1	38
Georgetown, 331 g	660	29	59	2	40
King Bullion, 352 g	636	26	55	1	42
Lawless Leadville, 352 g	629	26	56	1	42
Mother Lode, 500 g	999	56	58	1	63
Silver City, 380 g	870	53	58	1	44
• Tombstone, 362 g	617	24	55	1	44
Virginia City, 352 g	645	28	58	1	40

Silver Mine Subs (cont.)	Cal	Fat	Cbs	Fbr	Prtn
8" Hot Sub Sandwiches (on white bread)					
Boomtown, 295 g	809	46	55	1	42
Coeur D'Alene, 280 g	490	10	52	0	42
Cripple Creek, 337 g	708	31	58	1	42
Frontier, 321 g	679	23	67	1	41
Homestake, 344 g	547	15	61	3	41
Silver Plume, 358 g	710	30	58	1	41
Steam Engine, 387 g	804	43	61	2	43
8" Lowfat Sub Sandwiches (on white bread)					
Caribou, 276 g	380	4	58	2	25
Comstock, 308 g	440	7	54	1	34
Homestake, 314 g	440	7	60	3	33
King Bullion, 308 g	419	5	54	1	35
Lawless Leadville, 308 g	412	5	56	1	34
Pikes Peak Or Bust, 216 g	327	4	58	2	13
Silver Plume, 314 g	493	9	58	1	34
Tombstone, 318 g	400	3	55	1	36
Virginia City, 308 g	428	7	57	1	33
Bread and Tortilla Wraps					
Wheat - 11", 149 g	373	5	69	5	16
Wheat - 5", 75 g	187	3	35	3	8
Wheat- 8" 112 g	280	4	52	4	12
White - 11", 149 g	373	3	69	0	16
White bead - 5", 75 g	186	1	35	0	8
White bread - 8", 112 g	280	2	52	0	12
White Flour Tortilla Wrap - 10", 71 g	210	5	36	3	6
Cheeses (For 8" subs)					
Cheddar Cheese, 30 g	118	10	1	0	8
Provolone Cheese, 30 g	107	9	1	0	8
Desserts					
Chocolate Chunk Cookie, 85 g	387	15	59	1	5
Deluxe Fudge Brownie, 85 g	409	21	54	2	5
Kid's Sub's (on white bread) & Kids Related Items					
Fruit Snacks, 25 g	80	0	19	0	1
Goldfish Crackers, 21 g	100	4	14	1	2
Ham & Cheddar Cheese, 50 g	113	8	1	0	10
Ham & Provolone Cheese, 45 g	88	6	1	0	9
Turkey & Cheddar Cheese, 50 g	105	7	1	0	11
Turkey & Provolone Cheese, 45 g	80	5	1	0	10
Meats (For 8" subs)					
Bacon - 3 strips, 21 g	101	8	0	0	8
Bacon - 9 strips (boomtown), 63 g	302	23	0	0	23
Grilled Chicken - Grilled Chkn Salad, 84 g	135	5	2	0	14
Grilled Chicken - Silver Plume, 126 g	203	7	3	0	21
Ham, 120 g	138	5	3	0	20
Meatballs, 140 g	383	32	2	0	22
Pepperoni, 84 g	420	39	2	0	15
Philly Cheesesteak, 126 g	150	5	6	2	21
Roast Beef - cold, 120 g	150	5	0	0	21
Roast Beef - hot, 168 g	210	8	0	0	30
Salami, 120 g	493	45	0	0	21
Tuna Salad, 134 g	336	26	11	1	16
Turkey, 120 g	107	1	0	0	24

RESTAURANTS & FAST-FOOD CHAINS

Silver Mine Subs (cont.)

	Cal	Fat	Cbs	Fbr	Prtn
Salads & Salad Related Items					
Blue Cheese Dressing - 1 packet, 43 g	180	19	2	0	1
Chef Salad, 208 g	82	2	6	1	12
Croutons - 1 package, 14 g	35	0	4	0	1
Fat Free Ranch Dressing - 1 packet, 43 g	60	0	14	0	1
Garden Salad, 148 g	21	0	5	1	1
Golden Italian Dressing - 1 packet, 43 g	110	10	3	0	0
Grilled Chicken Salad, 232 g	156	5	7	1	15
Honey Mustard, 42 g	182	15	10	0	0
• Ranch Dressing - 1 packet, 43 g	250	26	2	0	0
• Romaine Lettuce Mix - Side Salad, 56 g	6	0	1	0	0
Romaine Lettuce Mix , 98 g	10	0	2	1	1
Side Salad, 81 g	11	0	3	1	1
Sandwich Dressings					
Avocado, 18 g	34	2	3	1	0
Dijon Mustard, 15 g	15	0	1	1	0
Honey Mustard, 15 g	65	6	4	0	0
• Mayonnaise, 14 g	110	12	0	0	0
Oil, 5 g	40	5	0	0	0
Oregano, 0 g	0	0	0	0	0
Ranch Dressing, 14 g	75	8	1	0	0
• Vinegar, 5 g	0	0	0	0	0
Yellow Mustard, 15 g	0	0	0	0	0
Sides					
Fruit Cup, 113 g	80	0	19	1	1
• Potato Salad, 156 g	270	15	33	3	3
• Whole Dill Pickle, 168 g	5	0	0	0	0
Soup & Chili & Related Items					
Broccoli Cheese, 8 oz. cup	160	8	17	0	5
• Chili, 8 oz. cup	280	13	26	7	18
• Oyster crackers, 1 package	60	2	10	0	1
Side of Wheat Bread, 75 g	187	3	35	3	8
Side of White Bread, 75 g	186	1	35	0	8
Veggie Sub Sandwiches (on white bread)					
• Pikes Peak Or Bust - large (11"), 398 g	906	47	78	3	40
Pikes Peak Or Bust - medium (8"), 290 g	651	33	59	2	28
• Pikes Peak Or Bust - small (5"), 188 g	396	19	39	1	16
Veggies (For 8" subs)					
• Black Olives, 44 g	69	7	3	0	0
Cucumbers, 28 g	4	0	1	0	0
Green Peppers, 22 g	5	0	1	0	0
Hot Banana Peppers, 18 g	3	0	1	0	0
Jalapeños, 20 g	3	0	1	1	0
Lettuce, 42 g	4	0	1	1	0
Mushrooms, 22 g	5	0	1	0	1
Onions, 18 g	8	0	2	0	0
• Pickle Slices, 44 g	0	0	0	0	0
Sprouts, 10 g	3	0	0	0	0
Tomato, 34 g	6	0	1	0	0

Skyline Chili

	Cal	Fat	Cbs	Fbr	Prtn
Bowls					
• Chili Bean Bowl	270	12	17	6	23
Chili Bowl	270	16	6	1	25

RESTAURANTS & FAST-FOOD CHAINS

Skyline Chili (cont.)	Cal	Fat	Cbs	Fbr	Prtn
Bowls (cont.)					
Chili Cheese Bowl	440	30	6	1	35
• Coney Bowl	870	69	9	2	54
Loaded Chili Bowl	580	40	18	4	38
Vegetarian Black Beans and Rice Bowl	320	9	46	8	12
Burritos					
All Chili Burrito	560	30	37	3	34
All Chili Burrito Deluxe	650	35	45	6	37
Black Bean Burrito	600	25	67	9	25
• Black Bean Burrito Deluxe	690	30	75	11	27
Chili Bean Mix Burrito	610	30	54	8	30
Chili Bean Mix Burrito Deluxe	700	36	62	10	33
• Chili Cheese Melt	350	16	33	2	17
Chili Spaghetti Dishes (Regular Size)					
3-Way	760	44	43	3	46
4-Way Bean	850	45	59	9	52
4-Way Onion	770	44	46	4	47
5-Way	840	45	58	9	51
Black Bean & Rice 3-Way	800	40	74	9	36
Black Bean & Rice 4-Way	810	40	77	9	37
• Black Bean & Rice 5-Way	880	40	89	14	41
Black Bean & Rice Spaghetti	490	12	79	9	16
• Chili Spaghetti	450	18	43	4	28
Chili Spaghetti Bean	520	17	61	9	30
Chili Spaghetti Bean & Onion	530	17	64	9	31
Chili Spaghetti Onion	470	17	51	4	26
Coneys					
• Cheese Coney	340	22	17	1	18
Chili Cheese Sandwich	290	17	17	1	19
• Regular Chili Sandwich (w/o cheese)	180	7	17	1	12
Regular Coney (w/o cheese)	220	12	17	1	11
Dressings					
Buttermilk Ranch Dressing	230	24	2	0	1
Chili Ranch Dressing	275	29	0	0	0
Dijon Honey Mustard Dressing	180	17	8	0	1
• Greek Salad Dressing	250	28	1	0	0
Honey French Dressing	210	18	14	0	0
• Light Italian Dressing	20	1	2	0	0
Light Ranch Dressing	70	4	8	0	1
Fresh Selects Salads (No Dressing)					
Buffalo Chicken Salad	150	7	7	2	17
Classic Chicken Salad	150	7	8	2	17
Garden Salad	80	5	6	2	5
Greek Chicken Salad	170	8	9	8	18
• Greek Salad	60	4	5	2	3
• SW Chicken Salad w/ Tortilla Chips	760	44	66	8	30
SW Chicken Salad w/o Tortilla Chips	460	16	18	5	25
Fresh Selects Wraps (No Dressing)					
Buffalo Chicken Wrap	520	21	55	3	31
Classic Chicken Wrap	510	21	55	3	31
• Greek Chicken Wrap	510	21	54	7	29
• Southwest Chicken Wrap	670	30	65	6	34
Fries					
French Fries	630	33	79	6	8

(• = most healthy • = least healthy)   **RESTAURANTS & FAST-FOOD • 319**

RESTAURANTS & FAST-FOOD CHAINS

Skyline Chili (cont.)

	Cal	Fat	Cbs	Fbr	Prtn
Kids Meals					
• 3-Way Special	380	22	22	2	23
Coney Special w/ Chz	330	22	16	1	17
Coney Special w/o Chz	210	12	15	1	10
Double Wiener Hot Doggy w/ Chz	360	26	16	0	15
Double Wiener Hot Doggy w/o Chz	250	17	15	0	8
P'sghetti Special	280	16	19	1	14
Single Wiener Hot Doggy w/ Chz	270	18	15	0	12
• Single Wiener Hot Doggy w/o Chz	160	9	14	0	5
Sides					
• Bowl of Crackers	100	3	20	1	3
• Cheddar Bread Full	520	39	32	0	12
Cheddar Bread Half	260	20	16	0	6
Garlic Bread Full	410	30	31	0	5
Garlic Bread Half	200	15	16	0	3
Side of Cheese	230	19	1	0	14
Side of Chili	130	8	3	1	12
Steamed Potatoes					
3-Way Potato	870	49	75	7	33
4-Way Potato	890	49	78	7	33
• 5-Way Potato	950	50	90	12	37
Cheddar Potato	740	41	72	6	21
Chili Potato	440	8	74	7	19
• Plain Potato	310	0	72	6	7
Sour Cream Potato	570	27	72	6	7

Smoothie King

	Cal	Fat	Cbs	Fbr	Prtn
Smoothies: Classic					
Açaí Adventure®, 20 oz.	437	5	93	4	5
Angel Food™, 20 oz.	370	0	89	6	6
Blackberry Dream™, 20 oz.	371	1	91	2	2
Blueberry Heaven®, 20 oz.	325	1	73	2	7
Celestial Cherry High™, 20 oz.	344	0	85	3	2
Coffee Smoothie Amaretto, 20 oz.	164	0	31	0	8
Coffee Smoothie French Roast, 20 oz.	187	0	39	0	8
• Coffee Smoothie French Vanilla, 20 oz.	164	0	31	0	8
Coffee Smoothie Hazelnut, 20 oz.	164	0	31	0	8
Coffee Smoothie Irish Creme, 20 oz.	164	0	31	0	8
Coffee Smoothie Mocha, 20 oz.	219	3	38	0	13
Cranberry Cooler™, 20 oz.	503	0	124	3	1
Cranberry Supreme®, 20 oz.	560	1	134	3	4
Gladiator®, 20 oz.	300	0	31	2	45
Go Goji™, 20 oz.	347	0	82	1	1
Green Tea Tango®, 20 oz.	368	4	72	3	8
Hearty Apple®, 20 oz.	405	1	86	2	9
High Protein Almond Mocha, 20 oz.	382	9	48	2	31
High Protein Banana, 20 oz.	322	9	32	4	27
High Protein Chocolate, 20 oz.	382	9	48	2	31
High Protein Lemon, 20 oz.	372	9	44	1	26
High Protein Pineapple, 20 oz.	315	9	29	2	27
Immune Builder®, 20 oz.	384	1	92	6	5
Instant Vigor™, 20 oz.	368	0	88	4	4
Island Impact®, 20 oz.	312	0	73	2	4
Island Treat®, 20 oz.	337	0	84	6	3

Smoothie King (cont.)	Cal	Fat	Cbs	Fbr	Prtn
Smoothies: Classic (cont.)					
Kiwi Island Treat®, 20 oz.	504	1	119	0	6
Low-Carb Banana, 20 oz.	268	9	7	1	39
Low-Carb Chocolate, 20 oz.	268	9	7	1	39
Low-Carb Strawberry, 20 oz.	268	9	7	1	39
Low-Carb Vanilla, 20 oz.	268	9	7	1	39
MangoFest™, 20 oz.	285	0	72	1	0
Mangosteen Madness™, 20 oz.	343	0	84	2	1
Muscle Punch Plus™, 20 oz.	379	1	90	6	6
Muscle Punch®, 20 oz.	380	1	90	6	6
Orange Ka-BAM®, 20 oz.	469	0	120	3	1
Passion Passport®, 20 oz.	399	0	99	2	2
Peach Slice™, 20 oz.	333	0	78	2	6
Pep Upper®, 20 oz.	413	0	98	3	4
Pineapple Pleasure®, 20 oz.	284	0	69	3	2
Pomegranate Punch™, 20 oz.	425	0	100	3	1
Power Punch Plus®, 20 oz.	518	1	119	6	10
Power Punch®, 20 oz.	446	1	107	6	6
Raspberry Collider™, 20 oz.	344	0	88	4	1
Raspberry Sunrise™, 20 oz.	399	0	99	2	2
Slim-N-Trim Chocolate™, 20 oz.	224	1	49	2	8
Slim-N-Trim Orange-Vanilla™, 20 oz.	215	1	46	0	7
Slim-N-Trim Strawberry™, 20 oz.	379	1	87	5	8
Slim-N-Trim Vanilla™, 20 oz.	256	1	56	3	7
Strawberry Kiwi Breeze™, 20 oz.	376	0	90	3	4
Super Punch Plus®, 20 oz.	461	0	117	6	2
Super Punch™, 20 oz.	395	0	100	6	2
The Activator Chocolate®, 20 oz.	422	1	89	5	20
The Activator Strawberry®, 20 oz.	575	1	127	8	21
The Activator Vanilla®, 20 oz.	425	1	89	5	20
The Hulk Chocolate™, 20 oz.	919	35	128	7	28
• The Hulk Strawberry™, 20 oz.	1065	35	163	8	27
The Hulk Vanilla™, 20 oz.	915	35	125	5	27
The Shredder - Chocolate™, 20 oz.	311	3	36	1	39
The Shredder - Strawberry™, 20 oz.	356	1	57	3	29
The Shredder - Vanilla™, 20 oz.	283	2	30	0	36
Youth Fountain™, 20 oz.	252	0	64	3	2
Smoothies: Power Meal™					
Banana Berry Treat®, 20 oz.	372	0	90	6	4
Banana Boat®, 20 oz.	554	14	98	6	12
Berry Punch™, 20 oz.	367	0	93	4	0
Caribbean Way®, 20 oz.	399	0	100	6	2
Cherry Picker®, 20 oz.	441	0	105	2	5
Coconut Surprise®, 20 oz.	493	7	100	3	10
Fruit Fusion™, 20 oz.	360	0	84	2	4
Grape Expectations II™, 20 oz.	551	0	136	6	2
Grape Expectations®, 20 oz.	401	0	98	3	2
Kids' Kups Berry Interesting™, 20 oz.	277	0	69	3	1
• Kids' Kups Choc-A-Laka™, 20 oz.	191	3	30	1	11
Kids' Kups CW, Jr.™, 20 oz.	270	0	68	5	1
Kids' Kups Gimme-Grape™, 20 oz.	265	0	64	2	1
Kids' Kups Lil' Angel™, 20 oz.	223	0	56	5	1
Kids' Kups Smarti Tarti™, 20 oz.	200	0	49	0	1
Lemon Twist Banana®, 20 oz.	361	0	90	3	2

RESTAURANTS & FAST-FOOD CHAINS

Smoothie King (cont.)

	Cal	Fat	Cbs	Fbr	Prtn
Smoothies: Power Meal™ (cont.)					
Lemon Twist Strawberry®, 20 oz.	442	0	110	3	1
Light & Fluffy®, 20 oz.	399	0	102	6	1
Malts, 20 oz.	771	39	87	0	19
Mo'cuccino™, 20 oz.	477	14	78	1	11
Peach Slice Plus®, 20 oz.	483	0	116	5	6
• Peanut Power Plus Grape™, 20 oz.	782	25	130	3	12
Peanut Power Plus Strawberry™, 20 oz.	732	25	120	6	13
Peanut Power®, 20 oz.	582	25	82	3	12
Piña Colada Island®, 20 oz.	632	10	120	3	17
Pineapple Surf®, 20 oz.	465	1	107	4	7
Shakes, 20 oz.	761	39	85	0	19
Strawberry X-Treme®, 20 oz.	369	0	93	6	1
Yogurt D-Lite®, 20 oz.	432	4	81	1	15

Sonic Drive-In

	Cal	Fat	Cbs	Fbr	Prtn
Add Ins (Medium)					
Blue Coconut, 18 g	35	0	9	0	0
Cherry, 23 g	50	0	14	0	0
• Chocolate Topping Add-In , 38 g	100	0	23	0	0
Diet Cherry, 19 g	10	0	2	0	0
Fresh Lemon Add-In, 18 g	5	0	2	0	0
• Fresh Lime Add-In, 14 g	5	0	1	0	0
Grape, 19 g	40	0	9	0	0
Orange, 18 g	40	0	10	0	0
Pineapple Topping, 35 g	60	0	14	0	0
Strawberry Topping, 35 g	70	0	17	1	1
Vanilla, 19 g	40	0	11	0	0
Watermelon, 19 g	45	0	12	0	0
Add Ons					
• Bacon, 13 g	70	5	0	0	4
Cheese, 18 g	60	5	2	0	3
• Chili, 33 g	50	4	2	1	3
Burgers					
Bacon Cheeseburger, 273 g	770	47	55	4	32
Burger w/ Ketchup, 235 g	540	25	54	4	24
Burger w/ Mayo, 242 g	630	37	53	4	24
Burger w/ Mustard, 235 g	540	25	52	4	24
Cheeseburger w/ Ketchup, 260 g	610	31	57	4	28
Cheeseburger w/ Mayo, 260 g	700	42	55	4	27
Cheeseburger w/ Mustard, 253 g	600	31	54	4	27
• Jr. Burger, 117 g	320	16	29	2	15
Jr. Cheeseburger, 135 g	380	21	30	2	18
SuperSONIC® Chzbrgr w/ Ketchup, 337 g	880	52	59	4	45
SuperSONIC® Chzbrgr w/ Mustard, 330 g	870	52	55	4	45
• SuperSONIC® Chzburger w/ Mayo, 337 g	970	63	56	4	45
Chicken					
• BBQ Sauce, 28 g	45	0	11	0	0
Breaded Chicken Sandwich, 255 g	670	33	66	6	26
• Chicken Strip Dinner, 4 pcs.	920	43	97	9	36
Grilled Chicken Sandwich, 204 g	340	12	32	2	27
Honey Mustard Sauce, 28 g	90	7	7	0	0
Jumbo Popcorn Chicken™ (Snack), 113 g	370	21	27	2	19
Ranch Sauce, 28 g	150	16	1	0	0

Sonic Drive-In (cont.)	Cal	Fat	Cbs	Fbr	Prtn
Coneys					
Corn Dog, 73 g	250	15	23	2	5
Extra-Long Cheese Coney, 237 g	600	33	54	4	24
Famous Slushes (Medium)					
Blue Coconut Slush, 20 oz.	290	0	76	0	0
Cherry Slush, 20 oz.	290	0	78	0	0
Grape Slush, 20 oz.	290	0	76	0	0
Lemon Fresh Fruit Slush, 20 oz.	290	0	78	0	0
• Lemon-Berry Fresh Fruit Slush, 20 oz.	310	0	83	1	1
Lime Fresh Fruit Slush, 20 oz.	290	0	78	0	0
Minute Maid® Apple Juice Slush, 20 oz.	280	0	76	0	0
Minute Maid® Cran Juice Slush, 20 oz.	290	0	77	0	0
• Mt. Blast® POWERADE® Slush, 20 oz.	280	0	76	0	0
Orange Slush, 20 oz.	290	0	77	0	0
Strawberry Fresh Fruit Slush, 20 oz.	310	0	82	1	1
Watermelon Slush, 20 oz.	290	0	78	0	0
Fresh Tastes® Salads					
Grilled Chicken Salad, 358 g	310	14	19	4	30
• Hidden Valley® Fat Free Golden Italian, 57 g	50	0	13	0	0
Hidden Valley® Honey Mustard, 57 g	240	21	14	0	1
Hidden Valley® Original Light Ranch, 57 g	120	7	14	0	1
Hidden Valley® Ranch Dressing, 57 g	260	28	0	0	0
• Jumbo Popcorn Chicken® Salad, 354 g	490	28	39	5	22
Santa Fe Grilled Chicken Salad, 406 g	380	15	29	6	32
Frozen Drinks & Desserts (Regular Size)					
Banana Cream Pie Shake, 14 oz.	690	23	113	1	8
Banana Malt, 14 oz.	560	20	89	1	8
Banana Shake, 14 oz.	550	19	87	1	8
Banana Split, 319 g	450	12	82	2	5
Barq's® Root Beer Float/Blended Float , 14 oz.	300	8	56	0	3
Blue Coconut CreamSlush® Treat, 14 oz.	430	13	76	0	5
Butterfinger® Sonic Blast®, 14 oz.	670	31	89	1	9
Cherry CreamSlush® Treat, 14 oz.	440	13	77	0	5
• Chocolate Cream Pie Shake, 14 oz.	750	23	127	1	8
Chocolate Malt, 14 oz.	630	20	102	0	8
Chocolate Shake, 14 oz.	610	19	101	0	7
Chocolate Sundae, 255 g	410	13	67	0	4
Coca-Cola® Float/Blended Float, 14 oz.	290	8	54	0	3
Coconut Cream Pie Shake, 14 oz.	680	24	108	1	8
Diet Coke® Float/Blended Float, 14 oz.	220	8	33	0	3
Diet Dr. Pepper® Float/Blended Float, 14 oz.	220	8	33	0	3
Dr. Pepper® Float/Blended Float, 14 oz.	310	8	58	0	3
Grape CreamSlush® Treat, 14 oz.	430	13	76	0	5
Hot Fudge Sundae, 253 g	440	18	63	1	4
Lemon CreamSlush® Treat, 14 oz.	430	13	77	0	5
Lemon-Berry CreamSlush® Treat, 14 oz.	460	12	85	1	5
Lime CreamSlush® Treat, 14 oz.	430	13	77	0	5
M&M's® Sonic Blast®, 14 oz.	660	28	95	1	8
Nuts Add-On, 4 g	20	2	1	0	1
Orange CreamSlush® Treat, 14 oz.	430	13	77	0	5
Oreo® Sonic Blast®, 14 oz.	660	28	94	1	8
Pineapple Malt, 14 oz.	590	20	93	0	8
Pineapple Shake, 14 oz.	570	19	92	0	7
Pineapple Sundae, 252 g	370	13	58	0	4

RESTAURANTS & FAST-FOOD CHAINS

Sonic Drive-In (cont.)

	Cal	Fat	Cbs	Fbr	Prtn
Frozen Drinks & Desserts (Regular Size) (cont.)					
Reese's PB Cups® Sonic Blast®, 14 oz.	620	22	96	1	10
Strawberry Cream Pie Shake, 14 oz.	720	23	120	1	8
Strawberry CreamSlush® Treat, 14 oz.	450	12	84	1	5
Strawberry Malt, 14 oz.	590	20	96	1	8
Strawberry Shake, 14 oz.	580	19	94	1	8
Strawberry Sundae, 252 g	380	13	61	1	4
• Vanilla Cone, 133 g	180	6	30	0	2
Vanilla Dish, 184 g	240	9	36	0	3
Vanilla Malt, 14 oz.	550	21	84	0	8
Vanilla Shake, 14 oz.	540	20	82	0	8
Watermelon CreamSlush® Treat, 14 oz.	440	13	77	0	5
Kids' Meals					
• Chicken Strips - 2 strips, 72 g	210	11	13	1	14
Corn Dog, 73 g	250	15	23	2	5
• Grilled Cheese, 118 g	390	17	45	2	14
Jr. Burger, 117 g	320	16	29	2	15
Jr. Cheeseburger, 135 g	380	21	30	2	18
Sides (Regular)					
• French Fries, 75 g	210	10	28	4	3
w/ cheese, 93 g	280	15	29	4	6
w/ chili & cheese, 122 g	300	18	31	5	9
Mozzarella Sticks, 135 g	410	21	35	2	19
• Onion Rings, 156 g	500	28	55	4	6
Tater Tots, 84 g	220	14	23	3	2
w/ cheese, 102 g	290	19	25	3	5
w/ chili & cheese, 131 g	310	21	26	3	8
Toaster® Sandwiches					
Bacon Cheeseburger Toaster®, 251 g	690	37	58	3	31
Chicken Club Toaster®, 265 g	690	35	64	4	32
Wraps					
Chicken Strip Wrap, 234 g	480	20	56	5	20
• FRITOS® Chili Cheese Wrap, 239 g	670	38	66	6	22
• Grilled Chicken Wrap, 253 g	380	11	44	4	28
Your Ultimate Drink Stop! (Medium)					
Apple Juice Limeade, 20 oz.	200	0	54	0	0
Cherry Limeade, 20 oz.	220	0	59	0	0
Cranberry Limeade , 20 oz.	200	0	53	0	0
• Ice Tea, 20 oz.	5	0	1	0	0
Limeade, 20 oz.	170	0	47	0	0
Lo-Cal Diet Cherry Limeade, 20 oz.	15	0	3	0	0
Lo-Cal Diet Limeade, 20 oz.	10	0	1	0	0
Ocean Water®, 20 oz.	200	0	53	0	0
Peach Ice Tea, 20 oz.	5	0	1	0	0
Raspberry Ice Tea, 20 oz.	5	0	2	0	0
• Strawberry Limeade, 20 oz.	230	0	60	1	1

Souper Salad

	Cal	Fat	Cbs	Fbr	Prtn
Beverages					
Lemonade, Mango Premium, 24 oz.	220	0	58	0	0
• Lemonade, Premium, 24 oz.	190	0	49	0	0
Lemonade, Raspberry Premium, 24 oz.	220	0	58	0	0
Lemonade, Strawberry Premium, 24 oz.	220	0	57	0	0
• Smoothie, Mango, Grande, 20 oz.	350	0	89	0	0

RESTAURANTS & FAST-FOOD CHAINS

Souper Salad (cont.)	Cal	Fat	Cbs	Fbr	Prtn
Beverages (cont.)					
Smoothie, Peach, Grande, 20 oz.	320	0	87	0	0
Smoothie, Raspberry, Grande, 20 oz.	320	0	87	0	0
Smoothie, Strawberry, Grande, 20 oz.	320	0	84	0	0
Bread					
Blueberry Bread, 1 piece	150	3	29	1	3
Bread, Cheese Drop Biscuit, 1 piece	70	3	8	0	2
Breadstick, Garlic, 1 piece	130	5	18	1	3
Cornbread, 1 piece	170	5	30	1	3
Gingerbread, 1 piece	180	6	30	1	2
Dessert					
Banana Pudding, 1/2 cup	160	6	26	0	2
Brownies, Prepared, 2 pcs.	120	5	21	0	1
Caramel Dessert Topping, 1 tbsp.	50	1	11	0	0
Chocolate Pudding, 1/2 cup	170	5	30	0	2
Chocolate Syrup, 1 tbsp.	50	0	12	0	0
Cottage Cheese, Lowfat, 1/2 cup	90	2	5	0	13
Oreo Crumbles, 1 tbsp.	30	1	4	0	0
Peaches, 1/2 cup	70	0	17	0	0
Pineapple Tidbits, 1/4 cup	60	0	15	1	0
Pineapple Topping, 1 tbsp.	35	0	9	0	0
Rainbow Sprinkles, 1 tbsp.	25	1	4	0	0
Sponge Cake, Yellow, 4 pcs.	80	2	14	0	1
Strawberries, Sliced, 1/2 cup	150	0	38	3	0
Strawberry Parfait, 1/2 cup	100	2	19	0	2
Vanilla Wafers, 4 pcs.	70	2	13	0	1
Whipped Topping, 1/2 cup	100	8	8	0	0
Dressing					
Balsamic Vinegar Dressing, 1 oz.	60	0	15	0	0
Bleu Cheese Dressing, 2 oz.	220	23	1	0	2
Caesar Dressing, 2 oz.	280	30	4	0	4
Chipotle Ranch Dressing, 2 oz.	280	28	6	0	0
Cranberry Vinaigrette, 2 oz.	100	0	24	0	0
French Dressing, Fat Free, 2 oz.	60	0	18	1	0
Green Goddess, 2 oz.	260	24	4	0	2
Honey Mustard, 2 oz.	240	26	2	0	0
House Vinaigrette, 2 oz.	220	22	4	0	0
• Italian Dressing w/ Chz, Fat Free, 2 oz.	30	0	6	0	0
Mayonnaise, 2 tbsp.	200	22	0	0	0
Olive Oil, 1 oz.	240	28	0	0	0
Peppercorn Ranch Dressing, 2 oz.	220	23	2	0	1
Ranch Dressing, 2 oz.	220	23	2	0	1
Ranch Dressing, Reduced Calorie, 2 oz.	120	11	3	0	0
Tangy Oriental, 2 oz.	160	12	10	0	2
• Thousand Island Dressing, 2 oz.	300	30	6	0	0
Featured Salad					
Apple Walnut Salad for Bar, 1 cup	130	11	7	1	3
Asian Chicken Salad, 1 cup	80	3	10	2	3
Asian Shrimp Salad, 1 cup	100	4	13	2	4
Buffalo Chicken Salad, 1 cup	70	6	3	1	3
Capri Salad, 1 cup	50	2	8	0	1
Chicago Chopped Salad, 1 cup	120	10	3	1	4
Chicken Caesar Salad, 1 cup	90	7	4	1	5
Chicken Salsa Caesar Salad, 1 cup	80	5	4	1	4

(•= most healthy •= least healthy)   **RESTAURANTS & FAST-FOOD • 325**

RESTAURANTS & FAST-FOOD CHAINS

Souper Salad (cont.)

	Cal	Fat	Cbs	Fbr	Prtn
Featured Salad (cont.)					
Cobb Salad, 1 cup	100	8	2	1	4
Green Goddess Crab Salad, 1 cup	70	5	4	1	2
Italian Antipasto Salad, 1 cup	70	5	3	1	2
Mango Berry Salad, 1 cup	110	6	13	1	1
• Marinated Tomato Salad, 1 cup	60	2	11	1	1
Salmon Medley Salad, 1 cup	70	2	10	1	4
Shrimp and Crab Louie, 1 cup	130	10	5	1	5
Shrimp Caesar Salad, 1 cup	90	7	3	1	4
Southwest Chicken Chipotle, 1 cup	90	7	4	1	3
Hot Bar					
Bacon Bits, Real, 2 tbsp.	80	7	0	0	5
Chicken Fajita, 1/3 cup	45	3	3	1	3
Chili Potato Topping, 2 oz.	70	3	5	2	4
Chipotle Pepper Sauce, 1/4 tsp.	0	0	0	0	0
Cholula Hot Sauce, 1/4 tsp.	0	0	0	0	0
Colby, Shredded, 2 oz.	110	9	1	0	7
Crackers, 1 package	30	1	4	0	0
Flour Tortilla, 1 piece	90	3	16	2	3
Jalapeño Cheese Sauce, 2 oz.	35	2	5	0	1
Melba Toast, 1 slice	45	1	8	0	1
• Parmesan, 1 tbsp.	20	1	2	0	2
• Potato, Baked, Plain, 1 piece	200	0	46	3	5
Red Pepper, Crushed, 1/4 tsp.	0	0	0	0	0
Rice, White, Prepared, 1/3 cup	70	0	15	0	1
Romano, 1 tbsp.	30	2	0	0	1
Saltine Crackers, 1 package	40	1	7	0	1
Sour Cream, Light, 2 tbsp.	40	3	3	0	1
Southwestern Quesadilla, 1 slice	90	5	9	1	4
Spanish Rice, prepared, 1/3 cup	80	2	17	1	1
Sriracha Hot Sauce, 1/4 tsp.	0	0	0	0	0
SW Beans w/ Roasted Corn, 1/3 cup	60	1	10	2	3
Whipped Margarine for Hot Bar, 1 tbsp.	40	5	0	0	0
Hot Pasta					
Alfredo Sauce for Pasta Bar, 1 1/2 tbsp.	45	4	2	0	2
Basil Pesto for Pasta Bar, 1 tbsp.	45	5	0	0	1
Bowtie for Pasta Bar, 1 cup	240	5	42	2	7
Chicken Alfredo, 1 cup	320	9	40	1	19
• Macaroni & Cheese, 1 cup	380	18	38	1	15
• Marinara for Pasta Bar, 1 1/2 tbsp.	10	0	2	0	0
Meaty Marinara for Pasta Bar, 1 1/2 tbsp.	20	1	2	0	1
Penne for Hot Pasta Bar, 1 cup	230	5	42	2	7
Spaghetti & Meatballs, 1 cup	280	9	38	2	11
Spaghetti for Pasta Bar, 1 cup	240	5	41	2	7
Tortellini for Pasta Bar, 1 cup	290	11	38	3	11
Pizza					
• Cheese Pizza, 1 slice	70	3	8	0	0
Garden Pizza, 1 slice	80	3	9	1	1
• Pepperoni Pizza, 1 slice	90	4	8	0	0
Sausage Pizza, 1 slice	80	4	9	1	1
Signature Salad					
Broccoli Coleslaw, 1/3 cup	80	6	6	1	1
California Chicken Salad, 1/3 cup	80	6	4	0	5
Chickpea Salad, 1/3 cup	110	6	11	4	3

Souper Salad (cont.)

	Cal	Fat	Cbs	Fbr	Prtn
Signature Salad (cont.)					
Edamame Salad, 1/3 cup	70	5	4	2	4
Fettuccine Pasta Salad, 1/3 cup	100	5	11	1	2
Fisherman's Kettle Shrimp & Crab Salad, 1/3 cup	120	8	9	0	3
Gazpacho Salad, 1/3 cup	30	3	3	1	0
• Marinated Mushrooms, 1/3 cup	60	7	1	0	1
• Marinated Oriental Cucumber, 1/3 cup	10	0	2	0	0
Melon Couscous Salad, 1/3 cup	50	1	10	1	1
Mustard Potato Salad, 1/3 cup	80	5	7	1	1
Paco's Taco Salad, 1/3 cup	100	5	12	2	3
Pasta de Garden, 1/3 cup	80	5	8	0	1
Pasta Primavera Salad, 1/3 cup	45	3	4	0	1
Red Potato Salad, 1/3 cup	50	4	5	1	1
Rice Florentine Salad, 1/3 cup	90	5	11	0	1
Roasted Vegetables, 1/3 cup	20	2	2	1	0
Rsted Mshrms & Artichokes w/ Feta Chz, 1/3 cup	40	3	3	1	1
Salad of the Sea, 1/3 cup	50	2	6	0	2
Santa Fe Corn Salad, 1/3 cup	100	4	13	3	4
Sweet Garden Slaw, 1/3 cup	35	2	4	1	0
Thai Chicken Pasta Salad, 1/3 cup	100	5	11	1	3
Tropical Tuxedo Salad, 1/3 cup	60	3	7	0	1
Tuna Fish Salad, 1/3 cup	70	5	1	0	6
Soup					
Adobe Rice and Chkn Soup, 5 oz. bowl	100	5	10	1	3
Alaskan Salmon Chowder, 5 oz. bowl	70	2	9	1	3
Beef Mushroom Barley, 5 oz. bowl	80	2	11	2	4
Beef Noodle Soup, 5 oz. bowl	80	3	10	1	4
Beef Shellini Soup, 5 oz. bowl	90	3	11	1	5
Beef Stroganoff, 5 oz. bowl	120	5	13	1	4
Black Bean Soup, 5 oz. bowl	80	2	20	11	8
Broccoli Cheese Soup, 5 oz. bowl	70	2	10	1	2
Cajun Gumbo Soup, 5 oz. bowl	110	4	13	1	5
Cauliflower Cheese Soup, 5 oz. bowl	70	2	11	1	2
Cheddar Chkn Broccoli Stew, 5 oz. bowl	140	6	15	2	6
Cherokee Joe's Cornbread Soup, 5 oz. bowl	70	2	13	2	2
Chicken Creole Soup, 5 oz. bowl	100	4	12	1	6
• Chicken Enchilada Soup, 5 oz. bowl	180	12	13	1	6
Chicken Gumbo Soup, 5 oz. bowl	90	4	10	1	4
Chicken Mshrm Barley Soup, 5 oz. bowl	80	3	9	1	5
Chicken Noodle Soup, 5 oz. bowl	80	3	8	1	4
Chicken Tetrazini Soup, 5 oz. bowl	120	5	13	1	6
• Chicken Tortilla Soup, 5 oz. bowl	60	2	7	1	4
Cream of Asparagus, 5 oz. bowl	140	10	7	1	2
Cream of Broccoli Soup, 5 oz. bowl	60	4	4	2	2
Cream of Cauliflower Soup, 5 oz. bowl	60	2	10	1	2
Cream of Chicken Soup, 5 oz. bowl	100	5	9	1	5
Cream of Mushroom Soup, 5 oz. bowl	80	4	10	1	2

Souplantation

	Cal	Fat	Cbs	Fbr	Prtn
Bakery					
Apple Cinnamon Bran Muffin, 1 piece	130	1	30	3	2
Apple Raisin Muffin, 1 piece	150	7	22	1	2
• Banana Crunch Muffin Top, 1 piece	120	5	19	1	3
Banana Nut Muffin, 1 piece	150	7	22	1	4

(• = most healthy • = least healthy)

RESTAURANTS & FAST-FOOD CHAINS

Souplantation (cont.)

	Cal	Fat	Cbs	Fbr	Prtn
Bakery (cont.)					
BBQ Chicken Focaccia, Honey Wheat Crust, 1 pc	200	8	23	2	9
Black Forest Muffin, 1 piece	230	9	36	1	2
Bruschetta Focaccia, 1 piece	140	7	15	1	4
Buffalo Chicken Focaccia, Honey Wht Crust, 1 pc	170	7	20	2	6
Buttermilk Biscuits, 1 biscuit	190	8	25	0	4
Buttermilk Cornbread, 1 piece	140	2	27	2	3
Cappuccino Chip Muffin, 1 piece	190	6	31	1	3
Caribbean Key Lime Muffin, 1 piece	170	6	28	1	2
Carrot Pineapple Muffin w/ Oat Bran, 1 piece	150	6	23	2	3
Cherry Nut Muffin, 1 piece	150	7	22	1	2
Chile Corn Muffin, 1 piece	140	3	27	2	3
Chipotle Lime Butter, 1 tbsp.	90	10	0	0	0
Chocolate Brownie Muffin, 1 piece	180	8	26	1	3
Chocolate Chip Muffin, 1 piece	170	8	22	1	3
Chocolate Peanut Butter Chip Muffin, 1 piece	220	10	31	1	3
Country Blackberry Muffin, 1 piece	170	6	27	1	2
Cranberry Orange Bran Muffin, 1 piece	130	1	30	3	2
Date N' Honey Bran, 1 piece	150	6	24	2	2
French Quarter Praline Muffin, 1 piece	250	10	35	1	4
Fruit Medley Bran Muffin, 1 piece	130	1	29	3	2
Garlic Asiago Focaccia, 1 piece	160	8	19	1	4
Georgia Peach Poppyseed Muffin, 1 piece	150	6	20	1	2
Grilled Cheese Focaccia, 1 piece	190	10	18	0	5
Indian Grain Bread (Low-Fat), 1 piece	200	2	35	0	11
Irish Soda Bread, 1 piece	180	5	29	0	4
Lemon Vanilla Butter, 1 tbsp.	90	8	3	0	0
Mango Tropics Muffin w/ Coconut, 1 piece	180	7	28	1	2
Maple Walnut Muffin, 1 piece	230	10	32	1	3
Old World Greek Focaccia, 1 piece	190	9	24	2	3
Pauline's Apple Walnut Cake, 1 piece	220	12	24	1	3
Pepperoni Focaccia, 1 piece	190	9	21	1	5
Pesto & Sun-Dried Tomato Focaccia, 1 piece	170	8	20	1	5
Pumpkin Raisin Muffin, 1 piece	150	6	25	1	2
Quattro Formaggio Focaccia, 1 piece	140	5	19	1	5
Roasted Potato Focaccia, 1 piece	150	6	17	2	6
Roasted Red Pepper, Honey Wht Focaccia, 1 piece	170	8	20	2	5
Sauteed Vegetable Focaccia, 1 piece	180	9	19	1	5
Sourdough Bread, 1 piece	150	1	27	0	9
Southwest Chipotle Focaccia, 1 piece	160	8	19	1	4
Spiced Pumpkin Muffin w/ Cranberries, 1 piece	180	7	29	1	2
Strawberry Buttermilk Muffin, 1 piece	140	6	21	1	2
Sweet Cherry Butter, 1 tbsp.	80	7	4	0	0
Sweet Orange & Cranberry Muffin, 1 pc	200	7	33	1	2
Sweet Strawberry Butter, 1 tbsp.	80	7	4	0	0
Taffy Apple Muffin, 1 piece	160	6	25	1	2
Tangy Lemon Muffin, 1 piece	140	4	24	1	2
Thai Chicken Focaccia w/ Peanuts, 1 piece	170	7	20	1	7
Wildly Blue Blueberry Muffin, 1 piece	140	5	22	1	2
Wowie Maui Focaccia w/ Ham, 1 piece	170	7	21	1	6
Zucchini Nut Muffin, 1 piece	150	7	22	1	2
Desserts					
Apple Cobbler, 1/2 cup	360	10	67	2	3
Apple Medley (Fat-Free), 1/2 cup	70	0	18	1	1

Souplantation (cont.)	Cal	Fat	Cbs	Fbr	Prtn
Desserts (cont.)					
Banana Pudding, 1/2 cup	160	4	27	1	4
Banana Royale (Fat- Free), 1/2 cup	80	0	20	1	1
Butterscotch Pudding (Low-Fat), 1/2 cup	140	3	24	0	4
Candy Sprinkles (Low-Fat), 1 tbsp.	70	3	11	0	0
• Caramel Apple Cobbler, 1/2 cup	390	12	68	2	3
Cherry Apple Cobbler, 1/2 cup	330	10	57	2	2
Chocolate Chip Cookie - 1 Small, 1 cookie	75	3	10	0	1
Chocolate Chip Cookie Bars, 1 piece	90	4	13	0	1
Chocolate Frozen Yogurt (Fat-Free), 1/2 cup	95	0	21	0	3
Chocolate Lava Cake, 1/2 cup	330	8	62	0	2
Chocolate PBCookie Cups, 1 piece	140	6	18	1	1
Chocolate Pudding (Low-Fat), 1/2 cup	150	3	25	0	4
Choco Pudding (No Sugar Added), 1/2 cup	90	2	21	0	4
Chocolate Syrup (Fat- Free), 2 tbsp.	70	0	18	0	0
Cranberry Apple Cobbler, 1/2 cup	370	10	58	3	3
Cran-Raspberry Gelatin (Fat-Free), 1/2 cup	100	0	26	0	1
Deep Chocolate Winter Mint Lava Cake, 1/2 cup	330	8	58	0	2
Gelatin (Fat-Free), 1/2 cup	80	0	20	0	1
• Gelatin (Sugar Free, Fat-Free), 1/2 cup	10	0	0	0	1
Granola Topping, 2 tbsp.	110	4	16	2	2
Green Tea Mousse, 1/2 cup	190	8	29	0	3
Holiday Cookies w/ Sprinkles, 1 cookie	80	4	12	0	0
Hot Lemon Lava Cake, 1/2 cup	320	11	51	1	2
Nutty Waldorf Salad (Low-Fat), 1/2 cup	90	3	14	3	1
Oatmeal Raisin Cookie - 1 small, 1 cookie	120	5	16	1	1
Pineapple Gelatin (Fat-Free), 1/2 cup	120	0	29	0	1
Pineapple Upside- Down Cake, 1/2 cup	270	10	42	1	2
Raspberry Apple Cobbler, 1/2 cup	380	11	67	2	3
Rice Pudding (Low- Fat), 1/2 cup	110	2	20	1	3
Shortcake, 1 piece	220	7	36	0	3
Strawberry Apple Cobbler, 1/2 cup	340	10	67	2	3
Sugar-free Chocolate Mousse, 1/2 cup	40	3	3	1	1
Sugar-free Lemon Mousse, 1/2 cup	40	3	4	1	1
Sugar-free Strawberry Mousse, 1/2 cup	40	3	4	1	1
Tapioca Pudding (Low-Fat), 1/2 cup	140	3	24	0	4
Vanilla Pudding, 1/2 cup	150	4	27	0	3
Vanilla Soft Serve (Reduced Fat), 1/2 cup	140	5	22	0	3
Warm Carrot Cake w/ Cream Chz Lava, 1/2 cup	320	15	40	1	3
Dressings					
Avocado Ranch Dressing, 2 tbsp.	150	14	4	0	1
Bacon Dressing, 2 tbsp.	110	11	7	0	0
• Balsamic Vinaigrette, 2 tbsp.	180	19	1	0	0
Basil Vinaigrette, 2 tbsp.	160	17	1	0	0
Blue Cheese Dressing, 2 tbsp.	130	13	3	0	1
Chow Mein Noodles, 1/4 cup	70	1	15	0	1
Cranberry Orange Vinaigrette (Low-Fat), 2 tbsp.	80	2	15	0	0
Creamy Italian Dressing, 2 tbsp.	120	13	0	0	0
Cucumber Dressing (Reduced Calorie), 2 tbsp.	70	7	3	0	0
Garlic Parmesan Seasoned Croutons, 5 pieces	80	5	6	0	2
Green Chili Ranch Dressing, 2 tbsp.	150	14	4	0	1
Honey Lime Cilantro Vinaigrette, 2 tbsp.	100	6	15	0	0
Honey Mint Lemonade, 2 tbsp.	130	7	19	0	0
Honey Mustard Dressing (Fat-Free), 2 tbsp.	45	0	10	0	0

RESTAURANTS & FAST-FOOD CHAINS

Souplantation (cont.)

	Cal	Fat	Cbs	Fbr	Prtn
Dressings (cont.)					
Honey Mustard Dressing, 2 tbsp.	150	13	8	0	0
• Italian Dressing (Fat- Free), 2 tbsp.	25	0	7	0	0
Kahlena French Dressing, 2 tbsp.	120	9	10	0	0
Monterey Blue Salad Dressing, 2 tbsp.	120	11	5	0	0
Parmesan Pepper Cream Dressing, 2 tbsp.	140	16	1	0	1
Pineapple Vinaigrette, 2 tbsp.	120	11	5	0	0
Plain Croutons, 5 pieces	50	2	7	0	1
Ranch Dressing (Fat- Free), 2 tbsp.	50	0	2	0	1
Ranch Dressing, 2 tbsp.	150	15	4	0	1
Roasted Garlic Dressing, 2 tbsp.	100	10	3	0	1
Smoky BBQ Vinaigrette, 2 tbsp.	110	10	5	0	0
Spicy Buffalo Ranch Dressing, 2 tbsp.	130	14	2	0	1
Sweet Maple Dressing, 2 tbsp.	180	17	6	0	0
Thousand Island Dressing, 2 tbsp.	90	9	3	0	0
Tomato Basil Croutons, 5 pieces	70	5	5	0	1
Warm Bacon Dressing, 2 tbsp.	110	10	5	0	0
Hot Pastas & Kitchen Favorites					
4 Cheese Alfredo (Vegetarian), 1 cup	390	13	50	3	19
Arizona Marinara (Vegetarian), 1 cup	360	11	47	3	17
Beefy Meatball Stroganoff, 1 cup	340	21	28	2	9
Broccoli Alfredo w/ Basil, 1 cup	380	17	45	1	12
Bruschetta, 1 cup	260	4	41	3	10
Carbonara Pasta w/ Bacon, 1 cup	290	10	43	2	8
• Chicken Tetrazzini, 1 cup	480	23	47	3	19
Cilantro Lime Pesto (Vegetarian), 1 cup	370	21	36	2	9
Creamy Bruschetta (Vegetarian), 1 cup	360	16	43	3	12
Creamy Herb Chicken, 1 cup	310	17	32	2	8
Curried Pineapple & Ginger, 1 cup	200	2	40	2	6
Fettuccine Alfredo (Vegetarian), 1 cup	390	18	41	2	15
Fire-Roasted Tomato Basil Alfredo, 1 cup	370	14	44	3	19
Garden Vegetable w/ Italian Sausage, 1 cup	300	10	42	3	12
Garden Vegetable w/ Meatballs, 1 cup	310	10	44	3	11
Greek Mediterranean (Vegetarian), 1 cup	290	8	45	2	10
Hand-Crafted Mexican Beans, 1 cup	260	2	47	9	14
Italian Sausage w/ Red Pepper Puree, 1 cup	250	10	35	2	6
Italian Vegetable Beef, 1 cup	290	9	43	4	10
Lemon Cream w/ Capers, 1 cup	390	21	44	1	6
Linguini w/ Clam Sauce, 1 cup	380	10	56	1	16
Macaroni & Cheese (Vegetarian), 1 cup	290	10	40	2	10
Nutty Mushroom (Vegetarian), 1 cup	390	20	42	2	12
Oriental Noodle & Green Bean, 1 cup	240	3	45	2	7
Pasta Florentine (Vegetarian), 1 cup	360	10	54	7	18
Penne Arrabbiatta (Vegetarian), 1 cup	340	10	43	3	18
Roasted Eggplant Marinara, 1 cup	340	10	43	3	18
Roasted Garlic & Asiago Alfredo, 1 cup	330	11	45	2	13
Roasted Mushroom Alfredo w/ Rosemary, 1 cup	380	14	44	2	19
Salsa de Lupe (Fat- Free, Vegan), 1/4 cup	30	0	6	0	1
• Sautéed Balsamic Vegetables, 1/2 cup	100	6	11	3	1
Smoked Salmon & Dill, 1 cup	360	16	41	2	13
Smoky BBQ Baked Beans, 1 cup	320	3	61	9	14
Spicy Italian Sausage & Peppers, 1 cup	360	11	43	3	19
Steamed Veggies w/ Lemon Herb Butter, 1/2 cup	130	9	10	3	1
Stuffing, 1/2 cup	211	12	20	1	5

RESTAURANTS & FAST-FOOD CHAINS

▶ Souplantation (cont.)

	Cal	Fat	Cbs	Fbr	Prtn
Hot Pastas & Kitchen Favorites (cont.)					
Tomato Spinach Whole Wheat, 1 cup	290	10	38	8	12
Tuscany Sausage w/Capers & Olives, 1 cup	240	10	29	2	10
Vegetable Ragu (Vegetarian), 1 cup	250	6	41	3	9
Vegetarian Marinara w/ Basil, 1 cup	260	4	44	3	10
Walnut Pesto (Vegetarian), 1 cup	310	9	42	2	10
Morning Menu					
Belgian Waffles, 1 piece	90	0	16	1	20
Blueberry Sauce / Blueberry Stir-In, 2 tbsp.	60	0	15	1	0
Country Ham & Egg Breakfast Burrito	210	10	21	2	10
Egg Scramble Focaccia w/ Bacon , 1 piece	180	8	20	1	7
French Toast (Plain), 1 piece	150	4	25	1	5
Homemade Oatmeal (Plain), 3/4 cup	110	2	19	3	3
Mediterranean Sunrise Pasta, 1 cup	210	12	19	2	6
Potatoes O'Brien, 1/2 cup	140	6	19	2	2
Scrambled Eggs, 1/2 cup	135	8	2	0	12
Strawberry Sauce/ Strawberry Stir-In, 2 tbsp.	60	0	14	0	0
Sweet Cinnamon Biscuits w/ Frosting, 1 piece	270	13	37	0	4
Sweet Maple Buttermilk Biscuit, 1 piece	240	9	39	1	3
Sweet Pepper & Sausage Egg Breakfast Burrito	210	11	20	2	9
Sweet Strawberry Buttermilk Biscuit, 1 piece	250	9	40	1	3
Tom's Country Gravy, 2 tbsp.	90	5	8	0	3
Zucchini Fritatta, 1 piece	160	6	22	4	7
Salads					
Ambrosia w/ Coconut (Vegetarian), 1/2 cup	190	9	30	2	1
Artichoke Rice (Vegetarian), 1/2 cup	190	12	19	1	1
• Aunt Doris' Red Pepper Slaw, 1/2 cup	70	0	18	3	1
Baja Bean & Cilantro, 1/2 cup	180	3	29	5	9
BBQ Potato (Vegetarian), 1/2 cup	170	9	21	2	2
Carrot Raisin, 1/2 cup	90	3	17	2	1
Chinese Krab, 1/2 cup	160	8	19	3	5
Citrus Noodles w/ Snow Peas, 1/2 cup	140	6	19	2	3
Confetti Avocado Slaw, 1/2 cup	140	9	12	3	2
Dijon Potato w/ Garlic Dill Vinaigrette, 1/2 cup	150	12	9	3	1
Field Corn & Very Wild Rice, 1/2 cup	170	9	19	3	4
German Potato, 1/2 cup	150	6	23	2	2
Italian White Bean, 1/2 cup	140	5	19	4	6
Jalapeño Potato, 1/2 cup	170	9	21	2	2
Joan's Broccoli Madness, 1/2 cup	180	14	11	3	2
Lemon Rice w/ Cashews, 1/2 cup	160	7	23	1	2
Mandarin Noodles w/ Broccoli, 1/2 cup	170	3	31	2	4
Mandarin Shells w/ Almonds, 1/2 cup	120	3	19	2	3
Old Fashioned Macaroni w/ Ham, 1/2 cup	200	13	18	2	4
Oriental Ginger Slaw w/ Krab, 1/2 cup	70	3	8	4	2
Pesto Pasta, 1/2 cup	180	9	21	2	4
Picnic Potato, 1/2 cup	190	14	11	2	2
Pineapple Coconut Slaw, 1/2 cup	150	10	14	2	1
Poppyseed Coleslaw, 1/2 cup	120	9	9	3	1
Red Potato & Tomato, 1/2 cup	170	11	17	3	2
Rstd Potato w/ Chipotle-Chile Vinaigrette, 1/2 cup	140	6	18	4	3
San Francisco Herb Rice, 1/2 cup	180	6	27	1	4
Shrimp & Seafood Shells, 1/2 cup	210	13	20	1	5
Smoky Ham & Cheddar Broccoli Slaw, 1/2 cup	260	18	21	3	5
Southern Black-Eyed Pea, 1/2 cup	130	6	18	3	2

RESTAURANTS & FAST-FOOD CHAINS

Souplantation (cont.)

Salads (cont.)	Cal	Fat	Cbs	Fbr	Prtn
Southern Dill Potato, 1/2 cup	120	3	20	2	4
Southwestern Rice & Beans, 1/2 cup	90	3	15	3	1
Spicy Cajun Shells (Vegetarian), 1/2 cup	300	13	40	3	5
Spicy Southwestern Pasta, 1/2 cup	130	3	21	4	5
Summer Barley w/ Black Beans, 1/2 cup	110	3	19	4	4
Sweet & Sour Broccoli Slaw, 1/2 cup	150	3	28	3	2
Sweet Marinated Vegetables, 1/2 cup	80	0	19	4	1
Tabouli (Vegan), 1/2 cup	200	10	24	5	3
Thai Citrus & Brown Rice, 1/2 cup	220	12	26	2	2
Thai Noodle w/ Chicken & Peanut Sauce, 1/2 cup	190	10	19	2	5
Three Bean Marinade, 1/2 cup	170	6	27	3	4
Tomato Cucumber Marinade, 1/2 cup	80	5	8	1	0
Tuna Tarragon, 1/2 cup	250	15	21	1	6
Turkey Chutney Pasta, 1/2 cup	240	12	20	1	8
Wheat Berry & Curry, 1/2 cup	210	5	36	5	6
Whole Grain Fiesta Couscous, 1/2 cup	280	11	39	8	8
• Wild Rice & Chicken, 1/2 cup	300	21	21	1	5
Zesty Tortellini, 1/2 cup	230	15	20	2	4
Soups					
8 Vegetable Chicken Stew, 1 cup	160	7	17	2	8
Albondigas Locas, 1 cup	210	11	19	2	8
• Asian Ginger Broth, 1 cup	50	2	6	0	1
Beef & Barley Stew, 1 cup	240	10	19	3	12
Better than Mom's Beef Stew, 1 cup	270	17	19	2	9
Big Chunk Chicken Noodle, 1 cup	170	3	19	1	15
Border Black Bean & Chorizo Soup, 1 cup	240	10	27	6	11
Broccoli Cheese, 1 cup	280	20	16	2	10
• Canadian Cheese w/ Smoked Ham, 1 cup	370	27	20	1	12
Cheese Stuffed Cappelletti, 1 cup	250	11	31	2	6
Chesapeake Corn Chowder, 1 cup	290	17	30	2	6
Chicken & Rice, 1 cup	160	5	18	1	10
Chicken Fajitas & Black Bean, 1 cup	280	7	37	7	22
Chicken Pot Pie Stew, 1 cup	310	21	21	2	8
Chili Cheeseburger, 1 cup	290	12	29	3	15
Chunky Potato Cheese w/ Thyme, 1 cup	240	11	25	2	8
Classic Creamy Tomato Soup, 1 cup	200	13	19	2	2
Classical French Onion, 1 cup	150	6	21	1	1
Classical Minestrone, 1 cup	120	2	20	3	4
Classical Shrimp Bisque, 1 cup	240	16	15	1	9
Continental Lentil & Spinach, 1 cup	160	2	28	10	7
Corned Beef & Cabbage, 1 cup	150	6	17	3	6
Country Corn & Red Potato Chowder, 1 cup	220	8	35	4	3
Cream of Broccoli (Vegetarian), 1 cup	260	19	19	3	4
Cream of Chicken, 1 cup	290	21	16	1	10
Cream of Mushroom, 1 cup	290	24	15	1	5
Cream of Rosemary Potato, 1 cup	320	22	26	2	3
Creamy Herbed Turkey, 1 cup	320	22	18	1	11
Creamy Vegetable Chowder, 1 cup	270	14	26	2	8
Curried Yellow Split Pea, 1 cup	230	2	40	12	12
Deep Kettle House Chili, 1 cup	230	3	26	7	15
Deep Kettle House Chili, 33% more meat!, 1 cup	250	8	26	7	15
Deep Kettle House Chili, 50% more meat!, 1 cup	290	11	29	6	18
El Paso Lime & Chicken, 1 cup	160	4	24	2	7

RESTAURANTS & FAST-FOOD CHAINS

Souplantation (cont.)

	Cal	Fat	Cbs	Fbr	Prtn
Soups (cont.)					
Field of Creams - Sweet Tomato Basil, 1 cup	220	15	20	2	3
Fire-Roasted Green Chile & Corn Chowder, 1 cup	240	15	21	1	5
Garden Fresh Vegetable, 1 cup	150	2	27	4	4
Garden of Eatin', 1 cup	150	3	25	6	5
Golden Yam Bisque, 1 cup	220	8	28	2	2
Green Chile Stew w/ Pork, 1 cup	170	6	18	2	9
Indian Lentil, 1 cup	160	3	25	9	8
Irish Potato Leek, 1 cup	260	16	23	2	5
Lemon Chicken Orzo, 1 cup	220	9	21	1	13
Loaded Baked Potato & Cheese w/ Bacon, 1 cup	290	18	24	2	9
Longhorn Beef Chili, 1 cup	190	6	25	4	10
Marvelous Minestrone w/ Bacon, 1 cup	220	8	31	4	7
Minestrone w/ Italian Sausage, 1 cup	220	12	17	4	9
Mulligatawny, 1 cup	240	14	17	2	10
Neighbor Joe's Gumbo, 1 cup	210	10	20	2	9
New Mexican Corn Tortilla w/ Chicken, 1 cup	200	10	19	2	8
New Orleans Jambalaya, 1 cup	210	11	18	3	11
Old Fashion Vegetable, 1 cup	100	2	18	5	2
Pinto Bean & Basil Barley, 1 cup	160	2	29	7	6
Posole w/ Pork, 1 cup	150	6	8	2	12
Potato Tomato & Spinach, 1 cup	150	2	28	2	2
Ratatouille Provencale, 1 cup	110	0	25	2	2
Roasted Mushroom w/ Sage, 1 cup	320	26	19	1	5
Rustic Tuscan Stew, 1 cup	140	2	25	4	6
Santa Fe Black Bean Chili, 1 cup	190	3	26	8	9
Savory Turkey Harvest, 1 cup	220	12	18	2	9
Smoky Pinto & Brown Rice, 1 cup	150	2	28	5	5
Southwest Tomato Cream, 1 cup	130	7	14	2	3
Southwest Turkey Chowder w/ Bacon, 1 cup	240	15	21	2	6
Spicy Sausage & Pasta, 1 cup	300	12	34	5	13
Spicy Vegetable Chili w/ Energy Boost, 1 cup	100	1	17	6	5
Split Pea & Potato Barley, 1 cup	200	2	37	10	8
Split Pea w/ Ham, 1 cup	290	10	36	8	14
Sweet Tomato Onion, 1 cup	90	3	13	2	2
Texas Red Chili, 1 cup	190	7	24	6	8
Three-Bean Turkey Chili, 1 cup	170	3	24	7	13
Tomato Chipotle Bisque, 1 cup	250	17	20	2	5
Tomato Parmesan & Vegetables, 1 cup	120	3	18	3	4
Turkey Cassoulet w/ Bacon, 1 cup	240	12	17	3	14
Turkey Vegetable, 1 cup	210	12	15	2	10
U.S. Senate Bean w/ Smoked Ham, 1 cup	150	4	20	3	7
Vegetable Bean & Barley Stew, 1 cup	150	2	0	5	4
Vegetable Medley, 1 cup	90	1	14	3	2
Vegetarian Harvest, 1 cup	200	10	23	4	4
White Bean & Lime Chicken Chili, 1 cup	220	5	29	6	15
Yankee Clipper Clam Chowder w/ Bacon, 1 cup	340	20	21	2	18
Sweet Tomatoes Extras					
Azteca Taco w/ Turkey, 1 cup	130	9	7	4	6
Bartlett Pear & Caramelized Walnut, 1 cup	180	12	13	2	4
BBQ Julienne Chopped w/ Chicken, 1 cup	210	11	23	3	5
BBQ Smokehouse Bacon & Peanuts, 1 cup	290	17	25	2	9
Buffalo Chicken, 1 cup	180	14	10	1	4
Caesar Salad Asiago, 1 cup	270	22	10	2	5

RESTAURANTS & FAST-FOOD CHAINS

Souplantation (cont.)

Sweet Tomatoes Extras (cont.)

	Cal	Fat	Cbs	Fbr	Prtn
California Cobb w/ Bacon, 1 cup	190	15	7	2	5
Cambay Curry w/ Almonds & Coconut, 1 cup	220	17	17	4	3
Cape Cod Spinach Walnuts & Bacon, 1 cup	170	14	6	4	4
Cherry Chipotle Spinach, 1 cup	160	8	20	4	1
Chicken Tortilla, 1 cup	180	10	16	2	6
• Classic Greek, 1 cup	120	9	4	2	3
Club Blue BLT w/ Bacon, 1 cup	270	17	20	3	6
Country French w/ Bacon, 1 cup	210	18	7	2	10
Crunchy Island Pineapple, 1 cup	160	8	20	2	1
Field of Greens: Citrus Vinaigrette, 1 cup	150	12	10	2	1
Field of Greens: Sweet Maple, 1 cup	180	15	10	2	1
• Green Chile Ranch Cornbread Bites, 1 cup	330	21	26	3	8
Honey Minted Fruit Toss, 1 cup	140	6	20	3	1
Mandarin Spinach w/ Caramelized Walnuts, 1 cup	170	11	14	3	3
Monterey Blue w/ Peanuts, 1 cup	270	17	25	2	5
Outrageous Orange w/ Cashews, 1 cup	210	15	16	2	2
Ragin' Cajun w/ Chicken, 1 cup	220	14	15	3	7
Ranch House BLT w/ Turkey & Bacon, 1 cup	190	13	11	6	6
Roasted Vegetables w/ Feta & Olives, 1 cup	190	15	12	2	2
Sedona Green Chile & Chipotle, 1 cup	220	16	15	3	2
Smoked Turkey & Spinach w/ Almonds, 1 cup	190	10	20	3	6
Sonoma Spinach w/ Dijon Vinaigrette, 1 cup	210	14	16	2	5
Spiced Pecan & Roasted Veggies w/ Bacon, 1 cup	200	13	15	2	5
Spinach Gorgonzola w/ Pecans & Bacon, 1 cup	230	19	9	3	5
Spinach w/ Pumpkin Seeds & Cranberries, 1 cup	200	15	11	6	6
Strawberry Fields w/ Caramelized Walnuts, 1 cup	130	8	15	3	3
Summer Lemon w/ Spiced Pecans, 1 cup	220	17	16	2	2
Sweet Tomato, Basil & Mozzarella, 1 cup	120	9	7	1	4
Thai Peanut & Red Pepper, 1 cup	220	11	23	5	7
Thai Udon & Peanut, 1 cup	220	13	19	3	5
Traditional Spinach w/ Bacon, 1 cup	190	13	11	3	5
Won Ton Chicken Happiness, 1 cup	170	9	15	2	6

Southern Tsunami

	Cal	Fat	Cbs	Fbr	Prtn
Blue Crab Roll, 251 g	674	14	112	8	20
California Roll, 270 g	628	5	129	5	15
Classic Miso Roll, 306 g	758	9	13	4	30
Cream Cheese Roll, 280 g	794	19	123	4	29
Crunchy Shrimp Roll, 294 g	773	18	129	8	26
Dragon Roll (FW Eel), 288 g	785	18	130	6	23
Dragon Roll (Sea Eel), 288 g	736	14	131	6	19
Eel Roll (FW Eel), 281 g	770	16	128	4	25
Eel Roll (Sea Eel), 281 g	713	11	130	4	20
Fullmoon Combo, 281 g	698	12	128	5	19
M&M Roll (Shrimp, Avocado), 214 g	609	4	125	5	16
M&M Roll (Tuna, Cucumber), 223 g	611	1	124	4	21
Marina Plate, 218 g	633	7	111	2	27
Meteor Special, 263 g	700	3	141	5	22
Nigiri (Egg Cake), 54 g	141	1	29	1	3
Nigiri (Fish Roe), 38 g	102	0	19	0	7
Nigiri (FW Eel), 45 g	149	5	20	1	6
• Nigiri (Octopus), 29 g	98	1	18	0	3
Nigiri (Salmon), 38 g	109	1	18	0	5

Southern Tsunami (cont.)

	Cal	Fat	Cbs	Fbr	Prtn
Nigiri (Sea Eel), 60 g	159	3	27	1	4
Nigiri (Shrimp), 45 g	112	0	25	0	3
Nigiri (Smoked Salmon), 53 g	136	1	25	0	5
Nigiri (Tilapia), 47 g	118	0	25	0	3
Nigiri (Tuna), 53 g	129	0	25	0	5
Nigiri (Yellowtail), 50 g	123	1	25	0	4
Ocean Crab Roll, 283 g	678	8	125	6	27
Orange Roll, 299 g	672	6	131	5	25
Rainbow Roll, 353 g	764	8	129	5	37
Red Chili Roll, 255 g	600	13	89	3	26
Seaside Combo (Tuna, Salmon), 238 g	684	4	124	3	31
Seaside Combo (Tuna, Salmon, Shrimp, Eel), 217 g	639	4	125	4	22
Sheroline Combo, 319 g	811	7	156	5	27
Snack Pack (Cucumber), 214 g	593	0	133	4	11
Snack Pack (Krab, Cucumber), 266 g	645	4	140	4	16
Spicy Roll (Baby Shrimp), 286 g	710	8	133	5	23
Spicy Roll (Salmon), 279 g	745	14	121	4	30
Spicy Roll (Tuna), 285 g	731	9	125	4	30
• Stardust Combo, 352 g	981	9	200	6	22
Tempura Roll, 315 g	806	11	146	4	30
Tsunami Roll, 260 g	734	12	133	5	24
Vegetable Combo (12 pcs.), 267 g	618	6	128	7	12
Vegetable Combo (24 pcs.), 331 g	877	3	191	8	17
Condiments					
• Green Horseradish, 4 g	7	0	1	0	0
Pickled Ginger, 13 g	9	0	24	0	0
• Soy Sauce, 7 g	16	0	2	0	2
Salads					
Edamame (Soybean), 75 g	90	5	3	8	9
• Edamame Salad, 113 g	124	7	9	1	7
• Seabreeze Salad, 113 g	13	3	23	0	0

Starbucks

	Cal	Fat	Cbs	Fbr	Prtn
Brewed Coffees - Grande					
• Caffe Misto/Café Au Lait, 16 fl.oz.	110	4	10	0	7
• Coffee of the Week, 16 fl.oz.	5	0	0	0	1
Decaf Coffee Of the Week, 16 fl.oz.	16	0	0	0	1
Iced Brewed Coffee, 16 fl.oz.	90	0	21	0	0
Brownies, Cookies & Bars					
Blueberry Oat Bar w/ Organic Blueberries, 103 g	390	15	59	3	5
Chocolate Chip Cookie, 85 g	350	15	54	3	5
Crispy Marshmallow Square, 92 g	360	9	68	0	3
• Mini Chocolate Chip Cookie, 28 g	120	5	18	1	2
Oatmeal Raisin Cookie, 85 g	350	12	56	3	5
Seasonal Cookie, 102 g	410	16	64	1	4
• Snickerdoodle Cookie, 99 g	410	17	62	1	5
Classic Favorites					
Apple Juice, 16 fl.oz.	250	0	64	0	0
Caramel Apple Spice - no whip, 16 fl.oz.	310	0	74	0	0
Caramel Apple Spice - whip, 16 fl.oz.	380	8	76	0	0
Chocolate Milk, 16 fl.oz.	350	11	52	2	18
Cinnamon Dolce Crème - no whip, 16 fl.oz.	280	7	40	0	12
Cinnamon Dolce Crème - whip, 16 fl.oz.	350	14	42	0	13
Hot Chocolate - no whip, 16 fl.oz.	300	9	47	2	14

RESTAURANTS & FAST-FOOD CHAINS

Starbucks (cont.)

	Cal	Fat	Cbs	Fbr	Prtn
Classic Favorites (cont.)					
Hot Chocolate - whip, 16 fl.oz.	370	16	49	2	14
Milk, 16 fl.oz.	260	10	25	0	17
Steamed Apple Juice, 16 fl.oz.	230	0	56	0	0
Vanilla Crème - no whip, 16 fl.oz.	260	7	36	0	12
• Vanilla Crème - whip, 16 fl.oz.	33	14	38	0	13
White Hot Chocolate - no whip, 16 fl.oz.	40	12	61	0	16
• White Hot Chocolate - whip, 16 fl.oz.	490	19	63	0	16
Croissants, Bagels & Breads					
Butter Croissant, 102 g	370	21	37	1	7
• Chocolate Croissant, 120 g	470	26	54	2	7
• Lowfat Eight Grain Roll, 112 g	270	2	56	5	8
Plain Bagel, 113 g	310	1	62	2	11
Pretzel, 113 g	290	5	52	2	8
Strawberry Jam Buttermilk Biscuit, 113	340	13	50	1	5
Doughnuts, Sweet Rolls & Danishes					
Cheese Danish, 111 g	390	24	36	1	7
• Cinnamon Roll, 167 g	500	15	83	3	8
Doughnuts, Sweet Rolls & Danishes, 113 g	480	25	60	2	5
Top Pot Apple Fritter, 123 g	490	22	65	1	4
Top Pot Glazed Old Fashioned Doughnut, 113 g	480	23	64	1	4
• Top Pot Glazed Old Fashioned Mini Doughnut, 34 g	150	7	19	0	1
Drink Extras					
Flavored Syrup, 1 pump 10 g	20	0	5	0	0
Mocha Syrup, 1 Pump 17 fl.oz.	25	1	6	0	1
Plus Energy, 15 fl.oz.	5	0	1	0	0
• Sugar Free Flavored Syrup, 1 pump 10 g	0	0	0	0	0
Toppings - Caramel, 15 g	15	1	2	0	0
Toppings - Chocolate, 4 g	5	0	1	0	0
• Whip Cream Grande & Venti Cold, 35 g	110	11	3	0	1
Whip Cream Grande & Venti Hot, 22 g	70	7	2	0	0
Espresso - Cold - Grande 2% Milk					
• Iced Caffe Americano, 16 fl.oz.	15	0	3	0	1
Iced Caffe Latte, 16 fl.oz.	130	5	13	0	8
Iced Caffe Mocha - no whip, 16 fl.oz.	200	6	35	2	9
Iced Caffe Mocha - whip, 16 fl.oz.	320	17	38	2	9
Iced Caramel Macchiato, 16 fl.oz.	230	6	33	0	10
Iced Doubleshot on Ice +Energy Bev, 16 fl.oz.	100	1	20	0	3
Iced Doubleshot on Ice Beverage, 16 fl.oz.	90	1	20	0	2
Iced Ppprmnt Wht Choc. Mocha no whip, 16 fl.oz.	400	9	72	0	9
• Iced Ppprmnt Wht Choc. Mocha - whip, 16 fl.oz.	510	20	75	0	10
Iced Sugar-Free Syrup Flavored Latte, 16 fl.oz.	110	4	12	0	7
Iced Syrup Flavored Latte, 16 fl.oz.	190	4	30	0	7
Iced Vanilla Latte, 16 fl.oz.	190	4	30	0	7
Iced White Chocolate Mocha - no whip, 16 fl.oz.	340	9	55	0	10
Iced White Chocolate Mocha - whip, 16 fl.oz.	450	20	58	0	11
Espresso - Hot - Grande					
• Caffe Americano, 16 fl.oz.	15	0	3	0	1
Caffe Latte, 16 fl.oz.	190	7	18	0	12
Caffe Mocha - no whip, 16 fl.oz.	260	8	41	2	13
Caffe Mocha - whip, 16 fl.oz.	330	15	43	2	13
Cappuccino, 16 fl.oz.	120	4	12	0	8
Caramel Macchiato, 16 fl.oz.	240	7	34	0	10
Cinnamon Dolce Latte - no whip, 16 fl.oz.	260	6	40	0	11

Starbucks (cont.)

	Cal	Fat	Cbs	Fbr	Prtn
Espresso - Hot - Grande (cont.)					
Cinnamon Dolce Latte - whip, 16 fl.oz.	330	13	42	0	12
Cinnamon Dolce Latte, Sugar-Free Syrup, 16 fl.oz.	180	6	18	0	12
Peppermnt White Choc. Mocha - no whip, 16 fl.oz.	460	11	78	0	14
Peppermnt White Choc. Mocha - whip, 16 fl.oz.	530	18	80	0	14
Syrup Flavored Latte, 16 fl.oz.	250	6	36	0	12
Vanilla Latte, 16 fl.oz.	250	6	36	0	12
White Choc. Mocha - no whip, 16 fl.oz.	400	11	61	0	15
White Choc. Mocha - whip, 16 fl.oz.	470	18	63	0	15
Frappuccino Blended Coffee - Grande 2% Milk					
Caffè Vanilla - no whip, 16 fl.oz.	310	3	67	0	5
Caffè Vanilla - whip, 16 fl.oz.	430	14	70	0	6
Caramel - no whip, 16 fl.oz.	270	4	53	0	5
Caramel - whip, 16 fl.oz.	380	15	57	0	6
Cinnamon Dolce - no whip, 16 fl.oz.	260	3	52	0	5
Cinnamon Dolce - whip, 16 fl.oz.	370	14	55	0	6
Coffee, 16 fl.oz.	240	3	48	0	5
• Espresso, 16 fl.oz.	190	3	38	0	4
Java Chip - no whip, 16 fl.oz.	340	8	64	2	7
• Java Chip - whip, 16 fl.oz.	460	19	67	2	7
Mocha - no whip, 16 fl.oz.	260	4	54	0	6
Mocha - whip, 16 fl.oz.	380	15	57	0	6
White Chocolate Mocha - no whip, 16 fl.oz.	300	5	59	0	6
White Chocolate Mocha - whip, 16 fl.oz.	410	16	62	0	7
Frappuccino Blended Crème - Grande 2% Milk					
• Chai - no whip, 16 fl.oz.	330	2	67	0	10
Chai - whip, 16 fl.oz.	440	13	71	0	11
Green Tea - no whip, 16 fl.oz.	380	3	78	1	11
Green Tea - whip, 16 fl.oz.	490	14	82	1	12
Double Chocolaty Chip - no whip, 16 fl.oz.	400	8	75	2	13
Double Chocolaty Chip - whip, 16 fl.oz.	510	19	78	2	14
Strawberries & Crème - no whip, 16 fl.oz.	440	3	92	1	12
• Strawberries & Crème - whip, 16 fl.oz.	570	15	95	1	12
Vanilla Bean - no whip, 16 fl.oz.	350	3	72	0	11
Vanilla Bean - whip, 16 fl.oz.	470	14	75	0	12
Frappuccino Light Blended Coffee - Grande					
Caffé Vanilla Light, 16 fl.oz.	190	1	42	3	6
Caramel Light, 16 fl.oz.	160	2	30	3	5
Cinnamon Dolce Light, 16 fl.oz.	140	1	29	3	5
Coffee Light, 16 fl.oz.	130	1	25	3	5
• Espresso Light, 16 fl.oz.	110	1	20	2	5
Java Chip Light, 16 fl.oz.	200	5	36	4	6
• Mint Mocha Chip Light no whip, 16 fl.oz.	210	4	40	4	6
Mocha Light, 16 fl.oz.	140	1	29	3	6
White Chocolate Mocha Light, 16 fl.oz.	180	2	34	3	6
Loaves & Coffee Cakes					
Banana Walnut Loaf, 128 g	410	17	60	2	6
Classic Coffee Cake, 113 g	420	18	61	1	5
• Crumble Coffee Cake, 122 g	500	25	65	1	5
Lemon Loaf, 128 g	430	19	62	0	6
No Sugar Added Banana Nut Cake, 124 g	480	28	63	3	7
Rdcd.-Fat Strwbrries & Crème Cake, 124 g	330	9	57	1	5
Reduced-Fat Blueberry Cake, 122 g	320	6	54	1	4
• Reduced-Fat Cinnamon Swirl Cake, 105 g	300	6	53	1	4

(•= most healthy •= least healthy)   **RESTAURANTS & FAST-FOOD • 337**

RESTAURANTS & FAST-FOOD CHAINS

Starbucks (cont.)

	Cal	Fat	Cbs	Fbr	Prtn
Loaves & Coffee Cakes (cont.)					
Reduced-Fat Lemon Blueberry Loaf, 136 g	360	10	63	1	5
Muffins & Scones					
Banana Bran Muffin, 149 g	410	14	69	6	8
• Blueberry Muffin, 170 g	500	19	75	2	8
Blueberry Scone, 120 g	400	17	54	2	5
Cranberry Orange Scone, 135 g	450	16	72	2	5
Lowfat Apricot Blueberry Muffin, 159 g	380	5	77	2	7
Maple Oat Nut Scone, 113 g	440	22	56	2	5
• Mini Blueberry Muffin, 68 g	200	8	30	1	3
Triple Berry Cobbler Muffin, 150 g	480	25	61	1	5
Zucchini Walnut Mini Muffin, 105 g	390	24	42	2	6
Oven-Toasted Breakfast Items					
Bcn, Avocado, Aged Cheddar & Egg Wrap, 153 g	380	24	26	7	20
Bacon, Egg & Cheddar Bkfst. Sandwich, 156 g	370	17	37	2	18
Forest Ham, Egg & Cheddar Bkfst. Sand, 173 g	360	15	37	2	20
• Sausage, Egg & Cheddar Bkfst. Sandwich, 184 g	440	23	37	2	20
Spinach, Rsted Tomato, Feta & Egg Wrap, 144 g	240	10	29	7	13
Special Treats					
Triple Chocolate Cupcake, 90 g	360	20	46	2	3
Vanilla Cupcake, 86 g	330	16	43	1	3
Tazo Tea - Grande					
Black Shaken Iced Tea Lemonade, 16 fl.oz.	130	0	33	0	0
Black Shaken Iced Tea, 16 fl.oz.	80	0	21	0	0
Chai Iced Tea Latte, 16 fl.oz.	240	4	44	0	7
Chai Tea Latte, 16 fl.oz.	240	4	44	0	7
Green Shaken Iced Tea Lemonade, 16 fl.oz.	130	0	33	0	0
Green Shaken Iced Tea, 16 fl.oz.	80	0	21	0	0
Green Tea Latte, 16 fl.oz.	240	5	41	1	8
• Iced Green Tea Latte, 16 fl.oz.	270	5	44	1	10
Lemonade Blended with Zen™ Green Tea, 16 fl.oz.	190	0	47	1	0
Passion™ Shaken Iced Tea Lemonade, 16 fl.oz.	130	0	33	0	0
Passion™ Shaken Iced Tea, 16 fl.oz.	80	0	21	0	0
• Tea, 16 fl.oz.	0	0	0	0	0
Vivanno Nourishing Blends - Grande					
Banana Choc. Blend w/ Espresso Shot, 16 fl.oz.	260	5	42	5	20
Banana Chocolate Blend, 16 fl.oz.	270	5	44	6	21
• Orange Mango Banana Blend w/ Matcha, 16 fl.oz.	290	2	57	6	16
• Orange Mango Banana Blend, 16 fl.oz.	250	2	46	6	16

Steak Escape

	Cal	Fat	Cbs	Fbr	Prtn
7" Sandwiches					
Cajun Chicken, 245 g	408	5	58	N/A	31
• Capicola Portion, 28 g	31	1	0	N/A	5
Chicken Portion, 112 g	120	4	0	N/A	21
• Classic Italian, 238 g	471	11	60	N/A	27
Grand Chicken, 266 g	410	6	60	N/A	32
Ham Portion, 84 g	75	1	3	N/A	8
Salami Portion, 28 g	105	9	0	N/A	6
Steak Portion, 112 g	130	5	0	N/A	19
The Grand Escape, 266 g	420	6	60	N/A	30
Turkey Club, 224 g	380	2	62	N/A	21
Turkey Portion, 84 g	75	1	3	N/A	8
Vegetarian, 252 g	311	1	65	N/A	13

Steak Escape (cont.)	Cal	Fat	Cbs	Fbr	Prtn
7" Sandwiches (cont.)					
Wild West BBQ, 273 g	455	6	60	N/A	29
Fries					
Fresh Cut Fries - 16 oz. cup, 224 g	651	34	87	N/A	10
Fresh Cut Fries - 32 oz. cup, 448 g	996	52	134	N/A	16
Kids Meal Fresh Cut Fries, 84 g	249	13	34	N/A	4
Loaded Fries - Bacon & Cheddar, 308 g	905	44	88	N/A	18
Loaded Fries - Ranch & Bacon, 308 g	1044	71	84	N/A	18
Kids Sandwiches					
Chicken, 110 g	205	7	29	N/A	12
Ham, 106 g	183	1	31	N/A	6
Steak, 110 g	210	3	29	N/A	9
Turkey, 106 g	183	1	31	N/A	6
Loaded Smashed Potatoes					
Bacon & Cheddar, 476 g	636	26	91	N/A	13
Ranch & Bacon, 476 g	692	34	87	N/A	14
Salad					
Side Salad, 168 g	40	1	8	N/A	3
with Chicken, 316 g	177	5	11	N/A	25
with Ham, 302 g	132	2	8	N/A	19
with Meatball, 546 g	561	24	58	N/A	27
with Portabello, 532 g	290	1	63	N/A	15
with Steak, 316 g	187	6	11	N/A	23
with Turkey, 302 g	132	2	8	N/A	19
Smashed Potatoes					
Plain, 392 g	246	0	53	N/A	11
with Chicken, 568 g	383	4	56	N/A	33
with Ham, 554 g	338	2	59	N/A	27
with Meatball, 546 g	561	24	58	N/A	27
with Portabello, 532 g	290	1	63	N/A	15
with Steak, 568 g	393	5	56	N/A	31
with Turkey, 554 g	338	2	59	N/A	27
Toppings					
Bacon, 28 g	32	3	2	N/A	0
Balsamic Vinaigrette, 42 g	90	9	3	N/A	0
BBQ Sauce, 28 g	40	0	9	N/A	0
Black Olives, 42 g	11	0	2	N/A	0
Bleu Cheese Dressing, 42 g	184	18	3	N/A	2
Brown Mustard, 28 g	0	0	0	N/A	0
Cheddar, 28 g	116	8	1	N/A	8
Italian Dressing, 14 g	51	5	1	N/A	0
Jalapeño Peppers, 42 g	11	N/A	N/A	N/A	N/A
Lettuce, 28 g	2	0	1	N/A	1
Margarine, 28 g	203	23	0	N/A	0
Mayonnaise, 28 g	101	11	0	N/A	0
Mild Peppers, 42 g	11	0	4	N/A	0
Parmesan, 7 g	30	2	0	N/A	3
Provolone, 21 g	80	6	0	N/A	5
Ranch Dressing, 14 g	83	9	0	N/A	0
Sour Cream, 28 g	61	6	1	N/A	1
Tomatoes, 56 g	24	0	2	N/A	2
White American, 28 g	101	9	3	N/A	6

RESTAURANTS & FAST-FOOD CHAINS

Sub Station II

	Cal	Fat	Cbs	Fbr	Prtn
Bologna & Cheese, 6"	658	47	44	N/A	18
Corned Beef & Cheese, 6"	613	39	40	N/A	25
• Genoa Salami, Pepperoni & Cheese, 6"	791	58	43	N/A	26
Ham & Cheese, 6"	582	36	42	N/A	19
Ham, Bologna & Cheese, 6"	645	44	42	N/A	20
Ham, Bologna, Cappicola & Cheese, 6"	624	42	41	N/A	20
• Ham, Cappicola & Cheese, 6"	580	36	42	N/A	21
Ham, Genoa Salami & Cheese, 6"	679	45	45	N/A	23
Ham, Genoa Salami, Pepperoni & Chz, 6"	789	55	48	N/A	28
Ham, Pepperoni & Cheese, 6"	720	49	48	N/A	24
Ham, Turkey & Cheese, 6"	606	37	49	N/A	22
Provolone, Swiss & American Cheese, 6"	700	49	40	N/A	25
Roast Beef & Cheese, 6"	631	40	44	N/A	26
Roast Beef, Ham & Cheese, 6"	608	38	42	N/A	24
Roast Beef, Ham, Turkey & Cheese, 6"	628	39	39	N/A	28
Roast Beef, Turkey & Cheese, 6"	603	38	41	N/A	25
Turkey & Cheese, 6"	601	37	48	N/A	24

Submarina

	Cal	Fat	Cbs	Fbr	Prtn
Salads					
Coleslaw, 1 side	170	12	14	2	1
Green Salad - large	31	0	6	4	2
• Green Salad - small	16	0	3	2	1
• Macaroni Salad, 1 side	230	13	23	2	3
Pasta Salad, 1 side	174	11	17	2	3
Potato Salad, 1 side	143	8	18	2	1
Specialities					
• Albacore Tuna, 6"	816	50	59	3	31
ATC, 6"	521	17	58	4	33
Avocado, Roast Beef & Cheese, 6"	542	18	61	4	32
California Sub, 6"	761	38	58	4	45
Chicken Caesar, 6"	611	26	60	6	35
Club Sub, 6"	712	32	57	2	44
East Coast Sub, 6"	632	26	57	2	38
Grilled Chicken, 6"	512	16	53	2	37
Italian Sub, 6"	666	31	59	2	34
Meatball & Cheese, 6"	648	29	67	4	33
NY Style Hot Pastrami, 6"	795	48	54	2	37
Santa Fe Chicken, 6"	716	36	58	4	45
• Triple Play, 6"	501	12	57	2	36
• Veggie, 6"	544	24	58	5	26

Subway

	Cal	Fat	Cbs	Fbr	Prtn
4" Subway® Minis					
• Ham, 137 g	180	3	30	4	11
Roast Beef, 147 g	190	4	30	4	13
• Tuna (with cheese), 156 g	320	18	30	4	13
Turkey Breast, 147 g	190	3	30	4	12
6" Breads , Rolls & Wraps					
• Deli Style Roll, 71 g	170	3	32	3	6
Flatbread, 94 g	250	5	43	2	8
Hearty Italian Bread, 75 g	220	2	41	2	8
Honey Oat, 88 g	250	4	48	5	10
Italian Herbs & Cheese, 82 g	251	5	41	2	10

RESTAURANTS & FAST-FOOD CHAINS

Subway (cont.)	Cal	Fat	Cbs	Fbr	Prtn
6" Breads , Rolls & Wraps (cont.)					
Italian (White) Bread, 71 g	200	2	38	1	7
Parmesan Oregano Bread, 75 g	220	3	41	2	8
Wheat Bread, 78 g	200	3	40	4	8
Monterey Cheddar, 82 g	240	5	39	1	10
Wrap, 103 g	310	8	51	1	8
6" Breakfast Sandwiches					
Cheese, 189 g	420	18	44	5	23
Chipotle Steak & Cheese, 281 g	600	32	49	6	34
Double Bacon & Cheese, 207 g	510	25	45	5	30
Honey Mustard Ham & Cheese, 238 g	470	19	52	5	28
Western with Cheese, 229 g	450	19	46	5	28
6" Double Meat Subs					
Double Chicken & Bacon Ranch (w/ chz), 377 g	710	35	48	6	55
Double Cold Cut Combo (w/ cheese), 320 g	550	28	49	5	31
Double Ham, 281 g	350	7	49	5	28
Double Italian BMT (w/ cheese), 306 g	630	35	49	5	34
• Double Meatball Marinara, 575 g	860	42	82	11	37
Double Oven Roasted Chicken, 309 g	400	8	51	6	38
Double Roast Beef, 281 g	360	7	46	5	29
Double Steak & Cheese, 632 g	540	18	52	7	46
Double Subway Club®, 347 g	420	8	50	5	39
Double Subway Melt® (w/ cheese), 330 g	490	17	51	5	40
Double Sweet Onion Chkn. Teriyaki, 373 g	480	7	65	6	43
Double Turkey Breast & Ham, 300 g	360	7	50	5	31
• Double Turkey Breast, 281 g	330	5	48	5	28
6" Jared Sandwiches					
Ham, 224 g	290	5	47	5	18
Oven Roasted Chicken Breast, 238 g	310	5	48	5	24
Roast Beef, 224 g	290	5	45	5	19
Subway Club®, 257 g	320	6	47	5	24
• Sweet Onion Chicken Teriyaki, 281 g	370	5	59	5	26
Turkey Breast & Ham, 234 g	290	5	47	5	20
Turkey Breast, 224 g	280	5	46	5	18
• Veggie Delite®, 167 g	230	3	44	5	9
6" Limited Time Subs					
• Barbecue Chicken, 238 g	310	6	52	5	16
Barbecue Rib Patty, 245 g	420	19	47	5	20
Buffalo Chicken, 274 g	380	18	46	5	25
Subway® Seafood Sensation (w/ cheese), 250 g	450	22	51	5	16
• The Feast (w/ cheese), 372 g	590	25	52	5	44
Veggie Patty, 252 g	390	8	56	8	24
6" Sandwiches					
• Chicken & Bacon Ranch, 297 g	580	30	47	6	36
Cold Cut Combo, 249 g	410	17	47	5	21
Italian BMT®, 243 g	450	21	47	5	23
Meatball Marinara, 377 g	560	24	63	8	24
Spicy Italian, 227 g	480	25	45	5	21
Steak & Cheese, 278 g	400	12	48	6	29
• Subway Melt®, 254 g	380	12	48	5	25
Tuna, 250 g	530	31	44	5	22
8" Pizza					
Cheese & Veggies, 381 g	740	25	100	5	36
• Cheese, 293 g	680	22	96	4	32

(•= most healthy •= least healthy) **RESTAURANTS & FAST-FOOD • 341**

Subway (cont.)

	Cal	Fat	Cbs	Fbr	Prtn
8" Pizza (cont.)					
Pepperoni, 323 g	790	32	96	4	38
• Sausage, 339 g	830	35	97	4	40
Cheese (amount on 6" sub, wrap or salad)					
• American, Processed, 11 g	40	4	1	0	2
Monterey Cheddar, Shredded, 14 g	50	5	1	0	3
• Natural Cheddar, 15 g	60	5	0	0	4
Pepperjack, 14 g	50	4	0	0	3
Provolone, 14 g	50	4	0	0	4
Swiss, 14 g	50	5	0	0	4
Cookies & Desserts					
• Apple Pie, 71 g	250	10	37	1	0
• Apple Slices - 1 package, 71 g	35	0	9	2	0
Chocolate Chip, 45 g	210	10	30	1	2
Chocolate Chunk, 45 g	220	10	30	1	2
Double Chocolate Chip, 45 g	210	10	30	1	2
M & M®, 45 g	210	10	32	1	2
Oatmeal Raisin, 45 g	200	8	30	1	3
Peanut Butter, 45 g	220	12	26	1	4
Raisins - 1 package, 43 g	140	0	33	2	2
White Chip Macadamia Nut, 45 g	220	11	29	1	2
Yogurt - Dannon® All-Natural Strawberry, 113 g	110	1	20	0	5
Fruizle Express (Small)					
Berry Lishus (w/ banana), 396 g	140	0	35	2	1
Berry Lishus, 369 g	110	0	28	1	1
• Peach Pizzazz, 341 g	100	0	26	0	0
• Pineapple Delight (w/ banana), 396 g	160	0	40	2	1
Pineapple Delight, 369 g	130	0	33	1	1
Sunrise Refresher, 341 g	120	0	29	1	1
Individual Meats (amount on 6" sub or salad)					
Chicken Patty, Roasted, 71 g	90	3	4	0	15
Chicken Strips, 71 g	80	2	0	0	16
Cold Cut Combo Meats, 71 g	140	11	2	0	10
Egg Patty, 85 g	110	8	3	1	9
Ham, 57 g	60	2	3	0	9
Italian BMT® Meats, 64 g	180	14	2	0	12
• Meatballs, 198 g	300	18	19	3	13
Roast Beef, 57 g	70	2	1	0	10
Seafood Sensation, 71 g	190	16	7	0	5
Subway Club® Meats, 90 g	100	3	3	0	15
Tuna, 71 g	260	24	0	0	10
• Turkey Breast, 57 g	50	1	2	0	9
Veggie Patty, 85 g	160	5	12	3	15
Jared Salads					
Ham, 371 g	120	3	14	4	12
Oven Roasted Chicken Breast, 385 g	140	3	11	4	19
Roast Beef, 371 g	120	3	12	4	13
Subway Club®, 404 g	150	4	14	4	18
• Sweet Onion Chicken Teriyaki, 427 g	210	3	26	4	20
Turkey Breast & Ham, 380 g	120	3	14	4	14
Turkey Breast, 371 g	110	3	13	4	12
• Veggie Delite®, 314 g	60	1	11	4	3
Salad Dressing					
Fat Free Italian, 57 g	35	0	7	0	1

Subway (cont.)

Subway (cont.)	Cal	Fat	Cbs	Fbr	Prtn
Salad Dressing (cont.)					
Ranch, 57 g	320	35	3	0	0
Sandwich Condiments (amount on 6" sub)					
Bacon (2 strips), 9 g	45	4	0	0	3
Chipotle Southwest Sauce, 21 g	96	10	1	0	0
Honey Mustard Sauce, Fat Free, 21 g	30	0	7	0	0
Light Mayonnaise (1 tbsp.), 15 g	50	5	1	0	0
Mayonnaise (1 tbsp.), 14 g	110	12	0	0	0
Mustard yellow or deli brown (2 tsp.), 10 g	5	0	1	0	0
Olive Oil Blend (1 tsp.), 7 g	45	5	0	0	0
Ranch Dressing, 21 g	120	13	1	0	0
Red Wine Vinaigrette, Fat Free, 21 g	29	0	6	0	0
Sweet Onion Sauce, Fat Free, 21 g	40	0	9	0	0
Vinegar (1 tsp.), 8 g	0	0	0	0	0
Soup					
Chicken and Dumpling, 10 oz.	170	5	23	2	8
Chili Con Carne, 10 oz.	290	8	35	12	19
Cream of Broccoli, 10 oz.	160	7	18	5	6
Cream of Potato with Bacon, 10 oz.	240	13	26	3	5
Golden Broccoli & Cheese, 10 oz.	200	12	17	3	5
Minestrone, 10 oz.	80	1	15	4	4
New England Style Clam Chowder, 10 oz.	150	5	20	4	6
Roasted Chicken Noodle, 10 oz.	80	2	11	1	6
Spanish Style Chicken with Rice, 10 oz.	110	2	17	1	6
Tomato Garden Vegetable w/ Rotini, 10 oz.	90	0	20	2	3
Vegetable Beef, 10 oz.	100	2	15	3	6
Wild Rice with Chicken, 10 oz.	210	11	21	2	6
Vegetables (amount on 6" sub)					
Banana Peppers (3 rings), 4 g	0	0	0	0	0
Cucumbers (3 slices), 17 g	5	0	1	0	0
Green Peppers (3 strips), 7 g	0	0	0	0	0
Jalapeño Peppers (3 rings), 4 g	5	0	0	0	0
Lettuce, 21 g	5	0	0	0	0
Olives (3 rings), 3 g	5	0	0	0	0
Onions, 14 g	5	0	1	0	0
Pickles (3 chips), 9 g	0	0	0	0	0
Tomatoes (3 wheels), 34 g	5	0	2	0	0

Sweet Tomatoes	Cal	Fat	Cbs	Fbr	Prtn
Bakery					
Apple Cinnamon Bran Muffin, 1 piece	130	1	30	3	2
Apple Raisin Muffin, 1 piece	150	7	22	1	2
Banana Crunch Muffin Top, 1 piece	120	5	19	1	3
Banana Nut Muffin, 1 piece	150	7	22	1	2
BBQ Chkn Focaccia, Honey Wheat Crust, 1 pc	200	8	23	2	9
Black Forest Muffin, 1 piece	230	9	36	1	2
Bruschetta Focaccia, 1 piece	140	7	15	1	4
Buffalo Chkn Focaccia, Honey Wht. Crust, 1 pc	170	7	20	2	6
Buttermilk Biscuits, 1 biscuit	190	8	25	0	4
Buttermilk Cornbread, 1 piece	140	2	27	2	3
Cappuccino Chip Muffin, 1 piece	190	6	31	1	3
Caribbean Key Lime Muffin, 1 piece	170	6	28	1	2
Carrot Pineapple Muffin w/ Oat Bran, 1 pc	150	6	23	2	3
Cherry Nut Muffin, 1 piece	150	7	22	1	2

RESTAURANTS & FAST-FOOD CHAINS

Sweet Tomatoes (cont.)

	Cal	Fat	Cbs	Fbr	Prtn
Bakery (cont.)					
Chile Corn Muffin, 1 piece	140	3	27	2	3
Chipotle Lime Butter, 1 tbsp.	90	10	0	0	0
Chocolate Brownie Muffin, 1 piece	180	8	26	1	3
Chocolate Chip Muffin, 1 piece	170	8	22	1	3
Chocolate Peanut Butter Chip Muffin, 1 piece	220	10	31	1	2
Country Blackberry Muffin, 1 piece	170	6	27	1	2
Cranberry Orange Bran Muffin, 1 piece	130	1	30	3	2
Date N' Honey Bran, 1 piece	150	6	24	2	2
• French Quarter Praline Muffin, 1 piece	250	10	35	1	4
Fruit Medley Bran Muffin, 1 piece	130	1	29	3	2
Garlic Asiago Focaccia, 1 piece	160	8	19	1	4
Georgia Peach Poppyseed Muffin, 1 piece	150	6	20	1	2
Grilled Cheese Focaccia, 1 piece	190	10	18	0	5
Indian Grain Bread, 1 piece	200	2	35	0	11
Irish Soda Bread, 1 piece	180	5	29	1	4
Lemon Vanilla Butter, 1 tbsp.	90	8	3	0	0
Mango Tropics Muffin w/ Coconut, 1 piece	180	7	28	1	2
Maple Walnut Muffin, 1 piece	230	10	32	1	3
Old World Greek Focaccia, 1 piece	190	9	24	2	3
Pauline's Apple Walnut Cake, 1 piece	220	12	24	1	3
Pepperoni Focaccia, 1 piece	190	9	21	1	5
Pesto & Sun-Dried Tomato Focaccia, 1 piece	170	8	20	1	5
Pumpkin Raisin Muffin, 1 piece	150	6	25	1	2
Quattro Formaggio Focaccia, 1 piece	140	5	19	1	5
Roasted Potato Focaccia, 1 piece	150	6	17	2	6
Roasted Red Pepper, Honey Wht. Focaccia, 1 piece	170	8	20	2	5
Sautéed Vegetable Focaccia, 1 piece	180	9	19	1	5
Sourdough Bread, 1 piece	150	1	27	0	9
Southwest Chipotle Focaccia, 1 piece	160	8	19	1	5
Spiced Pumpkin Muffin w/ Cranberries, 1 piece	180	7	29	1	2
Strawberry Buttermilk Muffin, 1 piece	140	6	21	1	2
Sweet Cherry Butter, 1 tbsp.	80	7	4	0	0
Sweet Orange & Cranberry Muffin, 1 piece	200	7	33	1	2
Sweet Strawberry Butter, 1 tbsp.	80	7	4	0	0
Taffy Apple Muffin, 1 piece	160	6	25	1	2
Tangy Lemon Muffin, 1 piece	140	4	24	1	2
Thai Chicken Focaccia w/ Peanuts, 1 piece	170	7	20	1	7
Wildly Blue Blueberry Muffin, 1 piece	140	5	22	1	2
Wowie Maui Focaccia w/ Ham, 1 piece	170	7	21	1	6
Zucchini Nut Muffin, 1 piece	150	7	22	1	2
Desserts					
Apple Cobbler, 1/2 cup	360	10	67	1	2
Apple Medley, 1/2 cup	70	0	18	1	1
Banana Pudding, 1/2 cup	160	4	27	1	4
Banana Royale, 1/2 cup	80	0	20	1	1
Butterscotch Pudding, 1/2 cup	140	3	24	0	4
Candy Sprinkles, 1 tbsp.	70	3	11	0	0
• Caramel Apple Cobbler, 1/2 cup	390	12	68	2	3
Cherry Apple Cobbler, 1/2 cup	330	10	57	2	2
Chocolate Chip Cookie Bars, 1 piece	90	4	13	0	1
Chocolate Chip Cookie, 1 cookie	75	3	10	0	1
Chocolate Frozen Yogurt , 1/2 cup	95	0	21	0	3
Chocolate Lava Cake, 1/2 cup	330	8	62	0	2

RESTAURANTS & FAST-FOOD CHAINS

Sweet Tomatoes (cont.)

	Cal	Fat	Cbs	Fbr	Prtn
Desserts (cont.)					
Chocolate Peanut Butter Cookie Cups, 1 piece	140	6	18	1	1
Chocolate Pudding, 1/2 cup	150	3	25	0	4
Choco Pudding, Lowfat, No Added Sugar 1/2 cup	90	2	21	0	4
Chocolate Syrup, 2 tbsp.	70	0	18	0	0
Cranberry Apple Cobbler, 1/2 cup	370	10	58	3	3
Cran-Raspberry Gelatin , 1/2 cup	100	0	26	0	1
Deep Chocolate Winter Mint Lava Cake, 1/2 cup	330	8	58	0	2
Green Tea Mousse, 1/2 cup	190	8	29	0	3
Holiday Cookies w/ Sprinkles, 1 cookie	80	4	12	0	0
Hot Lemon Lava Cake, 1/2 cup	320	11	51	1	2
Nutty Waldorf Salad, 1/2 cup	90	3	14	3	1
Oatmeal Raisin Cookie, 1 cookie	120	5	16	1	1
Pineapple Gelatin, 1/2 cup	120	0	29	0	1
Pineapple Upside- Down Cake, 1/2 cup	270	10	42	1	2
Raspberry Apple Cobbler, 1/2 cup	380	11	67	2	3
Rice Pudding, 1/2 cup	110	2	20	1	3
Shortcake, 1 piece	220	7	36	0	3
Strawberry Apple Cobbler, 1/2 cup	340	10	67	2	3
• Sugar-free Chocolate Mousse, 1/2 cup	40	3	3	1	1
Sugar-free Lemon Mousse, 1/2 cup	40	3	4	1	1
Sugar-free Strawberry Mousse, 1/2 cup	40	3	4	1	1
Tapioca Pudding, 1/2 cup	140	3	24	0	4
Vanilla Pudding, 1/2 cup	150	4	27	0	3
Vanilla Soft Serve, 1/2 cup	140	5	22	0	3
Warm Carrot Cake w/ Cream Chz Lava, 1/2 cup	320	15	40	1	3
Dressings					
Avocado Ranch Dressing, 2 tbsp.	150	14	4	0	1
Bacon Dressing, 2 tbsp.	110	11	7	0	0
• Balsamic Vinaigrette, 2 tbsp.	180	19	1	0	0
Basil Vinaigrette, 2 tbsp.	160	17	1	0	1
Blue Cheese Dressing, 2 tbsp.	130	13	3	0	1
Chow Mein Noodles, 1/4 Cup	70	1	15	0	1
Cranberry Orange Vinaigrette, 2 tbsp.	80	2	15	0	0
Creamy Italian Dressing, 2 tbsp.	120	13	0	0	0
Cucumber Dressing, 2 tbsp.	70	7	3	0	0
Garlic Parmesan Seasoned Croutons, 5 pieces	80	5	6	0	2
Green Chili Ranch Dressing, 2 tbsp.	150	14	4	0	1
Honey Lime Cilantro Vinaigrette, 2 tbsp.	100	6	15	0	0
Honey Mint Lemonade, 2 tbsp.	130	7	19	0	0
Honey Mustard Dressing, 2 tbsp.	150	13	8	0	0
Honey Mustard Dressing, 2 tbsp.	45	0	10	0	0
• Italian Dressing, 2 tbsp.	25	0	7	0	0
Kahlena French Dressing, 2 tbsp.	120	9	10	0	0
Monterey Blue Salad Dressing, 2 tbsp.	120	11	5	0	0
Parmesan Pepper Cream Dressing, 2 tbsp.	140	16	1	0	1
Pineapple Vinaigrette, 2 tbsp.	120	11	5	0	0
Plain Croutons, 5 pieces	50	2	7	0	1
Ranch Dressing, 2 tbsp.	150	15	4	0	1
Ranch Dressing Fat Free, 2 tbsp.	50	0	2	0	1
Roasted Garlic Dressing, 2 tbsp.	100	10	3	0	1
Smoky BBQ Vinaigrette, 2 tbsp.	110	10	5	0	0
Spicy Buffalo Ranch Dressing, 2 tbsp.	130	14	2	0	0
Sweet Maple Dressing, 2 tbsp.	180	17	6	0	0

RESTAURANTS & FAST-FOOD CHAINS

Sweet Tomatoes (cont.)

	Cal	Fat	Cbs	Fbr	Prtn
Dressings (cont.)					
Thousand Island Dressing, 2 tbsp.	90	9	3	0	0
Tomato Basil Croutons, 5 pieces	70	5	5	0	1
Warm Bacon Dressing, 2 tbsp.	110	10	5	0	0
Hot Pastas & Kitchen Favorites					
4 Cheese Alfredo, 1 cup	390	13	50	3	19
Arizona Marinara, 1 cup	360	11	47	3	17
Beefy Meatball Stroganoff, 1 cup	340	21	28	2	9
Broccoli Alfredo w/ Basil, 1 cup	380	17	45	1	12
Bruschetta, 1 cup	260	4	41	3	10
Carbonara Pasta w/ Bacon, 1 cup	290	10	43	2	8
• Chicken Tetrazzini, 1 cup	480	23	47	3	19
Cilantro Lime Pesto, 1 cup	370	21	36	2	9
Creamy Bruschetta, 1 cup	360	16	43	3	12
Creamy Herb Chicken, 1 cup	310	17	32	2	8
Curried Pineapple & Ginger, 1 cup	200	2	40	2	6
Fettuccine Alfredo, 1 cup	390	18	41	2	15
Fire-Roasted Tomato Basil Alfredo, 1 cup	370	14	44	2	19
Garden Vegetable w/ Italian Sausage, 1 cup	300	10	42	3	12
Garden Vegetable w/ Meatballs, 1 cup	310	10	44	3	11
Greek Mediterranean, 1 cup	290	8	45	2	10
Hand-Crafted Mexican Beans, 1 cup	260	2	47	9	14
Italian Sausage w/ Red Pepper Puree, 1 cup	250	10	35	2	6
Italian Vegetable Beef, 1 cup	290	9	43	4	10
Lemon Cream w/ Capers, 1 cup	390	21	44	1	6
Linguini w/ Clam Sauce, 1 cup	380	10	56	1	16
Macaroni & Cheese, 1 cup	290	10	40	2	10
Nutty Mushroom, 1 cup	390	20	42	2	12
Oriental Noodle & Green Bean, 1 cup	240	3	45	2	7
Pasta Florentine, 1 cup	360	10	54	7	18
Penne Arrabbiatta, 1 cup	340	10	43	3	18
Roasted Eggplant Marinara, 1 cup	340	10	43	3	18
Roasted Garlic & Asiago Alfredo, 1 cup	330	11	45	2	13
Roasted Mushroom Alfredo w/ Rosemary, 1 cup	380	14	44	2	19
Salsa de Lupe, 1/4 cup	30	0	6	0	1
• Sautéed Balsamic Vegetables, 1/2 cup	100	6	11	3	1
Smoked Salmon & Dill, 1 cup	360	16	41	2	13
Smoky BBQ Baked Beans, 1 cup	320	3	61	9	14
Spicy Italian Sausage & Peppers, 1 cup	360	11	43	3	19
Steamed Veggies w/ Lemon Herb Butter, 1/2 cup	130	9	10	3	1
Stuffing, 1/2 cup	210	12	20	1	5
Tomato Spinach Whole Wheat, 1 cup	290	10	38	8	12
Tuscany Sausage w/ Capers & Olives, 1 cup	240	10	29	2	10
Vegetable Ragu, 1 cup	250	6	41	3	9
Vegetarian Marinara w/ Basil, 1 cup	260	4	44	3	10
Walnut Pesto, 1 cup	310	9	42	2	10
Morning Menu					
• Belgian Waffles, 1 piece	90	0	16	1	20
Blueberry Sauce, 2 tbsp.	60	0	15	1	0
Country Ham & Egg Breakfast Burrito, 1 burrito	210	10	21	2	10
Egg Scramble Focaccia w/ Bacon, 1 piece	180	8	20	1	7
French Toast (Plain), 1 piece	150	4	25	1	5
Homemade Oatmeal (Plain), 3/4 cup	110	2	19	3	3
Mediterranean Sunrise Pasta, 1 cup	210	12	19	2	6

RESTAURANTS & FAST-FOOD CHAINS

Sweet Tomatoes (cont.)

	Cal	Fat	Cbs	Fbr	Prtn
Morning Menu (cont.)					
Potatoes O'Brien, 1/2 cup	140	6	19	2	2
Scrambled Eggs, 1/2 cup	135	8	2	0	12
Strawberry Sauce, 2 tbsp.	60	0	14	0	0
Sweet Cinnamon Biscuits w/ Frosting, 1 piece	270	13	37	0	4
Sweet Maple Buttermilk Biscuit, 1 piece	240	9	39	1	3
Sweet Strawberry Buttermilk Biscuit, 1 piece	250	9	40	1	3
Swt. Pepper & Sausage Egg Bkfst. Burrito	210	11	20	2	9
Tom's Country Gravy, 2 tbsp.	90	5	8	0	3
Zucchini Fritatta, 1 piece	160	6	22	4	7
Salads					
Ambrosia w/ Coconut, 1/2 cup	190	9	30	2	1
Artichoke Rice, 1/2 cup	190	12	19	1	1
Aunt Doris' Red Pepper Slaw, 1/2 cup	70	0	18	3	1
Baja Bean & Cilantro, 1/2 cup	180	3	29	5	9
BBQ Potato, 1/2 cup	170	9	21	2	2
Carrot Raisin, 1/2 cup	90	3	17	2	1
Chinese Krab, 1/2 cup	160	8	19	3	5
Citrus Noodles w/ Snow Peas, 1/2 cup	140	6	19	2	3
Confetti Avocado Slaw, 1/2 cup	140	9	12	3	2
Dijon Potato w/ Garlic Dill Vinaigrette, 1/2 cup	150	12	9	3	1
Field Corn & Very Wild Rice, 1/2 cup	170	9	19	3	4
German Potato, 1/2 cup	150	6	23	2	2
Greek Couscous w/ Feta & Pinenuts, 1/2 cup	210	10	25	4	5
Italian White Bean, 1/2 cup	140	5	19	4	6
Jalapeño Potato, 1/2 cup	170	9	21	2	2
Joan's Broccoli Madness, 1/2 cup	180	14	11	3	2
Lemon Rice w/ Cashews, 1/2 cup	160	7	23	1	2
Mandarin Noodles w/ Broccoli, 1/2 cup	170	3	31	2	4
Mandarin Shells w/ Almonds, 1/2 cup	120	3	19	2	3
Old Fashioned Macaroni w/ Ham, 1/2 cup	200	13	18	2	4
Oriental Ginger Slaw w/ Krab, 1/2 cup	70	3	8	4	2
Penne Pasta w/ Chkn & Citrus Vinaigrette, 1/2 cup	130	3	20	2	5
Pesto Pasta, 1/2 cup	180	9	21	2	4
Picnic Potato, 1/2 cup	190	14	17	2	2
Pineapple Coconut Slaw, 1/2 cup	150	10	14	2	1
Poppyseed Coleslaw, 1/2 cup	120	9	9	3	1
Red Potato & Tomato, 1/2 cup	170	11	17	3	2
Rstd Potato w/ Chipotle-Chile Vinaigrette, 1/2 cup	140	6	18	4	3
San Francisco Herb Rice, 1/2 cup	180	6	27	1	4
Shrimp & Seafood Shells, 1/2 cup	210	13	20	1	5
Smoky Ham & Cheddar Broccoli Slaw, 1/2 cup	260	18	21	3	5
Southern Black-Eyed Pea, 1/2 cup	130	6	18	3	2
Southern Dill Potato, 1/2 cup	120	3	20	2	4
Southwestern Rice & Beans, 1/2 cup	90	3	15	3	1
Spicy Cajun Shells, 1/2 cup	300	13	40	3	5
Spicy Southwestern Pasta, 1/2 cup	130	3	21	4	5
Summer Barley w/ Black Beans, 1/2 cup	110	3	19	4	4
Sweet & Sour Broccoli Slaw, 1/2 cup	150	3	28	3	2
Sweet Marinated Vegetables, 1/2 cup	80	0	19	4	1
Tabouli, 1/2 cup	200	10	24	5	3
Thai Citrus & Brown Rice, 1/2 cup	220	12	26	2	2
Thai Noodle w/ Chicken & Peanut Sauce, 1/2 cup	190	10	19	2	5
Three Bean Marinade, 1/2 cup	170	6	27	3	4

(•= most healthy •= least healthy)

RESTAURANTS & FAST-FOOD CHAINS

Sweet Tomatoes (cont.)

	Cal	Fat	Cbs	Fbr	Prtn
Salads (cont.)					
Tomato Cucumber Marinade, 1/2 cup	80	5	8	1	0
Tuna Tarragon, 1/2 cup	250	15	21	1	6
Turkey Chutney Pasta, 1/2 cup	240	12	20	1	8
Wheat Berry & Curry, 1/2 cup	210	5	36	5	6
Whole Grain Fiesta Couscous, 1/2 cup	280	11	39	8	8
• Wild Rice & Chicken, 1/2 cup	300	21	21	1	5
Zesty Tortellini, 1/2 cup	230	15	20	2	4
Soups					
8 Vegetable Chicken Stew, 1 cup	160	7	17	2	8
Albondigas Locas, 1 cup	210	11	19	2	8
• Asian Ginger Broth, 1 cup	50	2	6	0	1
Beef & Barley Stew, 1 cup	240	10	19	3	12
Better Than Mom's Beef Stew, 1 cup	270	17	19	2	9
Big Chunk Chicken Noodle, 1 cup	170	3	19	1	15
Border Black Bean & Chorizo Soup, 1 cup	240	10	27	6	11
Broccoli Cheese, 1 cup	280	20	16	2	10
• Canadian Cheese w/ Smoked Ham, 1 cup	370	27	20	1	12
Cheese Stuffed Cappelletti, 1 cup	250	11	31	2	6
Chesapeake Corn Chowder, 1 cup	290	17	30	2	6
Chicken & Rice, 1 cup	160	5	18	1	10
Chicken Fajitas & Black Bean, 1 cup	280	7	37	7	22
Chicken Pot Pie Stew, 1 cup	310	21	21	2	8
Chicken Tortilla w/ Jalapeño & Tomatoes, 1 cup	100	3	11	1	6
Chili Cheeseburger, 1 cup	290	12	29	3	15
Chunky Potato Cheese w/ Thyme, 1 cup	240	11	25	2	8
Classic Creamy Tomato Soup, 1 cup	200	13	19	2	2
Classical French Onion, 1 cup	150	6	21	1	1
Classical Minestrone, 1 cup	120	2	20	3	4
Classical Shrimp Bisque, 1 cup	240	16	15	1	9
Continental Lentil & Spinach, 1 cup	160	2	28	10	7
Corned Beef & Cabbage, 1 cup	150	6	17	3	6
Country Corn & Red Potato Chowder, 1 cup	220	8	35	4	3
Cream of Broccoli, 1 cup	260	19	19	3	4
Cream of Chicken, 1 cup	290	21	16	1	10
Cream of Mushroom, 1 cup	290	24	15	1	4
Cream of Rosemary Potato, 1 cup	320	22	26	2	3
Creamy Herbed Turkey, 1 cup	320	22	18	1	11
Creamy Vegetable Chowder, 1 cup	270	14	26	2	8
Curried Yellow Split Pea, 1 cup	230	2	40	12	12
Deep Kettle House Chili, 1 cup	230	3	26	7	15
Deep Kettle House Chili, 33% more meat!, 1 cup	250	8	26	7	15
Deep Kettle House Chili, 50% more meat!, 1 cup	290	11	29	6	18
El Paso Lime & Chicken, 1 cup	160	4	24	2	7
Field of Creams - Cauliflower w/ Cheese, 1 cup	280	21	17	1	5
Field of Creams - Sweet Tomato Basil, 1 cup	220	15	20	2	3
Fire-Roasted Green Chile & Corn Chowder, 1 cup	240	15	21	1	5
Garden Fresh Vegetable, 1 cup	150	2	27	4	4
Garden of Eatin', 1 cup	150	3	25	6	5
Golden Yam Bisque, 1 cup	220	8	28	4	2
Green Chile Stew w/ Pork, 1 cup	170	6	18	2	9
Indian Lentil, 1 cup	160	3	25	9	8
Irish Potato Leek, 1 cup	260	16	23	2	5
Lemon Chicken Orzo, 1 cup	220	9	21	1	13

RESTAURANTS & FAST-FOOD CHAINS

Sweet Tomatoes (cont.)

	Cal	Fat	Cbs	Fbr	Prtn
Soups (cont.)					
Loaded Baked Potato & Cheese w/ Bacon, 1 cup	290	18	24	2	9
Longhorn Beef Chili, 1 cup	190	6	25	4	10
Marvelous Minestrone w/ Bacon, 1 cup	220	8	31	4	7
Minestrone w/ Italian Sausage, 1 cup	220	12	17	4	9
Moroccan Garbanzo & Lentil Bean, 1 cup	230	2	40	12	13
Mulligatawny, 1 cup	240	14	17	2	10
Neighbor Joe's Gumbo, 1 cup	210	10	20	2	9
New Mexican Corn Tortilla w/ Chicken, 1 cup	200	10	19	2	8
New Orleans Jambalaya, 1 cup	210	11	18	3	11
Old Fashion Vegetable, 1 cup	100	2	18	5	2
Pinto Bean & Basil Barley, 1 cup	160	2	29	7	6
Posole w/ Pork, 1 cup	150	6	8	2	12
Potato Tomato & Spinach, 1 cup	150	2	28	2	2
Ratatouille Provencale, 1 cup	110	0	25	4	2
Roasted Mushroom w/ Sage, 1 cup	320	26	19	1	5
Rustic Tuscan Stew, 1 cup	140	2	25	4	6
Santa Fe Black Bean Chili, 1 cup	190	3	26	8	9
Savory Turkey Harvest, 1 cup	220	12	18	2	9
Smoky Pinto & Brown Rice, 1 cup	150	2	28	5	5
Southwest Tomato Cream, 1 cup	130	7	14	2	3
Southwest Turkey Chowder w/ Bacon, 1 cup	240	15	21	2	6
Spicy Sausage & Pasta, 1 cup	300	12	34	5	13
Spicy Vegetable Chili w/ Energy Boost, 1 cup	100	1	17	6	5
Split Pea & Potato Barley, 1 cup	200	2	37	10	8
Split Pea w/ Ham, 1 cup	290	10	36	8	14
Sweet Tomato Onion, 1 cup	90	3	13	2	2
Texas Red Chili, 1 cup	190	7	24	6	8
Three-Bean Turkey Chili, 1 cup	170	3	24	7	13
Tomato Chipotle Bisque, 1 cup	250	17	20	2	5
Tomato Parmesan & Vegetables, 1 cup	120	3	18	3	4
Turkey Cassoulet w/ Bacon, 1 cup	240	12	17	3	14
Turkey Vegetable, 1 cup	210	12	15	2	10
U.S. Senate Bean w/ Smoked Ham, 1 cup	150	4	20	3	7
Vegetable Bean & Barley Stew, 1 cup	150	2	0	5	4
Vegetable Medley, 1 cup	90	1	14	3	2
Vegetarian Harvest, 1 cup	200	10	23	4	4
White Bean & Lime Chicken Chili, 1 cup	220	5	29	6	15
Yankee Clipper Clam Chowder w/ Bacon, 1 cup	340	20	21	2	18
Tossed Salads					
Azteca Taco w/ Turkey, 1 cup	130	9	7	4	6
Bartlett Pear & Caramelized Walnut, 1 cup	180	12	13	2	4
BBQ Julienne Chopped w/ Chicken, 1 cup	210	11	23	3	5
BBQ Smokehouse Bacon & Peanuts, 1 cup	290	17	25	2	9
Buffalo Chicken, 1 cup	180	14	10	1	4
Caesar Salad Asiago, 1 cup	270	22	10	2	5
California Cobb w/ Bacon, 1 cup	190	15	7	2	5
Cambay Curry w/ Almonds & Coconut, 1 cup	220	17	17	4	3
Cape Cod Spinach Walnuts & Bacon, 1 cup	170	14	6	4	4
Cherry Chipotle Spinach, 1 cup	160	8	20	4	1
Chicken Tortilla, 1 cup	180	10	16	2	6
Classic Greek, 1 cup	120	9	4	2	3
Club Blue BLT w/ Bacon, 1 cup	270	17	20	3	6
Country French w/ Bacon, 1 cup	210	18	7	2	10

RESTAURANTS & FAST-FOOD CHAINS

▶ Sweet Tomatoes (cont.)

	Cal	Fat	Cbs	Fbr	Prtn
Tossed Salads (cont.)					
Crunchy Island Pineapple, 1 cup	160	8	20	2	1
Field of Greens: Citrus Vinaigrette, 1 cup	150	12	10	2	1
Field of Greens: Sweet Maple, 1 cup	180	15	10	2	1
• Green Chile Ranch Cornbread Bites, 1 cup	330	21	26.	3	8
Honey Minted Fruit Toss, 1 cup	140	6	20	3	1
Mandarin Spinach w/ Caramelized Walnuts, 1 cup	170	11	14	3	3
Monterey Blue w/ Peanuts, 1 cup	270	17	25	2	5
Outrageous Orange w/ Cashews, 1 cup	210	15	16	2	2
Ragin' Cajun w/ Chicken, 1 cup	220	14	15	3	7
Ranch Maple BLT w/Turkey, 1 cup	190	13	11	6	6
Roasted Veggies w/ Feta & Olives, 1 cup	190	15	12	2	2
Sedona Green Chile & Chipotle, 1 cup	220	16	15	3	2
Smoked Turkey & Spinach w/ Almonds, 1 cup	190	10	20	3	6
Sonoma Spinach w/ Dijon Vinaigrette, 1 cup	210	14	16	2	5
Spiced Pecan & Rsted Veggies w/ Bacon, 1 cup	200	13	15	2	5
Spinach Gorgonzola w/ Pecans & Bacon, 1 cup	230	19	9	3	5
Spinach w/ Pumpkin Seeds & Cranberries, 1 cup	200	15	11	6	6
Strawberry Fields w/ Caramelized Walnuts, 1 cup	130	8	15	3	3
Summer Lemon w/ Spiced Pecans, 1 cup	220	17	16	2	2
Sweet Tomato, Basil & Mozzarella, 1 cup	120	9	7	1	4
Thai Peanut & Red Pepper, 1 cup	220	11	23	5	7
Thai Udon & Peanut, 1 cup	220	13	19	3	5
Traditional Spinach w/ Bacon, 1 cup	190	13	11	3	5
Won Ton Chicken Happiness, 1 cup	170	9	15	2	6

▶ Swiss Chalet

	Cal	Fat	Cbs	Fbr	Prtn
Desserts					
Baked Apple Blossom, 160 g	470	28	52	6	5
Carrot Cake, 156 g	740	48	70	5	8
• Chocolate Eruption Cheesecake, 200 g	820	55	72	3	9
Classic Apple Pie, 136 g	330	14	49	2	3
Coconut Cream Pie, 106 g	310	20	23	1	3
Colossal Caramel Fudge Cheesecake, 200 g	700	39	78	2	10
• Lemon Meringue Pie, 113 g	295	9	65	1	3
Perfect Pecan Pie, 120 g	530	28	66	4	5
Sauce - Butterscotch, 34 g	100	0	24	0	0
Sauce - Chocolate, 34 g	80	0	20	0	1
Sauce - Strawberry, 34 g	40	0	10	0	0
Swiss Alps Chocolate Layer Cake, 125 g	590	39	55	4	6
From The Grill					
Feature Cut BBQ Ribs, 150 g	420	26	3	2	44
Grilled Chkn Breast (w/ rice and flatbread), 330 g	500	8	70	3	37
• Grilled Chkn Breast (w/o rice & flatbread), 115 g	130	2	1	0	28
Grilled Chicken Caesar (w/out flatbread), 285 g	490	34	16	9	34
• Large Cut BBQ Ribs, 452 g	1270	77	9	4	131
Regular Cut BBQ Ribs, 226 g	630	38	4	2	66
Kids' Meals (not including sides)					
Cheesy Pizza, 150 g	370	13	45	2	17
Chicken Strips, 3 strips	310	16	24	1	19
Chkn Thigh & Drumstick (w/ Skin), 139 g	310	19	2	2	35
• Grilled Cheese, 138 g	510	33	42	2	11
Mini Burgers (2), 138 g	360	18	32	2	22
• Mini Chicken Sandwiches (2), 151 g	281	8	30	2	23

⟩ Swiss Chalet (cont.)	Cal	Fat	Cbs	Fbr	Prtn
Rotisserie Chicken					
Chicken Pot Pie, 428 g	580	33	42	3	31
Double Leg (w/ skin), 278 g	630	38	4	4	70
Half Chicken (w/ skin), 298 g	610	31	5	5	82
Quarter Chicken Breast (skinless), 124 g	210	7	0	0	38
Quarter Chicken Breast (w/ skin), 149 g	300	11	3	3	47
Quarter Chicken Leg (skinless), 116 g	230	11	1	1	32
Quarter Chicken Leg (w/ skin), 139 g	310	19	2	2	35
Salad Dressings & Dips					
Famous Chalet Sauce, 100 ml	30	1	5	0	0
Asian Sesame Dressing, 15 ml	30	1	5	0	1
Balsamic Vinaigrette, 15 ml	40	4	2	0	0
Blue Cheese Dip, 15 ml	70	7	1	0	0
Caesar Dressing, 15 ml	90	9	1	0	0
Cajun Sauce Dip, 57 ml	100	9	3	0	2
Chalet Dressing, 15 ml	80	7	3	0	0
Fat-Free Raspberry Vinaigrette, 15 ml	15	0	3	0	0
Greek Dressing, 15 ml	70	7	1	0	0
Light Italian Dressing, 15 ml	35	4	1	0	0
Light Mayonnaise, 15 ml	45	5	1	0	0
Ranch Dressing, 15 ml	50	6	1	0	0
Salsa, 50 g	20	0	4	0	1
Tangy Plum Sauce, 28 g	50	0	24	0	0
Sides					
Baked Potato, 284 g	220	0	48	5	0
Butter, 10 g	70	8	0	0	0
Chinese Noodles, 160 g	230	2	44	0	10
Corn, 170 g	140	2	24	4	0
Flatbread, 46 g	140	4	22	2	4
Fresh Corn Chips, 28 g	140	7	19	2	2
Fresh Cut Fries (Fried in Trans Fat-Free Oil), 168 g	470	25	56	5	7
Fresh Vegetables, 170 g	80	1	15	7	0
Gravy, 113 g	45	2	7	0	1
Mashed Potatoes, 140 g	100	4	17	2	1
Oven-baked Roll (Homestyle White), 51 g	130	1	27	1	5
Oven-baked Roll (Multigrain), 56 g	150	2	28	2	6
Ramekin of Coleslaw, 64 g	70	5	5	1	1
Rice Pilaf, 170 g	240	3	48	1	5
Sautéed Mushrooms, 170 g	220	16	11	4	6
Side Caesar Salad, 100 g	210	19	9	5	4
Side Garden Salad (w/out dressing), 122 g	15	0	4	2	0
Side Greek Salad, 107 g	130	11	5	2	3
Sour Cream & Chives, 43 ml	70	5	3	0	2
Traditional Coleslaw, 180 g	200	14	15	3	2
Starters					
Caesar Salad, 170 g	360	32	15	9	6
Chalet Chicken Soup, 355 ml	160	4	17	2	14
Chalet Chicken Wings, 8 Mild Wings	640	44	16	1	40
Chicken Spring Rolls, 2 pieces	460	13	53	2	32
Dry Ribs, 400 g	920	64	4	0	76
Garden Salad (no dressing), 162 g	30	0	6	3	2
Greek Salad, 183 g	220	18	9	3	5
Perogies (7 pieces), 196 g	420	10	69	4	12
Sundried Garlic Cheese Loaf, 276 g	910	57	78	5	28

Swiss Chalet (cont.)

	Cal	Fat	Cbs	Fbr	Prtn
Starters (cont.)					
Sundried Garlic Loaf (no cheese), 219 g	700	39	75	5	15
Wholesome Choices					
Garden Fresh Quarter Chkn Breast Dinner, 368 g	360	11	14	8	50
Oriental Chkn Salad, no dressing or noodles, 460 g	300	11	14	3	37
• Oriental Noodles, 28 g	130	6	16	1	4
Santa Fe Grilled Chkn Salad (no dressing), 354 g	300	4	35	5	34
• Spinach Chkn Salad, no dressing or tortillas, 428 g	370	10	19	6	46
Tortillas, 26 g	150	10	13	1	2
Vegetable Stir Fry (no rice or noodles), 432 g	270	3	54	6	7
with Grilled Chicken (no rice or noodles), 547 g	400	4	55	6	35
Wraps, Sandwiches & Burgers					
Bacon Cheese Burger (w/out bun), 200 g	630	42	2	0	45
• Bacon Cheese Burger (with bun), 285 g	870	46	45	1	55
Chicken Club Wrap, 364 g	840	40	61	4	56
Chicken on a Kaiser (dark meat), 241 g	570	15	44	2	57
Chicken on a Kaiser (white meat), 222 g	440	8	31	1	53
Chicken Quesadilla, 290 g	590	18	73	7	33
Grilled Santa Fe Chicken Sandwich, 240 g	380	4	49	3	42
Hamburger (w/out bun), 165 g	490	38	1	0	35
Hamburger (with bun), 250 g	730	49	44	1	45
Messy Chicken Sandwich (dark meat), 344 g	540	18	41	2	50
Messy Chicken Sandwich (white meat), 344 g	490	12	40	1	56
• Veggie Burger (w/out bun), 90 g	190	9	8	5	18
Veggie Burger (with bun), 175 g	430	13	51	6	28

T.J. Cinnamons

	Cal	Fat	Cbs	Fbr	Prtn
Original Gourmet Cinnamon Roll					
Cinnamon Roll, 149 g	507	10	73	4	10
Pecan Sticky Bun					
Cinnamon Roll, 1 piece, 149 g	507	10	73	4	10
Sticky Bun Smear w/ pecans, 1 piece, 35 g	181	12	18	1	1
T.J. Cinnamons Mocha Chill					
Mocha Chill, 340 g	264	4	46	1	11
Whipped Cream, 14 g	43	3	1	0	0
T.J. Icing					
Cream Cheese Icing, 28 g	117	5	18	0	1
Twists					
Chocolate Twist, 71 g	250	12	34	2	4
Cinnamon Twist, 71 g	260	14	33	1	3

Taco Time

	Cal	Fat	Cbs	Fbr	Prtn
Burrito					
Big Juan, Chicken, 13 oz.	594	19	68	10	35
Big Juan, Seasoned Ground Beef, 13 oz.	651	26	71	12	30
Big Juan, Shredded Beef, 13 oz.	633	25	67	10	33
Casita, Chicken, 12 oz.	494	18	43	5	34
Casita, Seasoned Ground Beef, 12 oz.	552	25	46	6	29
Casita, Shredded Beef, 12 oz.	533	25	42	5	31
• Cheddar Melt, 3 oz.	250	12	25	4	11
Chicken & Black Bean, 10 oz.	476	16	51	9	30
• Chicken B.L.T., 10 oz.	721	41	44	8	41
Chicken Ranchero, 11 oz.	654	32	52	7	36
Crisp Chicken, 6 oz.	336	10	32	2	27

Taco Time (cont.)

	Cal	Fat	Cbs	Fbr	Prtn
Burrito (cont.)					
Crisp Meat (Seasoned Ground Beef), 6 oz.	450	22	36	4	23
Crisp Pinto Bean, 6 oz.	394	16	50	6	13
Soft Meat (Seasoned Ground Beef), 7 oz.	426	16	43	8	23
Soft Pinto Bean, 7 oz.	377	11	54	10	14
Veggie, 11 oz.	534	18	74	12	18
Desserts					
Churro w/ cinn & sugar, 2 oz.	245	15	26	0	2
Crustos, 4 oz.	294	6	58	3	6
Empanada, Apple, 4 oz.	234	7	40	2	4
Empanada, Cherry, 4 oz.	240	7	41	2	4
Empanada, Pumpkin, 4 oz.	256	8	42	2	6
Plain Churro, 2 oz.	205	15	16	0	2
Extras					
Chicken Filling, 3 oz.	102	0	1	0	21
Chipotle Ranch, 1 oz.	165	18	1	0	1
Guacamole, 1 oz.	50	5	2	1	0
Mild Cheddar, 2 oz.	223	18	1	0	14
Ranch, 1 oz.	181	20	1	N/A	1
Salsa Nuevo, 1 oz.	8	0	2	0	0
Salsa Verde, 1 oz.	6	0	2	0	0
Seasoned Ground Beef Filling, 3 oz.	143	7	4	2	13
Shredded Ground Beef Filling, 3 oz.	124	7	0	0	16
Sour Cream, 2 oz.	85	7	1	0	1
Taco Shells, 1 oz.	103	7	8	0	1
Thousand Island, 1 oz.	132	12	5	0	0
Tortilla Salad Bowl, 10", 2 oz.	259	13	31	2	5
Tortilla Salad Bowl, 8", 3 oz.	155	9	17	1	3
Salad					
Taco, Regular - Chicken, 9 oz.	351	15	24	2	27
Taco, Regular - Seasoned Ground Beef, 8 oz.	396	23	24	4	22
Taco, Regular - Shredded Beef, 8 oz.	377	22	21	2	25
Tostada Delight, Chicken, 11 oz.	565	29	36	4	37
Tostada Delight, Seasoned Ground Beef, 11 oz.	623	36	39	6	32
Tostada Delight, Shredded Beef, 11 oz.	604	36	35	5	35
Sides					
Chips, Taco, 2 oz.	150	3	27	1	3
Fries, Cheddar - Medium, 8 oz.	529	36	43	4	12
Fries, Mexi - Medium, 7 oz.	418	27	42	4	4
Fries, Stuffed - Medium, 7 oz.	463	9	42	4	11
Mexi-Rice, 4 oz.	87	1	19	0	2
Nachos, Grande, 17 oz.	1132	57	114	11	39
Refritos w/ chips, 7 oz.	304	11	35	6	14
Refritos w/o chips, 7 oz.	285	11	32	6	13
Taco					
1/2 lb. Soft, Chicken, 9 oz.	401	11	43	7	30
1/2 lb. Soft, Seasoned Ground Beef, 9 oz.	459	18	46	9	25
1/2 lb. Soft, Shredded Beef, 9 oz.	440	18	42	7	28
Crisp, Seasoned Ground Beef w/ Sour Cream, 5 oz.	254	14	13	2	15
Crisp, Seasoned Ground Beef, 4 oz.	225	12	12	2	15
Super Soft, Chicken - Wheat Tortilla, 12 oz.	586	19	27	6	37
Super Soft, Chicken, 11 oz.	540	18	56	10	35
Super Soft, Snd. Ground Beef - Wht. Tortilla, 12 oz.	644	26	30	8	32
Super Soft, Seasoned Ground Beef, 11 oz.	598	25	59	12	30

(•= most healthy •= least healthy)   **RESTAURANTS & FAST-FOOD • 353**

RESTAURANTS & FAST-FOOD CHAINS

▶ Taco Time (cont.)

Taco (cont.)	Cal	Fat	Cbs	Fbr	Prtn
Super Soft, Shredded Beef - Wheat Tortilla, 12 oz.	626	26	26	6	34
Super Soft, Shredded Beef, 11 oz.	579	25	55	10	32
Value Soft, 5 oz.	314	13	28	6	18

▶ Taco Bell

Big Bell Value Menu®	Cal	Fat	Cbs	Fbr	Prtn
• 1/2 lb. Beef & Potato Burrito, 252 g	530	23	66	6	15
1/2 lb. Beef Combo Burrito, 241 g	440	18	51	8	21
1/2 lb. Cheesy Bean & Rice Burrito, 227 g	470	20	58	6	13
Caramel Apple Empanada, 85 g	290	14	37	1	3
Cheesy Fiesta Potatoes, 135 g	290	17	29	2	4
Double Decker® Taco, 156 g	320	13	38	6	14
Grande Soft Taco, 206 g	430	20	43	5	19
Spicy Chicken Burrito, 191 g	400	17	48	3	14
• Spicy Chicken Soft Taco, 113 g	170	6	20	2	10
Burritos					
7-Layer Burrito, 283 g	490	18	65	9	17
Bean Burrito, 198 g	350	9	54	8	13
Burrito Supreme® - Beef, 248 g	420	17	51	7	17
Burrito Supreme® - Chicken, 248 g	400	13	49	6	20
Burrito Supreme® - Steak, 248 g	390	14	49	6	18
Fiesta Burrito - Beef, 184 g	370	13	49	4	14
Fiesta Burrito - Chicken, 184 g	350	10	47	3	18
• Fiesta Burrito - Steak, 184 g	340	11	47	3	15
• Grilled Stuft Burrito - Beef, 325 g	680	30	76	9	27
Grilled Stuft Burrito - Chicken, 325 g	640	23	73	7	34
Grilled Stuft Burrito - Steak, 325 g	630	25	72	7	30
Chalupas					
• Baja - Beef, 153 g	410	27	30	4	13
Baja - Chicken, 153 g	390	23	29	3	17
Baja - Steak, 153 g	390	24	28	3	15
Nacho Cheese - Beef, 153 g	370	22	32	3	12
Nacho Cheese - Chicken, 153 g	350	18	30	2	16
• Nacho Cheese - Steak, 153 g	340	19	30	2	14
Supreme - Beef, 153 g	380	23	30	3	14
Supreme - Chicken, 153 g	360	20	29	2	17
Supreme - Steak, 153 g	360	21	28	2	15
Gordita					
• Gordita Baja® - Beef, 153 g	340	19	29	4	13
Gordita Baja® - Chicken, 153 g	320	16	28	3	17
Gordita Baja® - Steak, 153 g	320	17	27	3	15
Gordita Nacho Cheese - Beef, 153 g	300	14	31	3	12
Gordita Nacho Cheese - Chicken, 153 g	280	11	29	2	16
• Gordita Nacho Cheese - Steak, 153 g	270	12	29	2	14
Gordita Supreme® - Beef, 153 g	310	16	29	3	14
Gordita Supreme® - Chicken, 153 g	290	12	28	2	17
Gordita Supreme® - Steak, 153 g	290	13	28	2	15
Nachos and Sides					
Cinnamon Twists, 35 g	170	7	26	1	1
Mexican Rice, 128 g	180	7	23	1	6
• Nachos BellGrande®, 305 g	770	44	77	12	19
Nachos Supreme, 191 g	440	26	41	7	12
Nachos, 99 g	330	21	32	2	4

Taco Bell (cont.)	Cal	Fat	Cbs	Fbr	Prtn
Nachos and Sides (cont.)					
Pintos 'n Cheese, 128 g	160	6	19	7	9
New Fresco Menu					
Fresco Bean Burrito, 213 g	330	7	54	9	12
Fresco Burrito Supreme® - Chicken, 241 g	330	8	49	7	18
Fresco Burrito Supreme® - Steak, 241 g	330	8	48	7	16
Fresco Crunchy Taco, 92 g	150	8	13	3	7
Fresco Fiesta Burrito - Chicken, 198 g	330	8	48	3	16
Fresco Grilled Steak Soft Taco, 128 g	160	5	20	2	10
Fresco Ranchero Chicken Soft Taco, 135 g	170	4	21	3	12
Fresco Soft Taco - Beef, 113 g	180	7	21	3	8
Fresco Zesty Chkn. Border Bowl no drssing, 397 g	350	8	51	10	19
Regional Menu Items					
Cheese Quesadilla, 142 g	470	26	39	3	19
Chili Cheese Burrito, 156 g	370	16	40	3	16
Tostada, 170 g	240	10	27	7	11
Specialties					
Chicken Fiesta Taco Salad without Shell, 479 g	430	18	38	11	30
Chicken Fiesta Taco Salad, 544 g	790	38	77	13	37
Chicken Grilled Taquitos, 128 g	310	11	37	2	18
Chicken Quesadilla, 184 g	520	28	40	3	28
Crunchwrap Supreme®, 254 g	560	24	68	5	17
Enchirito® - Beef, 213 g	360	17	34	7	18
Enchirito® - Chicken, 213 g	340	13	33	6	22
Enchirito® - Steak, 213 g	330	14	33	6	20
Express Taco Salad, 475 g	610	32	56	14	25
Fiesta Taco Salad without Shell, 479 g	470	24	41	13	23
• Fiesta Taco Salad, 544 g	840	45	80	15	30
Guacamole Side, 43 g	70	5	5	2	1
Mexican Pizza, 213 g	530	30	46	6	20
Meximelt®, 128 g	280	14	22	3	15
Salsa Side, 43 g	15	0	3	0	0
Sour Cream Side, 43 g	80	7	3	0	1
Southwest Steak BORDER BOWL®, 443 g	600	24	68	9	28
Spicy Chicken Crunchwrap Supreme®, 254 g	540	23	67	4	19
• Steak Grilled Taquitos, 128 g	310	11	36	2	16
Steak Quesadilla, 184 g	520	28	39	3	26
Zesty Chicken Border Bowl no dressing, 376 g	440	15	57	10	21
Zesty Chicken Border Bowl, 418 g	640	35	60	10	22
Tacos					
Crunchy Taco Supreme®, 113 g	210	13	15	3	9
• Crunchy Taco, 78 g	170	10	13	3	8
• Double Decker® Taco Supreme®, 191 g	370	17	40	7	14
Grilled Steak Soft Taco, 128 g	270	16	20	2	12
Ranchero Chicken Soft Taco, 135 g	270	14	21	2	14
Soft Taco - Beef, 99 g	200	9	21	3	10
Soft Taco Supreme® - Beef, 135 g	250	13	23	3	11

❯ Taco Cabana	Cal	Fat	Cbs	Fbr	Prtn
Breakfast Tacos					
• Barbacoa, 1 ea.	307	15	2	N/A	22
Bacon & Egg, 1 ea.	246	12	22	N/A	13
Chorizon & Egg, 1 ea.	248	12	22	N/A	12
• Potato & Egg, 1 ea.	234	10	27	N/A	10

(•= most healthy •= least healthy)   **RESTAURANTS & FAST-FOOD • 355**

RESTAURANTS & FAST-FOOD CHAINS

Taco Cabana (cont.)

	Cal	Fat	Cbs	Fbr	Prtn
Burritos					
• Bean & Cheese, 1 ea.	710	27	85	N/A	28
• Beef, 1 ea.	353	24	76	N/A	30
Black Bean, 1 ea.	559	11	95	N/A	16
Chicken, 1 ea.	665	26	74	N/A	31
Fajitas					
• Beef, 4 oz.	245	12	3	N/A	31
Chicken Clark, 4 oz.	236	11	2	N/A	33
• Chicken White, 4 oz.	191	6	3	N/A	30
Grilled Chicken					
• 1/4 Chicken Dark, 5 oz.	298	18	1	N/A	33
• 1/4 Chicken no Skin, 4 oz.	167	3	0	N/A	35
1/4 Chicken White, 5 oz.	295	14	1	N/A	42
1/4 Dark no Skin, 3 oz.	170	7	1	N/A	26
Sides					
6" flour tortilla, 1 ea.	129	3	22	N/A	3
6" corn tortilla, 1 ea.	70	1	11	N/A	2
Black Beans, 4 oz.	111	1	21	N/A	6
Borracho Beans, 4 oz.	108	3	17	N/A	4
Calabacita, 4 oz.	78	5	6	N/A	2
Chips, 2 oz.	285	14	36	N/A	5
Elotes, 1 ea.	220	11	26	N/A	7
• Guacamole, 1 oz.	48	4	2	N/A	0
Queso, 3 oz.	184	12	7	N/A	9
Refried Beans, 4 oz.	171	6	21	N/A	7
Sour Cream, 1 oz.	57	5	1	N/A	1
Spanish Rice, 4 oz.	181	5	30	N/A	3
• Tortilla Soup Large, 19 oz.	371	13	32	N/A	33
Tortilla Soup Small, 9 oz.	249	8	26	N/A	18
Tacos					
• Bean & Cheese, 1 ea.	292	12	35	N/A	12
Black bean, 1 ea.	216	5	37	N/A	14
Carne gulsada, 1 ea.	202	8	20	N/A	14
• Crispy beef, 1 ea.	148	7	13	N/A	9
Soft Chicken, 1 ea.	217	9	21	N/A	13

Taco Del Mar

	Cal	Fat	Cbs	Fbr	Prtn
Almost Jumbo Burritos					
• Beef, Refried, 1 burrito	500	14	70	6	24
Cheese, Refried, 1 burrito	460	13	69	5	16
Chicken, Refried, 1 burrito	490	12	69	6	24
• Fish, Refried, 1 burrito	450	16	60	7	17
Pork, Refried, 1 burrito	490	13	70	6	22
Almost Super Burritos					
• Beef, Refried, 1 burrito	610	23	73	7	28
Chicken, Refried, 1 burrito	590	21	72	6	28
Fish, Refried, 1 burrito	520	24	57	6	20
Pork, Refried, 1 burrito	590	21	73	6	26
• Veggie, Refried, 1 burrito	510	17	72	6	17
Baja Bowls					
Beef, Refried, 1 bowl	830	35	81	10	44
• Chicken, Refried, 1 bowl	790	31	79	9	44
• Fish, Refried, 1 bowl	880	41	95	9	31
Pork, Refried, 1 bowl	790	33	81	9	40

Taco Del Mar (cont.)	Cal	Fat	Cbs	Fbr	Prtn
Breakfast Menu					
Almost Jumbo Brkfst Burrito, Refried, 1 burrito	590	27	60	6	28
Almost Super Brkfst Burrito, Refried, 1 burrito	640	31	62	7	29
Breakfast Taco, Flour, Refried, 1 taco	260	15	18	1	13
Egg & Cheese Brkfst Burrito, Refried, 1 burrito	490	19	59	6	22
Egg & Cheese Taco, Flour, Refried, 1 taco	200	10	17	1	9
Eggs, 2 oz. scoop	90	7	1	0	7
Hash Browns, 1 triangle	110	6	13	2	1
Jumbo Breakfast Burrito, Refried, 1 burrito	1080	50	105	11	52
Potatoes Diced, 2 oz. scoop	60	1	11	1	2
Sausage, 1 oz. scoop	100	8	1	0	6
Super Breakfast Burrito, Refried, 1 burrito	1190	59	110	13	54
Carbohydrate Modified Items					
Carb Modified Almost Burrito, Beef, 1 burrito	340	17	26	12	29
Carb Modified Almost Burrito, Chicken, 1 burrito	320	15	25	11	29
Carb Modified Almost Burrito, Pork, 1 burrito	320	16	26	11	27
Carb Modified Baja Bowl, Beef, 1 bowl	450	28	15	5	33
Carb Modified Baja Bowl, Chicken, 1 bowl	410	25	13	4	34
Carb Modified Baja Bowl, Pork, 1 bowl	410	26	14	4	29
Carb Modified Quesadilla, Beef, 1 quesadilla	510	31	25	10	38
Carb Modified Quesadilla, Chicken, 1 quesadilla	490	29	24	10	39
Carb Modified Quesadilla, Pork, 1 quesadilla	490	30	25	10	36
Desserts					
• Butter Cookie, 1 cookie	220	10	31	0	2
Chocolate Chip Cookie, 1 cookie	240	12	34	1	2
Chocolate Chip/nut Cookie, 1 cookie	240	13	30	2	3
Milk Chocolate Cookie, 1 cookie	240	12	31	0	3
Oatmeal/Raisin/Walnut Cookie, 1 cookie	240	11	35	1	3
• Oreo Brownie, 1 brownie	400	17	59	1	4
Peanut Butter Cookie, 1 cookie	240	13	27	0	4
Triple Chocolate Cookie, 1 cookie	230	12	31	1	3
White Chocolate Cookie, 1 cookie	270	16	30	0	3
Enchiladas					
• Beef, 1 enchilada	1030	37	115	13	55
• Cheese, 1 enchilada	820	27	112	12	31
Chicken, 1 enchilada	990	33	113	12	55
Pork, 1 enchilada	990	35	114	12	51
Jumbo Burritos					
• Beef, Refried, 1 burrito	960	27	133	12	47
Cheese, Refried, 1 burrito	870	24	130	10	30
Chicken, Refried, 1 burrito	920	23	130	11	47
• Fish, Refried, 1 burrito	840	30	110	12	32
Pork, Refried, 1 burrito	920	24	132	11	43
Kids Menu					
• Kids Bean & Cheese Burrito & Chips, 1 meal	760	31	95	9	24
Kids Bean & Cheese Burrito, 1 burrito	480	17	58	7	20
Kids Chips & Cheese, 1 tray	400	22	38	2	10
Kids Quesadilla & Chips, 1 meal	600	27	71	4	17
Kids Quesadilla, 1 quesadilla	320	14	34	2	13
Kids Taco, Beef, 1 taco	270	15	16	1	17
• Kids Taco, Chicken, 1 taco	250	13	15	1	17
Kids Taco, Pork, 1 taco	250	14	16	1	15
Nachos & Chips					
Chips & Salsa, 1 tray	590	27	78	5	8

RESTAURANTS & FAST-FOOD CHAINS

Taco Del Mar (cont.)

	Cal	Fat	Cbs	Fbr	Prtn
Nachos & Chips (cont.)					
Super Nachos, Refried, 1 tray	1190	65	110	12	37
Quesadillas					
• Beef, 1 quesadilla	800	37	66	6	49
• Cheese, 1 quesadilla	710	35	63	4	32
Chicken, 1 quesadilla	770	33	64	5	49
Pork, 1 quesadilla	770	35	65	5	45
Sauces					
Enchilada Sauce, 3 oz.	35	0	7	0	1
• Green Sauce, 2 tbsp.	5	0	1	0	0
Guacamole, 1 oz scoop	40	4	2	1	1
Habanero Sauce, 2 tbsp.	10	0	1	0	0
Red Sauce, 2 tbsp.	5	0	1	0	0
Salsa, 3 oz. scoop	15	0	4	1	1
Sour Cream, 1 oz scoop	70	6	2	0	1
• White Sauce, 2 tbsp.	120	13	1	0	0
Sides					
Beans, Black, 4 oz. spoon	140	2	24	8	7
Beans, Refried, 4 oz. spoon	160	4	24	5	7
• Beans, Whole Pinto, 4 oz. spoon	90	0	20	6	6
Beef, 4 oz. scoop	200	11	4	1	24
Cheese, 1 scoop	110	9	1	0	7
Chicken, 4 oz. scoop	170	7	1	0	24
Cod, 2 pieces	120	4	13	0	10
Pork, 4 oz. scoop	170	8	3	0	20
Rice & Black Beans, 1 tray	370	5	69	9	12
• Rice & Refried Beans, 1 tray	390	7	69	6	12
Rice & Whole Pinto Beans, 1 tray	320	3	66	8	10
Rice, 1 scoop	230	3	45	1	4
Super Burritos					
• Beef, Refried, 1 burrito	1180	44	138	13	55
Chicken, Refried, 1 burrito	1140	40	136	12	55
Fish, Refried, 1 burrito	1060	48	116	14	41
Pork, Refried, 1 burrito	1150	42	138	12	51
• Veggie, Refried, 1 burrito	980	33	136	12	32
Taco Salads					
Beef, Refried	930	49	75	12	47
• Chicken, Refried	900	45	73	11	47
• Fish, Refried	1040	61	89	11	34
Pork, Refried	900	46	74	11	43
Tacos					
Hard, Beef, 1 taco	270	15	17	1	17
Hard, Chicken, 1 taco	260	13	16	1	17
Hard, Fish, 1 taco	270	15	23	1	10
Hard, Pork, 1 taco	260	14	17	1	15
Soft, Beef, 1 taco	280	11	28	4	18
• Soft, Chicken, 1 taco	260	9	27	3	19
Soft, Fish, 1 taco	270	11	34	3	12
Soft, Pork, 1 taco	260	10	28	3	16
• Soft, Veggie, 1 taco	310	8	49	5	11
Tortillas					
Carb Modified Tortilla, 1 tortilla	110	3	19	10	12
Corn Tortillas, 2 each	120	2	24	3	3
Flour Tortilla 10", 1 each	210	5	33	2	7

RESTAURANTS & FAST-FOOD CHAINS

Taco Del Mar (cont.)

	Cal	Fat	Cbs	Fbr	Prtn
Tortillas (cont.)					
Flour Tortilla 13", 1 each	350	9	57	3	11
Flour Tortilla 6", 1 each	100	3	15	0	3
Spinach Tortilla 13", 1 each	350	10	56	5	10
Taco Salad Shell, 1 each	280	16	29	1	4
Taco Shell, 1 each	110	5	14	0	2
Tomato Tortilla 13", 1 each	350	10	56	5	10
Whole Wheat Tortilla 13", 1 each	300	5	54	8	12
Vegan Burritos					
Almost Vegan, Refried, 1 burrito	430	11	70	6	13
Vegan Burrito, Refried, 1 burrito	800	19	133	12	24

Taco John's

	Cal	Fat	Cbs	Fbr	Prtn
10 g or less of Fat					
Bean Burrito, 7 oz.	320	7	53	10	11
Chicken Softshell Taco, 4 oz.	190	6	19	4	14
• Crispy Taco, 3 oz.	180	10	13	3	9
Mexican Rice, 6 oz.	240	8	36	1	4
• Refried Beans, 9 oz.	340	9	49	11	15
Softshell Taco, 4 oz.	230	10	20	3	11
Taco Burger, 5 oz.	250	9	30	3	13
Texas Style Chili, 8 oz.	210	8	26	4	11
Breakfast Menu					
Bravo Scrambler® (Bacon), 9 oz.	520	25	53	8	20
Bravo Scrambler® (Sausage), 10 oz.	675	44	48	5	18
Breakfast Burrito (Bacon), 8 oz.	515	25	52	8	20
Breakfast Burrito (Sausage), 9 oz.	620	32	55	8	20
Breakfast Egg Burrito, 7 oz.	400	19	39	6	20
Breakfast Quesadilla (Bacon), 9 oz.	665	41	41	7	34
Breakfast Quesadilla (Sausage), 9 oz.	735	45	42	7	33
Breakfast Quesadilla, 8 oz.	570	34	41	7	27
• Breakfast Taco (Bacon), 4 oz.	270	13	25	2	10
Breakfast Taco (Sausage), 4 oz.	320	17	26	2	10
Scrambler Burrito (Bacon), 9 oz.	520	25	53	8	20
Scrambler Burrito (Sausage), 9 oz.	620	32	52	8	20
Super Olés Scrambler (Bacon), 14 oz.	960	62	75	8	27
• Super Olés Scrambler (Sausage), 16 oz.	1120	72	76	8	29
Burritos					
• Bean Burrito, 7 oz.	380	10	53	10	15
Beef Grilled Burrito, 8 oz.	590	30	49	9	27
Beefy Burrito, 7 oz.	430	20	41	8	22
Chicken & Potato Burrito, 8 oz.	460	20	54	8	18
Chicken & Rice Burrito, 10 oz.	520	20	68	6	22
Chicken Grilled Burrito, 8 oz.	590	30	47	8	33
Combination Burrito, 7 oz.	400	15	47	9	18
Crunchy Chicken and Potato Burrito, 9 oz.	590	30	62	8	20
Meat & Potato Burrito, 8 oz.	490	20	55	9	15
Steak & Potato Burrito, 8 oz.	460	20	53	10	17
Steak & Rice Burrito, 10 oz.	520	20	67	8	20
• Steak Grilled Burrito, 8 oz.	600	35	46	11	31
Super Burrito, 9 oz.	450	20	49	10	19
Desserts					
Apple Grande, 3 oz.	240	10	41	0	5
• Choco Taco, 4 oz.	385	20	48	1	5

RESTAURANTS & FAST-FOOD CHAINS

Taco John's (cont.)

	Cal	Fat	Cbs	Fbr	Prtn
Desserts (cont.)					
Churro, 2 oz.	235	10	31	1	2
• Giant Goldfish® Grahams, 1 bag	120	5	19	1	1
Local Favorites					
• Chili Cheese Potato Olés®, 11 oz.	610	36	59	7	13
Chili Enchilada, 8 oz.	315	16	24	5	18
Mexi Rolls® - 2 Piece w/o Nacho Cheese, 2 oz.	155	7	16	6	8
• Nacho Cheese, 2 oz.	60	5	2	0	2
Ranch Burrito (Beef), 7 oz.	420	22	41	8	17
Ranch Burrito (Chicken), 7 oz.	390	18	40	7	19
Smothered Burrito, 11 oz.	505	21	55	11	23
Sides					
Chili, 8 oz.	270	10	26	4	15
Mexican Rice, 6 oz.	250	5	45	0	5
Nachos, 5 oz.	380	20	38	1	6
• Potato Olés® (Medium), 7 oz.	620	35	67	6	5
Potato Olés® with Nacho Cheese, 8 oz.	550	35	52	5	7
Refried Beans, 10 oz.	395	15	50	11	18
• Side Salad w/o dressing, 4 oz.	80	5	6	1	3
Specialties					
Cheese Quesadilla, 6 oz.	480	30	39	6	20
• Chicken Festiva Salad w/o dressing, 11 oz.	400	25	24	4	24
Chicken Quesadilla, 7 oz.	540	30	41	7	29
Chicken Super Nachos, 12 oz.	780	45	62	2	31
Chicken Taco Salad w/o dressing, 13 oz.	540	30	44	4	28
Crunchy Chkn Festiva Salad w/o dressing, 11 oz.	580	35	35	3	27
Crunchy Chicken Taco Salad w/o dressing, 14 oz.	710	40	56	3	31
Crunchy Chicken w/ Ketchipotle, 5 oz.	485	30	30	0	29
Crunchy Chicken, 5 oz.	455	30	24	0	29
Steak Festiva Salad w/o dressing, 11 oz.	410	25	23	7	22
Steak Quesadilla, 7 oz.	545	30	40	9	28
Steak Taco Salad w/o dressing, 13 oz.	545	30	43	6	26
Super Nachos, 13 oz.	830	50	73	5	22
• Super Potato Olés®, 17 oz.	1060	70	91	11	23
Taco Salad w/o dressing, 13 oz.	580	30	46	4	24
Tacos					
Chicken Softshell Taco, 4 oz.	190	5	19	4	14
• Crispy Taco, 3 oz.	180	10	13	3	9
Softshell Taco, 4 oz.	220	10	21	4	11
Steak Softshell Taco, 4 oz.	190	10	19	6	13
• Taco Bravo®, 7 oz.	340	15	39	8	15
Taco Burger, 5 oz.	280	10	28	3	14

Taco Mayo

	Cal	Fat	Cbs	Fbr	Prtn
Burritos					
Bean Burrito, 238 g	496	16	71	12	21
• Beef Burrito, 238 g	492	23	41	3	30
Beef N Bean Burrito, 238 g	494	19	56	8	25
• Super Burrito, 285 g	539	23	57	8	26
Drinks					
Piña Colada Chill, 560 g	479	25	59	0	2
Strawberry Chiller, 560 g	378	7	79	0	2
Favorites					
Beef Soft Taco, 119 g	229	11	17	2	14

RESTAURANTS & FAST-FOOD CHAINS

Taco Mayo (cont.)

	Cal	Fat	Cbs	Fbr	Prtn
Favorites (cont.)					
Chicken Soft Taco, 105 g	184	6	16	1	15
Taco Burger, 161 g	303	13	28	2	19
Taco, 77 g	161	9	10	1	9
Tostada, 147 g	295	13	37	9	12
Fresh Grilled					
Cheese Quesadilla, 257 g	592	35	45	4	25
Chicken Burrito Supreme, 194 g	407	16	39	2	25
Chicken Quesadilla, 313 g	672	37	46	4	39
Fajita Chicken Quesadilla, 327 g	698	39	47	5	40
Fajita Steak Quesadilla, 327 g	725	40	47	5	42
Mexicali-Chicken Grill Burrito, 238 g	607	30	54	2	30
Mexicali-Steak Grill Burrito, 238 g	633	32	54	2	30
Steak Burrito Supreme, 194 g	434	18	39	2	27
Steak Quesadilla, 313 g	698	38	46	4	41
Fresh Grilled					
Chicken Mexicali Bowl, 572 g	1152	59	115	20	47
DoSmoChili-Beef, 547 g	955	40	100	15	49
DoSmoChili-Chicken, 519 g	879	32	99	14	48
DoSmoChili-Steak, 519 g	905	34	99	14	50
DoSmoQueso-Chicken, 519 g	883	32	101	13	48
DoSmoQueso-Steak, 519 g	910	34	101	13	50
DoSmoVerde-Chicken, 519 g	856	31	101	13	45
DoSmoVerde-Steak, 519 g	883	32	101	13	47
• Fajita-Chicken Grill Burrito, 224 g	492	23	42	3	27
Fajita-Steak Grill Burrito, 224 g	519	25	42	3	29
• Steak Mexicali Bowl, 557 g	1158	60	115	20	45
Tamale Grande Platter, 439 g	714	31	78	13	31
Nachos					
• Classic-Cheese Nachos, 135 g	377	19	45	4	6
Classic-Chicken Nacho Supreme, 313 g	510	26	48	4	21
Classic-Nacho Supreme, 342 g	719	37	70	12	28
Classic-Steak Nacho Supreme, 313 g	537	27	48	4	23
FB-Cheese Nachos, 123 g	505	31	40	3	18
FB-Chicken Nacho Supreme, 306 g	638	37	43	3	33
FB-Nacho Supreme, 335 g	846	49	65	11	40
FB-Steak Nacho Supreme, 306 g	664	39	43	3	35
Queso-Cheese Nacho, 142 g	407	21	45	3	12
Queso-Chicken Nacho Supreme, 320 g	539	27	47	3	27
Queso-Nacho Supreme, 345 g	748	38	70	12	34
Queso-Steak Nacho Supreme, 320 g	566	28	47	3	29
• Ultimate Nacho, 523 g	968	49	102	17	29
Salads					
Chicken Acapulco Salad, 350 g	678	50	35	5	23
• Chicken Taco Salad, 334 g	438	23	30	3	27
• Steak Acapulco Salad, 350 g	705	51	35	5	25
Steak Taco Salad, 320 g	444	25	30	3	26
Taco Salad, 460 g	705	38	57	13	37
Sides					
Guac N' Chips, 163 g	386	21	45	7	4
• Mexicali Rice, 140 g	160	1	36	2	4
• Potato Loco-Lg, 196 g	586	37	55	7	7
Potato Loco-Sm, 133 g	379	24	36	5	5
Queso N' Chips, 170 g	449	22	49	3	14

(•= most healthy •= least healthy) **RESTAURANTS & FAST-FOOD · 361**

RESTAURANTS & FAST-FOOD CHAINS

Taco Mayo (cont.)

	Cal	Fat	Cbs	Fbr	Prtn
Sides (cont.)					
Refried Beans, 168 g	294	9	43	14	15

Tacone

	Cal	Fat	Cbs	Fbr	Prtn
Breakfast					
El Grande Wrap, 149 g	280	16	20	1	15
Venice Beach Wrap, 354 g	630	31	46	4	40
Desserts					
Fresh Fruit Salad, 227 g	80	0	21	2	2
Farm Fresh Salads					
• Caesar, 307 g	500	46	18	5	9
• Fiesta, 310 g	340	19	18	5	27
T.J. Cobb, 272 g	430	30	6	3	36
Flavor Sides					
• Grilled Veggies + Feta, 4 oz.	170	14	6	1	6
Spa Salad, 225 g	190	9	22	3	7
• Sweet Potato Fries, 109 g	190	9	23	3	2
Global Grill Platter					
Empire Steak, 468 g	380	21	14	5	34
Napa Valley Chicken, 355 g	320	15	10	3	36
• Rotisserie Chicken, 595 g	830	37	37	2	81
• Tradewind Shrimp, 457 g	250	12	14	5	26
Gourmet Wraps					
Baja Wrap with Chicken, 238 g	420	13	47	5	27
Baja, 215 g	370	11	54	8	14
• Buffalo Kickin' Chicken Wrap, 1/2 wrap	460	12	43	3	44
Campfire, 213 g	340	2	41	2	19
Kickin' Fried Chicken, 151 g	280	11	22	1	22
Kingston, 1/2 wrap	320	10	41	1	16
Malibu Melt, 173 g	360	17	25	1	27
Mambo, 146 g	220	7	26	1	16
Perfect Ten Wrap, 1/2 wrap	360	17	43	4	10
Pilgrim, 158 g	260	14	21	1	12
Spa, 136 g	200	9	26	2	5
Thai Cone, 177 g	300	9	35	1	20
• Try Our Lo-Carb Whole Wheat Tortilla, 90 g	180	6	33	1	9
Grilled Sandwiches					
• Angus Khan Burger, 411 g	1150	69	56	2	74
Chick-a-Boom, 256 g	570	38	25	2	32
Great Gobbler, 237 g	470	24	40	2	25
United Steak of America, 196 g	560	40	23	2	27
• Veggie Caprese, 115 g	310	18	29	1	9
Kids					
• Grilled Cheese + Tortilla Chips, 68 g	220	11	20	1	11
Kickin' Fried Chicken Jr., 142 g	250	24	7	1	1
• Quesadilla Jr., 122 g	420	22	35	0	19
Quesadillas					
4 Cheese, 85 g	210	11	18	1	10
• Apollonia, 225 g	640	39	39	1	32
BBQ Chicken, 136 g	300	13	28	2	18
Smoothies & Desserts					
Bikini Blast, 617 g	410	2	94	5	9
Blue Voodoo, 583 g	400	1	93	6	7
• Orangabang, 539 g	360	1	84	4	8

RESTAURANTS & FAST-FOOD CHAINS

Tacone (cont.)

	Cal	Fat	Cbs	Fbr	Prtn
Smoothies & Desserts (cont.)					
Palm Peach, 834 g	500	2	116	7	12
• Pink Flamingo, 658 g	520	1	125	7	9
Tacone® Sides					
Black Beans + Jack Cheese, 4 oz.	210	5	27	14	14
Down-Home Coleslaw, 4 oz.	35	1	7	3	2
• Homemade Tortilla Chips + Salsa, 142 g	300	12	42	3	5
Seasoned French Fries, 108 g	200	9	29	3	3
Seasoned Potato Chips, 86 g	160	8	21	2	2
Tacone® Rice, 170 g	240	1	51	1	5
Tacone® Side Salad, 100 g	140	11	9	2	3
• Thai Cucumber Salad, 122 g	20	0	5	1	1

Tastee-Freez

	Cal	Fat	Cbs	Fbr	Prtn
For Tastee-Freez nutritional information, please see Wienerschnitzel on pg. 384					

TCBY

	Cal	Fat	Cbs	Fbr	Prtn
Hand-Scooped Frozen Yogurt & Sorbet					
Butter Pecan Perfection, 4 fl.oz.	110	5	14	1	4
Chocolate Chocolate Swirl, 4 fl.oz.	120	4	19	1	4
Chocolate Chunk Cookie Dough, 4 fl.oz.	160	6	24	0	3
Cookies & Cream, 4 fl.oz.	140	4	22	0	3
Cotton Candy, 4 fl.oz.	120	4	20	0	3
Mint Chocolate Chunk, 4 fl.oz.	140	5	22	0	3
Mocha Almond, 4 fl.oz.	150	5	22	1	3
No Sugar Added Choco Choco Swirl, 4 fl.oz.	90	1	23	6	4
No Sugar Added Vanilla Fudge Brownie, 4 fl.oz.	100	2	22	5	4
• No Sugar Added (NSA) Vanilla, 4 fl.oz.	80	1	19	5	4
Pralines & Cream, 4 fl.oz.	140	5	23	0	3
• Psychedelic Sorbet, 4 fl.oz.	290	0	75	0	0
Rainbow Cream, 4 fl.oz.	120	4	20	0	3
Rocky Road, 4 fl.oz.	220	7	36	1	3
Strawberries & Cream, 4 fl.oz.	120	3	21	0	2
Vanilla Bean, 4 fl.oz.	120	4	19	0	3
Vanilla Chocolate Chunk, 4 fl.oz.	140	5	22	0	3
Smoothies					
Berrylicious, 16 fl.oz.	290	3	65	3	3
• Black 'n Blueberry, 16 fl.oz.	280	3	63	2	3
Mango Tango, 16 fl.oz.	330	3	76	2	3
Mangolada, 16 fl.oz.	340	6	70	2	3
Mondo Mango, 16 fl.oz.	310	3	70	2	3
• Pina Paradise, 16 fl.oz.	350	12	58	1	3
Pink Pineapple, 16 fl.oz.	340	9	63	2	3
Straight-Up Strawberry, 16 fl.oz.	280	4	64	1	3
Strawberry Bananza, 16 fl.oz.	320	4	74	2	3
Strawberry Fling, 16 fl.oz.	340	3	78	2	3
Soft Serve Creamy Frozen Yogurt & Fruity Sorbet					
• 96% Fat Free Frozen Yogurt, 97 g	140	3	23	0	4
Low Carb Frozen Yogurt, 92 g	110	7	16	7	3
• No Sugar Added Nonfat Frozen Yogurt, 96 g	90	0	20	0	4
NonFat & NonDairy Sorbet, 97 g	100	0	24	0	0
NonFat Frozen Yogurt, 98 g	110	0	23	0	4

RESTAURANTS & FAST-FOOD CHAINS

The Coffee Bean & Tea Leaf

	Cal	Fat	Cbs	Fbr	Prtn
Coffee Ice Blended® Drinks					
Blk Forest No Sgr Added Pwder & Soy Mlk, 16 oz.	270	5	46	1	10
Black Forest No Sugar Added Powder, 16 oz.	270	5	47	1	11
Black Forest Soy Milk, 16 oz.	490	11	90	1	11
• Black Forest, 16 oz.	500	10	91	1	12
Caramel NSA Powder & Soy Milk, 16 oz.	290	4	57	0	9
Caramel NSA Powder, 16 oz.	300	3	57	0	10
Caramel Soy Milk, 16 oz.	530	11	98	0	11
Caramel, 16 oz.	540	11	99	0	12
Extreme Caramel NSA Powder, 16 oz.	270	3	54	0	7
Extreme Caramel, 16 oz.	510	11	95	0	9
• Extreme Mocha NSA Powder, 16 oz.	110	1	21	0	8
Extreme Mocha, 16 oz.	340	7	65	0	8
Extreme Ultimate Mocha NSA Powder, 16 oz.	160	5	27	1	8
Extreme Ultimate Mocha, 16 oz.	390	10	71	1	9
Extreme Ultimate Vanilla NSA Powder, 16 oz.	170	4	28	1	8
Extreme Ultimate Vanilla, 16 oz.	410	12	70	1	10
Extreme Vanilla NSA Powder, 16 oz.	120	1	22	0	7
Extreme Vanilla, 16 oz.	360	9	63	0	9
Mocha NSA Powder & Soy Milk, 16 oz.	130	2	23	0	9
Mocha NSA Powder, 16 oz.	140	1	24	0	10
Mocha Soy Milk, 16 oz.	360	8	67	0	10
Mocha, 16 oz.	370	7	68	0	11
Ultimate Mocha NSA Powder & Soy Milk, 16 oz.	190	5	30	1	10
Ultimate Mocha NSA Powder, 16 oz.	190	5	31	1	11
Ultimate Mocha Soy Milk, 16 oz.	410	11	74	1	11
Ultimate Mocha, 16 oz.	420	10	75	1	12
Ultimate Vanilla NSA Powder & Soy Milk, 16 oz.	200	5	31	1	9
Ultimate Vanilla NSA Powder, 16 oz.	200	4	32	1	10
Ultimate Vanilla Soy Milk, 16 oz.	440	13	72	1	11
Ultimate Vanilla Ice, 16 oz.	440	12	73	1	13
Vanilla Ice NSA Powder & Soy Milk, 16 oz.	140	2	25	0	8
Vanilla Ice NSA Powder, 16 oz.	150	1	25	0	10
Vanilla Ice Soy Milk, 16 oz.	380	10	66	0	10
Vanilla Ice, 16 oz.	390	9	67	0	12
White Chocolate Dream® Soy Milk, 16 oz.	440	19	66	0	5
White Chocolate Dream®, 16 oz.	450	18	67	0	6
Espresso & Coffee Hot Drinks					
Americano, 16 oz.	10	0	1	0	0
Brewed Coffee, 16 oz.	5	0	0	0	1
Café Caramel NSA Powder & Soy Milk, 16 oz.	220	3	43	0	5
Café Caramel NSA Powder, 16 oz.	220	2	44	0	6
Café Caramel Soy Milk, 16 oz.	300	6	57	0	6
Café Caramel, 16 oz.	300	5	58	0	6
Café Latté Nonfat Milk, 16 oz.	160	0	24	0	16
Café Latté Soy Milk, 16 oz.	150	5	20	0	9
Café Latté Whole Milk, 16 oz.	270	14	24	0	14
Café Mocha NSA Powder & Soy Milk, 16 oz.	110	2	18	0	7
Café Mocha NSA Powder, 16 oz.	110	1	19	0	9
Café Mocha Soy Milk, 16 oz.	270	6	49	0	7
Café Mocha, 16 oz.	270	5	50	0	8
Café Vanilla NSA Powder & Soy Milk, 16 oz.	120	2	19	0	7
Café Vanilla NSA Powder, 16 oz.	120	1	20	0	8
Café Vanilla Soy Milk, 16 oz.	280	7	48	0	8

RESTAURANTS & FAST-FOOD CHAINS

The Coffee Bean & Tea Leaf (cont.)

	Cal	Fat	Cbs	Fbr	Prtn
Espresso & Coffee Hot Drinks (cont.)					
Café Vanilla, 16 oz.	290	7	48	0	9
Café White Chocolate Soy Milk, 16 oz.	330	14	49	0	4
Café White Chocolate, 16 oz.	330	14	49	0	5
Cappuccino Double Nonfat Milk, 12 oz.	70	0	10	0	6
Cappuccino Double Soy Milk, 12 oz.	60	2	9	0	4
Cappuccino Double Whole Milk, 12 oz.	110	6	10	0	6
Cappuccino Single Nonfat Milk, 12 oz.	80	0	11	0	8
Cappuccino Single Soy Milk, 12 oz.	70	2	10	0	4
Cappuccino Single Whole Milk, 12 oz.	130	7	11	0	7
Caramel Latté NSA Powder & Soy Milk, 16 oz.	320	6	57	0	11
Caramel Latté NSA Powder, 16 oz.	330	2	60	0	17
Caramel Latté Soy Milk, 16 oz.	400	9	72	0	11
Caramel Latté, 16 oz.	420	5	75	0	17
Double Espresso Macchiato Nonfat Milk, 4 oz.	10	0	2	0	1
Double Espresso Macchiato Soy Milk, 4 oz.	10	0	2	0	0
Double Espresso Macchiato Whole Milk, 4 oz.	15	1	2	0	1
Mocha Latté NSA Powder & Soy Milk, 16 oz.	210	5	32	0	13
Mocha Latté NSA Powder, 16 oz.	230	1	36	0	20
Mocha Latté Soy Milk, 16 oz.	370	9	64	0	13
Mocha Latté, 16 oz.	380	5	67	0	19
Single Espresso Macchiato Nonfat Milk, 4 oz.	10	0	1	0	1
Single Espresso Macchiato Soy Milk, 4 oz.	10	0	1	0	0
Single Espresso Macchiato Whole Milk, 4 oz.	10	1	1	0	1
• Single Espresso, 4 oz.	5	0	0	0	0
Vanilla Latté NSA Powder & Soy Milk, 16 oz.	220	5	33	0	13
Vanilla Latté NSA Powder, 16 oz.	230	1	37	0	19
Vanilla Latté Soy Milk, 16 oz.	390	10	63	0	13
Vanilla Latté, 16 oz.	400	7	66	0	19
White Chocolate Dream® Latté Soy Milk, 16 oz.	430	17	64	0	9
• White Chocolate Dream® Latté, 16 oz.	450	14	67	0	15
Fru Tea™ Ice Blended® Drinks					
• Lemon Zest FruTea™, 16 oz.	320	0	83	1	0
Mucho Mango FruTea™, 16 oz.	240	0	60	0	0
• Pomegranate FruTea™, 16 oz.	210	0	58	0	0
Hot Tea & Tea Lattés					
• Hot Tea, 16 oz.	5	0	1	0	0
Tea Latté w/ Choco & NSA Pwdr & Soy Milk, 16 oz.	110	2	19	0	7
Tea Latté w/ Choco Powder NSA Powder, 16 oz.	110	1	20	0	9
Tea Latté w/ Choco Powder Soy Milk, 16 oz.	270	6	50	0	7
Tea Latté w/ Chocolate Powder, 16 oz.	270	5	51	0	8
Tea Latté w/ Vanilla NSA Powder, Soy Milk, 16 oz.	120	2	20	0	6
Tea Latté w/ Vanilla Powder NSA Powder, 16 oz.	120	1	21	0	7
Tea Latté w/ Vanilla Powder Soy Milk, 16 oz.	280	7	49	0	7
• Tea Latté w/ Vanilla Powder, 16 oz.	290	7	50	0	8
Iced Espresso & Coffee Drinks					
Iced Cappuccino Nonfat Milk, 16 oz.	60	0	9	0	5
Iced Cappuccino Soy Milk, 16 oz.	50	2	7	0	3
Iced Cappuccino, 16 oz.	90	5	9	0	5
Iced Caramel Latté NSA & Soy Milk, 16 oz.	270	5	51	0	11
Iced Caramel Latté NSA Powder, 16 oz.	280	2	53	0	11
Iced Caramel Latté Soy Milk, 16 oz.	350	7	65	0	8
• Iced Caramel Latté, 16 oz.	360	5	67	0	11
Iced Coffee, 16 oz.	10	0	1	0	0

RESTAURANTS & FAST-FOOD CHAINS

The Coffee Bean & Tea Leaf (cont.)

	Cal	Fat	Cbs	Fbr	Prtn
Iced Espresso & Coffee Drinks (cont.)					
Iced Latte Nonfat Milk, 16 oz.	100	0	14	0	9
Iced Latte Soy Milk, 16 oz.	90	3	12	0	5
Iced Latte, 16 oz.	160	8	14	0	8
Iced Mocha Latte NSA Powder & Soy Milk, 16 oz.	150	3	24	0	10
Iced Mocha Latte NSA Powder, 16 oz.	160	1	26	0	13
Iced Mocha Latte Soy Milk, 16 oz.	310	7	55	0	9
Iced Mocha Latte, 16 oz.	320	5	57	0	12
• Iced Tea, 16 oz.	0	0	1	0	0
Iced Vanilla Latte NSA Powder & Soy Milk, 16 oz.	160	3	25	0	9
Iced Vanilla Latte NSA Powder, 16 oz.	170	1	27	0	13
Iced Vanilla Latte Soy Milk, 16 oz.	320	8	54	0	10
Iced Vanilla Latte, 16 oz.	330	7	56	0	13
Kid Friendly! Non Coffee & Non Tea					
Hot Chocolate NSA Powder & Soy Milk, 16 oz.	230	6	34	0	15
Hot Chocolate NSA Powder, 16 oz.	250	1	39	0	22
Hot Chocolate Soy Milk, 16 oz.	380	10	66	0	14
Hot Chocolate, 16 oz.	400	5	69	0	21
• Hot Vanilla NSA Powder & Soy Milk, 16 oz.	230	5	35	0	14
Hot Vanilla NSA Powder, 16 oz.	250	1	40	0	22
Hot Vanilla Soy Milk, 16 oz.	400	11	64	0	15
• Hot Vanilla, 16 oz.	420	7	68	0	22
Non Coffee Ice Blended® Drinks					
Banana Caramel NSA Powder, 16 oz.	330	3	69	0	6
• Banana Caramel, 16 oz.	570	11	110	0	8
• Chai Ice NSA Powder, 16 oz.	110	1	20	0	6
Chai, 16 oz.	350	9	62	0	8
Green Tea Soy Milk, 16 oz.	480	11	81	0	15
Green Tea, 16 oz.	480	10	82	0	18
Malibu Dream™ NSA Powder, 16 oz.	200	1	41	2	7
Malibu Dream™, 16 oz.	440	9	82	2	9
Pomegranate Blueberry NSA Powder, 16 oz.	220	1	46	0	7
Pomegranate Blueberry, 16 oz.	460	9	87	0	9
Pure Chocolate NSA Powder & Soy Milk, 16 oz.	160	3	26	0	10
Pure Chocolate NSA Powder, 16 oz.	160	1	28	0	13
Pure Chocolate Soy Milk, 16 oz.	390	9	70	0	11
Pure Chocolate, 16 oz.	390	7	72	0	14
Pure Vanilla NSA Powder & Soy Milk, 16 oz.	170	3	27	0	10
Pure Vanilla NSA Powder, 16 oz.	170	1	29	0	13
Pure Vanilla Soy Milk, 16 oz.	410	11	69	0	12
Pure Vanilla, 16 oz.	410	9	70	0	15

The Great American Bagel

	Cal	Fat	Cbs	Fbr	Prtn
Bagels					
4-Grain Honey, 5 oz., 1 bagel	390	4	80	6	13
Apple Cinnamon Oat Bran, 5 oz., 1 bagel	370	4	73	4	12
Apple Cinnamon Sugar, 5 oz., 1 bagel	390	4	78	4	12
Apple Crumb, 9 oz., 1 bagel	620	11	118	5	16
Asiago w/ Bl & Gr Olives, 7 oz., 1 bagel	540	20	70	4	22
Asiago, 6 oz., 1 bagel	520	16	72	3	23
Banana Nut, 5 oz., 1 bagel	410	9	69	3	14
Blueberry Crumb, 9 oz., 1 bagel	630	10	122	5	14
Blueberry, 5 oz., 1 bagel	370	4	75	4	12
Cheddar Bacon, 7 oz., 1 bagel	600	23	71	3	28

RESTAURANTS & FAST-FOOD CHAINS

The Great American Bagel (cont.)	Cal	Fat	Cbs	Fbr	Prtn
Bagels (cont.)					
Cheddar Herb, 5 oz., 1 bagel	390	8	66	3	15
Cheddar Onion, 6 oz., 1 bagel	500	13	75	3	20
Cheddar Salsa, 7 oz., 1 bagel	500	17	68	3	22
Cheddar Twist, 9 oz., 1 bagel	800	27	107	4	35
Chocolate Chip, 5 oz., 1 bagel	420	8	78	3	12
Cinnamon Delight, 7 oz., 1 bagel	640	18	108	4	14
Cinnamon Raisin, 5 oz., 1 bagel	380	4	76	3	12
Egg, 5 oz., 1 bagel	370	5	70	3	13
Everything, 5 oz., 1 bagel	380	5	73	3	13
French Toast, 5 oz., 1 bagel	430	8	77	3	12
Garlic, 5 oz., 1 bagel	390	4	75	3	14
Harvest 10-grain, 5 oz., 1 bagel	410	8	73	6	14
Hot Tomazzor, 8 oz., 1 bagel	520	13	77	4	25
Jalapeño Cheddar, 5 oz., 1 bagel	370	7	63	3	14
Onion, 5 oz., 1 bagel	380	4	74	3	13
PB Chocolate Chip, 5 oz., 1 bagel	420	8	76	3	12
Pesto, 5 oz., 1 bagel	360	5	67	3	13
Plain, 5 oz., 1 bagel	360	4	71	3	13
Poppy, 5 oz., 1 bagel	390	6	72	3	14
Provolone, 6 oz., 1 bagel	460	11	72	3	20
Pumpernickel, 5 oz., 1 bagel	360	4	71	4	13
Salt, 5 oz., 1 bagel	360	4	71	3	13
Sesame, 5 oz., 1 bagel	390	6	72	4	14
Sourdough Baguette, 4 oz.	300	2	56	2	11
Spinach Herb, 5 oz., 1 bagel	350	4	70	3	12
Strawberry Crumb, 9 oz., 1 bagel	630	10	123	4	14
Strawberry, 5 oz., 1 bagel	380	4	76	3	12
Stuffed Pepperoni, 9 oz., 1 bagel	570	17	78	4	27
Stuffed Spinach, 9 oz., 1 bagel	640	20	86	4	30
Sun-dried Tomato Basil, 5 oz., 1 bagel	390	4	74	3	14
Swiss Cheese, 6 oz., 1 bagel	470	12	72	3	21
Tomazzor, 8 oz., 1 bagel	520	13	77	4	25
Veggie, 5 oz., 1 bagel	310	4	61	3	11
• Whole Wheat Baguette, 4 oz.	290	4	56	6	11
Whole Wheat, 5 oz., 1 bagel	370	4	74	5	13
Cream Cheese Flavors					
Apple Cinnamon, 1 oz.	60	5	4	0	2
Blue Berry, 1 oz.	60	4	4	0	2
Chocolate Chip, 1 oz.	70	4	8	0	2
Cream Apple, 1 oz.	70	4	7	0	2
Cucumber, 1 oz.	60	5	1	0	3
Garlic Herb, 1 oz.	60	5	1	0	3
Lox, 1 oz.	60	5	1	0	3
Pineapple Walnut, 1 oz.	70	6	2	0	2
Plain, 1 oz.	60	5	1	0	3
Salsa, 1 oz.	50	5	1	0	2
Scallion, 1 oz.	50	5	1	0	2
• Spinach, 1 oz.	50	4	1	0	2
Strawberry, 1 oz.	55	5	1	0	3
Vegetable, 1 oz.	62	5	1	0	3
• Walnut Raisin, 1 oz.	80	6	6	0	2

(•= most healthy •= least healthy)   **RESTAURANTS & FAST-FOOD • 367**

RESTAURANTS & FAST-FOOD CHAINS

Tim Horton's	Cal	Fat	Cbs	Fbr	Prtn
Bagels					
Blueberry, 1 bagel	270	1	55	2	10
Cinnamon Raisin, 1 bagel	270	1	55	3	10
Cream Cheese - Garden Vegetable, 1.5 oz.	120	11	3	0	2
Cream Cheese - Light Plain, 1.5 oz.	85	6	3	0	4
Cream Cheese - Plain, 1.5 oz.	130	12	2	0	2
Cream Cheese - Strawberry, 1.5 oz.	120	10	6	0	2
Everything, 1 bagel	280	2	53	3	10
Flax Seed, 1 bagel	290	5	53	4	10
Onion, 1 bagel	260	2	53	3	9
• Plain, 1 bagel	260	2	52	2	9
Poppy Seed, 1 bagel	270	2	53	3	9
Sesame Seed, 1 bagel	270	3	53	3	9
Sun Dried Tomato, 1 bagel	310	4	59	2	9
• Twelve Grain, 1 bagel	330	9	52	6	10
Breakfast					
Bacon, Egg, Cheese	410	25	31	1	16
Bagel B.E.L.T.	450	14	58	3	21
Egg, Cheese	360	21	30	1	13
• Hash Brown	100	5	12	1	1
• Sausage, Egg, Cheese	520	37	30	1	19
Cookies					
Caramel Chocolate Pecan, 1 cookie	230	11	32	1	3
Chocolate Chip, 1 cookie	230	9	34	1	3
• Oatmeal Raisin Spice, 1 cookie	220	8	35	1	3
• Peanut Butter Chocolate Chunk, 1 cookie	260	15	28	2	5
Triple Chocolate, 1 cookie	250	13	31	2	3
White Chocolate Macadamia Nut, 1 cookie	240	12	31	1	3
Donuts					
Angel Cream, 1 donut	310	13	46	1	4
Apple Fritter, 1 donut	300	11	49	2	4
Blueberry Fritter, 1 donut	330	10	55	2	6
Blueberry, 1 donut	230	8	36	1	4
Boston Cream, 1 donut	250	9	38	1	4
Canadian Maple, 1 donut	260	9	41	1	4
Chocolate Dip, 1 donut	210	9	30	1	4
Chocolate Glazed, 1 donut	260	10	39	2	4
Honey Cruller, 1 donut	320	19	37	0	1
Honey Dip, 1 donut	210	8	33	1	4
• Maple Dip, 1 donut	210	8	31	1	4
Old Fashion Glazed, 1 donut	320	19	35	1	3
Old Fashion Plain, 1 donut	260	19	20	1	3
Sour Cream Plain, 1 donut	270	17	27	1	3
Strawberry, 1 donut	230	8	36	1	4
• Walnut Crunch, 1 donut	360	23	35	1	4
Muffins					
Blueberry Bran, 1 muffin	300	10	53	5	6
Blueberry, 1 muffin	330	11	55	2	4
• Chocolate Chip Plain, 1 muffin	430	16	69	2	5
Cranberry Blueberry Bran, 1 muffin	290	10	51	5	4
Cranberry Fruit, 1 muffin	350	12	59	2	4
Fruit Explosion, 1 muffin	360	11	61	2	4
• Lowfat Blueberry, 1 muffin	290	3	62	2	4
Lowfat Cranberry, 1 muffin	290	3	62	2	4

RESTAURANTS & FAST-FOOD CHAINS

Tim Horton's (cont.)	Cal	Fat	Cbs	Fbr	Prtn
Muffins (cont.)					
Raisin Bran, 1 muffin	360	10	65	6	6
Strawberry Sensation, 1 muffin	350	11	61	1	4
Wheat Carrot, 1 muffin	400	19	55	4	6
Sandwiches					
B.L.T. (w/ mayonnaise), 1 piece	450	18	53	2	18
Chicken Salad (with lettuce & tomato)	380	9	55	3	21
Country Bun – white	240	1	49	2	9
Country Bun – whole wheat	230	1	46	4	10
Egg Salad (with lettuce)	390	13	52	2	17
Ham & Swiss (w/ Tim's Own dressing), 1 piece	440	12	56	3	28
Toasted Chicken Club (w/ bacon), 1 piece	460	7	70	2	30
Turkey Bacon Club (w/ honey mustard), 1 piece	440	8	63	2	30
Turkey Breast (w/ Tim's Own dressing), 1 piece	390	5	59	4	27
Soups & Chili					
Beef Stew, 10 oz.	236	8	25	3	17
Chicken Noodle, 10 oz.	120	2	18	1	5
Chili, 10 oz.	300	16	18	5	21
Cream of Broccoli, 10 oz.	160	9	16	1	6
Creamy Field Mushroom, 10 oz.	150	3	28	1	3
Hearty Vegetable, 10 oz.	70	0	14	3	4
Minestrone, 10 oz.	120	3	24	2	4
Potato Bacon, 10 oz.	180	6	30	2	3
Split Pea with Ham, 10 oz.	150	3	27	5	8
Turkey Rice, 10 oz.	120	2	21	1	3
Vegetable Beef Barley, 10 oz.	110	2	21	2	4
Specialty Baked Goods					
Butter Croissant, 1 croissant	340	18	38	1	7
Cheese Croissant, 1 croissant	370	20	37	0	9
Cherry Cheese Danish, 1 danish	330	13	46	1	5
Chocolate Danish, 1 danish	430	24	51	1	4
• Cinnamon Roll – Frosted, 1 roll	470	25	57	2	4
Cinnamon Roll – Glazed, 1 roll	420	23	50	2	4
Maple Pecan Danish, 1 danish	380	20	46	1	4
• Plain Tea Biscuit, 1 biscuit	250	9	35	1	5
Raisin Tea Biscuit, 1 biscuit	290	10	45	2	6
Timbits®					
• Apple Fritter, 1 timbit	50	2	9	0	1
Banana Cream, 1 timbit	60	2	9	0	1
Blueberry, 1 timbit	60	2	10	0	1
Chocolate Glazed, 1 timbit	70	3	10	0	1
Honey Dip, 1 timbit	60	2	9	0	1
Lemon, 1 timbit	60	2	9	0	1
Old Fashion Plain, 1 timbit	70	5	5	0	1
• Sour Cream Glazed, 1 timbit	90	5	12	0	1
Strawberry, 1 timbit	60	2	10	0	1
Yogurt & Berries					
Lowfat Creamy Vanilla Yogurt w/ Berries, 6 oz.	160	3	32	2	4
Lowfat Strawberry Yogurt w/ Berries, 6 oz.	150	3	32	2	4

▶ Topz	Cal	Fat	Cbs	Fbr	Prtn
Aero Fries, Rings & Nuggets					
Aero Fries, 158 g	380	14	58	7	6
• Aero Onion Rings, 166 g	298	11	46	4	4

(•= most healthy •= least healthy) **RESTAURANTS & FAST-FOOD • 369**

RESTAURANTS & FAST-FOOD CHAINS

Topz (cont.)

	Cal	Fat	Cbs	Fbr	Prtn
Aero Fries, Rings & Nuggets (cont.)					
• Chili Cheese Fries, 301 g	589	27	66	8	14
Dessertz					
Brownie, 105 g	350	5	67	4	7
• Chocolate Chip Cookie, 105 g	385	9	67	4	7
• Lowfat Ice Cream w/ Choc. Syrup, 162 g	255	7	43	0	6
Oatmeal Raisin Cookie, 105 g	385	9	67	4	7
Fresh Gourmet Salads					
• Chinese Chicken Salad, 392 g	322	14	17	7	33
Dijon Deli Chopped Salad, 382 g	229	13	9	7	19
Ginger Grilled Ahi Salad, 392 g	312	15	10	7	36
• Small Dijon Deli Salad, 21 g	101	6	3	2	6
Fruit Shakez					
• Chocolate Banana Shake, 472 g	460	8	80	3	17
Chocolate Shake, 372 g	360	9	55	0	16
Raspberry Shake, 427 g	404	9	64	1	16
• Strawberry Shake, 427 g	356	9	54	2	17
Gourmet Hot Dogs					
• Beef Chili Dog, 269 g	485	24	49	3	21
Double Turkey Dog, 242 g	390	8	60	7	20
Hebrew National Beef Dog, 230 g	450	21	52	3	19
• Turkey Chili Dog, 255 g	355	9	53	3	15
Gourmet Lean Burgers					
1/2 lb. Black Angus Burger w/o Sauce, 392 g	672	34	37	3	49
• 1/2 lb. Black Angus Burger, 415 g	735	40	40	3	49
1/4 lb. Black Angus Burger, w/o sauce, 278 g	444	19	37	3	28
1/4 lb. Black Angus Burger, 301 g	507	25	40	3	28
1/4 lb. Black Angus Chili Burger, 318 g	489	21	42	3	34
• Garden Burger, 228 g	355	12	46	6	17
Turkey Burger, 301 g	449	19	40	3	31
Kidz Mealz					
• Kidz Grilled Cheese, 62 g	207	9	24	1	8
• Kidz Beef Dog, 145 g	405	21	40	2	15
Kidz Burger, 184 g	408	19	33	2	27
Kidz Turkey Dog, 131 g	275	7	44	2	13
Signature Chili					
Signature Chili, 291 g	329	17	17	2	28
Signature Lean Sandwiches					
Classic Grilled Cheese Sandwich, 123 g	414	18	47	1	16
• Ginger Grilled Ahi Sandwich, 268 g	384	11	37	3	33
• Grilled Cheese & Tomato Sandwich, 144 g	418	18	48	1	16
Grilled Chicken Breast Sandwich, 290 g	396	10	39	3	33

Tropical Smoothie

	Cal	Fat	Cbs	Fbr	Prtn
Cheeses					
American, 2/3 oz.	53	4	0	0	3
Lowfat Mozzarella, 3 oz.	80	5	1	0	8
Pepper Jack, 2/3 oz.	50	5	0	0	3
Provolone	50	4	1	0	4
• Shredded Cheddar, 1/3 cup	177	15	1	0	11
• Shredded Parmesan, 1 oz.	50	3	0	0	4
Swiss, 2/3 oz.	55	4	0	0	4
Dessert Smoothies: w/ Splenda					
Beach Bum (Chocolate)	366	5	75	5	5

Tropical Smoothie (cont.)	Cal	Fat	Cbs	Fbr	Prtn
Dessert Smoothies: w/ Splenda (cont.)					
Beach Bum (Vanilla)	370	6	66	5	4
Chocolate Chiller	356	7	68	0	6
Coconut Royale	531	11	105	7	3
Mocha Madness	447	12	77	0	8
Peanut Butter Cup	638	24	92	5	13
• Tropi-colada	299	6	61	3	1
Kid's Menu					
Cheese Quesadilla	559	26	53	2	28
• Cheese Quesadilla w/Chicken	611	27	54	2	38
Ham and American Sandwich	257	7	32	1	17
Ham and American Wrap	422	14	53	2	22
• Turkey and American Sandwich	268	6	32	1	21
Turkey and American Wrap	433	13	53	2	26
Kids Smoothies: w/ Splenda					
• Chocolate Chimp	160	3	32	1	2
• Jetty Jr.	85	0	20	3	1
Orange Delight	100	3	17	1	3
Lowfat Smoothies: w/ Splenda					
Blimey Limey	210	0	52	1	0
• Blue Lagoon	130	1	30	5	1
Cool Breeze	209	1	49	3	3
Hawaiian Breeze	160	0	38	0	2
Island Fever	253	1	61	4	2
Jetty Punch	169	1	39	5	2
Kiwi Quencher	217	0	52	2	3
Mango Magic	203	0	47	2	3
Orange Passion	250	0	59	3	3
Paradise Point	263	1	62	6	2
Peaches n' Silk	182	1	43	4	1
• Raspberry Rush	384	1	90	9	3
Rockin' Raspberry	213	1	50	8	2
Strawberry Beach	151	0	34	5	3
Sunny Day	301	1	72	4	2
Sunrise Sunset	191	0	46	3	1
Toucan Delight	232	1	54	6	2
Power Smoothies: w/ Splenda					
Fat Buster	173	1	41	5	2
Health Nut	418	11	54	8	27
• Lean Machine	173	1	40	5	2
Morning After	241	1	57	4	2
Muscle Blaster	397	3	69	5	24
• Peanut Paradise	610	22	69	5	34
Salads					
Caesar Salad, 1 salad	116	1	8	3	18
Chef Salad, 1 salad	172	2	11	4	27
• Garden Classic Salad, 1 salad	59	1	10	5	4
• Sesame Chicken Salad, 1 salad	417	10	53	5	28
Thai Chicken Salad, 1 salad	353	4	54	6	26
Sauces					
Balsamic Vinaigrette Dressing, 1 oz.	61	5	4	0	0
Caesar Dressing, 1 oz.	160	17	1	0	1
• Chipotle Dressing, 1 oz.	180	20	2	0	0
• Fat Free Italian, 1 oz.	8	0	2	0	0

(• = most healthy • = least healthy)

RESTAURANTS & FAST-FOOD CHAINS

Tropical Smoothie (cont.)	Cal	Fat	Cbs	Fbr	Prtn
Sauces (cont.)					
Franks Red Hot Sauce, 1 oz.	10	0	1	0	0
Jamaican Jerk Sauce, 1 oz.	40	0	9	0	1
Light Ranch, 1 oz.	100	10	1	0	1
Light Ranch, 1/2 oz.	50	5	1	0	1
Mango Habanero Sauce, 1 oz.	30	0	7	0	0
Mayonnaise, Lowfat 1 oz.	50	5	1	0	0
Mayonnaise, Reduced Calorie, 1 oz.	80	7	4	0	0
Salsa, 1 oz.	10	0	3	0	0
Sesame Dressing, 1 oz.	90	5	11	0	0
Texas Petal Sauce, 1 oz.	160	17	1	0	0
Texas Petal Sauce, 1/2 oz.	80	9	1	0	0
Thai Peanut Dressing, 1 oz.	74	3	10	0	1
Specialty Breads					
Focaccia, 1 pc.	295	3	60	3	8
Specialty Sandwiches					
American Albacore	725	29	85	4	31
Cheese BLT Sandwich	717	37	72	3	24
Chicken Caesar Sandwich	624	25	66	3	34
Chipolte Chicken Sandwich	660	27	71	5	34
Club	703	26	77	3	41
Ham and Cheese	604	19	78	3	31
Roast Beef	681	30	63	3	40
• The Italian	748	39	71	4	30
Turkey Bacon Ranch	669	23	69	3	46
• Tuscan Turkey	439	13	67	3	13
Splendid Dessert Smoothies: w/ Splenda					
Chocolate Banana	410	7	81	3	6
Orange Dream	377	5	79	1	4
Splendid Smoothies: w/ Splenda					
• Citrus Split	196	1	47	3	1
Cranberry Crush	184	0	45	1	1
Pineapple Delight	181	0	44	2	1
• Strawberry Light	139	0	31	5	3
Supercharged Smoothies: w/ Splenda					
Banana Berry Boost	197	2	45	5	1
Get Up and Goji	225	0	53	4	3
Island Intensity	202	2	45	6	2
Mango Moxie	253	0	60	4	3
• Pomegranate Plunge	275	0	67	3	1
• Strawberry Stamina	197	1	45	4	2
Tortillas					
Garlic Herb Tortilla, 1 pc.	299	8	49	2	8
White Tortilla, 1 pc.	312	8	51	2	8
Wraps					
Breakfast Wrap (Bacon)	537	23	55	2	29
• Breakfast Wrap (Ham)	524	18	57	2	35
Buffalo Chicken	566	21	61	3	34
Chicken Cordon Bleu	610	26	56	2	37
Chicken Mango Habanero	654	14	95	3	38
Cool Tuna Wrap	646	27	71	4	30
Early Bird	672	34	56	2	35
Jamaican Jerk	579	13	79	4	36
King Caesar	557	26	55	3	25

Tropical Smoothie (cont.)

	Cal	Fat	Cbs	Fbr	Prtn
Wraps (cont.)					
Popeyes Favorite	578	20	60	3	39
Salsa Sunrise	594	24	57	2	39
Sesame Chicken	754	24	103	4	33
Thai Chicken Wrap	744	15	116	8	36
Totally Turkey	653	27	58	3	45
Veggie Veggie	615	26	72	5	24
Western Wrap	537	18	59	3	36

Tubby's

	Cal	Fat	Cbs	Fbr	Prtn
Regular: Burger Subs					
American Cheeseburger	810	48	56	4	39
• Big Tub	671	56	55	4	34
Burger Special	898	59	59	6	39
Cheeseburger	911	60	59	9	42
Mushroom Burger	868	59	53	5	38
• Pizza Burger	929	60	62	10	43
Taco	827	47	67	5	39
Regular: Burger Wraps					
American Cheeseburger	660	48	19	6	38
Burger Special	748	58	22	8	38
Cheeseburger	969	61	67	14	48
Mushroom Burger	776	59	24	11	43
• Pizza Burger	988	61	70	15	49
Taco	734	48	38	12	44
• Tub	579	57	26	11	39
Regular: Chicken Subs					
Chicken & Broccoli	552	23	56	5	35
Chicken & Cheddar	543	23	54	4	34
• Chicken Club	705	41	53	4	37
Chicken Fajita	445	12	57	4	33
• Chicken Parmesan	426	14	51	4	32
Grilled Chicken	346	5	52	4	28
Regular: Chicken Wraps					
Chicken & Broccoli	552	23	56	5	35
Chicken & Cheddar	451	24	25	11	39
• Chicken Club	613	42	24	11	42
Chicken Fajita	353	12	28	11	38
Chicken Parmesan	334	15	22	11	37
• Grilled Chicken	254	5	23	11	32
Regular: Deli Subs					
• Club Sub	701	41	53	4	36
Famous	664	39	55	4	26
• Ham & Cheese	568	30	54	4	27
Turkey & Cheese	598	32	51	4	29
Turkey Club	678	38	52	4	34
Regular: Deli Wraps					
Club Sub	591	41	23	11	38
Famous	570	40	26	11	33
• Ham & Cheese	476	31	25	11	32
Turkey & Cheese	534	32	22	11	40
• Turkey Club	614	38	23	11	45
Regular: Specialty Subs					
BLT	636	42	50	4	21

RESTAURANTS & FAST-FOOD CHAINS

Tubby's (cont.)	Cal	Fat	Cbs	Fbr	Prtn
Regular: Specialty Subs (cont.)					
Cold Veggie	462	14	66	8	23
• Italian Sausage	729	45	56	4	32
• Tuna	417	18	47	4	38
Veggie Stir Fry	652	27	89	8	21
Regular: Steak Subs					
Mushroom Steak	833	26	52	4	13
Pepper Steak	709	46	52	4	29
• Philly Cheesesteak	685	40	49	4	37
• Pizza Steak	986	57	85	7	42
Portabella Mushroom	801	48	54	5	43
Steak & Cheddar	833	56	52	4	37
Steak & Cheese	823	56	51	4	36
Steak Special	746	46	58	6	31
Regular: Steak Wraps					
Mushroom Steak	738	56	23	11	42
Pepper Steak	617	46	23	11	34
• Philly Cheesesteak	593	40	20	11	43
• Pizza Steak	750	56	25	12	42
Portabella Mushroom	709	48	25	12	48
Steak & Cheddar	741	57	23	11	42
Steak & Cheese	731	56	22	11	41
Steak Special	654	46	29	13	36

Una Mas	Cal	Fat	Cbs	Fbr	Prtn
Burritos					
Bean & Cheese (The Works), 527 g	1063	57	91	13	48
Bean & Cheese Burrito, 442 g	923	44	85	10	47
Butternut Squash Burrito (The Works), 641 g	842	44	97	12	28
Butternut Squash Burrito, 556 g	701	31	91	8	26
• Carnitas Burrito (The Works), 626 g	1560	100	84	13	83
Carnitas Burrito, 525 g	1367	83	78	10	77
Foghead Burrito, 584 g	876	36	102	8	37
Fresca Burrito (The Works), 598 g	774	29	105	14	26
Fresca Burrito, 499 g	581	12	99	11	21
Gallito Griller (The Works), 527 g	1085	63	63	6	69
Gallito Griller, 499 g	1024	57	62	6	68
Grilled Fajita Burrito-Chicken, 587 g	766	31	87	11	37
Grilled Fajita Burrito-Steak, 587 g	851	36	88	11	48
Grilled Fajita Burrito-Veggie, 502 g	666	28	86	11	22
Lobster Burrito (The Works), 570 g	1029	50	93	8	53
Lobster Burrito, 527 g	915	40	92	8	49
Mahi-Mahi Burrito (The Works), 587 g	937	53	81	8	38
Mahi-Mahi Burrito, 487 g	744	35	75	5	33
• Nino Burrito, 255 g	403	12	58	5	16
Pineapple Burrito, 390 g	660	19	87	5	35
Roasted Pasilla Veggie (The Works), 556 g	710	32	89	11	23
Roasted Pasilla Veggie Burrito, 528 g	649	26	88	11	22
San Lucas Fish Baja Style (The Works), 550 g	948	53	84	7	34
San Lucas Fish Burrito-Baja Style, 451 g	755	36	78	4	29
San Lucas Fish Cabo Style (The Works), 514 g	841	46	75	8	34
San Lucas Fish Burrito-Cabo Style, 415 g	648	29	69	4	29
Una Mas Burrito- Chicken (The Works), 570 g	779	32	89	10	36
Una Mas Burrito-Chicken, 471 g	587	15	84	7	31

Una Mas (cont.)	Cal	Fat	Cbs	Fbr	Prtn
Burritos (cont.)					
Una Mas Burrito- Steak (The Works), 570 g	864	36	90	10	47
Una Mas Burrito-Steak, 471 g	671	19	84	7	41
Vera Cruz Shrimp Baja Style (The Works), 520 g	1149	74	82	7	37
Vera Cruz Shrimp Burrito-Baja Style, 491 g	1082	67	81	7	36
Vera Cruz Shrimp Cabo Style (The Works), 558 g	940	50	88	10	37
Vera Cruz Shrimp Burrito-Cabo Style, 516 g	826	40	86	10	33
Wet Style Burrito, 669 g	960	45	92	11	47
Dinner Plates					
Fajitas Plato Combo, 723 g	846	35	81	10	54
Mahi-Mahi Dinner Plate, 707 g	874	45	77	11	43
Pescado Ranchero Dinner Plate, 707 g	859	46	75	10	38
Enchiladas					
Enchiladas Rojas, 435 g	532	24	50	7	31
Nachos					
Mas Nachos with Chicken, 765 g	1949	106	189	28	55
Mas Nachos with Steak, 765 g	2033	110	189	28	65
Mas Nachos, 680 g	1850	102	188	28	39
Nachos Ninos, 227 g	564	31	52	6	17
Quesadillas					
Monterey Butternut Squash Quesadilla, 458 g	925	57	67	6	39
Monterey Quesadilla- Chicken, 429 g	958	57	61	5	53
Monterey Quesadilla- Steak, 429 g	1042	61	61	5	64
Monterey Shrimp Quesadilla, 446 g	1073	67	63	5	55
Nino Quesadilla, 242 g	524	26	50	3	23
Quesadilla Chica, 157 g	447	24	38	1	20
Salad Dressings					
Lime-Jalapeño Vinaigrette, 1 oz.	133	15	1	0	0
Tangy Lime Vinaigrette, 1 oz.	153	17	1	0	0
Sides					
Bottomless Bskt of Chips/Salsa Fresca, 340 g	1104	48	158	17	1
Chipotle Sauce, 1 tbsp	82	9	0	0	0
Corn Salsa, 1/4 cup	22	0	5	1	1
Frijoles Negros, 1/2 cup	138	2	24	6	8
Frijoles Picantes, 1/2 cup	132	1	24	9	9
Guacamole, 1/4 cup	133	12	8	6	2
Mexican Fried Rice, 1/2 cup	70	2	12	1	2
Nacho Style Fried Tortilla Chips, 1 oz.	135	6	19	2	0
Pinto Beans, 1/2 cup	152	2	26	6	9
Roasted Pineapple Salsa, 1/4 cup	32	1	6	1	0
Salsa Barrio, 1/4 cup	26	1	5	2	1
Salsa Blanca, 1/4 cup	376	40	2	0	2
Salsa Fresca, 1/4 cup	12	0	3	1	1
Salsa Picante, 1/4 cup	62	5	5	1	1
Salsa Ranchera, 1/4 cup	20	1	3	1	1
Salsa Roja, 1/4 cup	13	0	3	0	0
Salsa Verde, 1/4 cup	21	0	4	1	1
Soups & Salads					
Caesar Salad with Chicken, 511 g	886	58	53	6	33
Crispy Taco Salad, 426 g	500	26	48	107	19
w/ Chicken, 511 g	600	30	49	11	34
w/ Steak, 511 g	684	34	50	11	44
Crispy Taco & Soup, 1 Taco/8 oz. Soup	728	39	64	10	36
Margarita Salad, 554 g	892	70	55	11	21

(• = most healthy • = least healthy)

RESTAURANTS & FAST-FOOD CHAINS

Una Mas (cont.)

	Cal	Fat	Cbs	Fbr	Prtn
Soups & Salads (cont.)					
w/ Chicken, 724 g	1078	73	57	11	57
• w/ Steak, 724 g	1260	86	58	11	73
Spicy Chipotle Chicken Breast Salad, 511 g	571	36	18	3	42
• Tortilla Soup (Small), 8 oz.	194	11	10	3	16
Verde Salad, 284 g	434	37	22	5	9
Tacos					
Crispy Chicken Taco Plate, 224 g	327	17	30	6	16
Flautas Puebla (Chicken) Plate, 619 g	784	38	86	15	30
Flautas Puebla (Chicken) Side Order, 256 g	362	20	35	6	13
• Flautas Puebla (Steak) Plate, 619 g	915	52	86	15	31
Flautas Puebla (Steak) Side Order, 256 g	405	25	32	5	14
Mahi-Mahi Taco (The Works), 259 g	494	33	32	6	18
Mahi-Mahi Taco, 188 g	341	20	28	4	14
San Lucas Fish Taco-Baja Style (The Works), 259 g	579	40	38	5	16
San Lucas Fish Taco-Baja Style, 188 g	426	26	34	4	12
San Lucas Fish Cabo Style (The Works), 223 g	472	33	29	5	16
San Lucas Fish Taco-Cabo Style, 153 g	319	19	26	4	11
Taco-Butternut Squash, 137 g	218	11	27	4	7
Taco-Carnitas, 180 g	460	27	28	4	27
• Taqueria Taco (per taco), 86 g	136	7	9	2	9
Taqueria Taco Combo Basket (/w Beans), 229 g	320	15	27	6	20
Taqueria Taco Combo Basket (/w Rice), 229 g	308	16	24	4	18
Una Mas Taco - Steak, 180 g	278	9	33	5	17
Una Mas Taco- Chicken (The Works), 222 g	320	14	36	7	15
Una Mas Taco- Chicken, 180 g	250	8	33	5	14
Una Mas Taco- Steak (The Works), 222 g	348	16	36	7	18
Una Mas Taco- Veggie (The Works), 279 g	304	13	40	8	10
Una Mas Taco- Veggie, 236 g	234	6	37	6	9
Vera Cruz Shrimp Baja Style (The Works), 222 g	549	39	33	5	16
Vera Cruz Shrimp Taco-Baja Style, 151 g	396	26	29	4	11
Vera Cruz Shrimp Cabo Style (The Works), 239 g	493	34	32	6	17
Vera Cruz Shrimp Taco-Cabo Style, 168 g	339	20	28	4	12

Village Inn

	Cal	Fat	Cbs	Fbr	Prtn
Breakfast					
• Cinnamon Raisin French Toast	370	11	57	4	8
Fruit & Nut Multigrain Pancakes	490	10	91	7	10
• Veggie Omelette	490	16	69	5	20
Entrees					
3-Course Sirloin Steak	640	22	70	3	38
• Chicken Stir-Fry Dinner Skillet	710	24	83	4	35
• Grilled Tilapia	630	20	64	2	47
Sandwiches					
• Grilled Chicken Sandwich	460	16	46	3	33
• Half Sandwich & Soup	290	9	27	2	24
Soup & Salads					
• Chicken Caesar Salad	380	16	25	7	34
• Chicken Noodle Soup	80	2	10	0	5
Garden Grand Salad	350	20	25	5	19
Minestrone Soup	100	2	17	3	5
Side Salad	80	4	8	2	4
Vegetable Beef Soup	140	7	12	3	8

RESTAURANTS & FAST-FOOD CHAINS

Wahoo's Fish Taco	Cal	Fat	Cbs	Fbr	Prtn
Appetizers					
Baja Rolls	475	20	49	3	27
Banzai Burrito					
Blackened Chicken	680	14	89	10	51
Blackened Fish	590	11	89	10	42
Carne Asada	675	18	87	10	42
• Carnitas	735	23	87	10	45
Charbroiled Chicken	675	14	87	10	50
Charbroiled Fish	585	11	87	10	42
Shrimp	600	11	87	10	39
• Vegetarian	520	9	96	11	17
Classic Burrito					
Blackened Chicken	545	17	51	4	46
Blackened Fish	460	14	53	4	38
Carne Asada	515	20	49	4	35
Carnitas	595	26	49	4	41
Charbroiled Chicken	540	17	49	4	46
Charbroiled Fish	455	14	51	4	38
• Mushroom	415	17	57	6	14
Shrimp	470	14	51	4	35
• Veggie	600	14	98	12	21
Combo Platters: #1 w/1 Taco					
• Blackened Chicken	750	11	121	18	41
Blackened Fish	715	9	122	18	37
Carne Asada	735	12	121	18	36
Carnitas	770	14	121	18	39
Charbroiled Chicken	745	10	121	18	41
Charbroiled Fish	710	9	121	18	37
• Mushroom	690	10	124	19	27
Shrimp	725	9	122	18	37
Veggie	740	9	136	21	29
Combo Platters: #2 w/2 Tacos					
2 Blackened Chicken	960	16	140	20	61
Blackened Chicken, Carne Asada	945	17	139	20	55
Blackened Chicken, Carnitas	980	20	139	20	59
Blackened Chicken, Mushroom	900	16	143	21	46
Blackened Chicken, Shrimp	935	15	140	20	57
Blackened Chicken, Veggie	950	15	154	23	49
Blackened Fish, Blackened Chicken	920	15	141	21	57
2 Blackened Fish	885	14	142	21	54
Blackened Fish, Carne Asada	905	16	140	20	52
Blackened Fish, Carnitas	945	19	140	20	55
Blackened Fish, Mushroom	865	15	143	21	43
Blackened Fish, Shrimp	895	14	141	21	54
Blackened Fish, Veggie	910	13	155	23	45
2 Carne Asada	930	18	138	20	50
Carne Asada, Carnitas	965	21	138	20	53
Carne Asada, Mushroom	885	17	142	21	41
Carne Asada, Shrimp	920	16	140	20	52
Carne Asada, Veggie	935	16	154	23	43
• 2 Carnitas	1005	24	138	20	56
Carnitas, Mushroom	925	20	142	21	44
Carnitas, Shrimp	955	19	139	20	55
Carnitas, Veggie	970	19	154	23	46

(•= most healthy •= least healthy) **RESTAURANTS & FAST-FOOD • 377**

RESTAURANTS & FAST-FOOD CHAINS

Wahoo's Fish Taco (cont.)

	Cal	Fat	Cbs	Fbr	Prtn
Combo Platters: #2 w/2 Tacos (cont.)					
Chicken, Blackened Chicken	955	16	139	20	61
Chicken, Blackened Fish	920	15	140	20	57
Chicken, Carne Asada	940	17	138	20	55
Chicken, Carnitas	975	20	138	20	58
Chicken, Chicken	950	16	138	20	61
Chicken, Mushroom	900	16	142	21	46
Chicken, Shrimp	930	15	139	20	57
Chicken, Veggie	945	15	154	23	49
Fish, Blackened Chicken	920	15	140	20	57
Fish, Blackened Fish	885	14	141	21	54
Fish, Carne Asada	905	16	139	20	52
Fish, Carnitas	940	19	139	20	55
Fish, Chicken	915	15	139	20	57
Fish, Fish	880	13	140	20	53
Fish, Mushroom	860	15	143	21	42
Fish, Shrimp	895	14	140	20	53
Fish, Veggie	910	13	155	23	45
• 2 Mushroom	845	16	145	22	32
Shrimp, Mushroom	875	15	143	21	43
Shrimp, Shrimp	905	14	141	20	54
Shrimp, Veggie	925	13	140	23	45
Veggie, Mushroom	890	14	157	24	34
2 Veggie	940	13	169	26	37
Combo Platters: #3 Classic Burrito					
Blackened Chicken	1085	22	154	20	67
Blackened Fish	1000	19	155	20	59
Carne Asada	1055	25	152	19	56
Carnitas	1135	31	152	19	62
Charbroiled Chicken	1080	22	152	19	67
Charbroiled Fish	995	19	154	20	59
• Mushroom	955	21	160	0	34
Shrimp	1010	19	154	20	56
• Veggie	1140	19	201	28	42
Combo Platters: #3 Banzaiai Burrito					
Blackened Chicken	1220	19	192	26	72
Blackened Fish	1130	15	192	26	63
Carne Asada	1215	22	190	25	63
• Carnitas	1275	27	190	25	66
Charbroiled Chicken	1215	19	190	25	71
Charbroiled Fish	1125	15	190	25	63
Shrimp	1140	16	190	25	60
• Vegetarian	1060	14	199	27	38
Combo Platters: #4 Burrito, Taco					
Blackened Chicken Banzaiai Burrito	680	14	89	10	51
Blackened Chicken Burrito	545	17	51	4	46
Blackened Chicken Taco	210	6	19	2	20
Blackened Fish Banzai Burrito	590	11	89	10	42
Blackened Fish Burrito	460	14	53	4	38
Blackened Fish Taco	175	4	19	3	16
Carne Asada Banzaiai Burrito	675	18	87	10	42
Carne Asada Burrito	515	20	49	4	35
Carne Asada Taco	195	7	18	2	15
• Carnitas Banzaiai Burrito	735	23	87	10	45

Wahoo's Fish Taco (cont.)	Cal	Fat	Cbs	Fbr	Prtn
Combo Platters: #4 Burrito, Taco (cont.)					
Carnitas Burrito	595	26	49	4	41
Carnitas Taco	230	10	18	2	18
Charbroiled Chicken Banzaiai Burrito	675	14	87	10	50
Charbroiled Chicken Burrito	540	17	49	4	46
Charbroiled Chicken Taco	205	6	18	2	20
Charbroiled Fish Banzai Burrito	585	11	87	10	42
Charbroiled Fish Burrito	455	14	51	4	38
Charbroiled Fish Taco	170	4	19	2	16
Mushroom Burrito	415	17	57	6	14
Mushroom Taco	150	5	21	3	6
Rice Beans	540	5	103	16	21
Shrimp Banzai Burrito	600	11	87	10	39
Shrimp Burrito	470	14	51	4	35
Shrimp Taco	180	5	19	2	16
Vegetable Banzai Burrito	520	9	96	11	17
Veggie Burrito	600	14	98	12	21
Veggie Taco	200	4	33	5	8
Combo Platters: #6 Maui Bowl					
Maui Bowl	1115	19	163	17	69
Combo Platters: #7 Chicken Bowl					
Blackened Chicken	1050	15	145	17	78
• Charbroiled Chicken	1035	15	143	16	78
• Teriyaki Chicken	1140	15	163	17	85
Combo Platters: #8 Wahoo Bowl					
Blackened Fish	913	10	145	17	66
• Charbroiled Fish	900	10	143	16	65
Shrimp	980	11	143	16	72
• Teriyaki Fish	1040	10	170	17	75
Combo Platters: #9 and #10					
#9 Veggie Bowl	995	8	195	21	39
#10 Kalua Pig Bowl	1230	28	163	16	78
Combo Platters: #11 Banzaiai Bowl					
Blackened Chicken	1080	13	172	20	67
Blackened Fish	990	9	172	20	59
Carne Asada	1049	15	171	20	56
• Carnitas	1130	21	171	20	62
Charbroiled Chicken	1075	13	171	20	67
• Charbroiled Fish	980	9	171	20	59
Shrimp	995	10	171	20	56
Kid's Bowl					
• Bean & Cheese Burrito	635	26	71	12	30
Blackened Chicken	435	5	66	12	30
Blackened Fish	395	4	66	12	27
Carne Asada	430	7	65	12	26
Carnitas	455	9	65	12	28
Charbroiled Chicken	430	5	65	12	30
• Charbroiled Fish	390	4	65	12	26
Shrimp	405	4	66	12	26
Kid's Sides					
Beans	445	2	80	29	30
Rice	475	6	94	1	9
Kid's Taco With Rice & Beans					
Carne Asada	570	10	89	12	29

(• = most healthy • = least healthy)   **RESTAURANTS & FAST-FOOD • 379**

RESTAURANTS & FAST-FOOD CHAINS

Wahoo's Fish Taco (cont.)

	Cal	Fat	Cbs	Fbr	Prtn
Kid's Taco With Rice & Beans (cont.)					
• Carnitas	590	12	89	12	30
Charbroiled Chicken	570	9	89	12	32
• Charbroiled Fish	535	8	90	12	28
Shrimp	540	8	90	12	27
Soup					
Chicken Tortilla Soup	140	4	8	2	19
Taco					
Blackened Chicken	210	6	19	2	20
Blackened Fish	175	4	19	3	16
Carne Asada	195	7	18	2	15
• Carnitas	230	10	18	2	18
Charbroiled Chicken	205	6	18	2	20
Charbroiled Fish	170	4	19	2	16
• Mushroom	150	5	21	3	6
Shrimp	180	5	19	2	16
Veggie	200	4	33	5	8
Wahoo's Salad (-chips)					
Blackened Chicken	565	28	16	5	64
Blackened Fish	430	23	16	5	52
Carne Asada	555	33	13	4	52
• Carnitas	640	41	13	4	57
Charbroiled Chicken	550	27	13	4	64
Charbroiled Fish	415	22	13	4	51
• Sautee'd Veggies	345	20	32	7	15
Shrimp	500	24	14	4	59
Veggie	490	22	56	12	21
Wahoo's Sandwich					
Blackened Chicken	650	25	58	3	47
Blackened Fish	570	22	58	3	40
Carne Asada	645	28	57	3	40
• Carnitas	695	33	57	3	43
Charbroiled Chicken	640	25	57	3	47
Charbroiled Fish	560	22	57	3	40
• Sautee'd Veggies	520	20	68	5	18
Shrimp	575	22	57	3	37

Wendy's

	Cal	Fat	Cbs	Fbr	Prtn
Chicken Temptations and Fish					
10-piece Chicken Nuggets, 150 g	460	22	24	0	24
Chicken Club, 246 g	540	7	48	2	34
Crispy Chicken Deluxe, 180 g	400	25	35	1	20
• Crispy Chicken Sandwich, 285 g	660	25	68	2	32
• Grilled Chicken Go Wrap, 122 g	260	16	23	1	17
Homestyle Chicken Fillet, 220 g	430	30	48	2	25
Homestyle Chicken Go Wrap, 252 g	630	11	57	2	31
Premium Fish Fillet Sandwich, 177 g	450	29	47	1	16
Spicy Chicken Go Wrap, 128 g	320	20	28	2	17
Spicy Chicken Sandwich, 223 g	440	16	46	3	28
Ultimate Chicken Grill, 211 g	320	16	36	2	28
Frosty					
• Frosty™ Float, 467 g	380	7	75	0	7
M&M® Twisted Frosty™, 269 g	560	19	86	1	10
Medium Original Choco Frosty™, 298 g	411	11	68	0	11

RESTAURANTS & FAST-FOOD CHAINS

Wendy's (cont.)	Cal	Fat	Cbs	Fbr	Prtn
Frosty (cont.)					
Medium Vanilla Frosty™, 596 g	820	21	135	0	21
Nestlé® Cookie Dough Twisted Frosty™, 257 g	480	16	77	1	10
Oreo® Twisted Frosty™, 247 g	450	14	72	1	10
Small Chocolate Fudge Frosty™ Shake, 329 g	410	11	69	0	9
Small Strawberry Frosty™ Shake, 325 g	390	11	67	0	7
Small Vanilla Bean Frosty™ Shake, 322 g	380	11	65	0	7
Garden Sensation Salads					
Chicken BLT Salad w/ Homestyle Chkn, 417 g	780	53	42	3	37
Chicken Caesar Salad w/ Grilled Chkn, 318 g	490	33	20	3	31
Mandarin Chicken® Salad w/ Grilled Chkn, 402 g	540	25	50	5	31
Southwest Taco Salad, 520 g	640	39	44	9	30
Hot Stuffed Baked Potatoes					
Bacon and Cheese Potato, 366 g	450	13	67	7	19
Broccoli and Cheese Potato, 397 g	320	2	69	8	10
Sour Cream and Chives Potato, 308 g	320	4	63	7	8
Side Dishes					
4-piece Nuggets, Kids' Meal, 60 g	190	12	10	0	10
5-piece Crispy Chicken Nuggets, 75 g	230	15	12	0	12
Bacon and Cheese Potato, 366 g	450	13	67	7	19
Broccoli and Cheese Potato, 397 g	320	2	69	8	10
Caesar Side Salad, 142 g	260	19	14	2	8
Chili, Chips and Cheese, 0 g	305	10	29	7	14
Chocolate Chip Cookie, 57 g	270	12	37	1	4
Mandarin Oranges, 142 g	80	0	19	1	1
Medium French Fries, 142 g	430	20	56	5	6
Side Salad, 225 g	130	8	11	3	3
Small Chili, 227 g	190	6	19	5	14
Sour Cream and Chives Potato, 308 g	320	4	63	7	8
Super Value Menu					
5-piece Crispy Chicken Nuggets, 75 g	230	15	12	0	12
Caesar Side Salad, 142 g	260	19	14	2	8
Crispy Chicken Sandwich, 142 g	330	14	34	1	16
Jr. Bacon Cheeseburger, 136 g	310	16	25	1	17
Side Salad, 225 g	130	8	11	3	3
Small Chili, 227 g	190	6	19	5	14
Small French Fries, 113 g	340	16	45	4	4
Small Original Chocolate Frosty™, 227 g	320	8	52	0	9
Sour Cream and Chives Potato, 308 g	320	4	63	7	8
Wendy's Old Fashioned Hamburgers					
1/2 lb. Double with Cheese, 318 g	700	40	38	2	47
1/4 lb. Deluxe Double Stack, 184 g	400	22	28	2	23
1/4 lb. Double Stack, 143 g	360	18	26	1	23
1/4 lb. Single, 226 g	430	20	37	2	25
3/4 lb. Triple with Cheese, 410 g	960	60	39	2	69
Baconator™, 276 g	830	51	35	1	56
Double Jr. Cheeseburger Deluxe, 186 g	390	20	28	2	23
Jr. Bacon Cheeseburger, 136 g	310	16	25	1	17
Jr. Cheeseburger Deluxe, 152 g	300	14	28	2	15
Jr. Cheeseburger, 109 g	260	11	26	1	15
Jr. Hamburger, 98 g	220	8	26	1	13
Stack Attack™ Double Cheeseburger, 135 g	380	20	26	1	23
Triple Stack, 178 g	490	28	26	1	34

RESTAURANTS & FAST-FOOD CHAINS

We're Rolling Pretzel Company

	Cal	Fat	Cbs	Fbr	Prtn
Pretzel					
Cinnamon Sugar Pretzel, 1 pretzel	492	5	102	3	10
Garlic Pretzel, 1 pretzel	448	10	78	3	9
• Plain Pretzel, 1 pretzel	368	1	78	3	9
Pretzel Rod 10 packs, 1 pretzel	641	8	125	4	15
Pretzel Rod 15 packs, 1 pretzel	962	12	188	6	23
• Pretzel Rod 20 packs, 1 pretzel	1282	16	250	8	30
Pretzel w/Butter & Salt, 1 pretzel	401	5	78	3	9
Raisin Pretzel, 1 pretzel	473	5	97	3	10
Sandwiches					
• Chicken Salad	574	20	70	3	27
Classic Italian	573	17	69	3	33
Ham & Swiss	491	10	69	3	31
• Turkey & Swiss	439	6	71	3	24

Wetzel's Pretzels

	Cal	Fat	Cbs	Fbr	Prtn
Pretzels					
Wetzel's Original w/o Butter, 1 pretzel	336	1	N/A	N/A	N/A
Wetzel's Original w/ Butter, 1 pretzel	384	4	N/A	N/A	N/A

Whataburger

	Cal	Fat	Cbs	Fbr	Prtn
Breakfast					
• Biscuit	300	17	32	1	5
Biscuit and Gravy	530	36	52	1	9
Biscuit Sandwich w/ bacon, egg & cheese	500	32	33	1	16
Biscuit Sandwich w/ egg & cheese	450	28	33	1	13
Biscuit Sandwich w/ sausage, egg & cheese	690	49	33	1	26
Biscuit w/ bacon	350	20	32	1	8
Biscuit w/ sausage	540	37	32	1	18
Breakfast On A Bun® w/ bacon	380	22	29	1	17
Breakfast On A Bun® w/ sausage	570	39	29	1	17
Breakfast Platter w/ bacon	740	45	53	2	24
• Breakfast Platter w/ sausage	930	62	53	2	34
Egg Sandwich	330	18	29	1	14
Honey Butter Chicken Biscuit	610	38	51	1	14
Pancakes w/ bacon	630	12	112	5	20
Pancakes w/ sausage	820	29	112	5	30
Pancakes, plain	580	8	112	5	17
Taquito w/ bacon & egg	380	21	27	3	17
Taquito w/ bacon, egg, & cheese	420	24	27	3	19
Taquito w/ potato & egg	430	23	37	3	15
Taquito w/ potato, egg & cheese	470	27	37	3	17
Taquito w/ sausage & egg	410	24	27	3	17
Taquito w/ sausage, egg, & cheese	450	28	27	3	19
Burgers					
• Justaburger®	320	16	30	1	15
Whataburger Jr.®	330	16	32	1	15
Whataburger®	640	32	61	3	30
Whataburger® with bacon & cheese	800	45	62	3	40
Whataburger®, Double Meat	890	51	61	3	47
• Whataburger®, Triple Meat	1140	70	61	3	65
Chicken and Fish					
• Chicken Strips, 2 pieces	380	24	22	0	18
Chicken Strips, 4 pieces (with gravy)	840	54	53	0	37

RESTAURANTS & FAST-FOOD CHAINS

Whataburger (cont.)	Cal	Fat	Cbs	Fbr	Prtn
Chicken and Fish (cont.)					
Grilled Chicken Sandwich	450	18	45	6	33
Whatacatch® Dinner, 2 piece	1580	92	161	8	29
Whatacatch® Sandwich	480	30	42	2	17
Whatachick'n® Sandwich	530	20	61	7	32
Kid's Menu					
Kid's Meal Chicken Strips	770	51	53	2	22
Kid's Meal Justaburger®	570	29	60	3	19
Desserts					
Cinnamon Roll	400	7	80	2	6
Cookie, Chocolate Chunk	230	11	33	1	2
Cookie, White Chocolate Chunk Macadamia Nut	250	14	30	0	3
Hot Apple Pie	230	11	29	2	3
Hot Peach Pie	280	14	36	2	3
Drinks (Medium)					
Chocolate Malt	1050	25	188	3	21
Chocolate Shake	1000	26	171	3	22
Strawberry Malt	1040	24	188	0	19
Strawberry Shake	990	26	171	0	20
Vanilla Malt	940	27	155	0	21
Vanilla Shake	890	28	139	0	22
Salads					
Chicken Strips	570	38	34	4	21
Garden	60	0	12	4	3
Grilled Chicken	230	7	19	4	23
Sides					
French Fries (Medium)	400	20	47	4	6
Hash Brown Sticks (4 each)	200	12	20	1	2
Onion Rings (Medium)	420	28	36	3	5
Texas Toast, 1 slice	180	8	25	1	4
White Peppered Gravy, 1 gravy	60	5	8	0	0

White Castle	Cal	Fat	Cbs	Fbr	Prtn
Beverages - Medium					
Chocolate Shake - Chicago region, 32 g	600	7	125	0	9
Chocolate Shake - Cincinnati region, 32 g	830	24	134	0	19
Chocolate Shake - Columbus & Detroit regions, 32 g	650	18	103	0	18
Chocolate Shake - Indianapolis region, 32 g	620	16	100	3	19
Chocolate Shake - New Jersey region, 32 g	890	23	148	0	23
Chocolate Shake - New York region, 32 g	740	20	128	0	13
Chocolate Shake - St. Louis region, 32 g	690	21	109	0	15
Chocolate Shake Louisville region, 32 g	810	23	134	6	17
Chocolate Shake Nashville region, 32 g	860	23	143	0	19
Strawberry Shake - Chicago region, 32 g	610	7	127	0	9
Strawberry Shake - Cincinnati region, 32 g	840	24	136	0	19
Strawberry Shake - Columbus/Detroit regions, 32 g	730	18	124	0	18
Strawberry Shake - Minneapolis region, 32 g	790	21	146	0	5
Vanilla Shake - Chicago region, 32 g	490	7	99	0	9
Vanilla Shake - Cincinnati region, 32 g	840	24	136	0	19
Vanilla Shake - Columbus/Detroit regions, 32 g	620	18	97	0	18
Vanilla Shake - Minneapolis regions, 32 g	680	21	118	0	5
Vanilla Shake - New Jersey region, 32 g	860	23	140	0	23
Vanilla Shake - New York region, 32 g	720	20	121	0	13
Vanilla Shake Nashville region, 32 g	790	23	126	0	19

RESTAURANTS & FAST-FOOD CHAINS

White Castle (cont.)

	Cal	Fat	Cbs	Fbr	Prtn
Cheeses					
• American Cheese Slice, 7 g	25	2	0	0	1
Cheddar Cheese Sauce - New York region, 43 g	70	5	6	0	0
Cheddar Cheese Sauce - St Louis region, 43 g	40	3	3	0	0
• Cheese Sauce, 43 g	130	10	6	0	3
Jalapeño Cheese Slice, 9 g	35	3	1	0	2
Nacho Cheese Sauce, 47 g	50	4	3	0	1
Sandwiches					
Bacon Cheeseburger, 71 g	200	11	15	1	10
Cheeseburger, 65 g	170	9	15	1	7
Chicken Breast Sandwich w/Cheese, 82 g	200	8	21	1	12
Chicken Ring Sandwich w/Cheese, 69 g	200	10	19	1	8
Chicken Ring Sandwich, 62 g	180	8	19	1	7
Chicken Supreme , 88 g	230	10	21	1	14
• Double Bacon Cheeseburger, 130 g	370	22	23	1	19
Double Cheeseburger, 118 g	300	17	23	1	14
Double Jalapeño Cheeseburger, 122 g	320	19	23	1	15
Double White Castle, 104 g	250	13	22	1	11
Fish w/Cheese, 77 g	180	8	19	1	9
Jalapeño Cheeseburger, 67 g	180	10	15	1	8
Surf & Turf, 157 g	390	22	28	1	20
• White Castle, 58 g	140	7	14	1	6
Sides					
Chicken Rings: 6 Rings, 110 g	340	23	15	0	18
Clam Strips: Regular, 113 g	250	22	5	0	8
Fish Nibblers: Regular, 117 g	280	16	24	5	19
French Fries: Regular, 108 g	310	15	39	4	4
Homestyle Onion Rings: Regular, 96 g	430	24	49	1	4
Mozzarella Cheese Sticks: 5 Sticks, 132 g	420	23	37	2	17
• Onion Chips: Regular, 112 g	480	23	62	2	7
• Onion Rings: Regular, 96 g	210	10	28	1	2

Wienerschnitzel

	Cal	Fat	Cbs	Fbr	Prtn
Breakfast					
• Biscuit, 81 g	260	11	35	1	6
with Bacon, 97 g	330	17	35	1	10
with Egg & Bacon, 154 g	390	21	36	1	16
with Egg & Sausage, 181 g	490	30	40	1	17
with Egg, 138 g	320	15	36	1	12
with Egg, Bacon & Cheese, 168 g	440	25	36	1	18
with Egg, Sausage & Cheese, 195 g	540	34	40	1	19
with Sausage, 124 g	430	26	39	1	11
Biscuit & Gravy, 138 g	350	17	42	1	8
Breakfast Platter with Bacon, 267 g	600	40	40	3	20
• with Sausage, 293 g	700	49	44	3	21
Burrito with Egg, Bacon & Cheese, 244 g	490	25	39	1	24
Burrito with Egg, Sausage & Chz, 271 g	590	34	43	1	25
Chili Cheese Burrito, 261 g	470	21	43	2	25
Country Breakfast, 294 g	640	40	47	1	24
Croissant with Egg, Bacon & Chz, 172 g	520	31	40	1	19
with Egg, Sausage & Cheese, 199 g	620	40	44	1	20
French Toast Sticks, 148 g	490	29	49	5	6
Hash Browns, 80 g	290	25	14	2	1
Sandwich with Egg, Bacon & Chz, 144 g	300	15	26	1	16

RESTAURANTS & FAST-FOOD CHAINS

Wienerschnitzel (cont.)	Cal	Fat	Cbs	Fbr	Prtn
Breakfast (cont.)					
with Egg, Sausage & Cheese, 171 g	400	24	30	1	17
Burgers & Sandwiches					
Bacon Ranch Chicken Sandwich, 200 g	430	21	37	2	23
Chili Cheese Fries Burrito, 196 g	470	21	53	3	14
Chili Cheeseburger, 159 g	350	13	32	1	25
Chipotle Ranch Pupsters, 147 g	440	24	43	2	23
Deluxe Cheeseburger, 235 g	450	23	33	2	23
Deluxe Hamburger, 221 g	400	19	33	2	21
Double Chili Cheeseburger, 260 g	560	24	35	2	45
Italian Sausage Sandwich, 156 g	350	17	31	2	17
• Original Burger, 150 g	290	9	29	1	20
Pastrami Burger, 202 g	510	26	30	1	34
• Pastrami Sandwich, 221 g	580	35	38	2	30
Polish Sausage Sandwich, 208 g	490	29	39	3	22
Ranch Dressing, 35 g	120	12	2	0	1
Desserts					
Apple Pie, 92 g	310	19	31	1	2
Fries & Sides					
• Chili Cheese Fries, 231 g	540	38	39	4	12
Jalapeño Poppers, 65 g	210	11	21	2	6
Large Fries, 181 g	470	34	39	4	4
Onion Straws, 98 g	430	35	25	3	3
• Ranch Dressing, 35 g	120	12	2	0	1
Regular Fries, 131 g	340	25	28	3	3
Hot Dogs					
All Beef Chili Cheese Dog Pretzel Bun, 214 g	570	28	59	2	22
All Beef Chili Cheese Dog, 175 g	430	25	33	1	19
All Beef Chili Dog Pretzel Bun, 200 g	520	24	59	2	19
All Beef Chili Dog, 161 g	380	21	33	1	16
All Beef Deluxe Dog Pretzel Bun, 238 g	510	23	58	2	17
All Beef Deluxe Dog, 200 g	370	20	32	2	14
All Beef Kraut Dog Pretzel Bun, 201 g	500	23	56	2	17
All Beef Kraut Dog, 162 g	360	20	30	1	14
All Beef Mustard Dog Pretzel Bun, 176 g	490	23	56	1	17
All Beef Mustard Dog, 137 g	350	20	30	1	14
All Beef Relish Dog Pretzel Bun, 192 g	500	23	58	1	17
All Beef Relish Dog, 154 g	360	20	32	1	14
Chicago Dog, 290 g	410	20	43	2	15
Chili Cheese Dog Pretzel Bun, 179 g	480	20	57	2	17
Chili Cheese Dog, 140 g	340	17	31	1	14
Chili Dog on a Pretzel Bun, 165 g	430	16	57	2	14
Chili Dog, 126 g	290	13	31	1	11
Deluxe Dog on a Pretzel Bun, 203 g	410	15	56	2	12
Deluxe Dog, 165 g	270	12	30	2	9
Kraut Dog on a Pretzel Bun, 166 g	400	15	54	2	12
Kraut Dog, 127 g	260	12	28	1	9
Mustard Dog on a Pretzel Bun, 141 g	400	15	54	1	12
Mustard Dog, 102 g	260	12	28	1	9
• Pastrami Dog, 245 g	640	34	57	2	26
Relish Dog on a Pretzel Bun, 157 g	410	15	56	1	12
Relish Dog, 119 g	270	12	30	1	9
Stadium Dog, 157 g	370	20	32	1	14
Turkey Chili Cheese Dog, 143 g	320	15	31	1	15

(•= most healthy •= least healthy)

RESTAURANTS & FAST-FOOD CHAINS

Wienerschnitzel (cont.)

	Cal	Fat	Cbs	Fbr	Prtn
Hot Dogs (cont.)					
Turkey Chili Dog, 129 g	270	11	31	1	12
Turkey Deluxe Dog, 168 g	250	10	30	2	10
Turkey Kraut Dog, 130 g	250	10	28	1	10
• Turkey Mustard Dog, 106 g	240	10	28	1	10
Turkey Relish Dog, 122 g	250	10	30	1	10
Kids Bags					
• Corn Dog, 82 g	250	17	15	1	7
Hamburger, 199 g	290	8	31	1	20
• Mini Corn Dogs (6-pack), 99 g	320	22	22	1	8
Mustard Dog, 102 g	260	12	28	1	9
Tastee-Freez Desserts					
• Banana Split, 450 g	820	24	149	8	13
Cone, 4 oz. Kids Chocolate Dipped, 122 g	400	25	43	2	5
• Cone, 4 oz. Kids Plain, 94 g	210	7	34	1	4
Cone, 6 oz. Chocolate Dipped, 166 g	490	29	57	2	7
Cone, 6 oz. Plain, 138 g	300	11	49	1	6
Freezee, Butterfinger, 279 g	620	24	100	3	13
Freezee, M&M, 279 g	630	25	99	2	13
Freezee, Oreo, 279 g	630	25	99	3	13
Freezee, Reese's Peanut Butter Cup, 279 g	630	26	97	3	14
Old Fashion Sundae, Caramel, 181 g	400	14	66	1	7
Old Fashion Sundae, Chocolate, 181 g	390	14	64	2	7
Old Fashion Sundae, Hot Fudge, 181 g	400	16	63	1	7
Old Fashion Sundae, Pineapple, 181 g	370	14	59	1	7
Old Fashion Sundae, Strawberry, 181 g	370	14	59	1	7
Shake, Chocolate, 311 g	650	23	110	3	13
Shake, Strawberry, 312 g	650	23	111	2	13
Shake, Vanilla, 312 g	650	23	110	2	13

Winchell's

	Cal	Fat	Cbs	Fbr	Prtn
Baked Products					
Croissant	260	17	28	N/A	5
Cake Products					
Chocolate Iced Cake	230	15	28	N/A	2
Traditional Cake	215	14	26	N/A	2
Yeast Raised Products					
Chocolate Bar	240	16	29	N/A	4
• Chocolate Round	240	16	29	N/A	4
Chocolate Twist	240	16	29	N/A	4
• Glazed Round	230	15	27	N/A	2
Glazed Twist	230	15	27	N/A	2

WingStreet

	Cal	Fat	Cbs	Fbr	Prtn
Bone In Wings					
• All American (2 pieces), 48 g	170	13	7	1	8
Buffalo Burnin Hot (2 pieces), 65 g	210	13	14	1	8
Buffalo Medium (2 pieces), 65 g	210	13	14	1	8
Buffalo Mild (2 pieces), 65 g	210	13	14	1	8
Cajun (2 pieces), 65 g	210	13	15	1	9
Garlic Parmesan (2 pieces), 56 g	210	16	8	1	9
• Honey BBQ (2 pieces), 70 g	230	13	20	1	9
Spicy Asian (2 pieces), 70 g	220	13	19	1	9
Spicy BBQ (2 pieces), 70 g	220	13	18	1	8

RESTAURANTS & FAST-FOOD CHAINS

WingStreet (cont.)

Bone In Wings (cont.)	Cal	Fat	Cbs	Fbr	Prtn
Teriyaki (2 pieces), 74 g	230	13	20	1	9
Bone Out Wings					
All American (2 pieces), 61 g	190	10	11	1	13
Buffalo Burnin Hot (2 pieces), 78 g	220	11	18	1	13
Buffalo Medium (2 pieces), 78 g	220	11	18	2	13
Buffalo Mild (2 pieces), 78 g	220	11	18	1	13
Cajun (2 pieces), 78 g	220	10	19	1	13
Garlic Parmesan (2 pieces), 69 g	220	14	12	1	13
Honey BBQ (2 pieces), 84 g	240	10	24	1	13
Spicy Asian (2 pieces), 84 g	230	10	23	1	13
Spicy BBQ (2 pieces), 84 g	230	10	22	1	13
Teriyaki (2 pieces), 87 g	240	10	24	1	13
Sides					
Apple Pie (2 pies), 105 g	370	17	50	2	3
Fried Cheese Sticks, 96 g	310	19	23	1	10
Taters, 227 g	790	52	74	6	7
Traditional Wings					
All American (2 pieces), 41 g	80	5	0	0	8
Buffalo Burnin Hot (2 pieces), 58 g	110	6	7	1	8
Buffalo Medium (2 pieces), 58 g	120	6	7	1	8
Buffalo Mild (2 pieces), 58 g	120	6	7	1	8
Cajun (2 pieces), 58 g	120	6	8	1	9
Garlic Parmesan (2 pieces), 49 g	120	9	1	0	9
Honey BBQ (2 pieces), 63 g	140	6	13	0	9
Spicy Asian (2 pieces), 63 g	130	6	12	0	9
Spicy BBQ (2 pieces), 63 g	130	6	11	0	8
Teriyaki (2 pieces), 67 g	110	6	6	0	8

Yard House

Appetizers	Cal	Fat	Cbs	Fbr	Prtn
Apple Plum Sauce, 1 tbsp.	20	1	2	0	0
Blue Crabs Cakes	540	46	18	3	14
Buffalo Chicken Wings w/o sauce	1050	66	20	4	98
California Roll	545	28	48	7	26
Chicken Nachos	1980	120	148	26	89
Chilled Edamame	300	9	27	12	24
Chinese Garlic Noodle	865	57	75	1	16
Coconut Shrimp	600	25	71	3	27
Firecrackers Chicken Wings	1370	83	55	3	101
Fried Calamari w/o sauce	665	39	31	3	48
Fried Chicken Strips - 4 strips	920	64	54	0	34
w/o sides and sauce	470	27	26	0	30
Grilled Artichoke w/ mayo	855	84	27	0	7
w/o chips & aioli mayonnaise	300	27	13	0	4
Grilled Korean BBQ Beef Ribs	870	42	55	2	64
Hawaiian Poke Stack	650	47	36	9	26
Jamaican Jerks Wings	1075	56	40	2	98
Lettuce Wraps with Chicken	1140	58	82	8	85
Lettuce Wraps with Mushrooms	1030	62	92	10	45
Lettuce Wraps with Shrimp	1060	53	82	8	78
Lobster Dip with Pita & Chips	1230	54	148	10	42
Moo Shu Egg Rolls	725	31	65	4	48
w/o carrots and sauce	270	8	25	2	24

RESTAURANTS & FAST-FOOD CHAINS

Yard House (cont.)

	Cal	Fat	Cbs	Fbr	Prtn
Appetizers (cont.)					
Onion Ring Tower w/o dressing	1380	70	170	8	16
Roasted Garlic Aioli, 1 tbsp.	70	7	2	0	0
Seared Ahi Sashimi	400	22	24	3	28
w/o dressing	195	4	13	3	27
Soy Vinaigrette, 1 tbsp.	50	5	3	0	0
Spicy Tuna Roll	625	38	38	8	37
Spinach Cheese Dip	945	53	88	6	30
Dressing					
• Balsamic Vinaigrette, 1 tbsp.	80	8	2	0	0
Bleu Cheese Dressing, 1 tbsp.	75	8	1	0	1
Caesar Dressing, 1 tbsp.	75	8	0	0	1
• Thai Peanut Vinaigrette, 1 tbsp.	45	2	5	0	1
Dressings					
Buttermilk Ranch Dressing, 1 tbsp.	55	6	1	0	0
• Caesar Dressing, 1 tbsp.	75	8	0	0	1
Chipotle Ranch Dressing, 1 tbsp.	50	5	1	0	0
Gorgonzola Dressing, 1 tbsp.	65	6	0	0	1
Soy Vinaigrette, 1 tbsp.	50	5	3	0	0
• Thai Peanut Vinaigrette, 1 tbsp.	45	2	5	0	1
Entrée Salads					
Ahi Crunchy Salad	815	51	58	11	36
w/o dressing	205	4	12	7	30
• BBQ Chicken Salad	1655	106	108	22	72
w/o fr. onions, tortilla strips & dressing	710	25	61	15	63
Caesar Salad with Ahi	525	39	9	6	34
w/o dressing	220	7	8	5	31
Caesar Salad with Chicken	755	52	11	6	59
w/o dressing	445	20	10	6	56
Caesar Salad with Shrimp	610	49	10	6	33
w/o dressing	305	17	8	6	30
Grilled Hearts of Romaine	600	52	22	8	15
w/o dressing	225	15	20	8	7
• w/o dressing & walnuts	60	2	8	7	5
Roasted Turkey Cobb Salad	1065	84	17	9	62
w/o dressing and bacon	420	25	14	9	37
Steak Salad w/o dressing & chips	760	51	23	15	56
Thai Chicken Salad	845	28	99	9	55
w/o dressing	490	8	56	6	47
Grilled Burgers (burger only)					
Avocado & Swiss Burger	1225	81	65	6	59
BBQ Bacon & Cheese Burger	1400	81	94	1	67
• Bearnaise Burger	1930	151	85	2	58
Chile Pepper Jack Burger	1285	85	63	4	64
Classic Cheese Burger	1160	75	62	2	58
• Grilled Portabella Burger	875	53	77	9	25
Hawaiian Burger	1390	81	99	1	63
Turkey Burger	1255	78	80	6	63
Healthy Dining Menu					
Ahi Crunchy Salad (w/o dressing)	205	4	12	7	30
BBQ Chicken Pizza, 2 slices	325	13	34	1	17
Caesar Dressing, 1 tbsp.	75	8	0	0	1
Caesar Salad with Ahi (w/o dressing)	220	7	8	5	31
Caesar Salad with Chicken (w/o dressing)	445	20	10	6	56

RESTAURANTS & FAST-FOOD CHAINS

Yard House (cont.)	Cal	Fat	Cbs	Fbr	Prtn
Healthy Dining Menu (cont.)					
Caesar Salad with Shrimp (w/o dressing)	305	17	8	6	30
California Roll	545	28	48	7	26
Chopped Salad, no bacon, 1/4 avocado	255	16	24	10	5
Edamame Appetizer, 1/2 order	150	5	14	6	12
Margherita Pizza, 2 slices	250	10	29	1	11
Soy Vinaigrette, 1 tbsp.	50	5	3	0	0
Spicy Tuna Dynamite Roll, 1/2 order	315	19	19	4	18
Thai Chicken Pizza, 2 slices	340	16	32	2	18
Thai Chicken Salad (w/o dressing)	490	8	56	6	47
Thai Peanut Vinaigrette, 1 tbsp.	45	2	5	0	1
House Favorites					
Angel Hair Pasta	1535	113	96	11	44
Chicken Enchilada Stack	1810	128	73	11	100
• Chicken Garlic Noodles	1410	93	84	6	63
Chicken Rice Bowl	1445	78	133	11	60
Jerk Chicken with Shrimp Stack	1520	96	67	8	101
Macaroni and Cheese	1780	120	95	5	81
Maui Chicken	1510	77	141	10	67
Orange Peel Chicken	1815	84	197	6	68
Parmesan Crusted Chicken	1415	71	106	8	78
Penne with Roasted Chicken w/o bread	1645	116	87	9	65
Southern Fried Chicken Breast	1485	110	78	6	43
• Turkey Pot Pie	2020	125	132	4	91
Kids Klub					
Cheese Burger only	840	49	56	0	42
Chicken Fingers w/o sides & sauce	470	27	26	0	30
Fish and Chips w/o sides & sauce	275	14	18	1	19
• Four Cheese Pizza, 2 slices	235	10	26	1	9
Fries	555	35	54	7	6
Grilled Cheese w/o sides	670	42	55	3	20
Hot Dog only	380	14	48	2	16
• Mac and Cheese	890	59	54	3	37
Pasta	720	49	59	1	12
Pepperoni Cheese Pizza, 2 slices	350	21	27	1	14
Ranch Dressing, 1 tbsp.	55	6	1	0	0
Sundae	325	15	48	0	5
Tartar Sauce, 1 tbsp.	75	8	1	0	0
Pizza					
BBQ Chicken Pizza, 2 slices	325	13	34	1	17
Four Cheese Pizza, 2 slices	280	14	26	1	12
Ham & Pineapple Pizza, 2 slices	275	12	29	1	13
• Margherita Pizza, 2 slices	250	10	31	1	11
• Pepperoni & Mushroom Pizza, 2 slices	350	21	27	1	13
Thai Chicken Pizza, 2 slices	340	16	32	2	18
Sandwiches (sandwiches only)					
Ahi Steak Sandwich	695	35	42	6	54
• w/o mayo	520	16	40	6	53
Blue Crab Cake Hoagie	1165	71	98	10	38
Cuban Roast Pork Dip Sandwich	1355	77	79	6	83
Grilled Chicken and Avocado Sandwich	1230	76	64	9	72
Grilled Pastrami Sandwich	980	56	71	4	58
• New York Steak Sandwich	1620	93	121	9	74
Portabello BLT Sandwich	870	62	61	9	20

(• = most healthy • = least healthy)

RESTAURANTS & FAST-FOOD CHAINS

Yard House (cont.)

	Cal	Fat	Cbs	Fbr	Prtn
Sandwiches (sandwiches only) (cont.)					
Roast Beef Dip	1135	55	66	0	90
Roasted Turkey Club	1125	58	94	10	61
w/o mayo & bacon	755	19	92	10	57
Roasted Turkey Melt Sandwich	1000	56	69	4	58
w/o mayo & butter	700	22	68	4	58
Spicy Chicken Breast Sandwich	1175	68	71	4	69
Seafood					
Crab Crusted Swordfish	1320	93	58	9	63
• Fried Fish w/o fries	550	28	36	1	38
Fries with fish	1110	70	109	14	11
Ginger Crusted Salmon	1440	93	97	11	58
Grilled Jumbo Shrimp	1330	75	107	5	61
• Linguine and Clams	1500	113	79	5	41
Lobster Garlic Noodles	1065	56	80	8	63
Miso Chilean Sea Bass	1200	49	126	6	60
Orzo Scallops	1305	82	78	7	66
Pan Seared Ahi	980	40	89	4	65
Porcini Mushroom Crusted Halibut	1360	105	46	6	59
Shrimp Rice Bowl	1370	74	133	11	52
Vodka Shrimp Pasta	1200	72	73	4	53
Sides & Sauces					
Chipotle Ranch Dressing, 1 tbsp.	50	5	1	0	0
Cocktail Sauce, 1 tbsp.	15	0	4	0	0
Cole Slaw, 5 oz.	202	16	16	3	2
French Fries, 6 oz.	665	42	65	9	7
• Pickle, half	6	0	1	0	0
• Potato Chips, 3 cups	440	25	50	4	4
Ranch Dressing, 1 tbsp.	55	6	1	0	0
Sourdough Bread, 3 oz.	235	3	44	2	7
Sweet Potato Fries, 6 oz.	525	30	60	5	3
Tartar Sauce, 1 tbsp.	75	8	1	0	0
Starters					
Baby Leaf Spinach Salad	645	55	25	5	17
w/o dressing	330	24	16	5	17
Caesar Salad	395	36	9	6	9
w/o dressing	90	4	8	5	6
Chopped Salad	470	36	31	15	13
w/o bacon and only 1/4 avocado	255	16	27	10	5
Clam Chowder	340	20	39	4	7
French Onion Soup	485	36	23	2	16
House Salad	390	21	46	8	11
w/o dressing	220	12	25	7	7
• w/o dressing and wontons	65	2	10	5	5
Iceberg Wedge	550	51	20	4	9
w/o dressing	85	3	13	4	5
Mixed Fields Greens	395	34	22	4	4
w/o dressing	80	2	12	4	3
• Summer Salad	815	66	56	16	10
w/o dressing	580	43	50	16	10
w/o dressing and walnuts	235	16	25	14	4
Walnut Pear Salad	665	53	41	6	12
w/o dressing	345	22	31	6	11
w/o dressing and walnuts	186	9	20	5	9

RESTAURANTS & FAST-FOOD CHAINS

Yard House (cont.)

Steaks, Ribs, Chops	Cal	Fat	Cbs	Fbr	Prtn
• BBQ Baby Back Ribs	2275	115	206	9	106
BBQ Pork Tenderloin	1445	86	98	10	70
Grilled Ribeye Steak	1195	77	47	6	79
New York Steak	1135	63	46	6	95
New Zealand Lamb Chops	1630	128	77	6	51
Ribeye Steak and Grilled Shrimp	1410	90	48	6	103
Three Peppercorn Beef Tenderloin	1450	108	58	7	66
• Top Sirloin Steak	960	43	58	4	85

Yoshinoya

Bowls	Cal	Fat	Cbs	Fbr	Prtn
Combo Bowl (Bf & Ckn) No Skin, 25 oz.	1043	28	171	7	54
Combo Bowl (Beef & Chicken)	1220	36	171	7	54
• Kids Meal Beef Bowl	340	11	48	3	13
Kids Meal Chicken Bowl	370	9	53	2	20
Regular Beef Bowl	840	30	109	4	32
Regular Beef Bowl With Vegetables	770	23	114	5	26
Regular Chicken Bowl (Teriyaki or Spicy)	760	15	125	5	33
Regular Chicken Bowl No Skin, 17 oz.	608	7	125	5	33
Regular Vegetable Bowl	530	4	116	6	9
• Shrimp & Beef Combo Bowl	1280	44	184	8	39
Shrimp & Chicken Combo Bowl	1260	35	191	7	45
Shrimp Bowl	910	29	143	6	20

Desserts	Cal	Fat	Cbs	Fbr	Prtn
Cheesecake	280	15	31	1	7
• Chocolate Cake	330	17	44	2	4
• Flan	230	7	35	1	7
Strawberry Shortcake	290	15	37	0	2

Side Orders	Cal	Fat	Cbs	Fbr	Prtn
Beef	370	28	6	1	25
Chicken and Vegetables only	300	12	21	2	26
Rice	460	3	104	3	7
Vegetables	60	1	12	3	2

Z'Tejas Southwestern Grill

	Cal	Fat	Cbs	Fbr	Prtn
Grilled Cilantro Pesto-Rubbed Ruby Trout	530	25	31	3	45
• Grilled Miso Salmon	645	27	48	21	49
• Jerk Chicken Salad	515	24	27	5	45
Voodoo Blackened Tuna	540	19	41	9	49

Zero's Subs

6 " Sandwiches	Cal	Fat	Cbs	Fbr	Prtn
BLT	411	19	48	3	12
BLT no Mayo	330	12	43	3	12
Cosmo Vegetarian	469	23	46	4	20
• no cheese, no oil and no vinegar	216	2	45	4	6
Cosmo Vegetarian Deluxe	488	25	48	4	21
no cheese, no oil and no vinegar	235	3	47	4	7
Grilled Veggie Sub	394	14	52	6	19
no cheese, no oil and vinegar	244	3	51	6	8
Grinder	557	31	48	3	23
Grinder multigrain	559	32	50	4	20
no cheese, no oil & vinegar	401	18	49	3	12

Zeros (cont.)

	Cal	Fat	Cbs	Fbr	Prtn
6" Sandwiches (cont.)					
no cheese, no oil & vinegar	399	17	47	3	15
Ham & Cheese	439	19	44	3	24
no cheese, no oil & vinegar	286	5	43	3	17
• Hot Italian Sausage	663	37	45	3	35
Meatball & Cheese	565	30	50	4	22
no cheese	465	22	50	4	15
Pepperoni & Cheese	545	31	48	2	26
no Cheese	346	15	41	2	11
Philly Chicken & Cheese	402	10	48	3	32
no cheese	319	4	45	3	27
w/ M&GP	410	10	49	4	32
w/M&GP, no cheese	328	4	47	4	28
Philly Steak & Cheese	492	21	49	3	27
w/ M&GP	500	21	50	4	28
w/ M&GP, no cheese	418	15	48	3	23
no cheese	409	15	46	3	23
Roast Beef & Cheese	460	19	45	3	29
no cheese, no oil & vinegar	307	5	45	3	21
The Club	514	23	44	3	31
no cheese, no oil & vinegar	361	10	43	3	24
Tuna & Cheese	519	26	47	3	26
no cheese, no oil & vinegar	366	12	46	3	19
Turkey & Cheese	454	17	44	3	30
no cheese, no oil & vinegar	301	3	43	3	22

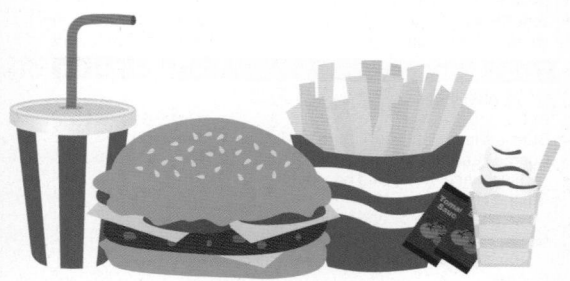

AKERY & BREAD

Bagels	Cal	Fat	Cbs	Fbr	Prtn
Lender's Bagels					
Blueberry, 4 oz.	300	3	61	2	11
Cinnamon Rasin, 4 oz.	310	4	60	2	10
Onion, 4 oz.	300	3	61	2	11
Plain, 4 oz.	310	3	62	2	11
Poppy Seed, 4 oz.	310	3	61	3	11
Sesame Seed, 4 oz.	310	3	60	4	11
Stuffed Bagel w/ Plain Cream Cheese, 4 oz.	320	11	46	3	10
Wheat, 4 oz.	310	3	61	5	11
Pepperidge Farm					
100% Whole Wheat, 1 bagel	250	2	49	6	11
Cinnamon Raisin, 1 bagel	270	1	57	3	8
Everything, 1 bagel	260	2	53	2	9
Plain, 1 bagel	260	1	54	3	9
Sesame, 1 bagel	280	3	53	4	10
Whole Grain White, 1 bagel	250	2	51	5	11

Breakfast Loaves	Cal	Fat	Cbs	Fbr	Prtn
Pepperidge Farm					
Breakfast Bread Apple & Grains, 1 slice	90	2	18	3	4
Breakfast Bread Raisin & Grains, 1 slice	100	2	19	3	5
• Brown Sugar Cinnamon Swirl, 1 slice	110	0	21	1	3
Cinnamon Swirl, 1 slice	80	2	15	1	2
Whole Grain Cinnamon Swirl, 1 slice	100	2	18	2	4

Chilled and Frozen Dough	Cal	Fat	Cbs	Fbr	Prtn
New York Garlic Bread					
• 6 Carb Texas Garlic Bread, 28 g	120	8	8	2	N/A
Five Cheese Texas Toast, 48 g	180	9	20	1	5
Garlic Bread, 57 g	180	7	25	1	5
Garlic Breadsticks, 50 g	170	6	24	1	5
Lite Texas Garlic Toast, 40 g	130	5	18	1	3
Texas Cheese Toast, 48 g	170	10	16	1	5
Texas Garlic Toast, 40 g	150	9	15	1	3
Pepperidge Farm					
• Five Cheese Garlic Bread, 2.25" slice	190	8	24	2	5
Garlic Bread, 2.5" slice	170	7	24	2	4
Garlic Breadsticks, 1 Bread Stick	160	5	25	1	5
Texas Toast Garlic, 1 slice	150	7	18	2	3
Whole Grain Texas Toast, 1 slice	150	8	14	2	4

English Muffins	Cal	Fat	Cbs	Fbr	Prtn
Pepperidge Farm					
100% Whole Wheat, 1 Muffin	140	2	26	3	6
Original English, 1 Muffin	130	2	25	1	5

Hamburger Buns	Cal	Fat	Cbs	Fbr	Prtn
Pepperidge Farm					
Classic 100% Whole Wheat, 1 Bun	120	2	18	2	6
Classic Hamburger Buns, 1 Bun	120	2	22	1	5
• Classic Onion Buns with Poppy Seeds, 1 Bun	150	3	28	1	6
Classic Buns with Sesame Seeds, 1 Bun	130	3	22	1	5
• Classic Whole Grain White, 1 Bun	100	1	18	2	6

(• = most healthy • = least healthy)

POPULAR BRANDS

BAKERY & BREAD

Hot Dog Buns

	Cal	Fat	Cbs	Fbr	Prtn
Pepperidge Farm					
Classic Hot Dog Buns, 1 Bun	140	3	26	1	5
Classic Whole Grain White, 1 Bun	110	1	21	2	6

Muffins

	Cal	Fat	Cbs	Fbr	Prtn
Bays English Muffins					
Honey Wheat, 57 g	130	2	25	2	5
Original, 57 g	140	2	27	1	5
Sourdough, 57 g	130	2	26	1	5
Zen Bakery					
Bran Muffins					
Apple Bran, 67 g	110	3	19	5	3
Blueberry Oat Bran, 68 g	135	3	23	4	4
Blueberry Raspberry Oat Bran, 68 g	135	3	23	4	4
Peach Bran, 68 g	110	3	21	5	3
Fiber Cakes					
• Apple Cranberry Fiber Cake, 57 g	80	2	22	13	5
• Banana Nut Muffin, 64 g	160	3	31	5	3
Blueberry Fiber Cake, 57 g	80	2	22	13	5
Carrot Cake Muffin, 60 g	110	2	23	3	3

Pizza Crust

	Cal	Fat	Cbs	Fbr	Prtn
Boboli					
Pizza Crusts					
12" 100% Whole Wheat Thin Crust, 57 g	150	3	27	5	6
• 12" Original Crust, 50 g	140	3	24	1	5
12" Thin Crust, 57 g	170	4	28	1	6
Value Packs					
• 8" Original Crust Party Pack, 71 g	200	5	32	1	7
12" Original Crust Value Pack, 67 g	150	3	27	1	5
12" Thin Crust Value Pack, 85 g	190	4	33	2	6

Rolls

	Cal	Fat	Cbs	Fbr	Prtn
Pepperidge Farm					
• Farmhouse Premium Wheat Rolls, 1 Roll	220	5	36	1	8
Hot & Crusty French Rolls, 1 Roll	100	1	19	1	3
Hot & Crusty Sourdough Rolls, 1 Roll	100	1	21	1	4
• Parkerhouse Dinner Rolls, 1 Roll	80	2	14	1	3
Soft Country Style Dinner Rolls, 1 Roll	90	2	17	1	3

Sandwich Bread

	Cal	Fat	Cbs	Fbr	Prtn
Pepperidge Farm					
Farmhouse Soft 100% Whole Wheat, 1 slice	110	2	19	3	5
Farmhouse Whole Grain White, 1 slice	110	2	21	3	4
Hot & Crusty Italian Bread, 2" slices	150	2	29	1	5
• Hot & Crusty Thin Sliced French, 2 slice	150	2	30	1	4
Italian Bread, 1 slice	90	1	17	1	3
• Oatmeal Bread, 1 slice	70	1	12	1	2
Original White Bread, 1 slice	70	1	13	1	2
Pumpernickel Bread, 1 slice	80	1	15	1	3
Very Thin Soft 100% Whole Wheat, 3 slices	110	2	20	3	4
Very Thin Whole Grain White Bread, 3 slices	110	2	21	3	4
White Sandwich Bread, 2 slices	130	3	23	1	4

BAKERY & BREAD

Sandwich Bread (cont.)

	Cal	Fat	Cbs	Fbr	Prtn
Pepperidge Farm					
Whole Grain 100% Whole Wheat, 1 slice	110	2	20	3	4
Whole Grain Rye with Seeds, 1 slice	70	1	14	2	3
Whole Grain White Bread, 2 slices	110	2	22	3	4

BAKING

Baking Chocolate

	Cal	Fat	Cbs	Fbr	Prtn
Baker's Chocolate and Coconut					
Chocolate - White Squares, 14 g	80	5	8	0	1
Chocolate - Semi-sweet, 14 g	40	5	8	1	1
Chocolate - Unsweetened Squares, 4 g	70	7	4	2	2
M&M's Bakery					
Milk Chocolate, 1 oz.	70	30	10	0	1
Semi-Sweet, 1 oz.	70	30	9	1	1
Nestle Toll House					
Baking					
• Choco Bake, 1/2 oz.	80	8	4	2	1
• Cocoa, 5 g	15	1	3	1	1
Unsweetened Choc Baking Bar, 1/2 oz.	70	7	4	1	1
Morsels					
Milk Chocolate and PB Swirled Morsels, 14 g	75	5	8	N/A	1
Milk Chocolate Morsels, 14 g	70	4	9	0	1
Semi-Sweet Chocolate Chunks, 12 g	60	4	8	1	1

Baking Coconut

	Cal	Fat	Cbs	Fbr	Prtn
Baker's Chocolate and Coconut					
Coconut - Angel Flake Sweetened, 15 g	70	5	6	1	1

Baking Flour

	Cal	Fat	Cbs	Fbr	Prtn
Aunt Jemima					
Self Rising Flour, 27 g	90	0	20	1	3

Baking Mix

	Cal	Fat	Cbs	Fbr	Prtn
Aunt Jemima					
Coffee Cake, 1/4 cup	140	5	27	1	2
Corn Bread, 1/3 cup	140	5	24	1	2
Betty Crocker					
Biscuits					
Complete Buttermilk Biscuits, 35 g	150	6	21	1	3
Heart Smart, 40 g	140	3	27	1	3
Original, 40 g	160	5	26	1	3
Bread					
Quick Bread Mix Banana, 1/12 Packing	130	3	25	N/A	2
Quick Bread Mix Cinnamon Streusel, 37 g	160	4	28	N/A	2
Quick Bread Mix Cran. Orange, 1/12 Packing	150	3	29	1	2
Brownies					
• Brownie Mix Fudge Brownies, 26 g	100	1	22	1	1
Brownie Mix Lowfat Fudge, 1/18 pkg.	130	3	27	1	2
• Warm Delights PB Fudge Brownie, 93 g	400	14	63	2	7
Cakes					
Angel Food White, 38 g	140	0	32	N/A	3
Pineapple Upside-Down Cake Mix, 102 g	350	9	65	N/A	2

(•= most healthy •= least healthy)

BAKING

Baking Mix (cont.)	Cal	Fat	Cbs	Fbr	Prtn
Betty Crocker (Cont.)					
Cakes (cont.)					
SuperMoist White, 43 g	170	4	33	0	2
Cookies					
Pouch Mix Oatmeal Cookie Mix, 28 g	100	2	22	1	2
Pouch Mix Rainbow Cookie, 28 g	110	2	22	N/A	1
Pouch Mix Sugar Cookie Mix, 28 g	120	3	22	N/A	1
Muffins					
Muffin Mix Apple Streusel, 46 g	180	3	37	1	2
Muffin Mix Banana Nut, 37 g	150	4	27	1	3
Authentic Cornbread & Muffin Mix, 31 g	110	1	24	1	2
Pancakes					
Heart Smart, 40 g	140	3	27	1	3
Original, 40 g	160	5	26	1	3
Shake 'n Pour Buttermilk, 63 g	220	3	42	1	6
Bisquick					
Complete Buttermilk Biscuits, 35 g	150	6	21	1	3
Complete Cheese Garlic Biscuits, 37 g	160	7	22	1	2
Complete Three Cheese Biscuits, 36 g	160	7	22	1	3
Bruce Food Products					
Sweet Potato Biscuit Mix, 37 g	140	4	25	1	3
Sweet Potato Muffin Mix, 36 g	150	4	25	1	2
Sweet Potato Pancake Mix, 65 g	230	3	47	2	5
Martha White					
Biscuits					
Cheese Garlic, 1/3 cup	190	N/A	21	1	3
Extra Rich Butter Milk, 1/3 cup	190	N/A	22	1	3
Homestyle Butter, 1/3 cup	190	N/A	22	1	3
Brownies					
Fudge, 1/20 Package	130	N/A	27	1	1
Walnut, 1/20 Package	130	N/A	23	1	2
Corn Meal					
Buttermilk, 31 g	110	1	22	2	2
Corn Meal White, 31 g	110	1	22	2	2
White Self-rising Oatmeal, 31 g	100	1	22	2	2
Yellow Cornmeal Mix, 31 g	110	1	22	2	2
Cornbreads					
Cornbreads Buttermilk, 34 g	130	N/A	23	1	2
Mexican Style, 28 g	110	N/A	18	1	1
Yellow Corn Bread, 37 g	140	N/A	25	1	3
Lowfat Varieties					
Lowfat Apple Cinnamon, 1/4 cup	130	N/A	27	1	1
Lowfat Blueberry, 1/4 cup	130	N/A	27	1	1
Lowfat Strawberry, 1/4 cup	130	N/A	27	1	1
Muffins					
Apple Cinnamon, 1/4 cup	140	N/A	24	N/A	1
Banana Nut, 1/4 cup	150	N/A	25	1	2
Honey Bran, 35 g	140	N/A	26	3	2
Strawberry Cheesecake, 1/4 cup	150	N/A	22	N/A	2
Other Products					
Deep Pan Pizza, 1/5 Package	140	1	28	1	1
Flap Stax, 1/2 cup	240	N/A	44	1	5

BAKING

Baking Mix (cont.)

	Cal	Fat	Cbs	Fbr	Prtn
Martha White (Cont.)					
Other Products (cont.)					
Pizza Crust Mix, 1/4 Package	160	1	32	1	5
Whole Grain Varieties					
Whole Grain Apple Cinnamon, 1/4 cup	140	4	24	1	2
Wholegrain Banana Nut, 1/4 cup	150	5	25	2	2
Pillsbury					
Brownies - Chocolate Fudge, 39 g	112	6	24	1	2
Brownies - Triple Chocolate Chunk, 39 g	160	6	24	1	2
Simply Bake PB Choco Chunk Bars, 40 g	110	9	23	0	2
Simply Bake Turtle Supreme Bars, 40 g	110	9	23	1	2
Zatarain's					
Crab Cake Mix, 4 tbsp.	110	1	23	2	4
Salmon Cake Mix, 33 g	110	1	23	2	4
Tuna Cake Mix, 33 g	110	1	23	2	4

Bread Crumbs

	Cal	Fat	Cbs	Fbr	Prtn
Progresso					
• Garlic & Herb, 28 g	110	2	20	1	4
Italian Style, 28 g	110	2	20	1	4
• Parmesan, 28 g	110	2	19	1	4
Plain, 28 g	110	2	20	1	4

Chilled & Frozen Dough

	Cal	Fat	Cbs	Fbr	Prtn
Pillsbury					
Biscuits					
Buttermilk, 64 g	150	2	29	1	4
Flaky Layer, 64 g	160	4	28	1	4
Golden Homestyle Buttermilk, 34 g	100	35	14	0	2
Golden Layers Honey Butter, 34 g	110	5	14	0	2
Bread Crusts					
Bread Country Italian Loaf, 47 g	110	2	21	1	4
Bread Crusty French Loaf, 52 g	120	2	24	1	4
Breadsticks Cornbread Twists, 41 g	140	6	18	0	3
Breadsticks, 52 g	240	3	25	1	4
Crescent Rolls					
Big N Buttery, 48 g	170	15	20	1	3
Big N Flaky, 48 g	180	15	20	1	3
Butterflake, 28 g	110	6	11	0	2
Original, 28 g	110	6	11	0	2
Reduced Fat, 28 g	90	5	12	0	2
Dinner Rolls - Freezer to Oven					
Dinner Rolls Butterflake, 48 g	160	7	21	0	4
Dinner Rolls Garlic, 38 g	140	6	17	1	3
Dinner Rolls Soft White, 35 g	110	4	17	1	3
• Dinner Rolls Whole Wheat, 35 g	90	1	17	3	4
Freezer to Oven Biscuits					
Buttermilk, 57 g	200	10	24	1	4
Cheddar Garlic, 59 g	190	9	22	1	4
Southern Style, 29 g	180	9	21	1	4
Grands! Biscuits					
Buttermilk Reduced Fat, 58 g	170	6	26	1	4

(•= most healthy •= least healthy)

BAKING

Chilled & Frozen Dough (cont.)	Cal	Fat	Cbs	Fbr	Prtn
Pillsbury (Cont.)					
Grands! Biscuits (cont.)					
Buttermilk, 58 g	190	8	24	1	4
Extra Rich, 61 g	210	10	26	1	4
Homestyle, 58 g	190	3	24	1	4
Grands! Sweet Rolls					
Grands! Cinnamon with Cream Cheese Icing, 99 g	310	9	54	1	5
Grands! Cinnamon with Icing, 99 g	310	9	54	1	5
Grands! Cinnamon with Buttercream Icing, 99 g	320	10	54	1	5
• Grands! Flaky Supreme with Chocolate Icing, 99 g	380	20	47	1	4
Sweet Rolls					
Caramel, 49 g	170	7	24	1	2
Cinnamon Rolls with Cream Cheese Icing, 44 g	150	5	23	1	2
Cinnamon Rolls with Icing Reduced Fat, 44 g	140	4	24	1	2
Cinnamon Rolls with Icing, 44 g	150	5	23	1	2

Condensed/Powdered Milk	Cal	Fat	Cbs	Fbr	Prtn
Magnolia					
Dulce de Leche, 39 g	120	2	24	0	2
• Evaporated Milk, 30 ml.	40	2	3	N/A	2
• Sweetened Condensed Milk, 39 g	130	3	23	0	3

Cookie Dough	Cal	Fat	Cbs	Fbr	Prtn
Nestle Toll House					
Chocolate Chip Cookie Dough, 1 oz.	130	6	18	1	1
Chocolate Chunk Cookie Dough, 25 g	120	6	15	1	1
Oatmeal Raisin Cookie, 39 g	160	6	24	1	2
Sugar Cookie Dough, 39 g	170	8	23	0	2
PB Choc. Chips & Chunks, 38 g	180	9	23	1	2
• Ultimates - White Choc. Mac. Nut, 38 g	190	10	22	1	2
• Walnut Chocolate Chip, 25 g	70	6	15	1	1
Pillsbury					
Create 'n Bake Cookies					
Chocolate Chip Cookies, 29 g	120	5	18	1	1
Gingerbread Cookies, 31 g	140	7	18	0	1
Oatmeal Chocolate Chip Cookies, 29 g	130	6	17	1	1
Peanut Butter Cookies, 29 g	130	6	16	0	2
Ready to Bake Cookies					
Chocolate Chip, 38 g	170	9	22	1	2
Chocolate Chunk & Chip, 38 g	180	9	22	1	2
S'mores, 38 g	160	7	23	1	1
Shape Bunny, 26 g	120	6	15	0	1
Shape Snowman, 26 g	120	6	15	0	1
Sugar, 38 g	170	9	22	0	2

Flour	Cal	Fat	Cbs	Fbr	Prtn
Gold Medal					
• All Purpose Flour, 30 g	100	0	22	1	3
Harvest King Better for Bread, 30 g	110	0	22	1	4
Organic Flour, 30 g	100	0	22	1	3
Self-Rising Flour, 30 g	100	0	23	1	3
Unbleached All Purpose Flour, 30 g	100	0	22	1	3

AKING

Flour (cont.)

	Cal	Fat	Cbs	Fbr	Prtn
Martha White					
All Purpose Flour, 32 g	110	0	N/A	N/A	N/A
Self Rising Flour, 32 g	110	N/A	23	1	3
Purity Foods					
Non-Organic White Spelt Flour, 30 g	100	1	21	1	4
Non-Organic Whole Grain Flour, 34 g	110	1	23	2	5
Organic White Spelt Flour, 30 g	100	1	21	1	4
Organic Whole Grain Spelt Flour, 34 g	110	1	23	2	5

Frosting & Icing

	Cal	Fat	Cbs	Fbr	Prtn
Betty Crocker					
Frost Mix Homestyle Fluffy White, 26 g	100	0	24	N/A	1
Frost Rich & Creamy Butter Cream, 33 g	140	5	23	N/A	0
Frost Whipped Choc Mousse, 24 g	90	5	14	1	0
Frost Whipped Vanilla, 24 g	110	5	15	N/A	0

Marshmallows

	Cal	Fat	Cbs	Fbr	Prtn
Jet-Puffed					
Chocomallows, 31 g	100	0	25	N/A	1
Marshmallows, 30 g	100	0	24	N/A	1
Miniature, 28 g	90	0	23	N/A	1
Strawberrymallows, 30 g	100	0	24	N/A	1
Toasted Coconut, 44 g	170	5	31	0	1

Pie Crusts & Pastry Shells

	Cal	Fat	Cbs	Fbr	Prtn
Betty Crocker					
Pie Crust Mix, 20 g	110	7	9	N/A	1
Honey Maid					
Pie Crust Graham Pie Crust, 28 g	150	8	18	0	1
Keebler					
Chocolate 6 oz., 21 g	100	5	14	1	1
Graham Cracker Crumbs, 18 g	70	2	13	1	1
Shortbread 6 oz., 21 g	110	5	14	0	1
Nilla Wafers					
Nilla Pie Crust Pie Crust, 28 g	140	8	18	0	1
Oreo					
Pie Crust, 28 g	130	7	19	1	1
Pillsbury					
Pet-Ritz Pie Crsts Dp Dish All Veggie, 21 g	90	5	11	0	1
Pet-Ritz Pie Crusts Deep Dish, 21 g	90	5	11	0	1
Pet-Ritz Pie Crusts Regular, 18 g	80	4	9	0	1
Pie Crusts All Ready Rolled, 27 g	110	7	12	0	1

Pie Filling

	Cal	Fat	Cbs	Fbr	Prtn
Libby's Pumpkin					
Easy Pumpkin Pie Mix, 1/3 cup	90	1	20	3	1
Lucky Leaf					
Coconut Creme, 1/3 cup	110	2	25	3	1
Lite Apple, 1/3 cup	30	N/A	7	N/A	N/A
Peach, 1/3 cup	80	N/A	21	N/A	N/A
Premium Apple, 1/3 cup	90	N/A	22	2	N/A
Premium Cherry, 1/3 cup	100	N/A	24	1	N/A

(• = most healthy • = least healthy)

POPULAR BRANDS

BAKING

Pie Filling (cont.)

	Cal	Fat	Cbs	Fbr	Prtn
Musselman's					
Banana Creme, 1/3 cup	110	N/A	28	N/A	N/A
Blueberry, 1/3 cup	90	N/A	22	1	N/A
Cherries Jubilee, 1/4 cup	80	N/A	20	1	N/A
Cherry, 1/3 cup	100	N/A	24	N/A	N/A
Chocolate Creme, 1/3 cup	100	N/A	25	N/A	N/A
Coconut Creme, 1/3 cup	110	1	25	N/A	N/A
None Such					
Classic Original Mincemeat, 98 g	200	0	48	1	1
Condensed Mincemeat, 43 g	150	1	36	1	0
• Mincemeat with Rum and Brandy, 99 g	200	1	47	0	0

Rolls & Pastry Dough

	Cal	Fat	Cbs	Fbr	Prtn
Pepperidge Farm					
Mini Puff Pastry Shells, 4 mini shells	180	9	15	1	3
Puff Pastry Sheets, 1/6 sheet	170	11	14	1	3
Puff Pastry Shells, 1 shell	190	13	16	1	3

Shake & Bake Coatings

	Cal	Fat	Cbs	Fbr	Prtn
McCormick					
• Cracker Meal Seafood Fry Mix, 32 g	130	1	24	N/A	3
Golden Dip® Breading Mix, 30 g	120	1	20	N/A	2
Golden Dip® Original Chkn Fry Mix, 14 g	50	0	9	N/A	0
Seafood Fry Mix, 18 g	60	0	13	N/A	1
Tempura Seafood Batter Mix, 28 g	100	0	21	N/A	2
Shake 'N Bake					
Extra Crispy, 10 g	35	1	7	0	1
• Garlic & Herb, 9 g	35	1	7	0	1
Hot & Spicy, 10 g	40	1	7	0	1
Italian, 10 g	35	1	7	0	1
Original Chicken, 10 g	40	1	7	0	1
Original Pork, 11 g	40	0	8	0	1
Ranch And Herb Crusted, 10 g	35	0	7	0	1
Zatarain's					
Crispy Seasoned Fish-Fri, 2 tbsp.	50	0	11	1	1
Garlic Fish-Fri, 1.5 tbsp.	40	0	9	N/A	1
Shrimp-Fri, 1.5 tbsp.	40	0	9	0	1
Wonderful Fish-Fri, 13 g	45	0	10	0	1

Sugar & Sweeteners

	Cal	Fat	Cbs	Fbr	Prtn
Equal					
Equal Granular, 1 tsp.	0	0	1	N/A	0

BEVERAGES

Fruit Flavored Drinks & Teas

	Cal	Fat	Cbs	Fbr	Prtn
Aquafina					
Aquafina Alive Peach Mango, 8 fl.oz.	10	0	3	3	0
Sparkling Citrust Twist, 8 fl.oz.	0	0	0	N/A	0
Wild Berry Flavor Splash, 8 fl.oz.	0	0	0	N/A	0
Baskin Robbins					
Medium					
Berry Pomegranate Fruit Blast, 24 fl.oz.	211	0	128	1	1

BEVERAGES

Fruit Flavored Drinks & Teas (cont.)	Cal	Fat	Cbs	Fbr	Prtn
Baskin Robbins (cont.)					
Medium (cont.)					
Strawberry Citrus Fruit Blast, 24 fl.oz.	480	1	122	4	2
Wild Mango Fruit Blast, 24 fl.oz.	470	2	116	2	1
Capri Sun					
Fruit Punch Pouches, 200 ml.	70	0	19	N/A	0
Grape Pouches, 200 ml.	70	0	19	N/A	0
Orange Pouches, 200 ml.	100	0	27	N/A	0
Splash Cooler Pouches, 200 ml.	70	0	19	N/A	0
Wild Cherry Pouches, 200 ml.	70	0	19	N/A	0
Celestial Seasonings					
African and Rooibos Teas					
African Orange Mango Rooibos Tea, 2 g	0	0	0	N/A	0
Madagascar Vanilla Red Rooibos Tea, 2 g	0	0	0	N/A	0
Peach Apricot Honeybush Tea, 2 g	0	0	0	N/A	0
Red Safari Spice® Rooibos Tea, 2 g	0	0	0	N/A	0
Black Teas					
Canadian Vanilla Maple Decaf Black Tea, 2 g	0	0	1	N/A	0
Devonshire English Breakfast Black Tea, 2 g	0	0	1	N/A	0
Tuscany Orange Spice Black Tea, 2 g	0	0	1	N/A	0
Victorian Earl Grey Black Tea, 2 g	0	0	0	N/A	0
Chai Teas					
Chocolate Caramel Enchantment® Chai, 3 g	0	0	0	N/A	0
Decaf India Spice Chai, 2 g	0	0	0	N/A	0
India Spice Chai, 2 g	0	0	0	N/A	0
Vanilla Ginger Green Tea Chai, 2 g	0	0	0	N/A	0
Drink Mixes: Ciders					
Apple Caramel Kiss® Cider, 21 g	80	0	21	N/A	0
Harvest Apple Spice® Cider, 21 g	80	0	21	0	0
Honey Vanilla Apple Cider, 21 g	80	0	21	0	0
Green Teas					
Blueberry Breeze® Green Tea, 2 g	0	0	0	N/A	0
Decaffeinated Green Tea, 2 g	0	0	0	N/A	0
Green Tea, 2 g	0	0	0	N/A	0
Raspberry Gardens® Green Tea, 2 g	0	0	0	N/A	0
Herbal Tea					
Acaí Mango Zinger®, 2 g	0	0	1	N/A	0
Caffeine Free Herbal Tea, 2 g	0	0	0	N/A	0
Chamomile, 2 g	0	0	0	N/A	0
Honey Vanilla Chamomile, 2 g	0	0	0	N/A	0
Lemon Zinger®, 2 g	0	0	0	N/A	0
Iced Teas					
Blueberry Ice Cool Brew Iced Tea, 2 g	0	0	0	N/A	0
Lemon Ice Cool Brew Iced Tea, 2 g	0	0	0	N/A	0
Peach Ice Cool Brew Iced Tea, 2 g	0	0	0	N/A	0
Raspberry Ice Cool Brew Iced Tea, 2 g	0	0	0	N/A	0
White Teas					
China Pearl™ Decaf White Tea, 2 g	0	0	0	N/A	0
Perfectly Pear® White Tea, 2 g	0	0	0	N/A	0
Vanilla Apple White Organic Tea, 2 g	0	0	0	0	0

(•= most healthy •= least healthy)

BEVERAGES

Fruit Flavored Drinks & Teas (cont.)	Cal	Fat	Cbs	Fbr	Prtn
Coca-Cola					
Dasani					
Grape, 8 fl.oz.	1	N/A	0	N/A	N/A
Lemon, 8 fl.oz.	2	N/A	0	N/A	N/A
Raspberry, 8 fl.oz.	1	N/A	0	N/A	N/A
Nestea					
Citrus Green Tea, 8 fl.oz.	85	0	23	N/A	0
Diet Citrus Green, 8 fl.oz.	3	0	0	N/A	0
Diet Lemon, 8 fl.oz.	2	0	0	N/A	0
Diet White Tea Berry Honey, 8 fl.oz.	3	0	0	N/A	0
Sweetened, 8 fl.oz.	63	0	17	N/A	0
Unsweetened, 8 fl.oz.	2	0	0	N/A	0
Crystal Light					
Lemon Tea Sugar Free, 8 fl.oz.	5	0	0	N/A	0
Pink Lemon Hydration Sugar Free, 8 fl.oz.	5	0	0	N/A	0
Rasp. Ice Sugar Free, 8 fl.oz.	5	0	0	N/A	0
Sunrise Classic Orange, 240 ml.	5	0	0	N/A	0
Sunrise - Ruby Red Grapefruit, 8 fl.oz.	5	0	0	0	0
Fruit 2 0					
Enhanced Water - Energy Rasp, 8 fl.oz.	0	0	0	N/A	0
Enhanced Water - Hydration Strawberry Tang, 8 fl.oz.	0	0	0	N/A	0
Natural Cherry, 8 fl.oz.	0	0	0	N/A	0
Natural Peach, 8 fl.oz.	0	0	0	N/A	0
Lipton					
Black Tea					
Decaf Iced Tea, 1 tea bag	0	0	0	N/A	0
Iced Tea, 1 tea bag	0	0	0	N/A	0
Flavored Black Tea					
Honey & Lemon Black Tea, 2 g	0	0	1	N/A	0
Spiced Chai Black Tea, 3 g	0	0	0	N/A	0
Green Tea					
100% Natural Decaf Green Tea, 1 g	0	0	0	N/A	0
100% Natural Green Tea, 3 g	0	0	0	N/A	0
Herbal Tea					
Lemon Herbal Tea, 2 g	0	0	1	N/A	0
Quietly Chamomile Herbal Tea, 2 g	0	0	1	N/A	0
Traditional Tea					
Earl Gray, 2 g	0	0	0	N/A	0
English Breakfast, 1 Tea Bag	0	0	0	N/A	0
Diet Raspberry Iced Tea, 2 g	5	0	1	N/A	0
Peach Iced Tea, 8 oz.	70	0	19	N/A	0
Sweetened Peach Iced Tea Mix, 20 g	80	0	19	N/A	0
Tuscan Lemon, 2 g	0	0	0	N/A	0
Paul Newman's Own					
Green Tea with Honey, 8 fl.oz.	70	0	18	0	N/A
Lightly Sweetened Lemonade, 8 fl.oz.	80	0	20	0	N/A
Orange Mango Tango, 8 fl.oz.	150	0	37	0	N/A
Razz-Ma-Tazz Raspberry, 8 fl.oz.	120	0	28	0	N/A
Snapple					
Acai Blackberry Juice Drink, 8 fl.oz.	120	0	30	N/A	0
Classic Black Tea Earl Grey, 240 ml.	35	0	8	N/A	0
Classic Black Tea English Breakfast, 240 ml.	40	0	10	N/A	0

BEVERAGES

Fruit Flavored Drinks & Teas (cont.)	Cal	Fat	Cbs	Fbr	Prtn
Snapple (cont.)					
Cranberry Raspberry Juice Drink, 8 fl.oz.	120	0	29	N/A	0
Decaf Tea, 8 fl.oz.	100	0	25	N/A	0
Diet Green Tea Original, 8 fl.oz.	0	0	0	N/A	0
Diet Lemon Tea, 8 fl.oz.	0	0	0	N/A	0
Diet Lemonade Iced Tea, 8 fl.oz.	10	0	2	N/A	0
Fruit Punch 100% Juiced, 340 ml.	170	0	42	N/A	0
Green Apple 100% Juiced, 340 ml.	160	0	41	N/A	0
Green Tea Original, 8 fl.oz.	60	0	15	N/A	0
Lemonade Iced Tea, 8 fl.oz.	110	0	28	N/A	0
Peach Tea, 8 fl.oz.	100	0	26	N/A	0
Raspberry Peach Juice Drink, 8 fl.oz.	120	0	29	N/A	0
Raspberry Tea, 8 fl.oz.	100	0	26	N/A	0
Strawberry Lime 100% Juiced, 340 ml.	180	0	45	N/A	0
Unsweetened Tea, 8 fl.oz.	0	0	0	N/A	0
Antioxidant Water					
Tropical Mango - Protect, 240 ml.	60	0	12	N/A	0
Dragonfruit - Awaken, 240 ml.	50	0	12	N/A	0
Raspberry Acerola - Defy, 240 ml.	45	0	11	N/A	0
Strawberry Acai - Awaken, 240 ml.	50	0	13	N/A	0
Special K					
Protein Water					
Lemon Twist, 473 ml.	50	0	13	5	5
Mixed Berry, 473 ml.	50	0	14	5	5
Strawberry Kiwi, 473 ml.	50	0	13	5	5
Welch's					
Cocktails & Drinks					
Apple Cranberry Juice Cocktail, 10 fl.oz.	180	0	45	N/A	0
Blueberry Kiwi Blast, 240 ml.	160	0	40	N/A	0
Cranberry Juice Cocktail, 240 ml.	140	0	35	N/A	0
Light Berry Juice Cocktail, 8 fl.oz.	70	0	17	N/A	0
Orange Pineapple Drink, 240 ml.	120	0	31	N/A	0
Pomegranate Pulse, 240 ml.	150	0	37	N/A	0
Strawberry Breeze Cocktail, 240 ml.	130	0	33	N/A	0

Juice	Cal	Fat	Cbs	Fbr	Prtn
Alta Dena					
Apple Juice, 240 ml.	120	0	28	0	0
Fruit Punch, 240 ml.	110	0	28	0	0
Orange Juice, 240 ml.	110	1	25	1	2
Apple Time					
Apple Juice, 8 fl.oz.	120	N/A	31	N/A	N/A
Cascadian Farm					
Juice Concentrate					
Apple Juice, 2 fl.oz.	120	0	29	N/A	0
Cranberry, 2 fl.oz.	120	0	32	N/A	0
Grape, 2 fl.oz.	150	0	38	N/A	0
Lemonade, 2 fl.oz.	110	0	28	N/A	0
Coca-Cola					
Fruitopia					
Cherry Vanilla Groove, 8 fl.oz.	110	0	30	N/A	0
Fruit Integration, 8 fl.oz.	110	0	30	N/A	0

(• = most healthy • = least healthy)

BEVERAGES

Juice (cont.)

	Cal	Fat	Cbs	Fbr	Prtn
Coca-Cola (cont.)					
Fruitopia (cont.)					
Kiwiberry Ruckus, 8 fl.oz.	110	0	29	N/A	0
Raspberry Dragonfruit Reflection, 8 fl.oz.	110	0	29	N/A	0
Minute Maid Juices					
Apple Juice, 8 fl.oz.	110	0	28	N/A	0
Lemonade, 8 fl.oz.	100	0	28	N/A	0
• Light Lemonade, 8 fl.oz.	5	0	1	N/A	0
Light Orangeade, 12 oz	10	0	2	N/A	0
Strawberry Raspberry Blend, 8 fl.oz.	120	0	33	N/A	0
Country Fresh					
Apple Juice, 240 ml.	120	0	29	0	0
Cranberry Apple Juice, 240 ml.	120	0	30	0	0
Orange Juice, 240 ml.	110	0	25	0	1
Orange Juice with Calcium, 240 ml.	120	0	29	0	1
Dean's					
Apple Juice, 240 ml.	120	0	29	0	0
Cranberry Apple Juice, 240 ml.	120	0	30	0	0
Orange Juice, 240 ml.	110	0	25	0	1
Orange Juice with Calcium, 240 ml.	120	0	29	0	1
Del Monte					
Tomato Juice, 240 g	50	0	10	1	2
Dole					
Pineapple Juice, 6 fl.oz.	110	0	26	0	1
Pineapple Orange, 6 fl.oz.	100	0	24	N/A	N/A
Pineapple Orange Banana, 6 fl.oz.	100	0	25	N/A	0
Land O'Lakes					
Apple Juice, 240 ml.	120	0	29	0	0
Cranberry Apple Juice, 240 ml.	120	0	30	0	0
Orange Juice with Calcium, 240 ml.	120	0	29	0	1
Orange Juice, 240 ml.	110	0	25	0	1
Lucky Leaf					
Lucky Leaf Premium Apple Juice, 8 fl.oz.	120	N/A	31	N/A	N/A
Lucky Leaf Sparkling Apple Cider, 8 fl.oz.	150	N/A	36	N/A	N/A
Minute Maid					
Orange Juice & Blends					
Multi-Vitamin, 8 fl.oz.	120	0	27	N/A	2
Original, 8 fl.oz.	110	0	27	N/A	2
Pulp Free, 8 fl.oz.	110	0	27	N/A	2
Lemonade & Punches					
Cherry Limeade, 8 fl.oz.	120	0	34	N/A	0
Lemonade, 8 fl.oz.	110	0	31	N/A	0
Pink Lemonade, 8 fl.oz.	100	0	28	N/A	0
Tropical Punch, 8 fl.oz.	110	0	30	N/A	0
Low Calorie Beverages					
Light Orange Juice Beverage, 8 fl.oz.	50	0	13	N/A	0
Light Orange Tangerine, 8 fl.oz.	15	0	4	N/A	0
Light Orangeade, 8 fl.oz.	110	0	29	N/A	0
Variety Juices & Juice Drinks					
Cranberry Apple Raspberry, 8 fl.oz.	120	0	33	N/A	0
Cranberry Grape, 8 fl.oz.	150	0	39	N/A	0
Grapefruit Juice, 8 fl.oz.	100	0	25	N/A	0

BEVERAGES

Juice (cont.)

	Cal	Fat	Cbs	Fbr	Prtn
Minute Maid (cont.)					
Variety Juices & Juice Drinks (cont.)					
Ruby Red Grapefruit, 8 fl.oz.	130	0	34	N/A	0
Musselman's					
Fresh Pressed Apple Cider, 8 fl.oz.	120	N/A	31	N/A	N/A
Ocean Spray					
Cranberry Blackcurrant, 250 ml	165	0	34	N/A	0
Cranberry Classic, 250 ml	124	0	31	N/A	0
Cranberry Light, 250 ml	20	0	5	N/A	0
Ruby Red Grapefruit, 250 ml	125	0	31	N/A	0
Sunny Delight					
Blends					
Orange Fused Mango, 8 fl.oz.	80	0	20	N/A	0
Orange Fused Peach, 8 fl.oz.	80	0	20	N/A	0
Orange Fused Pineapple, 8 fl.oz.	80	0	20	N/A	0
Orange Fused Strawberry, 8 fl.oz.	80	0	20	N/A	0
Original					
Fruit Punch, 8 fl.oz.	120	0	29	N/A	0
Mango, 8 fl.oz.	130	0	31	N/A	0
Smooth Style, 8 fl.oz.	130	0	32	N/A	0
SunnyD Reduced Sugar, 8 fl.oz.	60	0	15	N/A	0
SunnyD with Calcium, 8 fl.oz.	140	0	35	N/A	0
Tangy Original Style, 8 fl.oz.	120	0	29	N/A	0
Tropicana Juice					
Chilled Juices and Juice Beverages					
• Grape, 12 fl.oz.	230	0	58	0	0
Orchard Style Apple, 12 fl.oz.	170	0	43	0	0
Orchard Style Lemonade, 8 fl.oz.	120	0	31	0	0
Non-Refrigerated Juices & Juice Drinks					
100% Fruit Punch, 10 fl.oz.	170	0	40	0	1
100% Orange Juice, 8 fl.oz.	110	0	27	0	2
Grape, 8 fl.oz.	150	0	38	0	1
Light Apple, 10 fl.oz.	65	0	18	0	0
Light Mixed Berry, 10 fl.oz.	70	0	18	0	0
Pineapple Orange, 8 fl.oz.	130	0	32	0	1
Refrigerated Juice Drinks					
Fruit Punch, 8 fl.oz.	10	0	3	0	0
Light Fruit Punch, 8 fl.oz.	130	0	32	0	0
Tropicana Fruit Squeeze™					
Lime Raspberry, 8 fl.oz.	20	0	5	N/A	0
Pink Grapefruit, 8 fl.oz.	20	0	5	0	0
Tropical Tangerine, 8 fl.oz.	20	0	5	0	0
Tropicana Pure™					
Pomegranate Blueberry, 8 fl.oz.	130	0	33	0	0
Valencia Orange, 8 fl.oz.	110	0	26	0	2
Tropicana Pure Premium®					
Light 'n Healthy, 8 fl.oz.	50	0	13	0	1
Orange Juice, 8 fl.oz.	110	0	26	0	2
Tropicana® Organics, 8 fl.oz.	120	0	28	0	1
V8					
Diet V8 Splash® Juice Drink					
Diet Berry Blend, 8 oz.	10	0	3	0	0

(• = most healthy • = least healthy)

BEVERAGES

Juice (cont.)	Cal	Fat	Cbs	Fbr	Prtn
V8 (cont.)					
Diet V8 Splash® Juice Drink (cont.)					
Diet Tropical Blend, 8 oz.	10	0	3	0	0
V8® 100% Vegetable Juice					
100% Vegetable Juice, 8 oz.	50	0	10	2	2
Low Sodium V8, 8 oz.	50	0	10	2	2
Organic V8, 8 oz.	50	0	10	2	1
Spicy Hot V8, 8 oz.	50	0	10	2	1
V8® VFusion™ Juice					
Acai Berry, 8 oz.	110	0	27	0	0
Light Peach Mango, 8 oz.	50	0	13	0	0
Pomegranate Blueberry, 8 oz.	100	0	25	0	0
Strawberry Banana, 8 oz.	120	0	28	0	1
V8 Splash® Juice Drink					
Berry Blend, 8 oz.	70	0	18	0	0
Fruit Medley, 8 oz.	70	0	19	0	0
Mango Peach, 8 oz.	80	0	20	0	0
Welch's					
100% Juice					
Fruit Punch, 8 fl.oz.	120	0	30	N/A	0
Orange Juice, 8 fl.oz.	120	0	30	N/A	0
Raspberry Lime Twist, 12 fl.oz.	200	0	49	N/A	N/A
Tropical Passion Fruit, 296 ml	190	0	46	N/A	0
White Grape Cherry, 8 fl.oz.	140	0	35	N/A	0
White Grape Peach, 8 fl.oz.	160	0	39	N/A	0
Concentrates					
100% Juice Concentrates, 60 ml	160	0	41	N/A	0
Fruit Juice Cocktail Concentrates, 60 ml	150	0	38	N/A	0
Juices and Drinks					
100% Grape Juice With Fiber, 8 fl.oz.	180	0	45	N/A	0
100% Grape Juice, 8 fl.oz.	170	0	42	N/A	0
100% White Grape Juice, 240 ml	160	0	39	N/A	0
Lighter Options,					
Light Juice, 8 fl.oz.	70	0	17	N/A	N/A
Naturals, 296 ml.	100	0	26	N/A	0
Organic 100% Concord Grape Juice, 10 fl.oz.	210	0	53	N/A	0

Powdered Drink Mixes	Cal	Fat	Cbs	Fbr	Prtn
Accelerade					
Powder Fruit Punch, 31 g	120	1	21	0	5
Powder Lemonade, 31 g	120	1	21	0	5
Powder Orange, 31 g	120	1	21	0	5
Celestial Seasonings					
Go Stix					
Fruit Punch Go Stix™, 14 g	60	0	14	N/A	0
Orange Citrus Punch Go Stix™, 14 g	60	0	14	N/A	0
Triple Berry Go Stix™, 14 g	60	0	14	N/A	0
Wild Cherry Go Stix™, 14 g	60	0	14	N/A	0
Zingers To Go					
Blueberry Splash™, 1 g	60	N/A	N/A	N/A	N/A
Peach Delight®, 1 g	60	N/A	N/A	N/A	N/A
Tangerine Orange Wave®, 1 g	60	N/A	N/A	N/A	N/A

BEVERAGES

Powdered Drink Mixes (cont.)	Cal	Fat	Cbs	Fbr	Prtn
Celestial Seasonings (cont.)					
Zingers To Go (cont.)					
Wild Berry Chill®, 1 g	60	N/A	N/A	N/A	N/A
Country Time Drink Mix					
Lemonade, 17 oz.	60	0	16	N/A	0
Lemonade Iced Tea Classic, 23 oz.	90	0	22	N/A	0
Lemonade Iced Tea Raspberry, 23 oz.	90	N/A	22	N/A	0
Lemonade Lite, 9 oz.	35	0	0	N/A	8
Pink Lemonade, 17 oz.	60	0	16	N/A	0
Pink Lemonade Lite, 9 g	35	0	8	N/A	0
Raspberry Lemonade, 21 oz.	80	0	19	N/A	0
Strawberry Lemonade, 22 oz.	80	0	20	N/A	0
Crystal Light					
Fruit Drinks - Fusion Fruit Punch, 1 g	5	0	0	N/A	0
Iced Tea - Peach Sugar Free, 1 g	5	0	0	N/A	0
Lemonade - Pink Lemonade Sugar Free, 2 g	5	0	0	N/A	0
On The Go - Lemonade Sugar Free, 2 g	5	0	0	N/A	0
On The Go - Peach Tea Sugar Free, 1 g	5	0	0	N/A	0
On The Go - Sunrise Classic Orange, 2 g	5	0	0	N/A	0
General Foods International Coffee					
Chai					
Chai Latte, 15 g	70	2	12	N/A	0
Sugar Free Chai Latte, 5 g	30	2	2	N/A	0
Vanilla					
Sugar Free Vanilla Creme, 6 g	35	3	3	N/A	0
Vanilla Creme, 14 g	60	3	11	N/A	1
Kool Aid					
Cherry Sugar-sweetened, 17 g	60	0	16	N/A	0
Grape Sugar Free, 1 g	5	0	0	N/A	0
Lemonade Unsweetened, 8 fl.oz.	0	0	0	N/A	0
Orange Unsweetened, 1 g	0	0	0	N/A	0
Strawberry Sugar-sweetened, 17 g	60	0	16	N/A	0
Tropical Punch Sugar Free, 1 g	5	0	0	N/A	0
Lipton					
Chocolate, 28 g	120	2	21	N/A	3
• Original, 28 g	120	2	21	N/A	3
Vanilla, 28 g	120	2	21	N/A	3
Nutrasweet					
Hot Cocoa Mix With Nutrasweet®, 14 g	50	N/A	9	N/A	N/A
• Iced Tea Soft Drink Mix w/ Nutrasweet®, 1 g	2	N/A	0	N/A	N/A
Red Punch Soft Drink Mix w/ Nutrasweet®, 1 g	3	N/A	0	N/A	N/A
South Beach Living					
Strawberry Banana Drink Mix, 11 g	30	0	6	5	3
Tropical Breeze Drink Mix, 11 g	30	35	6	5	3
Special K					
Protein Water Mix Iced Tea, 17 fl.oz.	30	0	7	5	5
Protein Water Mix Pink Lemonade, 17 fl.oz.	30	0	6	5	5
Protein Water Mix Strawberry Kiwi, 17 fl.oz.	30	0	6	5	5
Tang					
Grape, 29 g	110	0	28	N/A	0
Orange, 25 g	90	0	23	0	0
Orange Pineapple, 8 fl.oz.	100	0	24	N/A	0

(•= most healthy •= least healthy)

POPULAR BRANDS

BEVERAGES

Powdered Drink Mixes (cont.)	Cal	Fat	Cbs	Fbr	Prtn
Tang (cont.)					
Orange Strawberry, 29 g	24	0	27	N/A	0
Orange Sugar Free, 2 g	5	0	0	N/A	0
Wild Berry, 11 g	40	0	10	N/A	0

Ready to Drink Coffee	Cal	Fat	Cbs	Fbr	Prtn
General Foods International Coffee					
Chocolate					
• Sugar Free Suisse Mocha, 6 g	30	2	2	N/A	0
Suisse Mocha, 13 g	60	2	10	N/A	0
Swiss White Chocolate, 16 g	70	3	12	N/A	0
Coffee					
Cafe Vienna, 16 g	70	2	12	N/A	0
Creme Caramel, 15 g	60	2	12	N/A	0
Hazelnut Belgian Café, 16 g	70	2	12	N/A	0
Italian Cappuccino, 13 g	50	2	10	N/A	0
Vanilla					
DeCaf French Vanilla Café, 14 g	60	2	10	N/A	0
French Vanilla Café, 14 g	60	3	10	N/A	0
Sugar Free French Vanilla Café, 6 g	30	3	2	N/A	0
Starbucks Beverages					
Doubleshots					
Energy + Coffee Vanilla	210	2	25	N/A	12
• Energy + Coffee	210	2	26	N/A	12
Light	70	4	5	N/A	3
Regular	140	6	17	N/A	4
Frappuccino					
Caramel	200	3	31	N/A	6
Dark Chocolate Mocha	190	4	33	N/A	7
Mocha Lite	100	3	11	N/A	6
Mocha	180	3	31	N/A	7
Vanilla	200	3	31	N/A	3

Smoothies	Cal	Fat	Cbs	Fbr	Prtn
Baskin Robbins					
Fruit Blast - Medium					
Berry Pomegranate Banana, 24 fl.oz.	710	1	172	3	7
Mango Fruit Blast, 24 fl.oz.	620	2	148	3	7
• Strawberry Banana, 24 fl.oz.	730	2	178	7	9
Clif Products					
Lime-ade Electrolyte Splash, 23 g	80	N/A	20	N/A	N/A
Watermelon Moons Energy Chews, 30 g	100	0	24	0	0
Dannon Light & Fit					
Berries & Cream, 7 fl.oz.	60	3	4	0	6
Mixed Berry, 7 fl.oz.	70	0	13	0	5
Peach Passion, 7 fl.oz.	70	0	13	0	5
Strawberry, 7 fl.oz.	70	0	13	0	5
Strawberry Banana, 7 fl.oz.	70	0	13	0	5
Strawberry Banana Cream, 7 fl.oz.	60	3	4	0	6
Strawberries & Cream, 7 fl.oz.	60	3	4	0	6
LightFull Foods					
Café Latte, 8 fl.oz.	90	1	37	5	5

BEVERAGES

Smoothies (cont.)	Cal	Fat	Cbs	Fbr	Prtn
LightFull Foods (cont.)					
Chocolate, 8 fl.oz.	90	1	36	5	5
Peachy Cream, 8 fl.oz.	90	0	37	5	5
Strawberry Bliss, 8 fl.oz.	90	0	37	5	5
Tropicana Juice					
Fruit Smoothies					
Mixed Berry, 11 fl.oz.	220	0	54	2	1
Strawberry Banana, 11 fl.oz.	220	0	53	2	2
Tropical Fruit, 11 fl.oz.	220	0	53	1	1
Twister®					
Cherry Berry Rev, 8 fl.oz.	70	0	16	N/A	0
Orange Strawberry banana Blast, 8 fl.oz.	70	0	16	N/A	0
White Grape Kiwi Twist, 8 fl.oz.	70	0	16	N/A	0
V8					
Strawberry Banana, 8 oz.	10	0	3	0	0
Tropical Colada, 8 oz.	100	0	21	1	3

Soda, Cola & Tonic	Cal	Fat	Cbs	Fbr	Prtn
7Up					
7Up Plus, 8 fl.oz.	10	0	2	N/A	0
7Up 100 % Natural Flavors, 8 fl.oz.	100	0	26	N/A	0
Diet 7Up, 8 fl.oz.	0	0	0	N/A	0
Coca-Cola					
Seagram's Mixers					
• Club Soda, 8 fl.oz.	0	N/A	0	N/A	N/A
Diet Ginger Ale, 8 fl.oz.	2	N/A	0	N/A	N/A
Diet Tonic Water, 8 fl.oz.	3	N/A	0	N/A	N/A
Ginger Ale, 8 fl.oz.	90	N/A	24	N/A	N/A
Original Seltzer, 8 fl.oz.	0	N/A	0	N/A	N/A
Tonic Water, 8 fl.oz.	83	N/A	22	N/A	N/A
Soft Drink					
• Barq's Floatz, 8 fl.oz.	127	0	34	N/A	0
Barq's root beer, 8 fl.oz.	111	0	30	N/A	0
Coca-Cola classic, 8 fl.oz.	97	0	27	N/A	0
Diet Barq's root beer, 8 fl.oz.	1	0	0	N/A	0
Diet Coke, 8 fl.oz.	1	0	0	N/A	0
Fanta Orange, 8 fl.oz.	111	0	35	N/A	0
Fresca, 8 fl.oz.	2	0	0	N/A	0
Full Throttle Energy Drink, 8 fl.oz.	111	N/A	29	N/A	N/A
Pibb Xtra, 8 fl.oz.	97	0	26	N/A	0
Pibb Zero, 8 fl.oz.	2	0	0	N/A	0
Sprite Zero, 8 fl.oz.	2	0	0	N/A	0
Sprite, 8 fl.oz.	96	0	26	N/A	0
Mountain Dew					
AMP, 8 fl.oz.	110	0	29	N/A	0
Baja Blast, 8 fl.oz.	110	0	30	N/A	0
Diet Mountain Dew, 8 fl.oz.	0	0	0	N/A	0
Livewire, 8 fl.oz.	110	0	31	N/A	0
Mountain Dew, 8 fl.oz.	110	0	31	N/A	0
Mug Root Beer					
Cream Soda, 8 fl.oz	120	0	32	N/A	0
Diet Cream Soda, 8 fl.oz	0	0	0	N/A	0

(• = most healthy • = least healthy)

BEVERAGES

Soda, Cola & Tonic (cont.)	Cal	Fat	Cbs	Fbr	Prtn
Mug Root Beer (cont.)					
Diet Mug, 8 fl.oz	0	0	0	N/A	0
Mug, 8 fl.oz	100	0	29	N/A	0
Pepsi Drinks					
Diet Pepsi, 8 fl.oz.	0	0	0	N/A	0
Pepsi, 8 fl.oz.	100	0	28	N/A	0

Sports & Energy Drinks	Cal	Fat	Cbs	Fbr	Prtn
Accelerade					
Accel Gel					
Citrus Orange, 41 g	100	0	20	0	5
Strawberry Kiwi, 41 g	100	0	20	0	5
Vanilla, 41 g	100	0	20	0	5
Ready to Drink					
Citrus Grape Fruit, 8 fl.oz.	80	0	15	N/A	4
Mountian Berry, 8 fl.oz.	80	0	15	N/A	4
Peach Mango, 8 fl.oz.	80	0	15	N/A	4
Clif Products					
Clif Shot Electrolyte Drink					
Cran Razz, 20 g	80	0	19	0	0
Crisp Apple, 20 g	80	0	19	0	0
• Hot Apple Cider, 40 g	150	N/A	38	N/A	N/A
Lemonade, 1 Scoop	80	0	19	0	0
Clif Shot Gel					
Apple Pie, 32 g	100	0	25	0	0
Chocolate, 32 g	100	1	25	0	0
Double Expresso, 32 g	100	0	25	0	0
Strawberry, 32 g	100	0	25	0	0
Vanilla, 32 g	100	0	25	0	0
Clif Shot Recovery Drink					
French Vanilla, 1 Scoop	150	0	31	0	6
Hot Chocolate, 40 g	140	2	23	2	6
Mango Orange, 40 g	140	0	31	0	5
Coca-Cola					
Energy Drinks					
Full Throttle, 8 fl.oz.	111	0	29	N/A	0
Full Throttle Fury, 8 fl.oz.	112	0	29	N/A	0
Sugar Free Full Throttle, 8 fl.oz.	5	0	0	N/A	0
Tab Energy, 8 fl.oz.	6	0	0	N/A	0
Hybrid Energy Sodas					
Vault, 8 fl.oz.	119	0	32	N/A	0
• Vault Zero, 8 fl.oz.	4	0	0	N/A	0
Powerade					
Advance Cherry Lime, 8 fl.oz.	66	0	17	N/A	0
Arctic Shatter, 8 fl.oz.	64	0	17	N/A	0
Black Cherry Lime, 8 fl.oz.	64	0	17	N/A	0
Option Lemon, 8 fl.oz.	10	0	2	N/A	0
Gatorade					
AM, 8 fl.oz.	50	0	14	N/A	0
Fierce, 8 fl.oz.	50	0	14	N/A	0
Frost, 8 fl.oz.	50	0	14	N/A	0
Rain, 8 fl.oz.	51	0	14	N/A	0

BEVERAGES

Sports & Energy Drinks (cont.)	Cal	Fat	Cbs	Fbr	Prtn
Gatorade (cont.)					
X-Factor, 8 fl.oz.	50	0	14	N/A	0

BREAKFAST

Breakfast Bars	Cal	Fat	Cbs	Fbr	Prtn
Post Cereal					
Banana Nut	140	4	24	1	2
Cranberry Almond	140	4	25	1	2
Oatmeal Raisin	130	3	25	2	2
South Beach Living					
High Protein Cereal Bar					
Chocolate, 35 g	140	5	15	3	10
Cinnamon Raisin, 35 g	140	5	15	3	10
Cranberry Almond, 35 g	140	5	15	3	10
Peanut Butter, 35 g	140	5	15	3	10

Cereal	Cal	Fat	Cbs	Fbr	Prtn
Cascadian Farm					
Cinnamon Raisin Granola, 55 g	210	3	42	3	5
Honey Nut Os, 30 g	120	2	24	2	3
Multi Grain Squares, 30 g	110	1	25	2	3
Oats & Honey Granola, 55 g	230	6	42	3	5
Purely O's, 30 g	110	2	22	3	3
Raisin Bran, 55 g	180	2	43	6	5
Chex					
Chocolate, 32 g	130	3	26	1	2
Corn, 31 g	120	1	26	1	2
Honey Nut, 32 g	120	1	28	1	2
Multi Bran, 47 g	160	2	39	6	3
Rice®, 27 g	100	1	23	0	2
Strawberry, 31 g	130	2	29	1	2
Wheat®, 47 g	160	1	38	5	5
Eggo					
French Toaster Sticks Original, 90 g	220	6	35	1	5
Stuffed French Sticks Maple Syrup, 59 g	150	4	27	1	3
General Mills Cereal					
Basic 4, 55 g	200	3	43	3	4
Boo Berry, 33 g	130	1	28	1	1
Cheerios, 28 g	100	2	20	3	3
Chex Corn, 31 g	120	1	26	1	2
Cinnamon Toast Crunch, 31 g	130	3	25	1	1
Cocoa Puffs, 27 g	110	2	23	1	1
Cookie Crisp, 26 g	100	1	22	1	1
• Fiber One, 30 g	60	1	25	14	0
French Toast Crunch, 31 g	130	1	24	1	2
Golden Grahams, 31 g	120	1	26	1	2
Kix, 30 g	110	1	25	3	2
Raisin Nut Bran, 49 g	180	3	38	5	4
Reese's Puffs, 29 g	120	3	22	1	2
Total Raisin Bran, 53 g	160	1	40	5	3
Total, 30 g	100	1	23	3	2
Trix, 32 g	120	2	28	1	1

(•= most healthy •= least healthy)

BREAKFAST

Cereal (cont.)	Cal	Fat	Cbs	Fbr	Prtn
General Mills Cereal (cont.)					
Wheaties, 27 g	100	1	22	3	3
Kellogg's Cereal					
Corn Flakes, 1 oz.	100	0	24	1	2
Corn Pops®, 1 oz.	110	0	26	0	1
Cracklin' Oat Bran®, 2 oz.	200	7	35	6	4
Froot Loops®, 1 oz.	110	1	25	1	1
Froot Loops® Reduced Sugar, 1 oz.	120	1	28	1	2
Frosted Flakes®, 1 oz.	110	0	27	1	1
Frosted Mini-Wheats® Bite Size, 2 oz.	200	1	48	6	6
Honey Smacks®, 1 oz.	100	1	24	1	2
Lowfat Granola without Raisins, 2 oz.	190	3	40	3	4
Mini-Wheats® Unfrosted Bite Size, 2 oz.	200	2	46	6	6
Raisin Bran®, 2 oz.	190	2	45	7	5
Smart Start® Maple & Brown Sugar, 2 oz.	220	3	47	2	6
Life Cereal					
Cinnamon Life, 32 g	120	2	25	2	3
Honey Graham Life, 32 g	120	2	25	2	3
Life Cereal, 32 g	120	2	25	2	3
Life Chocolate Oat Crunch, 51 g	190	3	40	3	5
Life Vanila Yogurt Crunch, 55 g	210	3	46	1	5
Malt O Meal					
Coco Roos, 30 g	120	2	26	1	1
Crispy Rice, 33 g	130	0	29	0	2
Frosted Flakes, 31 g	120	0	28	1	2
Golden Puffs, 27 g	110	0	24	0	2
Honey Buzzers, 29 g	110	1	26	1	1
Honey Graham Squares, 30 g	130	3	25	1	1
Mini Spooners, 55 g	190	1	45	6	5
Puffed Rice, 15 g	60	0	13	0	1
Raisin Bran, 59 g	220	2	49	6	5
Tootie Fruities, 32 g	130	1	28	1	2
Mom's Best					
Raisin Bran, 59 g	230	2	49	6	5
Toasted Wheat-fuls, 55 g	200	1	44	7	6
Toasted Whole Grain Oat Cereal, 30 g	120	2	23	3	4
Nature Valley					
Cereal Crunchy Cinnamon, 58 g	230	3	48	4	4
Cereal Crunchy Oats 'N Honey, 58 g	230	3	48	4	5
Organic Cereal Vanilla Nut, 50 g	190	2	41	3	4
Nutri-Grain					
Apple Cinnamon, 37 g	130	3	24	2	2
Blackberry, 37 g	130	3	24	2	2
Raspberry, 37 g	130	3	24	2	2
Strawberry, 37 g	130	3	24	2	2
Paul Newman's Own					
Flakes'N Strawberries Cereal, 30 g	100	1	25	2	2
Honey Flax Flakes Cereal, 30 g	100	1	24	4	3
Honey Nut O's Cereal, 30 g	100	2	22	2	3
Wheat Puffs Cereal, 27 g	100	1	22	1	3

REAKFAST

Cereal (cont.)	Cal	Fat	Cbs	Fbr	Prtn
Post Cereal					
Honey Bunches of Oats					
Almond, 31 g	130	3	25	2	2
Banana, 31 g	120	2	26	2	2
Honey Roasted, 31 g	120	2	25	2	2
Strawberry, 31 g	120	2	26	2	2
Post Healthy Classic					
Bran Flakes, 30 g	100	1	24	5	3
Fruit & Bran, 55 g	200	3	42	6	4
Grape Nut O's, 32 g	120	0	28	2	2
Grape Nuts Flakes, 29 g	110	1	24	3	3
Grape Nuts Trail Mix Crunch, 48 g	180	3	37	5	4
Raisin Bran, 31 g	190	1	46	8	4
Shredded Wheat Family, 47 g	160	1	37	6	5
Post Kids Cereal					
Cocoa Pebbles, 30 g	110	2	26	3	1
Fruity Pebbles, 30 g	110	1	26	3	1
Golden Crisp, 31 g	110	0	25	1	2
Honeycomb, 32 g	120	1	27	2	2
Oreo O's, 27 g	110	2	22	1	1
Waffle Crisp, 30 g	120	3	25	1	2
Post Selects					
Cranberry Almond Crunch®, 51 g	200	4	39	3	4
Banana Nut Crunch®, 59 g	240	6	44	4	5
Great Grains®-Raisins, 52 g	220	6	38	4	5
Maple Pecan Crunch®, 52 g	220	6	40	3	4
Purity Foods					
Vita-Spelt Toasted Flakes, 27 g	93	1	20	3	4
Red River Cereal					
Original, 40 g	154	3	27	6	6
Regular, 35 g	136	2	24	5	5
Maple & Brown Sugar, 40 g	153	2	29	5	5
Rice Krispies					
Berry Krispies™ cereal, 1 oz.	120	0	27	0	2
Cereal, 1 oz.	130	0	29	0	2
Cocoa Krispies® cereal, 1 oz.	120	1	27	1	1
Frosted Krispies® cereal, 1 oz.	110	0	27	0	1
Treats® Cereal, 1 oz.	120	2	26	0	1
South Beach Living					
Strawberry Harvest Crunch, 50 g	170	2	37	8	7
Vanilla Almond Crunch, 51 g	180	4	35	8	8
Special K					
Cereal, 1 oz.	120	1	22	1	7
Fruit & Yogurt cereal, 1 oz.	120	1	27	1	2
Low Carb Lifestyle Protein Plus, 1 oz.	100	3	14	5	10
Vanilla Almond Cereal, 1 oz.	110	2	25	1	2
Total Cereal					
Cranberry Crunch, 58 g	190	2	44	4	4
Total Honey Clusters®, 48 g	170	2	38	3	3
Total Raisin Bran, 53 g	160	1	40	5	3
Total Whole Grain, 30 g	100	1	23	3	2

(•= most healthy •= least healthy)

BREAKFAST

Granola	Cal	Fat	Cbs	Fbr	Prtn
Purity Foods					
Granola - Apple Cinnamon Raisin, 50 g	220	8	33	3	5
Granola - Cranberry Vanilla Walnut, 50 g	220	9	33	3	5
South Beach Living					
• Cherry Almond Granola Clusters, 30 g	130	4	18	6	0
Mixed Berry Granola Clusters, 30 g	130	4	18	6	6
Sunridge Farms					
Apple Blueberry Granola, 55 g	230	7	36	4	6
Cranberry Craze Granola, 55 g	240	8	36	4	6
Golden Nut and Honey Granola, 55 g	230	9	33	4	7
Organic Crunchy Lite Granola, 55 g	220	6	38	4	6
Organic Grandma Dave's Granola, 55 g	210	5	35	4	7
Organic Magic Muesli, 55 g	210	6	35	5	6
Organic Rolled Oats, 45 g	170	3	30	5	7
• Super Nut Crunch Granola, 55 g	240	9	35	4	6

Hot Cereal	Cal	Fat	Cbs	Fbr	Prtn
Malt O Meal					
Chocolate, 35 g	130	0	27	1	4
Creamy Hot Wheat, 35 g	130	0	27	1	4
• Maple & Brown Sugar, 45 g	170	0	37	1	4
Original, 35 g	130	1	27	1	5
Mom's Best					
Maple & Brown Sugar, 43 g	160	2	33	3	4
• Oats & Honey Blend, 30 g	120	2	25	1	2
Old Fashioned Oats, 40 g	150	3	27	4	5

Toaster Pastries	Cal	Fat	Cbs	Fbr	Prtn
Eggo					
Cereal Cinnamon Toast, 1 oz.	130	3	26	2	2
• Cereal Maple Syrup, 1 oz.	110	2	25	2	2
French Toaster Sticks Cinnamon, 90 g	230	6	38	1	4
Mrs. Butterworth's					
French Toast Sticks - Original, 4 oz.	250	12	31	1	4
French Toast Sticks - Thin, 5 oz.	230	4	41	2	7
Pepperidge Farm					
Apple Dumplings, 1 dumpling	230	11	29	1	3
Apple Turnovers, 1 turnover	270	15	31	1	4
Peach Dumplings, 1 dumpling	250	11	34	1	3
• Peach Turnovers, 1 turnover	280	15	34	1	4
Pillsbury					
Toaster Scramble					
Cheese, Egg & Bacon, 47 g	180	12	15	0	4
Cheese, Egg & Ham, 47 g	180	11	15	0	4
Reduced Fat Southwestern Style, 47 g	160	9	15	1	4
Toaster Strudel					
Brown Sugar Cinnamon, 54 g	200	9	28	1	3
Cream Cheese, 54 g	200	11	23	1	3
Strawberry Banana, 54 g	180	9	24	0	2
Strawberry, 54 g	190	9	26	1	3
Turnovers					
Turnovers Apple, 57 g	180	8	24	0	2

BREAKFAST

Toaster Pastries (cont.)	Cal	Fat	Cbs	Fbr	Prtn
Pillsbury (cont.)					
Turnovers (cont.)					
Turnovers Cherry, 57 g	180	8	24	0	2
Pop-Tarts					
Apple Strudel, 50 g	200	6	35	1	2
Blueberry, 52 g	210	6	37	1	2
Brown Sugar Cinnamon, 50 g	210	8	33	1	2
Chocolate Chip, 52 g	220	7	36	1	3
Frosted Cookies & Creme, 50 g	200	5	35	1	2
Lowfat Frosted Strawberry, 52 g	190	3	39	1	2
Whole Grain Brown Sugar Cinn., 50 g	200	7	34	3	3
Whole Grain Strawberry, 50 g	190	5	35	3	2

Waffles and Pancakes	Cal	Fat	Cbs	Fbr	Prtn
Aunt Jemima					
Butter Milk Complete, 1/3 cup	160	2	31	1	5
Original, 1/3 cup	150	1	33	1	4
Whole Wheat Blend, 1/4 cup	120	1	26	3	4
Eggo					
Pancakes					
Blueberry, 105 g	250	8	41	1	5
Buttermilk, 116 g	280	9	44	1	6
Jungle, 117 g	280	8	46	1	7
Minis, 110 g	260	8	42	1	5
Nutri-Grain®, 105 g	240	7	40	3	6
Waffles					
Apple Cinnamon, 70 g	190	6	29	1	4
Buttermilk, 70 g	180	6	26	1	5
Chocolate Chip, 70 g	210	7	32	1	4
• Cinnamon Toast, 92 g	300	11	45	1	5
French Toast, 45 g	140	6	19	1	3
Homestyle Waffles, 70 g	190	7	27	1	4
Minis Homestyle Waffles, 93 g	260	10	38	1	6
Mrs. Butterworth's					
Pancakes - Mini, 4 oz.	240	4	46	2	6
Pancakes - Original, 4 oz.	220	4	42	2	6
Waffles Jumbo Square, 3 oz.	200	6	32	1	5
Waffles Regular Square, 3 oz.	210	6	34	1	5
Pillsbury					
Pancakes Blueberry, 116 g	230	4	46	2	5
Pancakes Buttermilk, 116 g	240	4	47	2	6
Pancakes Maple Burst, 116 g	290	7	53	2	5
Pancakes Original, 116 g	250	4	49	2	6

CANDY

Chocolate	Cal	Fat	Cbs	Fbr	Prtn
Cadbury's					
Caramel Egg, 34 g	170	9	21	N/A	2
Caramello Candy Bar, 45 g	220	10	29	1	3
• Chocolate Egg, 34 g	150	5	25	N/A	1
Roast Almond, 39 g	210	13	21	1	4

CANDY

Chocolate (cont.)

	Cal	Fat	Cbs	Fbr	Prtn
Hershey Chocolates					
Cookies 'N' Créme Candy Bar, 34 g	170	9	21	N/A	3
Extra Creamy Chocolate & Caramel, 36 g	180	9	22	N/A	2
Hershey's Pretzel Bars, 20 g	100	5	13	N/A	1
Milk Chocolate, 43 g	210	13	26	1	3
Milk Chocolate With Almonds, 41 g	210	14	21	2	4
Special Dark Chocolate, 41 g	180	12	25	3	2
M&M's Bakery					
Almond, 1 oz.	200	100	21	2	3
Dark Chocolate, 2 oz.	240	100	33	2	2
M&M'S Minis, 1 oz.	150	60	21	1	1
Milk Chocolate, 2 oz.	240	90	34	1	2
Mint Crisp, 1 Bag	200	80	27	2	2
Peanut, 2 oz.	250	120	30	2	5
Peanut Butter, 2 oz.	240	120	26	2	5
Mauna Loa					
Candy Coated, 40 g	210	13	22	1	2
Dark Chocolate, 41 g	210	16	22	2	2
Milk Chocolate, 41 g	220	16	21	1	3
Snickers					
• Snickers, 2 oz.	280	14	35	1	4
Snickers Almond, 18 oz.	240	11	32	1	3
Snickers Dark, 2 oz.	250	13	30	2	4
Sorbee					
Chocolate Truffles, 40 g	180	12	22	2	3
Milk Chocolate Bar, 40 g	190	13	22	1	3
Peanut Butter Chocolates, 40 g	210	15	19	1	4
Peppermint Patties, 39 g	180	13	24	4	2
Stauffer's					
Almond, 1 oz.	230	15	19	2	4
Chocorooms, 1 oz.	160	8	20	1	2
Hello Panda Chocolate, 1 oz.	160	10	18	1	1
Pucca Regular Chocolate, 1 oz.	160	9	19	1	1
Sunridge Farms					
Chocolate Ginger, 40 g	170	7	28	1	1
Organic Chocolate Raisins, 40 g	160	6	27	1	2
Terry's					
Orange Dark, 44 g	240	13	28	3	1
Orange Milk, 44 g	230	12	27	1	3
Pure Milk, 44 g	230	12	27	0	3
Toblerone					
Swiss Choc w/ Honey & Almond Nougat, 33 g	170	9	21	1	2
Swiss White w/ Honey & Almond Nougat, 33 g	180	10	20	0	2
Truffle Peaks, 41 g	240	15	23	1	2

Various Kinds

	Cal	Fat	Cbs	Fbr	Prtn
Sorbee					
Hard Candies					
• Chocolate Lites, 13 g	25	0	13	N/A	0
Coffee Lites, 13 g	25	0	13	N/A	0
Fruit Flavors Lites, 13 g	25	0	13	N/A	0

CANDY

Various Kinds (cont.)	Cal	Fat	Cbs	Fbr	Prtn
Sorbee (cont.)					
Soft Candy					
Bursts, 40 g	120	3	34	N/A	0
Sunridge Farms					
Black Licorice Chews, 40 g	140	2	27	1	13
Black Licorice Scotties, 40 g	130	0	33	0	0
Natural Licorice Raspberry Hearts, 40 g	140	0	35	0	0
Organic Jolly Beans, 40 g	150	0	37	0	0
Organic Sunny Bears, 40 g	30	0	9	0	0
Wonka					
Chewy Gobstopper®, 15 g	50	0	14	N/A	0
Chewy Runts®, 15 g	60	1	14	N/A	0
Laffy Taffy® Rope, 1 rope	80	1	19	N/A	0
Laffy Taffy® Stretchy & Tangy Taffy, 1 bar	165	4	33	N/A	0
Nerds® Rope , 1 rope	90	0	22	N/A	0
Sour Mixups®, 43 g	160	2	36	N/A	0
Sour Sweetarts Variety, 9 g	30	0	8	N/A	0
Sweetarts Rope, 1 pkg	210	2	48	N/A	1
Sweetarts Squeeze, 1 tube	130	0	33	N/A	0

CHEESE

Cheese	Cal	Fat	Cbs	Fbr	Prtn
Alouette					
Alouette® Baby Brie®					
Original, 28 g	110	10	1	0	5
With Herbs, 28 g	100	8	1	0	5
Alouette® Reserve™					
Baby Brie® Cheese, 28 g	100	8	1	0	5
Chevre Style Cheese, 28 g	80	7	1	0	5
Havarti, 28 g	90	0	0	0	6
Swiss Style Cheese, 28 g	100	7	1	0	7
Alta Dena					
Cheese					
Mild Cheddar Cheese, 1 oz.	110	9	1	0	7
Monterey Jack Cheese, 1 oz.	100	8	0	0	6
Whipped Cream Cheese, 22 g	80	7	1	0	1
Cottage Cheese					
Cottage Cheese w/ Pineapple, 113 g	120	2	14	0	11
Lowfat Cottage Cheese, 105 g	100	3	4	0	14
Small Curd Cottage Cheese, 105 g	120	5	3	0	14
Athenos					
Blue Cheese Crumbled Natural, 32 g	110	9	2	1	7
Crumbled Reduced Fat, 34 g	90	7	2	1	7
Crumbled Traditional, 1 oz.	80	6	1	N/A	6
Gorgonzola Crumbled Natural, 32 g	110	9	2	1	7
Breakstone's					
Cottage Cheese					
Large Curd Lowfat 2% Milkfat, 119 g	90	3	6	0	11
Large Curd Smooth & Creamy 4% Milkfat, 120 g	120	5	6	0	12
Liveactive Lowfat With Mixed Berries, 113 g	120	2	18	3	8
Liveactive Lowfat With Pineapple, 113 g	110	2	17	3	8
Small Curd Fat Free, 126 g	80	0	8	0	12

(• = most healthy • = least healthy)

POPULAR BRANDS

CHEESE

Cheese (cont.)	Cal	Fat	Cbs	Fbr	Prtr
Breakstone's (cont.)					
Cottage Cheese (cont.)					
Small Curd Lowfat 2% Milkfat, 124 g	90	3	6	0	12
Small Curd Smooth & Creamy 4% Milkfat, 124 g	120	5	6	0	12
Cottage Doubles					
Blueberry Lowfat, 156 g	140	3	18	1	11
Raspberry Lowfat, 156 g	140	3	17	1	11
Strawberry Lowfat, 156 g	130	2	17	0	11
Country Fresh					
1% Lowfat Cottage Cheese, 113 g	90	2	5	0	13
2% Lowfat Cottage Cheese, 105 g	100	3	5	0	13
Cottage Cheese, 105 g	110	5	5	0	11
Fat Free Cottage Cheese, 113 g	80	0	6	0	14
Dean's					
1 % Lowfat Cottage Cheese, 113 g	90	2	5	0	13
2 % Lowfat Cottage Cheese, 2 g	100	3	5	0	13
Cottage Cheese, 105 g	110	5	5	0	11
Fat Free Cottage Cheese, 113 g	80	0	6	0	14
Deli Deluxe					
American 2% Milk Slices, 19 g	60	4	0	0	4
American Slices, 19 g	70	6	0	0	4
Colby Jack Slices, 23 g	90	7	0	0	5
Mild Cheddar Slices, 23 g	90	8	0	0	5
Mozzarella Slices Low Moisture, 21 g	60	4	0	0	6
Natural Swiss Slices, 21 g	80	7	0	0	6
Pepper Jack Spicy Slices, 23 g	90	7	0	0	5
Provolone Slices, 28 g	100	8	0	0	7
Sharp Cheddar 2% Milk Slices, 23 g	70	5	1	0	6
Sharp Cheddar Slices, 28 g	110	9	1	0	6
Swiss 2% Milk Reduced Fat Slices, 21 g	70	5	0	0	6
Swiss Slices, 28 g	90	7	1	0	6
Easy Cheese					
American, 32g	90	6	2	0	5
Cheddar, 32g	90	6	2	0	5
Cheddar 'N Bacon, 32g	90	7	2	0	5
Sharp Cheddar, 32g	80	6	2	0	4
Knudsen					
• Cottage Doubles Raspberry Lowfat, 156 g	150	3	20	1	11
Cottage Doubles Strawberry Lowfat, 156 g	140	3	19	0	11
Free Nonfat, 123 g	80	0	7	0	13
Lowfat & Pineapple, 123 g	120	2	15	0	10
Lowfat Small Curd, 122 g	100	3	6	0	14
Kraft Singles					
American 2% Milk, 21 g	50	3	2	0	4
American Fat Free, 19 g	30	0	2	0	4
Pepperjack 2% Milk, 21 g	50	3	2	0	4
Sharp Cheddar Fat Free, 21 g	30	0	2	0	5
Swiss Fat Free, 21 g	30	0	2	0	5
Swiss, 21 g	60	5	2	0	4
White American, 19 g	60	5	1	0	3
Land O'Lakes					
1% Lowfat Cottage Cheese, 113 g	90	2	5	0	13

CHEESE

Cheese (cont.)

	Cal	Fat	Cbs	Fbr	Prtn
Land O'Lakes (cont.)					
2% Lowfat Cottage Cheese, 105 g	100	3	5	0	13
Cottage Cheese, 105g	110	5	5	0	11
Fat Free Cottage Cheese, 113 g	80	0	6	0	14
Light N Lively					
Cottage Cheese - Fat Free, 125 g	80	0	8	0	12
Cottage Cheese - Lowfat, 113 g	80	1	5	0	11
Live Active					
Cottage Cheese - Breakstone's, 4 oz.	90	2	8	3	10
Cottage Cheese - Knudsen, 4 oz.	90	2	8	3	10
Natural Cheese					
Cheddar Bacon, 28 g	90	7	2	0	5
Colby, 28 g	110	9	1	0	6
Medium Cheddar, 28 g	120	10	0	0	6
Monterey Jack, 28 g	110	9	0	0	6
Mozzarella Low-moisture, 28 g	80	6	1	0	7
Sharp Cheddar, 28 g	120	10	0	0	6
Polly O					
Mozzarella Fat Free, 5 g	20	2	0	0	2
Mozzarella Part Skim, 64 g	70	3	3	0	8
Mozzarella Whole Milk, 28 g	80	7	0	0	5
Parmesan & Romano Grated, 43 g	120	10	0	0	7
Parmesan Grated, 5 g	20	2	0	0	2
Ricotta - Fat Free, 28 g	40	0	1	1	8
Ricotta - Lite, 28 g	60	3	1	0	7
Ricotta - Part Skim, 28 g	90	7	1	0	7
Ricotta Original, 63 g	110	6	2	0	8
Sargento					
Artisan Blends Shredded Cheese					
Mozzarella & Provolone, 28 g	90	9	0	0	6
Parmesan, 5 g	20	2	0	0	2
Swiss, 28 g	110	8	1	0	8
Bistro™ Blends Shredded Cheese					
Chipotle Cheddar Cheese, 28 g	100	8	1	0	6
Mozzarella & Asiago w/ Roasted Garlic, 28 g	80	5	2	0	7
Mozzarella w/ Sun-Dried Tomatoes & Basil, 28 g	90	6	1	0	7
Classic Fancy Shredded Cheese					
Cheddar Jack, 28 g	110	9	1	0	7
Mozzarella, 28 g	80	6	1	0	7
Sharp Cheddar, 28 g	110	9	1	0	7
Deli Style Sliced Cheeses					
Colby, 21 g	80	7	1	0	5
Colby-Jack Cheese, 19 g	70	6	0	0	4
Medium Cheddar, 28 g	80	6	0	0	5
Monterey Jack, 21 g	80	6	0	0	5
Mozzarella, 21 g	60	4	1	0	5
Muenster, 21 g	80	6	0	0	5
Pepper Jack Cheese, 21 g	80	6	0	0	4
Provolone, 21 g	70	6	0	0	5
Swiss, 19 g	70	5	0	0	5
Reduced Fat Deli Style Sliced Cheeses					
Reduced Fat Provolone, 19 g	50	4	0	0	5

(● = most healthy ● = least healthy)

CHEESE

Cheese (cont.)	Cal	Fat	Cbs	Fbr	Prtn
Sargento (cont.)					
Reduced Fat Deli Style Sliced Cheeses (cont.)					
Reduced Fat Swiss, 21 g	60	4	1	0	7
Reduced Fat Shredded Cheese					
4 Cheese Mexican, 28 g	80	6	1	0	8
Mild Cheddar, 28 g	80	6	1	0	7
Mozzarella, 28 g	80	5	1	0	8
Smart Balance					
Fat Free Slices, 1 slice	25	0	N/A	N/A	N/A
Cheese Product Shreds, 1 oz.	80	5	1	0	7
South Beach Living					
Lowfat Cottage Cheese, 4 oz.	80	1	6	0	11
The Laughing Cow					
Mini Baby Bel					
Gouda, 21 g	80	6	0	0	5
Light, 21 g	50	3	0	0	6
Mild Cheddar, 21 g	70	5	0	0	5
Original, 21 g	70	6	0	0	5
Wedges					
Light Garlic & Herb, 21 g	35	2	1	0	3
Light Swiss Original, 21 g	35	2	1	0	3
Original Creamy Swiss, 21 g	50	4	1	1	2
Velveeta					
2% Milk Cheese, 28 g	60	3	4	0	5
Mexican Mild Cheese, 28 g	80	6	3	0	5
Pepper Jack Cheese, 28 g	80	6	3	0	5
Regular Cheese, 28 g	80	6	3	0	5

Cheese Dips/Spreads	Cal	Fat	Cbs	Fbr	Prtn
Alouette					
Crème Spreadable Cheese					
Crème de Brie®, Fine Herbs, 28 g	90	8	1	0	4
Crème de Havarti™, Garlic & Herb, 28 g	70	7	1	0	3
Crème de Swiss™, Original, 28 g	80	7	1	0	3
Elégante®					
Roasted Garlic & Pesto, 28 g	100	9	2	0	2
Roasted Peppers & Olive Tapenade, 28 g	100	9	2	0	2
Sundried Tomatoes & Garlic, 28 g	100	9	2	0	2
Reserve™ Spreadable Cheese					
Original, 22 g	70	6	1	0	1
Vidalia Onion, 22 g	70	6	2	0	1
Spreadable Cheese					
Light Garlic & Herbs, 23 g	50	4	2	0	2
Savory Vegetable, 23 g	70	6	1	0	1
Sundried Tomato & Basil, 23 g	80	7	1	0	1
Cheese Whiz					
Light, 35 g	80	4	6	0	6
Original, 33 g	90	7	4	0	3
Salsa Con Queso, 33 g	90	7	4	0	3
Philadelphia Cream Cheese					
Cream Cheese					
Cream Swirls Peaches 'N Cream, 32 g	91	7	5	0	1

SE

Cheese Dips/Spreads (cont.)	Cal	Fat	Cbs	Fbr	Prtn
Philadelphia Cream Cheese (cont.)					
Cream Cheese (cont.)					
Fat Free, 28 g	30	0	2	0	4
Light, 31 g	70	5	2	0	2
Original, 28 g	100	10	1	0	2
Regular, 31 g	90	9	2	0	2
Salmon, 31 g	90	8	2	0	2
Whipped, 21 g	60	6	1	0	1
Rondele					
Bagel Temptations					
Garden Vegetable, 28 g	80	8	1	0	2
Original Plain, 28 g	110	10	1	0	2
Strawberry, 28 g	90	8	4	0	1
Dairy Box					
Blue Cheese, 25 g	80	8	1	0	1
Garden Vegetable, 27 g	70	7	1	0	1
Lite Garlic & Herbs, 28 g	60	5	2	0	3
Deli Cup					
Garden Vegetable, 23 g	70	7	1	0	1
Garlic & Herbs, 23 g	70	7	1	0	2
Toasted Onion, 23 g	70	7	2	0	1
Pub Cheese					
Cheddar Horseradish, 23 g	70	7	1	0	2
Sharp Cheddar, 23 g	80	7	1	0	2
Zesty Salsa, 23 g	30	6	1	0	1
Smart Balance					
Light Cream Cheese Spread, 30 g	70	5	3	0	0
Regular Cream Cheese Spread, 30 g	90	6	2	0	3

Snack Dip	Cal	Fat	Cbs	Fbr	Prtn
Athenos					
Artichoke & Garlic, 27 g	50	3	4	1	1
• Hummus Original, 27 g	50	3	5	1	1
Hummus Pesto, 27 g	50	3	5	1	1
• Roasted Eggplant, 27 g	45	2	5	1	1

CONDIMENTS, SPREADS & SPICES

Horseradish	Cal	Fat	Cbs	Fbr	Prtn
Zatarain's					
Prepared Horseradish, 1 tbsp.	15	0	2	N/A	N/A

Jalapeños and Peppers	Cal	Fat	Cbs	Fbr	Prtn
B&G Foods					
Peppers					
• Hot Cherry Peppers Red & Green, 1 oz.	28	3	0	N/A	0
Hot Chopped Roasted Peppers, 15 g	5	0	1	N/A	0
Peperoncini, 1 oz.	10	0	2	N/A	0
Pepper Toppers					
• Sliced Hot Jalapeños, 1 oz.	0	0	1	N/A	0
Sweet Bell Pepper, 1 oz.	20	0	5	N/A	0
Texas Pete					
Pepper Sauce, 4 g	5	0	0	N/A	0

(• = most healthy • = least healthy)

POPULAR BRANDS

CONDIMENTS, SPREADS & SPICES

Ketchup	Cal	Fat	Cbs	Fbr	Prtn
Annie's Naturals					
• Ketchup - Organic, 17 g	15	N/A	3	0	0
Del Monte					
Ketchup, 17 g	15	0	4	0	0
Quick Squeeze Ketchup, 17 g	15	0	4	0	0
Quick Squeeze Ketchup, 17 g	15	0	4	0	0
Heinz					
Ketchup 'With a Twist' Garlic, 100 g	97	0	22	1	1
Ketchup 'With a Twist' Sweet and Onion, 100 g	98	0	22	1	1
• Organic Tomato Ketchup, 100 g	113	0	26	1	1
Original Tomato Ketchup, 100 g	102	1	24	1	1
Reduced Sugar & Salt Tomato, 100 g	71	0	15	1	1
Muir Glen					
Tomato Ketchup, 17 g	20	0	4	N/A	0

Mayonnaise	Cal	Fat	Cbs	Fbr	Prtn
Best Foods					
Mayonnaise					
Light Mayonnaise, 14 g	45	5	1	N/A	0
Real Mayonnaise, 13 g	90	10	0	N/A	0
Reduced Fat Dressing, 15 g	20	2	2	N/A	0
Other Favorites					
Tartar Sauce, 30 g	80	7	4	N/A	0
Hellman's					
Light Mayonnaise, 14 g	45	5	1	N/A	0
Lowfat Mayonnaise Dressing, 15 g	15	1	2	0	0
Mayonnaise w/ Extra Virgin Olive Oil, 15 g	50	5	1	N/A	0
Real Mayonnaise, 13 g	90	10	0	N/A	0
Kraft Mayonnaise					
• Fat Free Dressing, 16 g	10	0	2	N/A	0
Light Mayonnaise, 15 g	40	4	2	0	0
• Real Mayonnaise Hot 'N Spicy, 14 g	100	11	0	0	0
Real Mayonnaise, 13 g	90	10	0	N/A	0
Smart Balance					
Omega Plus Light Mayonnaise, 15 g	50	5	2	N/A	0

Mustard	Cal	Fat	Cbs	Fbr	Prtn
Annie's Naturals					
Dijon Mustard - Organic, 5 g	0	0	0	N/A	0
Honey Mustard - Organic, 6 g	10	0	2	N/A	0
Yellow Mustard - Organic, 5 g	0	0	0	N/A	0
Best Foods					
Deli Mustard, 5 g	5	0	1	0	0
Dijonnaise™ Mustard, 5 g	5	0	1	0	0
Honey Mustard, 5 g	10	0	2	0	0
French's					
Bold N' Spicy Brown, 1 tsp.	5	0	0	0	0
• Classic Yellow®, 1 tsp.	0	0	0	0	0
Dijon, 1 tsp.	0	0	0	0	0
Sweet & Tangy Honey Mustard, 1 tsp.	10	0	1	0	0
Sweet 'N Zesty, 1 tsp.	5	0	1	0	0

CONDIMENTS, SPREADS & SPICES

▶ Mustard (cont.)	Cal	Fat	Cbs	Fbr	Prtn
Grey Poupon					
Country Dijon, 5 g	5	0	0	N/A	0
Dijon, 5 g	5	0	0	N/A	0
Hearty Spicy Brown, 4 g	0	0	0	N/A	0
Mild & Creamy, 5 g	0	0	1	N/A	0
Savory Honey, 5 g	10	0	1	N/A	0
Hellman's					
Deli Mustard, 5 g	5	0	1	0	0
Dijonnaise™ Mustard, 5 g	5	0	1	0	0
Honey Mustard, 5 g	10	0	2	0	0
Jack Daniel's					
Hickory Smoke Mustard, 5 g	5	0	0	0	0
Honey Dijon, 6 g	10	0	2	0	0
Horseradish Mustard, 5 g	5	0	0	0	0
Olde No. 7 Mustard, 5 g	5	0	0	0	0
Spicy Southwest Mustard, 5 g	0	0	1	0	0
Stone Ground Dijon Mustard, 5 g	5	0	0	0	0
Texas Pete					
• Honey Mustard, 37 g	45	0	11	N/A	0
Zatarain's					
Creole Mustard, 7 g	10	1	1	N/A	N/A

▶ Pickles, Relish & Olives	Cal	Fat	Cbs	Fbr	Prtn
B&G Foods					
Pickle Toppers					
Bread & Butter, 1 oz.	30	0	7	N/A	0
• Kosher Dill, 1 oz.	0	0	0	N/A	0
Pickles					
Dill, 1 oz.	0	0	0	N/A	0
Sweet Mixed, 1 oz.	35	0	9	N/A	0
Unsalted Kosher Dill, 1 oz.	10	0	2	N/A	0
Relish					
Dill Relish, 15 oz.	0	0	0	N/A	0
Sweet Relish, 15 g	15	0	4	N/A	0
Unsalted Relish, 15 g	20	0	5	N/A	0
Claussen Pickles					
Bread 'N Butter Chips, 28 g	20	0	4	N/A	0
Bread 'N Butter Slices, 34 g	5	0	5	N/A	3
Deli Style Kosher Dill Halves, 45 g	5	0	1	0	0
Hearty Garlic Deli Style Slices, 34 g	5	0	1	N/A	0
Hearty Garlic Deli Style Wholes, 28 g	20	5	1	N/A	0
Pickle Relish - Sweet Squeeze, 15 g	10	0	3	N/A	0
Pickle Relish - Sweet, 15 g	15	0	3	N/A	0
Sweet Gherkins, 28 g	5	0	1	N/A	0
Del Monte					
Pickles					
Genuine Dill Halves, 28 g	5	0	1	1	0
Hamburger Dill Chips, 28 g	0	0	0	0	0
Sweet Pickle Chips, 28 g	40	0	10	1	0
• Sweet Pickles, 28 g	40	0	10	1	0
Tiny Kosher Dills, 28 g	5	0	1	1	0

(• = most healthy • = least healthy)

CONDIMENTS, SPREADS & SPICES

Pickles, Relish & Olives (cont.)	Cal	Fat	Cbs	Fbr	Prtn
Del Monte (cont.)					
Relish					
Hamburger Style Relish, 17 g	20	0	5	1	0
Hot Dog Style Relish, 16 g	15	0	4	1	0
Sweet Pickle Relish, 16 g	20	0	5	0	0

Salt & Pepper	Cal	Fat	Cbs	Fbr	Prtn
Lawry's					
• Black Pepper Seasoned Salt, 1 g	0	0	0	0	0
Garlic Salt, 1 g	0	0	0	0	0
Lemon Pepper, 1 g	0	0	0	N/A	0
Seasoned Salt, 1 g	0	0	0	0	0
McCormick					
Asian Style Spiced Sea Salt, 1 g	0	0	0	N/A	0
Mediterranean Spiced Sea Salt, 1 g	0	0	0	N/A	0
Sicilian Sea Salt, 1 g	0	0	0	N/A	0
Pace Foods					
• Diced Green Chiles, 2 tbsp.	10	0	2	1	0
Jalapeños Nacho Sliced Peppers, 1 oz.	5	0	1	1	5

Sandwich Spreads	Cal	Fat	Cbs	Fbr	Prtn
Best Foods					
Sandwich Spread, 15 g	60	5	2	N/A	0
California Sun Dry					
Sun-Dried Tomato Spread, 2tbs	50	3	N/A	N/A	N/A
Hellman's					
Sandwich Spread, 15 g	60	5	2	N/A	0
• Tartar Sauce, 30 g	80	7	4	N/A	0
Miracle Whip					
All-out Squeeze! Miracle Whip, 15 g	35	3	2		0
• Free Nonfat, 16 g	15	0	3		0
Light Super Easy Squeeze, 16 g	20	2	2	N/A	0
Super Easy Squeeze, 15 g	40	3	2	N/A	0

Seasoning Powder/Mixes	Cal	Fat	Cbs	Fbr	Prtn
Lawry's					
Meat Tenderizer					
• Original, 1 g	0	0	0	N/A	0
Seasoned, 1 g	0	0	0	N/A	0
Seasoning Mixes					
Enchilada Sauce, 6 g	20	0	4	1	N/A
Fajitas, 5 g	10	0	3	N/A	0
Guacamole, 2 g	0	0	1	0	0
Meat Loaf, 10 g	30	0	7	1	1
Sloppy Joes, 7 g	20	0	5	N/A	0
Taco, 5 g	15	0	3	1	0
McCormick					
Bag 'n Season					
Beef Stew, 5 g	15	0	1	N/A	1
Chicken, 6 g	20	0	3	N/A	0
Herb Roasted Pork Tenderloin, 3 g	5	0	0	N/A	0
Pot Roast, 3 g	10	0	1	N/A	0

CONDIMENTS, SPREADS & SPICES

Seasoning Powder/Mixes (cont.)	Cal	Fat	Cbs	Fbr	Prtn
McCormick (cont.)					
Grill Mates					
Montreal Chicken Seasoning, 1 g	0	0	0	N/A	0
Montreal Steak Seasoning, 1 g	0	0	0	N/A	0
Salmon Seasoning, 1 g	0	0	0	N/A	0
Steamers					
Cheddar Cheese Veggie Steamers, 6 g	25	1	2	N/A	1
Garlic & Basil Veggie Steamers, 4 g	15	1	2	N/A	0
Italian Herb Potato Steamers, 8 g	30	1	4	N/A	0
Roasted Garlic & Rosemary Potato Steamers, 8 g	30	1	4	N/A	0
Pace Foods					
Taco Seasoning Mix, 2 tbsp.	10	0	3	1	0
Taco Bell Home Originals					
Taco Seasoning Mix - Chipotle Flavor, 6 g	20	0	3	N/A	1
Taco Seasoning Mix - Original, 6 g	20	0	3	N/A	1
Zatarain's					
Boiled Seafood					
Crab & Shrimp Boil - Pro Boil, 1 oz	20	1	2	1	N/A
Seasoning and Spices					
Creole Seasoning, 1/4 tsp.	0	0	0	0	0
Pinto Bean Seasoning Mix, 1/2 cup prepared	20	0	4	0	1
Red Bean Seasoning Mix, 1 tsp.	15	0	3	1	0
White Bean Seasoning Mix, 1 tsp.	15	0	3	0	0

DAIRY, FATS, & OILS

Butter & Margarine	Cal	Fat	Cbs	Fbr	Prtn
Alta Dena					
• Salted Butter, 14 g	100	11	0	N/A	0
Unsalted Sweet Butter, 14 g	100	11	0	N/A	0
Brummel & Brown					
• Spread, 14 g	45	5	0	N/A	0
Country Crock					
Limited Editions					
Cinnamon Apple, 11 g	60	6	2	N/A	0
Cinnamon Bluberry, 15 g	50	5	2	N/A	0
Cinnamon, 15 g	60	6	3	N/A	0
Maple, 15 g	60	6	3	N/A	0
Regular					
Churnstyle, 14 g	80	8	0	N/A	0
Plus Calcium And Vitamins, 14 g	50	5	0	N/A	0
Regular (Soft), 14 g	60	7	0	N/A	0
Spreadable Sticks, 14 g	60	7	0	N/A	0
Squeeze, 12 g	60	7	0	N/A	0
Spreads					
Omegaplus, 14 g	70	8	0	0	0
Spreadable Butter With Canolaoil, 11 g	80	9	0	N/A	0
Fleischmann's					
Light Margarine Sleeve, 1 tbs.	40	5	0	0	0
Olive Oil Sleeve, 1 tbs.	70	8	0	0	0
Original Margarine Sleeve, 1 tbs.	70	8	0	0	0
Parkay					
Light Margarine Sticks, 1 tbsp.	45	5	0	N/A	0

(• = most healthy • = least healthy)

POPULAR BRANDS

DAIRY, FATS, & OILS

Butter & Margarine (cont.)	Cal	Fat	Cbs	Fbr	Prtn
Parkay (cont.)					
Margarine Sticks, 1 tbsp.	80	9	0	0	0
Soft Margarine Sleeve, 1 tbsp.	60	7	0	N/A	0
Smart Balance					
Butter Blends Sticks					
Stick Regular, 14 g	100	11	0	N/A	0
Unsalted with Omega-3, 14 g	100	11	0	N/A	0
Buttery Spreads With Flax Oil					
Light With Flax Oil, 14 g	45	5	0	N/A	0
Regular With Flax Oil, 14 g	80	9	0	N/A	0
Omega-3 Buttery Spreads					
Extra Virgin Olive Oil Light, 14 g	50	5	0	N/A	0
Extra Virgin Olive Oil, 11 g	60	7	0	N/A	0
Omega-3 Bundle Light, 14 g	50	5	0	N/A	0
Omega-3 Bundle, 13 g	80	9	0	N/A	0
Original Buttery Spreads					
37% Light Buttery Spread, 14 g	45	5	0	N/A	0
67% Buttery Spread, 14 g	80	9	0	N/A	0
Low Sodium Buttery Spread, 11 g	65	7	0	N/A	0
Organic Buttery Spread, 11 g	80	9	0	N/A	0

Butter Alternatives	Cal	Fat	Cbs	Fbr	Prtn
I Can't Believe It's Not Butter					
Calcium, 14 g	50	5	0	N/A	0
• Fat Free, 14 g	5	0	0	N/A	0
Light, 14 g	50	5	0	N/A	0
Mediterranean Blend Light, 14 g	50	5	0	N/A	0
Mediterranean Blend, 14 g	80	8	0	N/A	0
• Original, 14 g	80	8	0	N/A	0

Cooking Oil & Sprays	Cal	Fat	Cbs	Fbr	Prtn
American Roland Food Corporation					
• Grapeseed Oil, 14 g	130	14	0	0	0
Hazelnut Oil, 14 g	130	14	0	0	0
Olive Oil, 15 g	120	14	0	0	0
Sesame Oil, 14 g	120	14	0	0	0
Truffle Oil, 15 g	120	14	0	0	0
Annie's Naturals					
Basil Oil, 15 ml.	120	14	0	N/A	N/A
Dipping Oil (8.1 oz. Bottle), 15 ml.	40	14	0	0	0
Roasted Garlic Extra Virgin Olive Oil, 15 ml.	120	14	0	0	0
Canola Info					
Canola oil, 14 g	120	14	0	N/A	0
Pam					
Grilling Spray, 1/3 second spray	7	1	0	N/A	0
Olive Oil Spray, 1/3 second spray	7	1	0	N/A	0
Original Canola Spray, 1/3 second spray	7	1	0	N/A	0
• Vegetable Spray, 1/3 second spray	7	1	0	N/A	0
Planters					
Peanut Oil, 14 g	120	14	N/A	N/A	N/A
Smart Balance					
Cooking Spray, 1 g	0	0	0	N/A	0

DAIRY, FATS, & OILS

Cooking Oil & Sprays (cont.)

	Cal	Fat	Cbs	Fbr	Prtn
Smart Balance (cont.)					
Omega Cooking & Salad Oil, 14 g	120	14	0	N/A	0
Wesson					
Canola Oil, 1 tbsp.	120	14	0	N/A	0
Corn oil, 1 tbsp.	120	14	0	N/A	0

Egg Nog

	Cal	Fat	Cbs	Fbr	Prtn
Alta Dena					
Holiday Eggnog, 118 ml.	230	10	29	0	6
Holiday Lite Eggnog, 118 ml.	170	4	29	0	6
Pumpkin Spice Eggnog, 120 ml.	230	10	29	0	6

Eggs

	Cal	Fat	Cbs	Fbr	Prtn
Alta Dena					
Eggs, 56 g	80	5	1	N/A	7
Egg Beaters					
Egg Beaters Egg Whites, 46 g	25	0	1	0	5
Egg Beaters Original, 61 g	30	0	1	0	6
Egg Beaters With Yolk, 61 g	40	2	1	0	6

Half N Half

	Cal	Fat	Cbs	Fbr	Prtn
Country Fresh					
Fat Free Half & Half, 15 ml.	20	0	3	0	1
Gourmet Half & Half, 15 ml.	35	4	1	0	5
Dean's					
Fat Free Half & Half, 30 ml.	20	0	3	0	1
Gourmet Half & Half, 30 ml.	35	4	1	0	1
Land O'Lakes					
Fat Half & Half, 30 ml.	20	0	3	0	1
Gourmet Half & Half, 30 ml.	35	4	1	0	1

Light/Reduced/Fat Free Spreads

	Cal	Fat	Cbs	Fbr	Prtn
Country Crock					
Light (soft), 14 g	50	5	0	N/A	0
OmegaPlus Light, 14 g	50	5	0	0	0

Milk

	Cal	Fat	Cbs	Fbr	Prtn
Alta Dena					
Chocolate Lowfat, 240 ml.	200	3	32	0	11
Chocolate Whole, 240 ml.	260	9	37	1	6
Fat Free Milk, 240 ml.	90	0	13	0	9
Half and Half, 30 ml.	40	3	1	0	1
Reduced Fat Milk (2% Milkfat), 240 ml.	130	5	13	0	10
Whole Milk, 240 ml.	150	8	13	0	8
Carnation Milk					
Evaporated Milk, 2 tbsp.	40	2	3	N/A	2
Fat Free Evaporated Milk, 2 tbsp.	25	0	4	N/A	2
Instant Nonfat Dry Milk, 240 ml.	80	0	12	N/A	8
Lowfat 2% Evaporated Milk, 2 tbsp.	25	1	3	N/A	2
Sweetened Condensed Milk, 2 tbsp.	130	3	22	N/A	3
Country Fresh					
1% Milk, 240 ml.	100	3	13	0	8
1/2 % Milk, 240 ml.	100	1	13	0	9

(•= most healthy •= least healthy)

Milk (cont.)

	Cal	Fat	Cbs	Fbr	Prtn
Country Fresh (cont.)					
2% Milk, 240 ml.	120	5	12	0	8
Skim Milk, 240 ml.	90	0	13	0	8
Whole Milk, 240 ml.	150	8	12	0	8
Dean's					
1 % Milk, 240 ml.	100	3	13	0	8
2 % Milk, 240 ml.	120	5	12	0	8
Skim Milk, 240 g	90	0	13	0	8
Whole Milk, 240 ml.	150	8	12	0	8
Eagle Brand					
Fat Free, 39 g	110	0	24	0	3
Lowfat Sweet Condensed Milk, 39 g	120	2	23	0	3
Original, 39 g	130	3	23	0	3
Land O'Lakes					
2% Milk, 240 ml.	120	5	12	0	8
Skim Chocolate Milk, 240 ml.	160	0	31	1	8
Skim Milk, 240 ml.	90	0	13	0	8
Strawberry Milk, 240 ml.	190	8	22	0	7
Whole Milk, 240 ml.	150	8	12	0	8
Skinny Cow Milk					
2% Reduced Fat Choc Milk, 236 ml.	150	0	26	0	11
Fat Free Whole Milk, 236 ml.	110	0	17	0	11
Smart Balance					
1% Lowfat Choc Milk, 240 ml.	150	1	26	N/A	9
1% Lowfat Milk, 240 ml.	130	3	14	N/A	10
Lactose-Free Fat Free Milk, 240 ml.	100	1	13	N/A	9

Milk Alternatives

	Cal	Fat	Cbs	Fbr	Prtn
Blue Diamond Almonds					
Original Almond Breeze					
• Chocolate, 8 fl.oz.	110	3	22	1	1
Original, 8 fl.oz.	60	3	8	1	1
Vanilla, 8 fl.oz.	90	3	16	1	1
Unsweetened Almond Breeze					
Chocolate - Unsweetened, 8 fl.oz.	45	4	3	1	2
Original - Unsweetened, 8 fl.oz.	40	3	2	1	1
Vanilla - Unsweetened, 8 fl.oz.	40	3	2	1	1
Taste the Dream					
Almond Dream Original, 8 fl.oz.	50	3	6	1	1
• Almond Dream Unsweetened, 8 fl.oz.	30	3	1	1	1

Non Dairy Creamers

	Cal	Fat	Cbs	Fbr	Prtn
Cremora					
Original, 2 g	10	1	1	0	0
• Lite & Creamy, 2 g	10	0	1	0	0
International Delight					
Amaretto Bottles, 15 ml.	40	2	7	0	0
Chocolate Caramel, 15 ml.	45	2	7	0	0
Chocolate Cream, 13 ml.	35	2	6	0	0
Dulce de Leche, 15 ml.	45	2	7	0	0
French Vanilla Bottles, 15 ml.	45	2	7	0	0
• Vanilla Hazelnut, 15 ml.	45	2	7	0	0

DAIRY, FATS, & OILS

Non Dairy Creamers (cont.)	Cal	Fat	Cbs	Fbr	Prtn
Silk Soymilk					
French Vanilla, 15 ml.	20	1	3	0	0
Hazelnut, 15 ml.	20	1	3	0	0
Original, 15 ml.	15	1	1	0	0

Rice Milk	Cal	Fat	Cbs	Fbr	Prtn
Taste the Dream					
Rice Dream® Refrigerated					
Enriched Original, 8 fl.oz.	120	3	23	0	1
Enriched Vanilla, 8 fl.oz.	130	3	26	0	1
Rice Dream® Shelf Stable					
Enriched Chocolate, 8 fl.oz.	160	3	34	1	2
Original, 8 fl.oz.	120	3	24	0	1
Vanilla, 8 fl.oz.	130	3	27	0	1

Sour Cream	Cal	Fat	Cbs	Fbr	Prtn
Alouette					
Cuisine™, Crème Fraîche, 28 g	110	11	1	0	1
Reserve™, 28 g	100	8	1	0	5
Alta Dena					
Creme Fraiche, 28 g	110	11	1	0	1
Light Sour Cream (2% Milkfat), 30 g	60	5	1	0	1
Sour Cream (4% Milkfat), 30 g	60	5	1	0	1
Breakstone's					
Sour Cream - All Natural, 30 g	60	5	1	0	1
Sour Cream - Free Fat Free, 32 g	30	0	5	0	1
Sour Cream - Reduced Fat, 31 g	40	3	2	0	1
Country Fresh					
Fat Free Sour Cream, 30 g	20	0	3	0	1
Light Sour Cream, 30 g	40	3	2	0	1
Sour Cream, 30 g	60	6	2	0	1
Dean's					
Fat Free Sour Cream, 30 g	20	0	3	0	1
Light Sour Cream, 30 g	40	3	2	0	1
Sour Cream, 30 g	60	6	2	0	1
Knudsen					
Fat Free, 32 g	30	0	5	0	2
Hampshire 100% Natural, 30 g	60	6	1	0	1
Light, 31 g	30	2	2	0	2
Land O'Lakes					
Sour Cream					
Fat Free Sour Cream, 30 g	20	0	3	0	1
Light Sour Cream, 30 g	40	3	2	0	1
Sour Cream, 30 g	60	6	2	0	1

Soy Milk	Cal	Fat	Cbs	Fbr	Prtn
8-th Continent					
Fat Free					
Original, 8 fl.oz.	60	0	8	0	6
Vanilla, 8 fl.oz.	70	0	11	0	6
Light					
Chocolate, 8 fl.oz.	90	2	12	1	7
Original, 8 fl.oz.	50	2	2	0	6

(●= most healthy ●= least healthy)

POPULAR BRANDS

DAIRY, FATS, & OILS

Soy Milk (cont.)

	Cal	Fat	Cbs	Fbr	Prtn
8-th Continent (cont.)					
Light (cont.)					
Vanilla, 8 fl.oz.	60	2	5	0	6
Original					
Chocolate, 8 fl.oz.	140	3	22	1	7
Original, 8 fl.oz.	80	3	7	0	6
Vanilla, 8 fl.oz.	100	3	11	0	6
Silk Soymilk					
Light					
Light Chocolate, 240 ml.	120	2	22	2	5
Light Plain, 240 ml.	70	2	8	1	6
Light Vanilla, 240 ml.	80	2	10	1	6
Unsweetened, 240 ml.	80	4	4	1	7
Original					
Chocolate, 240 ml.	140	4	23	2	5
Plain, 240 ml.	100	4	8	1	7
Vanilla, 240 ml.	100	4	10	1	6
Taste the Dream					
Soy Dream Refrigerated					
Classic Original, 8 fl.oz.	130	4	16	2	7
Enriched Original, 8 fl.oz.	100	4	9	2	8
Enriched Vanilla, 8 fl.oz.	120	4	14	2	8
Soy Dream Shelf Stable					
• Enriched Chocolate, 8 fl.oz.	150	4	21	3	7
Enriched Original, 8 fl.oz.	100	4	8	2	7
Enriched Vanilla, 8 fl.oz.	120	4	14	2	7

Whipped Cream

	Cal	Fat	Cbs	Fbr	Prtn
Alta Dena					
Heavy Whipping Cream, 15 ml.	50	5	0	0	0
• Whipped Light Cream, 6 g	15	1	1	0	0
Country Fresh					
Aersol Whipped Light Cream, 7 g	20	2	1	0	0
Heavy Whipping Cream, 15 ml.	50	5	0	0	0
Dean's					
Aersol Whipped Light Cream, 7 g	20	2	1	0	0
Heavy Wipping Cream, 15 ml.	50	5	0	0	0
Land O'Lakes					
Aerosol Whipped Light Cream, 7 g	20	2	1	0	0
• Heavy Whipping Cream, 15 ml.	50	5	0	0	0

Yogurt

	Cal	Fat	Cbs	Fbr	Prtn
Alta Dena					
All Natural Yogurt					
Black Cherry, 227 g	220	2	41	0	9
Peach, 227 g	220	2	41	0	9
Strawberry Banana, 227 g	210	3	39	1	9
Lowfat Yogurt					
Plain, 227 g	170	5	20	1	13
Nonfat Yogurt					
Plain, 227 g	110	0	16	0	11
Strawberry, 227 g	181	0	36	0	9

DAIRY, FATS, & OILS

Yogurt (cont.)

	Cal	Fat	Cbs	Fbr	Prtn
Alta Dena (cont.)					
Nonfat Yogurt (cont.)					
Vanilla, 227 g	160	0	30	0	10
Columbo Yogurt					
Banana Strawberry, 1 cup	230	2	47	N/A	7
Colombo Classic, 1 cup	220	2	42	N/A	7
Fat Free Light Yogurt, 1 cup	120	0	21	N/A	7
Lowfat Plain Flavour, 227 g	100	0	16	N/A	10
Lowfat Plain, 227 g	130	3	16	N/A	10
Lowfat French Vanilla, 227 g	180	3	32	N/A	8
Nonfat Vanila, 227 g	100	0	32	N/A	8
Strawberry, 227 g	190	3	33	N/A	8
Country Fresh					
Strawberry Lowfat Yogurt, 8 oz.	190	2	36	0	8
Strawberry Light Yogurt, 8 oz.	80	0	38	0	8
Dannon Light & Fit					
Carb & Sugar Control					
Blueberries & Cream, 4 oz.	60	3	3	0	5
Peaches & Cream, 4 oz.	60	3	3	0	5
Strawberries & Cream, 4 oz.	60	3	3	0	5
Vanilla & Cream, 4 oz.	60	3	3	0	5
Original					
• Blackberry, 6 oz.	60	0	10	0	5
Strawberry, 6 oz.	60	0	11	0	5
Vanilla, 6 oz.	60	0	10	0	5
White Chocolate Raspberry, 6 oz.	60	0	10	0	5
Land O'Lakes					
Strawberry Light Yogurt, 8 oz.	80	0	38	0	8
Strawberry Lowfat Yogurt, 8 oz.	190	2	36	0	8
Silk Soymilk					
Raspberry, 6 oz.	150	2	30	1	4
Strawberry, 6 oz.	160	2	31	1	4
Vanilla, 6 oz.	150	3	25	1	5

DELI FOODS

Deli Meats

	Cal	Fat	Cbs	Fbr	Prtn
Empire Kosher					
Deli Breasts					
Honey Smoked Turkey Breast, 56 g	45	0	3	0	11
Skinless All Natural Turkey Breast, 56 g	60	1	0	0	15
Smoked Turkey Breast, 57 g	45	0	0	0	9
Whole Turkey Pastrami, 56 g	70	4	0	0	9
Deli Slices					
Chicken Bologna, 45 g	80	6	1	0	5
Oven Prepared Turkey Breast, 57 g	50	0	1	0	11
Smoked Turkey Breast, 57 g	45	0	0	0	9
Turkey Salami, 64 g	90	5	0	0	12
Farmer John					
• Premium Oven Roasted Turkey Brst, 28 g	25	0	1	0	5
Sliced Cotto Salami, 56 g	140	11	3	0	7
Sliced Thick Bologna, 2 oz.	160	14	2	0	6
Sliced Bologna, 2 oz.	160	14	2	0	6

POPULAR BRANDS

DELI FOODS

Deli Meats (cont.)	Cal	Fat	Cbs	Fbr	Prtn
Hebrew National					
Beef Bologna, 1 slice	90	8	0	N/A	3
• Beef Bologna Chubs, 2 oz.	180	17	0	0	6
Beef Salami, 2 oz.	160	15	0	0	8
Sliced Bologna, 1 slice	90	8	0	N/A	3
Sliced Salami, 3 slices	170	15	0	N/A	8
Oscar Mayer					
Bologna					
Bologna 98% Fat Free, 28 g	25	1	3	N/A	3
Bologna Beef, 28 g	90	8	1	N/A	3
Bologna Light, 28 g	60	4	2	N/A	3
Deli Fresh					
Chicken Breast Oven Roasted, 65 g	70	2	1	N/A	11
Ham Cooked, 28 g	30	1	0	N/A	5
Ham Honey Shaved, 51 g	50	1	2	N/A	9
Salami Beef Deli Thin, 51 g	150	13	1	0	8
Turkey Breast Smoked Shaved, 51 g	45	1	1	N/A	8
Turkey Breast Smoked, 63 g	60	1	0	N/A	13
Ham					
Ham Baked, 63 g	60	2	1	0	10
Ham Honey, 63 g	70	2	2	N/A	11
Ham Smoked 96% Fat Free, 63 g	50	1	0	N/A	10
Turkey					
Turkey Honey Smoked Lean White, 28 g	35	2	2	N/A	3
Turkey Oven Roasted White, 28 g	30	1	1	N/A	4

Packaged Meals	Cal	Fat	Cbs	Fbr	Prtn
Carl Buddig					
Buddig Original Deli Pouches					
Beef, 2 oz.	90	5	1	N/A	10
Chicken, 2 oz.	110	7	1	N/A	12
Corned Beef, 2 oz.	90	5	1	N/A	10
Ham w/ Natural Juices, 2 oz.	120	7	1	N/A	12
• Honey Ham w/ Natural Juices, 2 oz.	120	7	3	N/A	12
Honey Turkey, 2 oz.	120	7	3	N/A	12
Oven-Roasted Turkey, 2 oz.	110	7	1	N/A	12
Pastrami, 2 oz.	90	5	1	N/A	10
Turkey, 2 oz.	110	7	1	N/A	12
Original Big Pak Deli Pouches					
Beef, 2 oz.	90	5	1	N/A	10
Chicken, 2 oz.	85	5	1	N/A	10
Corned Beef, 2 oz.	90	5	1	N/A	10
Ham w/ NaturalJuices, 2 oz.	85	5	1	N/A	10
Honey Ham w/ Natural Juices, 2 oz.	90	5	2	N/A	10
Honey Turkey, 2 oz.	90	5	2	N/A	9
Oven-Roasted Turkey, 2 oz.	90	5	1	N/A	9
Turkey, 2 oz.	90	5	1	N/A	9
Value Pack Deli Pouches					
Beef, 2 oz.	90	5	1	N/A	10
Chicken, 2 oz.	85	5	1	N/A	10
Corned Beef, 2 oz.	90	5	1	N/A	10
Ham w/ Natural Juices, 2 oz.	85	5	1	N/A	10

Packaged Meals (cont.)

	Cal	Fat	Cbs	Fbr	Prtn
Carl Buddig (cont.)					
Deli Cuts					
Baked Honey Ham, 2 oz.	80	3	3	N/A	10
Honey Roasted Cured Turkey Breast, 2 oz.	80	3	3	N/A	10
Oven Roasted Cured Chicken Breast, 2 oz.	70	3	1	N/A	10
Oven Roasted Cured Turkey Breast, 2 oz.	70	3	1	N/A	10
Smoked Turkey Breast, 2 oz.	70	3	1	N/A	10
Value Pack Deli Pouches (cont.)					
Honey Ham w/ Natural Juices, 2 oz.	90	5	2	N/A	10
Honey Turkey, 2 oz.	90	5	2	N/A	9
Turkey, 2 oz.	90	5	1	N/A	9

Sandwiches/Wraps

	Cal	Fat	Cbs	Fbr	Prtn
Oscar Mayer					
Deli Creations: Complete Sandwiches					
Oven Roasted Ham & Cheddar, 1 pk	460	16	51	3	29
Oven Roasted Ham & Cheddar, 1/2 pk	230	8	26	2	16
Steakhouse Cheddar, 1 pk	430	140	47	5	28
Turkey & Cheddar Dijon, 1 pk	430	15	48	5	26
Turkey Monterey, 1 pk	450	17	50	4	25
Deli Creations: Flatbread Sandwich					
Buffalo Style Ranch Chicken, 1 pk	310	11	30	1	22
Chicken & Bacon Ranch, 1 pk	320	13	30	1	22
Fajita Beef & Salsa, 1 pk	280	9	34	1	20
Steakhouse Beef, 1 pk	330	14	30	1	20
Sun Dried Tomato Chicken, 1 pk	300	13	31	1	23
South Beach Living					
Deli Ham & Turkey Ref. Wrap, 194 g	220	10	23	15	22
Grilled Chicken Caesar Ref. Wrap, 182 g	230	11	22	14	24
Sesame Chicken Ref. Wrap, 182 g	220	9	28	15	21
Southwestern Style Chicken Ref. Wrap, 222 g	240	11	26	15	25
Turkey & Bacon Club Ref. Wrap, 199 g	240	12	24	14	24
Tyson Chicken					
Asiago Roast Beef Wrap , 1 pc.	320	14	30	2	20
South of the Border Chicken Wrap, 1 pc.	390	21	30	2	19
Turkey Club Wrap, 1 pc.	390	23	28	2	19

Side Dishes

	Cal	Fat	Cbs	Fbr	Prtn
Country Crock					
Seasonal Side Dishes					
Deluxe Cornbread Stuffing, 100 g	150	5	22	1	4
Deluxe Homestyle Stuffing, 100 g	150	5	22	1	5
Deluxe Mashed Sweet Potatoes, 142 g	200	6	36	2	2
Side Dishes					
Deluxe Cheddar Broccoli Rice, 200 g	270	11	35	1	8
Deluxe Cinnamon Apples, 125 g	130	3	26	1	0
Deluxe Four Cheese Pasta, 230 g	380	17	41	2	15
Deluxe Loaded Mashed Potatoes, 142 g	200	11	22	2	4
Homestyle Mashed Potatoes, 142 g	180	9	23	2	2

(•= most healthy •= least healthy)

POPULAR BRANDS

DESSERTS

Cakes

	Cal	Fat	Cbs	Fbr	Prtn
Pepperidge Farm					
• Chocolate Coconut 3 Layer Cake, 1/8 cake	240	10	33	1	2
• Devil's Food 3 Layer Cake, 1/8 cake	220	9	34	1	2
Peppermint 3 Layer Cake, 1/8 cake	230	11	31	2	2

Cookies

	Cal	Fat	Cbs	Fbr	Prtn
100 Calorie Packs					
Cookie Crisps					
Alpha-bits Mini Cookies 6 Ct, 21 g	100	3	16	0	1
Chips Ahoy! 6 Ct, 23 g	100	3	18	1	1
Lorna Doone, 21 g	100	3	16	0	1
Planters Peanut Butter, 24 g	100	3	17	1	2
Variety Pack, 21 g	100	3	16	0	1
Chips Ahoy					
Big & Soft Chocolate Chunk, 39 g	170	7	27	1	1
Big & Soft Oatmeal Choc.Chunk, 39 g	180	8	26	1	2
Chewy Oatmeal Chocolate Chip, 27 g	120	6	18	1	1
Chewy, 27 g	120	6	18	1	1
Chocolate Chip Candy Blasts, 17 g	90	5	11	0	1
Chocolate Chip, 40 g	190	9	27	1	2
Chunky Chocolate, 17 g	80	5	11	1	1
Chunky White Fudge, 17 g	80	5	11	0	1
Mini Chocolate Chip Packs 2 Go!, 35 g	170	9	23	1	2
Peanut Butter Chunky, 17 g	90	5	10	0	1
Reduced Fat, 32 g	140	5	23	1	2
Famous Amos Cookies					
Chocolate Chip, 4 cookies	150	7	20	1	1
Oatmeal Raisin, 4 cookies	140	6	20	1	2
Peanut Butter Sandwich, 3 cookies	160	7	22	1	3
Vanilla Creme Sandwich, 4 cookies	170	7	25	1	2
Ginger Snaps					
Ginger Snaps, 28 g	120	3	23	0	1
Hershey Chocolates					
Caramel Cookies, 28 g	130	6	19	N/A	1
Hershey's With Almonds Cookies, 28 g	150	9	16	1	2
Sandwich Cookies, 28 g	130	6	1	N/A	1
Keebler					
Chips Deluxe					
Chocolate Lovers, 16 g	100	5	10	0	1
Original, 57 g	200	16	37	1	3
Peanut Butter Cups, 16 g	90	5	10	1	1
Soft 'n Chewy, 16 g	80	4	11	1	1
EL Fudge					
Double Stuffed, 35 g	180	9	24	1	2
Original, 18 g	90	4	13	1	1
Fudge Shoppe					
Caramel Filled, 30 g	160	8	20	0	1
Fudge Stripes, 21 g	150	7	21	1	1
Grasshopper, 29 g	140	7	19	1	1
Peanut Butter Filled, 30 g	170	10	16	1	3
Sandies					
Fudge Drops, 27 g	140	7	18	1	1

Cookies (cont.)

	Cal	Fat	Cbs	Fbr	Prtn
Keebler (cont.)					
Sandies (cont.)					
Simply Shortbread, 16 g	80	5	10	0	1
Vanilla Wafers					
Mini Vanilla Wafers, 30 g	140	6	21	1	1
Vanilla Wafers, 30 g	140	6	21	1	1
Mallomars					
Mallomars Cookies Pure Chocolate, 27 g	120	5	18	1	1
Mauna Loa					
Chocolate Chip, 28 g	150	9	17	1	1
Toffee Crunch, 28 g	150	9	17	1	1
Newtons					
Fig 100% Whole Grain, 37 g	130	3	26	3	1
Fig Newtons, 31 g	110	2	22	1	1
Fig Newtons Fat Free, 30 g	90	0	22	1	1
Fig Strawberry, 29 g	100	2	21	0	1
Nilla Wafers					
Mini, 30 g	140	6	21	0	1
Reduced Fat, 29 g	110	2	24	0	1
Wafers, 30 g	140	6	21	0	1
Nutter Butter					
Bites, 35 g	170	7	24	1	3
Bites - Milk Chocolate Covered PB, 36 g	180	9	24	1	2
Nutter Butter, 54 g	260	11	37	1	4
Sandwich Cookies, 28 g	130	6	19	1	2
Oreo					
• Chocolate, 57 g	270	11	41	2	3
Double Stuffed, 42 g	210	10	30	1	1
Original Golden, 35 g	170	7	25	0	1
Original Oreo, 34 g	160	7	25	1	2
Pure White Fudge Covered, 20 g	100	5	13	0	1
Reduced Fat, 34 g	150	5	27	1	1
Pepperidge Farm					
Black & White Milano, 3 cookies	180	10	21	1	2
Chocolate Fudge Pirouettes, 2 wafers	120	4	18	1	1
Chocolate Petite Truffle, 5 cookies	180	12	15	1	2
Dark Chocolate Drenched Milano, 1 cookie	90	6	10	0	1
French Vanilla Pirouettes, 2 wafers	120	5	18	0	1
Geneva Cookies, 3 cookies	160	9	19	1	2
Milano Cookies, 3 cookies	180	10	21	1	2
Mini Butter Cookies, 9 cookies	140	6	21	1	2
Mint Brussels Cookies, 3 cookies	190	10	22	1	2
Orange Milano Cookies, 2 cookies	130	7	16	1	1
Soft Baked Milk Chocolate, 1 cookie	150	7	21	1	1
Sugar Free Milano, 3 cookies	170	9	21	1	2
Tahiti Cookies, 2 cookies	170	10	17	2	2
Sargento					
Chocolate Dip & Cookie Sticks, 28 g	130	6	18	1	1
S'mores, 22 g	110	6	14	0	1
Strawberry Dip & Cookie Sticks, 28 g	130	5	19	0	1
Snack Wells					
• Devil's Food Fat Free, 7 oz.	50	0	12	0	1

(• = most healthy • = least healthy)

DESSERTS

Cookies (cont.)	Cal	Fat	Cbs	Fbr	Prtn
Snack Wells (cont.)					
Cakes Chocolate Mint, 7 oz.	50	1	12	0	1
Cookies Creme Sandwich, 8 oz.	110	3	20	0	1
Lemon Creme Sugar Free, 7 oz.	130	6	23	2	1
Shortbread Sugar Free, 7 oz.	130	6	21	2	2
Sorbee					
Animal Cookies, 28 g	100	3	21	0	1
Chocolate Chip, 25 g	110	6	16	0	1
Chocolate Sandwich Cookies, 25 g	110	5	19	0	19
Lemon Sandwich Cookies, 25 g	120	5	18	0	1
Oatmeal, 25 g	110	4	10	0	2
Peanut Butter, 25 g	110	7	10	0	3
South Beach Living					
Hazelnut Crème Wafer Sticks, 22 g	100	6	10	3	5
Peanut Butter Wafer Sticks, 22 g	100	6	10	3	5
Stauffer's					
Breakfast Animal Cookies, 1 oz.	140	6	21	1	2
Chocolate Chip Animal Cookies, 1 oz.	140	5	22	1	2
Cotton Candy Animal Cookies, 1 oz.	140	4	23	0	2
Lightly Iced Animal Cookies, 1 oz.	130	2	23	1	2
Assorted Cookies					
Coconut Crisps, 1 oz.	140	5	22	1	2
Ginger Snaps Bag, 1 oz.	120	4	22	1	2
Iced Animal Cookies, 2 oz.	210	6	38	1	3
Shortbread Cookies, 1 oz.	150	7	20	1	2
Snickerdoodles Box, 1 oz.	130	5	19	1	1
Sandwich Cremes					
Banana Sandwich Crèmes, 1 oz.	150	6	23	0	1
Chocolate Sandwich Crèmes, 1 oz.	150	5	23	1	1
Peanut Butter Sandwich Crèmes, 1 oz.	130	5	21	0	1
Strawberry Sandwich Crèmes, 1 oz.	150	6	23	1	1
Vanilla Sandwich Crèmes, 1 oz.	160	6	24	1	1
Sugar Wafers					
Chocolate Sugar Wafers, 1 oz.	160	9	22	1	1
Strawberry Sugar Wafers, 1 oz.	140	8	17	0	1
Vanilla Sugar Wafers, 1 oz.	140	8	17	0	1

Ice Cream Cakes & Pies	Cal	Fat	Cbs	Fbr	Prtn
Baskin Robbins					
Roll Ice Cream Cakes					
Mint Choc Chip Ice Crm/Choc, 117 g	290	14	36	2	5
• Vanilla Ice Crm/Choc, 117 g	270	14	39	2	4
Round Ice Cream Cakes					
• Choc Chip Cookie Dough Ice Crm/Devil's Food 6"	460	23	59	1	7
Pralines 'n Cream Ice Crm/White Sponge 9"	430	20	65	1	6
Vanilla & Choc Ice Crm/Fudge Crunch 9"	340	18	41	1	5
Sheet Ice Cream Cakes					
Pralines 'n Cream Ice Crm/White Sponge, 126 g	360	16	49	1	5
Vanilla & Choc Ice Crm/Fudge Crunch, 126 g	330	18	40	1	5
Very Strawberry Ice Crm/White Sponge, 126 g	310	13	44	1	4

Ice Cream Cones & Cups

Ice Cream Cones & Cups	Cal	Fat	Cbs	Fbr	Prtn
Comet Ice Cream Cones					
Ice Cream cups, 1 cup	20	0	4	0	0
Ice Cream cups - Rainbow, 1cup	20	0	4	N/A	0
Sugar Cones , 1 cone	50	0	11	N/A	1
Keebler					
Fudge Shoppe Cups, 8 g	35	2	6	0	0
Ice Cream Cups, 5 g	15	0	4	0	0
Sugar Cones, 13 g	50	1	10	0	1
Waffle Cones, 12 g	50	1	10	0	1
Oreo					
Chocolate Ice Cream Cones 12 Ct., 14 g	60	1	12	0	1

Ice Cream, Sorbet & Snacks

Ice Cream, Sorbet & Snacks	Cal	Fat	Cbs	Fbr	Prtn
Baskin Robbins					
Cappuccino Blasts®					
Caramel Medium, 24 fl.oz.	720	24	121	0	10
Mocha Medium, 24 fl.oz.	240	18	87	0	8
Oreo® N' Cookies Medium, 24 fl.oz.	800	31	118	2	13
Fruit Blast Bars					
Blue Raspberry Fruit Blast Bar, 1.75 fl.oz.	50	0	14	0	0
Mango Fruit Blast Bar, 1.75 fl.oz.	50	0	14	0	0
Strawberry Fruit Blast Bar, 1.75 fl.oz.	50	0	13	0	0
Grab-N-Go					
Choc Chip Cookie Dough Ice Crm, 73 g	200	10	23	0	3
Chocolate Ice Crm, 73 g	70	9	21	1	3
Jamoca® Almond Fudge Ice Crm, 76 g	180	10	21	1	4
Ice Cream: Classic Flavors					
French Vanilla Ice Cream, 4 oz.	280	18	26	0	4
Jamoca® Ice Cream, 4 oz.	240	13	26	0	5
Rocky Road Ice Cream, 4 oz.	290	15	36	1	5
Lighter Side: Lowfat, No Sugar Added					
Berries 'n Banana, 4 oz.	110	2	25	1	5
Chocolate Chocolate Chip, 4 oz.	150	5	31	1	6
Pineapple Coconut, 4 oz.	120	2	27	0	5
Nonfat Soft Serve Yogurt - No Sugar Added					
Truly Free® Cafe Mocha Nonfat Soft Serve, 88 g	90	0	18	1	4
Truly Free® Chocolate, 88 g	80	0	15	0	4
Truly Free® Vanilla, 88 g	90	0	17	1	4
Shakes					
Chocolate Oreo® Shake Medium, 633 g	1350	69	172	6	23
Strawberry Shake Medium, 24fl.oz	650	19	104	1	18
Vanilla Shake Medium, 24 fl.oz.	980	45	125	0	19
Sherbet					
Rainbow Sherbet, 4 oz.	160	2	34	0	1
Rock 'n Pop Swirl Sherbet, 4 oz.	190	4	37	0	1
Wild 'N Reckless Sherbet, 4 oz.	160	2	33	0	1
Sundaes					
Banana Royale Sundae, 316 g	630	27	91	5	9
Oreo® Sundae, 347 g	1030	47	147	3	11
• Peppermint Brownie Sundae, 512 g	1580	75	221	2	18
Sundae cups					
Oreo® Sundae cup, 1 cup	330	15	45	0	4

(•= most healthy •= least healthy)

Ice Cream, Sorbet & Snacks (cont.)	Cal	Fat	Cbs	Fbr	Prtn
Baskin Robbins (cont.)					
Sundae cups (cont.)					
Pralines 'n Cream Sundae Cup, 1 cup	330	16	43	1	4
Reese's® PB Sundae Cup, 1 cup	390	24	36	2	8
Ben & Jerry's					
Bars					
Cherry Garcia® Original Ice Cream, 1 bar	270	19	29	1	4
Vanilla Almond Original Ice Cream, 1 bar	340	23	30	2	5
Vanilla Original Ice Cream, 1 bar	300	20	26	1	4
Body & Soul™					
Cherry Garcia®, 1/2 cup	170	9	22	2	3
Choc Chip Cookie Dough, 1/2 cup	190	9	26	1	3
Chocolate Fudge Brownie™, 1/2 cup	180	7	25	2	4
Lowfat Frozen Yogurt					
Black Raspberry, 1/2 cup	140	2	28	1	3
Cherry Garcia®, 1/2 cup	170	3	32	1	4
Chocolate Fudge, 1/2 cup	190	3	35	1	5
Lowfat, 1/2 cup	170	3	33	1	5
Half Baked®, 1/2 cup	190	3	35	1	5
Vanilla Low, 1/2 cup	130	2	25	0	4
Novelties					
Wich Ice Cream Cookie Sandwich™	350	18	45	1	4
Organic Ice Cream					
Chocolate Fudge Brownie™, 1/2 cup	270	13	30	2	4
Strawberry, 1/2 cup	210	12	21	0	3
Sweet Cream & Cookies, 1/2 cup	250	15	24	0	4
Vanilla Organic Ice Cream, 1/2 cup	220	14	18	0	3
Original Ice Cream					
Black & Tan™, 1/2 cup	230	13	24	1	4
Chubby Hubby®, 1/2 cup	330	20	31	1	7
Oatmeal Cookie Chunk, 1/2 cup	270	15	31	1	4
Sorbet					
Berried Treasure™, 1/2 cup	110	0	29	1	0
Berry Berry Extraordinary™, 1/2 cup	100	0	27	1	0
Jamaican Me Crazy, 1/2 cup	130	0	33	4	0
Mango Lime, 1/2 cup	100	0	27	0	0
Strawberry Kiwi, 1/2 cup	110	0	27	1	0
Strawberry Kiwi Swirl, 1/2 cup	110	0	28	1	0
Blue Bunny Ice Cream					
Classics: Gelato					
Gelato Chocolate, 89 g	180	8	24	1	3
Gelato Hazelnut, 89 g	170	7	23	0	4
Gelato Italian Chocolate Chip, 64 g	130	7	16	0	2
Classics: Original					
Original Ice Cream Mint Chip, 66 g	140	7	17	0	2
Original Ice Cream Neapolitan, 66 g	130	6	16	0	2
Original Ice Cream Strawberry, 66 g	120	6	17	0	2
Classics: Premium					
All Natural Vanilla, 72 g	160	9	16	0	3
Double Strawberry, 74 g	140	6	20	0	2
Homemade Chocolate, 69 g	150	7	16	0	4

DESSERTS

Ice Cream, Sorbet & Snacks (cont.)	Cal	Fat	Cbs	Fbr	Prtn
Blue Bunny Ice Cream (cont.)					
Lighter Options: Ice Cream					
Peanut Butter Fudge, 69 g	150	10	15	4	3
Rocky Road, 71 g	130	6	21	2	4
Vanilla, 69 g	110	5	16	2	3
Lighter Options: Bars					
Sweet Freedom® Fudge Lites, 101 g	70	1	17	6	4
Sweet Freedom® Sugar Free Pops, 53 g	15	0	7	2	0
Sweet Freedom® Supremes® PB cup, 55 g	160	11	17	2	3
Lighter Options: No Sugar Added, Fat Free Ice Cream					
Brownie Sundae, 74 g	90	0	23	5	3
Caramel Toffee Crunch, 71 g	90	0	24	5	3
Vanilla, 71 g	80	0	20	5	4
Lighter Options: No Sugar Added, Fat Free Bars					
FrozFruit® Chunky Strawberry, 90 g	35	0	15	3	0
Health Smart® Rasp. & Orange Crème Bars, 63 g	70	0	17	4	1
Sugar Free Bomb Pop®, 53 g	25	0	8	2	0
Lighter Options: Personals®					
Bunny Tracks®, 68 g	130	5	21	3	3
Double Strawberry, 69 g	100	2	19	3	2
Super Fudge Brownie®, 67 g	120	3	22	3	3
Lighter Options: 100 Calorie Bars					
English Toffee Ice Cream Bars, 39 g	100	8	10	2	2
Orange & Raspberry Ice Cream Bars, 1 Bar	100	1	19	0	3
Pecan Ice Cream Bars, 39 g	100	7	10	2	2
Lighter Options: Hi Lite					
Cookies & Cream, 65 g	130	4	21	0	2
Homemade Vanilla, 67 g	110	4	18	0	3
Vanilla, 65 g	100	3	17	0	2
Lighter Options: Fat Free: Novelties					
FrozFruit® Chunky Strawberry, 90 g	70	0	18	1	0
FrozFruit® Double Lime, 120 g	90	0	22	0	0
FrozFruit® Superfruit® Raspberry Acai, 90 g	60	0	15	1	0
Lighter Options: Fat Free: Frozen Yogurt					
Brownie Fudge Fantasy, 74 g	110	0	24	0	3
Homemade Vanilla, 74 g	100	0	19	0	4
Strawberry Cheesecake, 74 g	100	0	21	0	3
Yogurt Varieties: Light No Sugar Added					
Black Cherry Burst, 170 g	80	0	11	0	7
Blueberry Bliss, 170 g	80	0	12	0	7
Key Lime Pie, 170 g	80	0	11	0	7
Yogurt Varieties: Light Superfruit					
Black Currant, 170 g	100	0	14	0	7
Mango Pomegranate, 170 g	100	0	14	0	7
Pomegranate Cherry, 170 g	100	0	14	0	7
Yogurt Varieties: Light Omega 3					
Blackberry Crème, 113 g	80	1	14	0	5
Raspberry Crème, 113 g	80	1	14	0	5
Strawberry Patch, 113 g	80	1	14	0	5
Yogurt Varieties: Light					
Key Lime Pie, 170 g	100	0	15	0	7
Strawberry Sensation, 170 g	100	0	15	0	7

(• = most healthy • = least healthy)

Ice Cream, Sorbet & Snacks (cont.)	Cal	Fat	Cbs	Fbr	Prtn
Blue Bunny Ice Cream (cont.)					
Yogurt Varieties: Light (cont.)					
Vanilla Crème, 170 g	100	0	16	0	7
Country Fresh					
Ice Cream,					
Light Vanilla Ice Cream, 65 g	100	3	17	0	3
Orange Sherbet, 90 g	130	2	28	0	2
Vanila Ice Cream, 68 g	150	8	17	0	2
Dean's					
Light Vanilla Ice Cream, 65 g	100	3	17	0	3
Orange Sherbet, 90 g	130	2	28	0	2
Vanilla Ice Cream, 68 g	150	8	17	0	2
Dreyer's Ice Cream					
Dibs					
Rocky Road w/ Choc Almond Coating, 26 pcs	400	29	29	2	5
Strawberry w/ Choc Coating, 26 pcs	370	26	30	1	3
Vanilla with NESTLÉ CRUNCH® Coating, 26 pcs	370	26	30	1	3
Fruit Bars					
Creamy Coconut, 1 Bar	120	3	21	1	3
Grape, 1 Bar	80	0	20	0	0
Strawberry, 1 Bar	120	N/A	29	1	N/A
Grand					
Chocolate, 1/2 cup	150	8	17	1	3
Coffee, 1/2 cup	140	8	15	0	2
Mint Chocolate Chip, 1/2 cup	170	9	18	0	3
Vanilla, 1/2 cup	150	10	14	0	2
Light					
Double Fudge Brownie, 1/2 cup	120	4	120	1	3
French Vanilla, 1/2 cup	100	4	15	0	3
Peanut Butter cup, 1/2 cup	130	6	17	0	3
Strawberry, 1/2 cup	110	3	18	0	2
Loaded					
Butter Finger, 1/2 cup	130	5	19	1	3
Chocolate Chip Cookie Dough, 1/2 cup	130	5	21	1	2
Cookies 'N Cream, 1/2 cup	110	4	18	1	2
No Sugar Added					
Butter Pecan, 1/2 cup	120	5	15	2	3
French Vanilla, 1/2 cup	100	3	14	2	3
Neapolitan, 1/2 cup	90	3	13	2	3
Triple Chocolate, 1/2 cup	110	4	17	2	3
Sherbet					
Berry Rainbow, 1/2 cup	130	2	29	N/A	1
Orange Cream, 1/2 cup	120	2	23	N/A	2
Swiss Orange, 1/2 cup	150	3	30	N/A	1
Yogurt Blends					
Berry Granola Crunch, 1/2 cup	120	4	19	0	3
Cappuccino Chip, 1/2 cup	110	4	18	0	2
Chocolate Fudge Brownie, 1/2 cup	120	4	19	1	3
Peach, 1/2 cup	100	2	17	0	2
Edy's Ice Cream					
Grand					
French Vanilla, 1/2 cup	151	9	16	0	2

DESSERTS

Ice Cream, Sorbet & Snacks (cont.)	Cal	Fat	Cbs	Fbr	Prtn
Edy's Ice Cream (cont.)					
Grand (cont.)					
Real Strawberry, 1/2 cup	130	6	16	0	2
Rocky Road, 1/2 cup	170	10	19	1	3
Spumoni, 1/2 cup	120	5	19	0	2
Light					
Cookie Dough, 1/2 cup	130	5	20	0	3
French Vanilla, 1/2 cup	100	4	15	0	3
Raspberry Chip Royale, 1/2 cup	120	4	18	0	3
Strawberry, 1/2 cup	110	3	18	0	2
No Sugar Added					
Coffee, 1/2 cup	90	3	13	2	3
Cookies 'N Cream, 1/2 cup	120	5	16	2	3
French Vanilla, 1/2 cup	100	3	14	2	3
Triple Chocolate, 1/2 cup	110	4	17	2	3
Yogurt Blends					
Berry Granola Crunch, 1/2 cup	120	4	19	0	3
Cappuccino Chip, 1/2 cup	110	4	18	0	2
Strawberry, 1/2 cup	100	3	17	0	2
Eskimo Pie					
Nestle Crunch Crisp & Butterfinger, 2 bars	250	17	21	0	2
Vanilla & Chocolate Snack Pack, 2 bars	200	16	18	1	3
Vanilla with Dark Chocolate Coating, 1 bar	160	11	14	1	2
Vanilla with Nestle Crunch Coating, 1 bar	210	14	18	0	2
Haagen-Dazs					
Bar					
Raspberry Sorbet & Vanilla Yogurt, 71 g	100	0	21	1	2
Vanilla & Almonds, 87 g	320	12	22	1	5
Vanilla & Milk Chocolate, 83 g	290	21	22	0	4
Classic Flavor					
Chocolate Peanut Butter, 109 g	360	24	27	2	8
Dulce De Leche, 106 g	290	17	28	0	5
Pineapple Coconut, 95 g	230	13	25	0	4
Frozen Yogurt					
Vanilla, 106 g	200	5	31	0	9
Vanilla Raspberry Swirl, 108 g	170	3	32	0	4
Wildberry, 106 g	180	2	34	0	7
Light					
Caramel Cone, 110 g	250	8	39	0	6
Dutch Chocolate, 106 g	190	5	33	1	4
Mint Chip, 109 g	230	8	34	0	6
Reserve					
Brazilian Açai Berry Sorbet, 106 g	120	2	25	1	0
Pomegranate & Dk Choco Ice Cream Bars, 84 g	280	18	27	1	3
Toasted Coconut Sesame Brittle Ice Cream, 102 g	300	18	31	1	4
Sorbet					
Coconut, 106 g	170	7	26	0	1
Mango, 114 g	120	0	37	0	0
Raspberry, 105 g	120	0	30	2	0
Healthy Choice					
Lowfat Fudge Bar, 1 bar	90	2	15	5	4
Sorbet Cream Bar, 1 bar	90	1	17	12	1

(• = most healthy • = least healthy)

Ice Cream, Sorbet & Snacks (cont.)	Cal	Fat	Cbs	Fbr	Prtn
Healthy Choice (cont.)					
Vanilla Ice Cream Sandwich, 1 Sandwich	130	2	25	2	3
Kool Aid					
Kool Pops Freezer Bars - Variety, 85 g	50	0	13	N/A	0
Land O'Lakes					
Ice Cream					
Light Vanilla Ice Cream, 65 g	100	3	17	0	3
Orange Sherbet, 90 g	130	2	28	0	2
Vanilla Ice Cream, 68 g	150	8	17	0	2
M&M's Bakery					
M&M'S Brand Ice Cream					
Cookie Dough Ice Cream, 1/2 cup	180	90	20	0	2
Cookie Ice Cream Sandwiches, 86 g	260	110	34	0	3
Ice Cream Cake, 4 fl.oz.	240	120	28	1	3
Ice Cream Cone, 79 g	250	110	33	1	3
Ice Cream Treats, 49 g	190	130	13	0	1
Taste the Dream					
Rice Dream® Non-Dairy Frozen Desserts - Novelties					
Chocolate Frozen Pies, 96 g	330	19	40	2	3
Mocha Frozen Pies, 96 g	330	19	40	2	3
Vanilla Bars with Chocolate Coating, 85 g	230	15	24	1	1
Rice Dream® Non-Dairy Frozen Desserts - Pints and Quarts					
Strawberry, 80 g	160	8	25	2	0
Vanilla Swiss Almond, 70 g	190	10	24	0	1
Vanilla, 70 g	150	6	23	1	0
Soy Dream® Non-Dairy Frozen Desserts					
Butter Pecan Pint, 70 g	150	9	19	1	1
Chocolate Quart, 70 g	120	6	17	1	1
Strawberry Swirl Quart, 70 g	140	7	20	1	1
Soy Dream® Non-Dairy Frozen Novelties					
Chocolate Lil' Dreamers, 40 g	100	5	15	1	1
Vanilla Lil' Dreamers, 40 g	100	4	15	0	1
Tropicana Juice					
Cherry Berry, 40 g	140	0	36	2	1
Orange Citrus, 40 g	140	0	36	2	1
Strawberry, 40 g	140	0	36	2	0
Smuckers					
Magic Shell					
Caramel, 34 g	220	17	14	0	2
Welch's					
Concord Grape No Sugar Added, 2 fl.oz.	30	0	8	N/A	0
Concord Grape, 3 fl.oz.	90	0	22	N/A	0
Strawberry Breeze - No Sugar Added, 2 fl.oz.	25	0	6	N/A	0
Strawberry Breeze, 2 fl.oz.	50	0	13	N/A	0
Wild Berry - No Sugar Added, 2 fl.oz.	25	0	6	N/A	0
Wild Berry, 2 fl.oz.	50	0	13	N/A	0

Ice Cream Toppings	Cal	Fat	Cbs	Fbr	Prtn
Smuckers					
Magic Shell					
• Caramel, 34 g	220	17	14	0	2
Chocolate, 34 g	210	16	17	1	1

DESSERTS
Ice Cream Toppings (cont.)

	Cal	Fat	Cbs	Fbr	Prtn
Smuckers (cont.)					
Magic Shell (cont.)					
Smores, 36 g	220	16	19	1	1
Turtle Delight, 34 g	210	15	17	1	1
Microwaveable Ice Cream Topping					
Chocolate Fudge, 40 g	130	2	28	1	0
Hot Fudge, 30 g	120	4	22	1	2
Specialty Ice Cream Topping					
Dove® Milk Chocolate, 38 g	130	4	21	1	2
Special Recipe Butterscotch Caramel, 42 g	140	1	31	0	1
Special Recipe Hot Fudge, 38 g	130	5	20	1	2
Special Recipe Triple Berry, 2 tbsp.	90	0	23	1	0
Spoonable Ice Cream Topping					
Butterscotch, 41 g	120	0	30	0	0
Dark Chocolate with Mint, 39 g	110	2	24	1	1
Dulce de Leche, 41 g	150	5	26	0	1
Hot Caramel, 41 g	140	4	27	0	1
Hot Fudge, 39 g	130	5	22	1	2
Light Hot Fudge, 39 g	90	0	23	2	2
Marshmallow, 40 g	110	28	28	N/A	0
Pecans in Syrup, 36 g	160	9	19	0	1
Strawberry, 40 g	100	0	26	N/A	0
Walnuts in Syrup, 36 g	150	7	20	1	2
Sugar Free Ice Cream Topping					
Caramel, 38 g	90	0	24	N/A	0
Hot Fudge, 38 g	90	0	24	1	19
• Strawberry, 33 g	25	0	9	N/A	0

Pudding & Gelatin

	Cal	Fat	Cbs	Fbr	Prtn
Snack Pack					
Banana Pudding, 1 pudding cup	110	4	19	0	1
Butterscotch Pudding, 1 pudding cup	120	4	21	0	1
Chocolate Butterscotch Pudding, 1 pudding cup	130	5	22	0	2
Chocolate Pudding, 1 pudding cup	120	4	21	1	2
Fat Free Chocolate Pudding, 1 pudding cup	90	0	20	0	2
Fat Free Vanilla Pudding, 1 pudding cup	80	0	18	0	1
No Sugar Added Cherry Gels, 1 pudding cup	10	0	2	1	0
No Sugar Added Chocolate Pudding, 1 pudding cup	60	3	8	1	1
No Sugar Added Vanilla Pudding, 1 pudding cup	60	4	8	0	1
Strawberry Gelatin Gels, 1 Gel cup	5	0	2	1	0
• Strawberry Orange Gelatin Gels, 1 Gel cup	100	0	25	0	0
Tapioca Pudding, 1 pudding cup	120	4	20	0	2
Vanilla Pudding, 1 pudding cup	120	4	20	0	1
Swiss Miss					
Chocolate/vanilla Swirl Pudding, 1 pudding cup	140	4	27	0	2
Classic Butterscotch Pudding, 1 pudding cup	130	4	22	0	2
Creamy Milk Chocolate Pudding, 1 pudding cup	150	4	27	0	3
Old Fashioned Tapioca Pudding, 1 pudding cup	140	4	24	0	2
• Triple Chocolate Dream Pudding, 1 pudding cup	150	4	26	1	3

POPULAR BRANDS

DESSERTS

Pudding & Gelatin Mix	Cal	Fat	Cbs	Fbr	Prtn
Uncle Ben's					
• Cinnamon & Raisins Rice Pudding, 42 g	160	1	37	0	2
• French Vanilla Rice Pudding, 33 g	120	0	28	1	2

Whipped Toppings	Cal	Fat	Cbs	Fbr	Prtn
Cool Whip					
• Chocolate, 2 tbsp.	25	2	2	N/A	0
French Vanilla, 2 tbsp.	25	2	2	N/A	0
Extra Creamy, 2 tbsp.	25	2	2	N/A	0
Regular, 2 tbsp.	25	2	2	N/A	0
Strawberry, 2 tbsp.	25	2	2	N/A	0
Sugar Free, 2 tbsp.	25	1	3	N/A	0
Topping - Lite, 2 tbsp.	20	1	3	N/A	0
Dream Whip					
• Whipped Topping Mix - Regular	10	0	2	N/A	0

FROZEN MEALS

Appetizers & Sides	Cal	Fat	Cbs	Fbr	Prtn
Cascadian Farm					
• Potatoes Country-Style Potatoes, 85 g	40	0	9	2	1
Potatoes Country-Style, 85 g	50	0	12	1	1
Potatoes Crinkle Cut French Fries, 3 oz.	130	4	21	2	2
Potatoes French Fries Straight Cut, 3 oz.	130	4	21	2	2
Potatoes Hash Browns, 85 g	60	0	14	1	2
Potatoes Oven Fries Wedge Cut, 3 oz.	110	3	21	2	2
Potatoes Shoe String Fries, 3 oz.	140	5	21	2	2
Potatoes Spud Puppies, 3 oz.	160	7	23	2	2
Empire Kosher					
Breaded Chicken Tenders, 85 g	220	3	26	1	21
Chicken Nuggets, 82 g	230	7	26	2	16
Frozen Appetizers					
Large Egg Rolls, 85 g	110	5	15	2	3
Mini Egg Rolls, 85 g	110	5	15	2	3
Mini Stuffed Cabbage, 113 g	90	2	9	1	9
Potato Pancakes, 56 g	120	5	19	1	1
Frozen Blintzes					
Apple Raisin Blintzes, 61 g	80	2	16	2	3
Blueberry Blintzes, 61 g	90	1	18	1	2
Cheese Blintzes, 61 g	80	2	13	2	6
Cherry Blintzes, 61 g	100	1	18	2	3
Potato Blintzes, 61 g	90	4	15	2	3
Green Giant					
Boxed Baby Brussels Sprouts & Butter, 104 g	60	1	9	3	3
Boxed Broccoli Spears & Butter, 4 oz.	40	2	6	2	2
Boxed Broccoli & Zesty Cheese, 109 g	60	2	8	1	2
Boxed Cheesy Rice & Broccoli, 283 g	270	5	50	2	7
Boxed Creamed Spinach, 109 g	70	3	9	1	3
Boxed Rstd Potatoes w/ Broccoli & Cheese, 122 g	110	3	18	2	3
Boxed Shoepeg White Corn & Butter Sauce, 112 g	110	2	22	2	2
Jimmy Dean					
Pancakes & Sausage Minis: Blueberry Sand, 72 g	260	18	19	0	5
Pancakes & Sausage Minis: Original, 72 g	260	18	19	0	5

FROZEN MEALS

Appetizers & Sides (cont.)	Cal	Fat	Cbs	Fbr	Prtn
Jimmy Dean (cont.)					
Pancakes & Sausage On A Stick: Blueberry, 71 g	230	13	23	0	6
Pancakes & Sausage On A Stick: Original, 71 g	220	13	21	0	6
Morningstar Farms					
New Products					
Asian Veggie Patties, 67 g	100	4	10	2	7
Ginger Teriyaki Veggie Cakes, 68 g	110	2	19	2	5
Southwestern Style Veggie Cakes, 68 g	130	3	21	2	6
Snacks					
Veggie Bites Broccoli Cheddar, 85 g	190	10	16	1	8
Veggie Bites Mushroom Mozzarella, 85 g	190	10	16	1	9
Veggie Bites Spinach Artichoke, 85 g	190	10	16	2	9
Mrs. Paul's					
Crab Cakes					
Deviled Crab Cakes, 82 g	220	12	12	3	20
Fish Sticks					
Crisp & Healthy Brded Fish Sticks, 104 g	140	1	24	1	9
Crunchy Breaded Sticks, 95 g	220	10	22	1	9
Original Breaded Sticks, 95 g	220	10	22	1	9
X-Large Fish Sticks, 96 g	220	11	22	1	9
Fish Tenders					
Battered Fish Tenders, 4 oz.	210	10	22	1	9
Beer Battered Tenders, 114 g	230	11	22	1	11
Popcorn Fish, 114 g	220	12	18	2	11
Select Cuts					
Fried Clams - 8 oz, 3 oz.	270	13	29	1	9
Fried Scallops - 7oz, 106 g	260	11	28	1	12
Lightly Breaded Flounder, 76 g	150	7	12	1	8
Lightly Breaded Tilapia, 113 g	240	11	17	1	16
Shrimp+Calamari					
Beer Battered Shrimp, 4 oz.	200	6	22	1	14
Breaded Popcorn Shrimp, 4 oz.	260	11	30	2	11
Butterfly Shrimp, 4 oz.	250	11	27	1	12
Fried Calamari, 4 oz.	270	13	26	1	10
Sweet Potatoes					
Candied Sweet Potatoes - 12 oz, 5 oz.	300	1	73	3	1
Candied Sweet Potatoes - 20 oz, 5 oz.	300	1	73	3	1
SeaPak					
Maryland Style Crab Cakes, 4 oz.	240	13	19	1	11
Butterfly Shrimp					
Breaded Butterfly Shrimp - Ready To Fry, 4 oz.	150	1	22	1	11
Butterfly Shrimp - Oven Crunchy, 3 oz.	210	10	20	1	10
Gourmet Breaded Shrimp - Ready To Fry, 4 oz.	170	2	23	1	14
Jumbo Butterfly Shrimp - Oven Crunchy, 3 oz.	210	10	20	1	10
Wild Amer Butterfly Shrimp - Oven Crunchy, 3 oz.	210	10	20	1	10
Popcorn Shrimp					
Firecracker Shrimp, 3 oz.	210	10	20	1	10
Jumbo Popcorn Shrimp, 3 oz.	210	10	20	1	10
Popcorn Shrimp, 3 oz.	210	10	20	1	10
Shrimp Poppers, 84 g	220	12	18	2	10
Shrimp Scampi					
• Butter and Garlic, Tails Off, 4 oz.	350	29	2	0	15

(•= most healthy •= least healthy)

FROZEN MEALS

Appetizers & Sides (cont.)	Cal	Fat	Cbs	Fbr	Prtn
SeaPak (cont.)					
Shrimp Scampi (cont.)					
Italian Parmesan, Tails Off, 4 oz.	330	29	2	0	15
Restaurant-Style, Tails On, 4 oz.	310	29	4	1	13
Wild American, Tails Off, 4 oz.	330	29	2	0	15
Specialty Shrimp					
Coconut Shrimp, 4 oz.	310	14	36	1	12
Crispy Light Shrimp, 3 oz.	190	10	13	0	10
Garlic Herb Marinated Shrimp, 4 oz.	130	4	3	0	17
Italian Garlic Shrimp, 3 oz.	180	11	11	1	10
Shrimp Alfredo, 3 oz.	210	15	5	0	14
Tempura Shrimp, 4 oz.	240	8	35	7	9
Simply Potatoes					
Homestyle Slices, 103 g	70	0	16	1	2
Red Potato Wedges, 81 g	50	0	10	2	2
Rosemary & Garlic Red Potato Wedges, 120 g	80	0	16	3	2
Tyson Chicken					
Frozen Bagged Items					
Any'tizers Pork Mini Ribs, 4 pieces	330	22	14	0	20
Fully Cooked Chicken Products					
Any'tizers BBQ Style Wings, 91 g	200	13	7	0	15
Any'tizers Buffalo Style Boneless Wings, 84 g	150	7	8	0	12
Any'tizers Cheddar & Bacon Bites, 90 g	240	14	12	0	16
Any'tizers Homestyle Fries, 90 g	230	11	19	1	13
Any'tizers Mini Bites, 85 g	270	18	15	1	13
Buffalo Style Hot Wings, 96 g	220	15	1	0	20
Buffalo Style Popcorn Bites, 82 g	170	8	11	1	14
Chicken Nuggets, 92 g	280	18	16	0	14
Italian Style Meatballs, 84 g	180	11	6	2	13
Popcorn Bites™, 89 g	250	12	22	2	14
Southwest Seas0oned Breast Strips, 84 g	110	3	2	0	18
Teriyaki Breast Fillets, 89 g	170	7	7	0	20
Teriyaki Flavored Wings, 4 pieces	200	12	4	0	19
Van de Kamp's					
Crisp Healthy					
C + H Breaded Fillets, 104 g	150	1.5	25	1	8
C + H Breaded Fish Sticks, 104 g	140	1	24	1	8
Fish Sticks					
Fish Sticks, 114 g	260	13	26	1	11
X-Large Sticks, 96 g	220	11	22	1	9
Shrimp + Calamari					
Beer Battered Shrimp, 113 g	200	6	22	1	14
Breaded Butterfly Shrimp, 113 g	250	11	27	1	12
Breaded Popcorn Shrimp, 113 g	260	11	30	2	11
Fried Calamari, 113 g	270	13	26	1	10
Tenders + Bites					
Battered Fish Tenders, 112 g	210	10	22	1	9
Breaded Popcorn Fish, 114 g	220	12	18	2	11

POPULAR BRANDS

FROZEN MEALS

Dinners & Meals	Cal	Fat	Cbs	Fbr	Prtn
Banquet					
Crock Pot Classics					
Beef Stew, 2/3 cup	140	6	15	4	12
Herb Chicken & Rice, 2/3 cup	200	3	34	4	11
Stroganoff with Beef & Noodles, 2/3 cup	300	14	29	5	14
Dinners					
Pepperoni Pizza Meal, 1 Meal	550	29	57	5	16
Salisbury Steak Meal, 1 Meal	300	16	25	5	14
Turkey Meal, 1 Meal	200	8	27	5	14
Hearty One					
Chicken Fried Steak, 1 Meal	750	42	66	5	26
Fried Chicken, 1 Meal	810	4	71	9	39
Turkey with Gravy, 1 Meal	430	16	43	9	29
Original					
Chicken Nuggets, 5 Nuggets	230	14	15	1	10
Crispy Chicken, 4 oz.	320	19	13	1	23
Pot Pies					
Beef Pot Pie, 1 Pie	450	27	36	2	14
Chicken Pot Pie, 1 Pie	370	21	34	2	10
Turkey Pot Pie, 1 Pie	390	21	36	2	10
Boca Meatless					
Wrap, Orig Sausage Egg Wh & Chz, 130 g	220	7	27	6	16
Wrap, S.W. Sausage Egg Wh & Chz, 130 g	200	7	25	6	14
Lasagna, Chky Tom & Hb w/ Boca Grd Bger, 298 g	290	5	42	5	21
Empire Kosher					
Chicken Continental, 177 g	380	16	30	1	27
Chicken Kiev, 117 g	590	43	24	0	27
Chicken Portobello, 177 g	370	17	27	1	27
Fully Cooked: Chicken					
Boneless Skinless Chicken Breasts, 84 g	250	7	26	1	19
Chkn Drumsticks & Thighs w/ Back Portions, 84 g	260	9	26	1	17
Split Chicken Breasts with Ribs, 84 g	250	7	26	1	19
Frozen Entrees					
Spaghetti & Meatballs, 369 g	400	13	48	4	23
Sweet & Sour Chicken Breast, 284 g	260	7	28	2	26
Teriyaki Turkey, 312 g	250	4	27	3	27
Turkey Meatloaf, 312 g	330	14	31	5	20
Frozen Meat Pies					
Frozen Chicken Pie, 227 g	460	23	43	10	21
Turkey Frozen Pie, 227 g	460	23	43	10	21
Farmer John					
Bacon, Egg & Cheese Burritos, 136 g	330	18	26	1	15
Sausage, Egg & Cheese Burritos, 136 g	350	21	28	1	13
S.W. Spicy Sausage, Egg & Cheese Burritos, 136 g	350	21	28	1	13
Green Giant					
Boxed Rice Medley, 283 g	240	4	47	3	7
Boxed Rice Pilaf, 283 g	200	3	40	3	6
Boxed White & Wild Rice, 283 g	260	5	48	3	6
Complete Skillet Meal Chkn & Chsy Pasta, 227 g	250	5	39	4	15
Complete Skillet Meal Chkn Alfredo, 227 g	240	5	37	3	16
Complete Skillet Meal Garlic Chkn Pasta, 227 g	230	6	33	4	13
Create a Meal! Stir-Fry Sesame, 215 g	100	5	12	4	4

(● = most healthy ● = least healthy) **POPULAR BRANDS • 447**

Dinners & Meals (cont.)	Cal	Fat	Cbs	Fbr	Prt
Green Giant (cont.)					
• Create A Meal! Stir-Fry Szechuan, 169 g	50	0	10	3	3
Create A Meal! Stir-Fry Teriyaki, 170 g	50	0	11	3	3
Healthy Choice					
Café Select Crmy Dill Salmon	240	6	26	5	19
Café Select Grl Basil Chkn	290	6	37	5	20
Café Select Rstd Chkn Chardonnay	270	6	30	4	22
Complete Select Country Breaded Chicken	370	9	53	6	15
Complete Select Lemon Pepper Fish	310	5	53	5	13
Complete Selections Meatloaf	300	8	40	9	15
Complete Select Sweet 'N Sour Chicken	430	9	69	5	16
Smpl Select Brded Chkn Brst Strip & Potatoes	200	3	31	5	11
Simple Select Chicken Enchilada	270	5	45	5	10
Simple Select Chicken Rigatoni	250	7	30	5	14
Simple Select Grilled Chicken With Potatoes	160	4	18	3	11
Simple Select Mandarin Chicken	240	3	39	5	13
Jimmy Dean					
Breakfast Bowls					
Eggs, Potato, & Ham, 227 g	390	23	23	3	24
Eggs, Potatoes, Bacon & Cheddar Cheese, 227 g	520	34	22	3	30
Eggs, Potatoes, Sausage & Cheddar Chz, 227 g	490	34	20	3	23
Pancake and Sausage Links, 244 g	710	31	93	3	13
Omelets					
Ham & Cheese, 122 g	250	19	4	0	16
Sausage & Cheese, 122 g	270	22	5	0	15
Three Cheese, 122 g	290	23	4	1	16
Western Style, 122 g	210	15	6	1	13
Sandwiches					
D-lights Croissant: Trky Sge, Egg Wh & Chz, 136 g	300	12	32	3	17
D-lights Sdwiches: Ca Bcn, Egg Wh & Chz, 128 g	230	6	30	2	15
D-lights Sdwiches: Tky Sge, Egg Wh & Chz, 145 g	260	7	30	2	18
Skillets					
Bacon, 127 g	230	13	14	2	10
Ham, 127 g	130	4	16	2	8
Smoked Sausage, 127 g	250	14	20	3	8
Southwest Style, 127 g	210	12	18	3	9
Kid Cuisine					
All American Fried Chicken Meal	480	20	47	6	25
All Star Chicken Breast Nuggets Meal	440	17	53	8	17
Bug Safari Chicken Breast Nuggets Meal	450	15	58	6	17
Cheese Blaster Mac & Cheese Meal	390	9	64	5	13
Cheeseburger Builder Meal	390	12	56	6	13
Magical Cheese Stuffed Crust Pizza Meal	420	11	62	10	17
Pop Star Popcorn Chicken Meal	430	13	64	9	13
Lean Cuisine					
Café Classics					
Bow Tie Pasta & Chicken, 10 oz.	230	5	32	3	16
Chicken Carbonara, 9 oz.	270	7	33	2	19
Chicken Marsala, 8 oz.	140	4	12	3	14
Fiesta Grilled Chicken, 9 oz.	250	5	31	2	19
Glazed Chicken, 9 oz.	220	4	25	1	21
Parmesan Crusted Fish, 9 oz.	290	8	40	4	15

FROZEN MEALS

Dinners & Meals (cont.)

	Cal	Fat	Cbs	Fbr	Prtn
Lean Cuisine (cont.)					
Café Classics (cont.)					
Shrimp Alfredo, 9 oz.	260	5	36	3	18
Steak Tips Portabello, 8 oz.	180	7	13	3	15
Sweet and Sour Chicken, 10 oz.	300	3	51	2	18
Teriyaki Steak, 11 oz.	280	6	37	3	19
Three Cheese Chicken, 8 oz.	210	10	10	3	21
Tortilla Crusted Fish, 8 oz.	330	9	45	3	16
Casual Eating™					
BBQ Recipe Chicken Pizza, 6 oz.	350	8	50	3	19
Chicken Philly Flatbread Melts, 7 oz.	330	8	41	5	21
Four Cheese Pizza, 6 oz.	360	8	55	2	17
Gourmet Mushroom Pizza, 6 oz.	320	7	49	2	15
Pepperoni French Bread Pizza, 5 oz.	290	8	43	3	15
Pepperoni Pizza, 6 oz.	370	9	53	4	20
Roasted Vegetable Pizza, 6 oz.	310	5	52	3	14
Steak, Cheddar & Mushroom Panini, 6 oz.	340	9	44	5	21
Comfort Classics					
Baked Chicken, 9 oz.	240	5	34	3	15
Glazed Turkey Tenderloins, 9 oz.	260	5	41	4	13
Herb Roasted Chicken, 8 oz.	180	4	20	3	18
Oven Roasted Beef, 9 oz.	210	8	18	2	16
Roasted Pork, 10 oz.	250	4	38	3	16
Roasted Turkey & Vegetables, 8 oz.	150	5	12	3	15
Salisbury Steak, 10 oz.	280	9	25	3	24
Dinnertime Selects™					
Balsamic Glazed Chicken, 12 oz.	350	9	43	6	24
Chicken Fettuccini, 12 oz.	400	8	48	6	33
Chicken Tuscan, 12 oz.	280	6	34	5	22
Grilled Chicken & Penne Pasta, 12 oz.	330	5	52	6	20
Orange Peel Chicken, 12 oz.	390	9	63	3	15
Salisbury Steak, 13 oz.	270	8	27	10	22
One Dish Favorites™					
Alfredo Pasta w/ Chicken & Broccoli, 10 oz.	250	6	33	3	17
Cheese Ravioli, 9 oz.	240	6	38	3	11
Chicken Fettuccini, 9 oz.	270	6	32	0	22
Chicken Florentine Lasagna, 10 oz.	290	6	37	3	21
Chicken Teriyaki Stir Fry, 10 oz.	300	5	49	3	17
Classic Five Cheese Lasagna, 12 oz.	320	8	44	4	19
Macaroni And Beef, 10 oz.	310	9	38	3	20
Spaghetti With Meatballs, 10 oz.	260	5	35	5	18
Stuffed Cabbage w/ Whipped Potatoes, 10 oz.	220	4	21	5	24
Spa Cuisine™ Classics					
Butternut Squash Ravioli, 10 oz.	350	9	56	6	13
Chicken In Peanut Sauce, 9 oz.	280	8	30	5	22
Chicken Pecan, 9 oz.	260	6	32	6	19
Ginger Garlic Stir Fry With Chicken, 10 oz.	290	4	46	4	17
Hunan Stir Fry With Beef, 9 oz.	270	7	37	2	15
Lemon Chicken, 9 oz.	300	9	40	3	15
Rosemary Chicken, 8 oz.	210	4	27	3	17
Salmon Mediterranean, 9 oz.	230	4	30	3	18
Salmon With Basil, 10 oz.	220	6	24	4	18

(•= most healthy •= least healthy)

FROZEN MEALS

Dinners & Meals (cont.)	Cal	Fat	Cbs	Fbr	Prtn
Marie Callender's					
• 1 Dish Classics Fettuccini Alfredo	870	51	76	8	25
1 Dish Classics Spaghetti w/ Meat Sauce	590	15	90	13	21
Beef Pot Pie, 1 cup	540	32	46	3	16
Beef Pot Roast	330	10	32	9	27
Beef Tips Dinner	360	12	35	6	26
Breaded Chicken Parmesan Dinner	650	29	66	5	31
Cheesy Chicken Pot Pie, 1 cup	600	37	46	3	17
Chicken Fried Beef	540	28	51	6	19
Chicken Pot Pie, 1 cup	530	31	48	3	14
Chicken Teriyaki	430	4	78	5	19
Chzy Chkn Breast, Rice w/ Broccoli	480	18	47	5	31
Country Fried Pork Chop	510	23	53	11	21
Creamy Mushroom & Chicken Pot Pie, 1 cup	560	35	45	3	15
Fried Chicken Tenderloins	470	19	52	5	21
Golden Battered Filet Dinner	450	16	53	4	22
Herb Roasted Chicken	460	25	26	5	30
Lasagna with Meat Sauce, 1 cup	240	8	28	4	13
Roast Beef Dinner	370	13	37	7	25
Salisbury Steak Dinner	400	16	38	7	27
Stuffed Pasta Medley	440	15	55	7	21
Swedish Meatballs	580	30	48	7	28
Sweet & Sour Chicken	600	18	88	10	22
Michelina's					
Creamy Parmesan Chicken, 227 g	220	5	37	2	13
Enchilada Bake, 241 g	300	8	47	6	12
Layered Lasagna with Meat Sauce, 227 g	310	6	49	8	15
Macaroni and Cheese, 255 g	270	4	47	2	10
Mandarin Chicken, 227 g	260	3	46	2	9
Meatloaf, 227 g	180	6	21	2	11
Penne Primavera, 227 g	280	6	43	3	11
Roasted Sirloin Supreme, 227 g	230	5	34	2	13
Santa Fe Style Rice and Beans, 241 g	330	9	55	4	8
Shrimp Scampi, 227 g	290	6	45	2	10
Morningstar Farms					
Breakfast Starters Classic Scramble, 78 g	60	1	8	1	6
Veggie Bites Country Scramble, 85 g	180	8	17	2	11
Veggie Bites Eggs Florentine, 85 g	180	8	17	2	10
Patio					
Beef Enchilada	380	12	55	5	11
Beef Tamale and Enchilada	460	14	69	5	13
Cheese Enchilada	390	13	58	10	12
Chicken Burrito	280	8	42	2	9
Chicken Enchilada	380	11	57	5	12
Hot Beef & Bean Burrito with Red Chili	310	11	42	4	9
Pepperidge Farm					
Chili w/ Beans & Cornbread 1 Dish Meal, 1 cup	360	17	40	3	11
Crmy Alfredo Chkn & Broc Premium Pot Pie, 1 cup	500	32	40	2	13
Roasted White Meat Chicken Pot Pie, 1 cup	510	32	43	3	13
Roasted White Meat Turkey Pot Pie, 1 cup	501	33	38	2	13

FROZEN MEALS

Dinners & Meals (cont.)

	Cal	Fat	Cbs	Fbr	Prtn
Rosetto Pasta					
All Natural					
Beef Ravioli	220	4	39	2	10
Cheese Ravioli	210	5	34	2	9
Whole Wheat Cheese Ravioli	200	5	33	6	10
Classic					
Beef Ravioli	240	4	40	2	9
Cheese Manicotti	270	11	30	1	13
Cheese Ravioli	230	4	37	2	10
Cheese Stuffed Shells	260	11	27	1	12
Cheese Tortellini	240	5	41	2	11
Chicken & Herb Ravioli	210	2	36	2	10
Gourmet					
Butternut Squash Ravioli	240	3	45	3	8
Pesto Ravioli with Walnuts	300	8	44	3	12
Steam 'n Eat					
Medium Square Cheese Ravioli	230	4	37	2	10
Eat Small Round Cheese Ravioli	230	4	36	2	10
SeaPak					
Artichoke Pesto Tilapia, 6 oz.	300	8	31	1	26
Herb Butter Salmon, 5 oz.	350	26	3	0	23
South Beach Living					
Caprese Style Chicken, 266 g	240	8	10	3	30
Chicken Fettuccini Alfredo, 263 g	240	7	20	7	26
Chicken in Roasted Red Pepper Sauce, 266 g	280	12	25	7	22
Garlic Herb Chicken, 232 g	240	10	10	3	23
Garlic Parmesan Chicken, 286 g	270	10	22	8	26
Garlic Sesame Beef, 255 g	210	9	15	3	15
Kung Pao Chicken, 235 g	250	9	14	4	25
Meatloaf with Gravy, 255 g	210	9	17	4	16
Roasted Turkey, 269 g	240	9	27	4	17
Savory Pork, 266 g	230	9	13	4	22
Tyson Chicken					
Meals and Entrees					
Chicken Cordon Bleu, 168 g	380	24	20	1	22
Chicken Kiev, 168 g	480	37	19	1	17
Chicken with Broccoli and Cheese, 168 g	310	16	23	2	17
Refrigerated					
Chkn Brst Medals in Italian Hrb Sauce, 140 g	120	2	7	0	18
Chkn Brst Medals in Sesame Teriyaki Sauce, 140 g	190	3	22	0	18
Chkn Brst Medals in Wh Wine & Grlc Sauce, 140 g	140	6	3	1	19
Van de Kamp's					
Battered Fillets, 100 g	190	9	20	1	8
Battered Haddock Fillets, 104 g	210	11	21	2	9
Beer Battered Fish Fillets, 60 g	120	6	12	1	6
Breaded Fish Fillets, 99 g	230	13	21	1	8
Lightly Breaded Tilapia, 113 g	240	11	17	1	16
Zatarain's					
Blackened Chkn & Yellow Rice	460	13	67	2	19
Blackened Chicken Alfredo	500	25	46	2	23
Chicken Jambalaya	400	5	69	2	18
Red Beans & Rice w/ Sausage	510	20	68	5	16

(• = most healthy • = least healthy)

POPULAR BRANDS

FROZEN MEALS

Dinners & Meals (cont.)	Cal	Fat	Cbs	Fbr	Prtn
Zatarain's (cont.)					
Sausage Jambalaya	480	14	77	3	13

Frozen Pizza	Cal	Fat	Cbs	Fbr	Prtn
California Pizza Kitchen					
Crispy Thin					
Crust BBQ Chicken Recipe, 139 g	290	9	35	2	17
Crust Garlic Chicken, 119 g	290	11	31	2	17
Crust Margherita, 121 g	290	13	31	2	13
Crust Sicilian Recipe, 120 g	310	14	30	2	17
Original					
BBQ Chicken, 122 g	270	2	33	2	16
BBQ Recipe Chicken, 132 g	310	9	38	2	17
Five Cheese & Tomato, 129 g	350	15	35	2	18
Hawaiian, 123 g	260	4	31	2	14
Sausage, Pepperoni & Mushroom, 118 g	290	13	30	2	14
Thai Recipe Chicken, 132 g	310	11	38	3	16
Digiorno Pizza					
Cheese Stuffed Crust Four Cheese, 150 g	360	14	41	3	19
• Digiorno For 1, Garlic Bread Crust Pepperoni, 274 g	840	44	81	4	30
Digiorno For 1, Thn Crst Grlled Chkn & Veg 240 g	520	17	64	4	28
For One Traditional Crust Supreme, 283 g	790	36	85	6	31
Garlic Bread Pizza Supreme, 121 g	290	13	31	3	14
Half & Half Rising Crust Pepperoni & Chz, 150 g	390	18	40	3	19
Harvest Wheat Thin Crispy Crust Supreme, 133 g	250	8	32	4	13
Rising Crust Supreme, 135 g	320	14	35	3	15
Rising Crust Supreme, 155 g	370	15	41	3	17
Thin Crispy Crust Supreme, 141 g	300	12	36	3	14
U S w/ Rsted Veggie-parm Focaccia Crust, 151 g	390	19	43	6	17
Ultimate Supreme Thin Crust, 150 g	360	17	34	3	17
Empire Kosher					
• Bagel Cheese Pizzas, 64 g	103	3	19	1	7
Four Cheese Pizza, 104 g	210	6	32	1	11
Mushroom Pizza, 104 g	210	4	32	1	6
Vegetable Supreme Pizza, 132 g	250	5	38	2	12
Healthy Choice					
French Bread Cheese Pizza, 1 Pizza	350	5	55	5	20
French Bread Pepperoni Pizza, 1 Pizza	350	5	54	5	22
French Bread Supreme Pizza, 1 Pizza	340	4	53	5	20
Jack's Pizza					
Half & Half Pepperoni/cheese, 170 g	440	23	38	3	20
Half & Half Sausage/pepperoni, 125 g	290	14	29	3	13
Naturally Rising The Works, 144 g	330	12	42	3	14
Naturally Rising Three Meat, 137 g	330	12	41	3	14
Original Cheese, 142 g	320	13	38	3	15
Original Pepperoni, 142 g	370	18	36	3	16
Original Sausage, 120 g	290	13	29	3	13
Original Spicy Italian Sausage, 158 g	380	17	38	3	18
Pizza Bursts - Pepperoni, 85 g	260	15	25	1	8
Pizza Bursts - Supreme, 85 g	260	14	25	1	8
Michelina's					
Five Cheese Pizza, 142 g	290	7	42	2	15

Frozen Pizza (cont.)

	Cal	Fat	Cbs	Fbr	Prtn
Michelina's (cont.)					
Pepperoni Pizza Snacks, 85 g	200	8	24	2	8
Pepperoni Pizza, 142 g	300	9	41	2	14
South Beach Living					
Deluxe, 192 g	340	11	37	10	30
Four Cheese, 178 g	340	11	37	10	31
Grilled Chicken & Vegetable, 192 g	330	10	37	10	30
Pepperoni, 178 g	350	12	36	9	31
Tombstone Pizza					
Brickoven Style Cheese, 151 g	350	15	38	3	17
Brickoven Style Deluxe, 134 g	280	12	30	2	14
Brickoven Style Supreme, 136 g	320	16	29	3	15
Garlic Bread Cheese, 130 g	350	14	40	3	15
Garlic Bread Pepperoni, 131 g	370	17	40	3	15
Half & Half Cheese/Sausage, 115 g	270	11	30	3	13
Half & Half Pepperoni & Cheese, 159 g	410	21	37	4	19
Half & Half Pepperoni/Sausage, 147 g	370	18	37	4	17
Harvest Wheat Thin Crust Supreme, 131 g	260	10	29	3	15
Light Veggie, 131 g	230	6	31	4	13
Original Deluxe, 124 g	270	12	29	3	13
Original Pepperoni, 113 g	280	14	28	3	13
Original Supreme, 130 g	300	14	31	3	14
Thin Crust Pepperoni, 128 g	320	18	28	3	15
Thin Crust Three Cheese, 134 g	310	15	28	3	16
Totino's Pizza Rolls					
Totino's Party Pizzas					
Cheese, 139 g	320	15	34	1	12
Combination, 152 g	380	21	34	1	14
Sausage, 153 g	360	19	34	1	14
Totino's Pizza Rolls					
Cheese, 85 g	190	6	26	1	8
Combination, 85 g	220	11	24	1	8
Pepperoni, 85 g	210	10	25	1	8
Mega Pizza Rolls Ultimate Pepperoni, 93 g	230	11	25	1	9

FRUITS

Fruits, Canned

	Cal	Fat	Cbs	Fbr	Prtn
Del Monte					
Apricots					
Apricot Halves, 127 g	100	0	26	1	0
Lite Apricot Halves, 122 g	60	0	16	1	0
Cherries Products					
Chunky Mixed Fruit in 100% Juice, 124 g	60	0	15	1	0
Dark Sweet Cherries, 120 g	100	0	24	1	1
Very Cherry Mixed Fruit, 124 g	90	0	22	1	1
Citrus Fruit Products					
Citrus Fruit Salad, 126 g	80	0	20	0	0
Mandarin Oranges, 126 g	80	0	19	1	0
Red Grapefruit, 126 g	90	0	21	1	1
SunFresh® Wh Grapefruit in Real Fruit Juice, 126 g	45	0	9	2	1
Fruit Cocktail Products					
Fruit Cocktail, 127 g	100	0	24	1	0

(•= most healthy •= least healthy)

▶ Fruits, Canned (cont.)	Cal	Fat	Cbs	Fbr	Prtn
Del Monte (cont.)					
Fruit Cocktail Products (cont.)					
Lite Fruit Cocktail, 124 g	60	0	15	1	0
Peaches Products: Freestone Peaches					
Freestone Slices, 127 g	100	0	24	1	0
Lite Freestone Slices, 124 g	60	0	14	1	0
Pear Products					
Cinnamon Flavored Pear Halves, 126 g	80	0	21	1	0
Lite Pear Halves, 124 g	60	0	15	1	0
Pear Halves, 127 g	100	0	24	1	0
Pineapple Products					
Pineapple Slices in Its Own Juice, 114 g	60	0	16	1	0
Pineapple Slices in Heavy Syrup, 117 g	90	0	23	1	0
Tropical Fruit Products					
Fruit Naturals® Tropical Medley, 124 g	70	0	18	1	0
SunFresh® Trop Mxd Frt in Lt Syrup, 126 g	80	0	21	1	0
Tropical Fruit Salad, 122 g	60	0	16	1	0
Yellow Cling Peaches					
Lite Peach Halves, 124 g	60	0	15	1	0
Peach Halves, 127 g	100	0	24	1	0
Dole					
Dates, 40 g	120	0	33	3	28
Diced Peaches, 113 g	70	0	18	1	1
Diced Pears, 113 g	80	0	19	N/A	0
Mandarin Oranges, 113 g	70	0	18	0	0
Mandarin Oranges, 122 g	80	0	19	1	0
Pineapple in 100% Juice, 114 g	60	0	15	1	0
Pineapple in Heavy Syrup, 123 g	90	0	24	1	1
Pineapple, 113 g	60	0	16	1	0
Prunes, 40 g	110	0	26	2	1
Raisins, 40 g	130	0	31	2	1
Tropical Mixed Fruit, 122 g	90	0	21	1	N/A
Luck's					
Fried Apples with Cinnamon, 1/2 cup	100	0	25	2	0
Fried Apples, 1/2 cup	110	0	29	2	0
Lucky Leaf					
Apple Sauce, 4 oz.	80	N/A	20	2	N/A
• Dutch Baked Apples, 1/2 cup	170	N/A	41	3	N/A
Lemon Creme Pie Filling, 1/3 cup	130	1	31	N/A	N/A
Lemon Pie Filling, 1/3 cup	120	1	29	N/A	N/A
Lite Strawberry Fruit 'N Sauce, 4 oz.	60	N/A	14	1	N/A
Unsweetened Apple Sauce, 1/2 cup	50	N/A	13	2	N/A
Musselman's					
Lite Mixed Berry Fruit'N Sauce, 4 oz.	60	N/A	14	1	N/A
Lite Strawberry Fruit'N Sauce, 4 oz.	60	N/A	14	1	N/A
Sesame Street Grape Apple Sauce, 4 oz.	80	N/A	20	1	N/A
Sesame Street Green Apple Sauce, 4 oz.	80	N/A	21	1	N/A
Sesame Street Watermelon Apple Sauce, 4 oz.	70	N/A	17	2	N/A
Sliced Apples, 1/2 cup	50	N/A	12	1	N/A
Ocean Spray					
• Jellied Cranberry Sauce, 10 g	16	0	4	N/A	0
Whole Berry Cranberry Sauce, 10 g	16	0	4	N/A	0

FRUITS

Fruits, Dried	Cal	Fat	Cbs	Fbr	Prtn
Ocean Spray					
Craisins®, 40 g	130	0	33	N/A	0
Sun-Maid					
Raisins					
California Apricots, 40 g	100	0	26	3	1
Cape Cod Cranberries, 30 g	120	4	22	1	1
Chocolate Yogurt Raisins, 30 g	130	5	21	1	1
Fruit Bits, 40 g	130	0	33	0	0
Jumbo Raisins, 40 g	130	0	31	2	1
Milk Chocolate Covered Raisins, 39 g	170	6	25	1	2
Peaches, 40 g	100	0	23	3	1
Pitted Plums, 40 g	100	0	26	3	1
Raisins, 40 g	130	0	31	2	1
Variety Pack					
Chopped Dates, 40 g	120	0	33	3	1
Goldens and Cherries, 40 g	130	0	31	2	1
Mixed Fruit, 40 g	100	0	26	3	1
Pitted Dates, 40 g	110	0	30	4	1
Sun-Maid Raisins, 28 g	90	0	22	2	1
Tropical Trio, 40 g	140	0	34	1	0
Vanilla Yogurt Raisins, 28 g	120	5	20	1	1
Sunridge Farms					
• Banana Chips, 40 g	210	13	23	3	1
California Pitted Prunes, 40 g	100	0	26	3	1
Dried Cranberries, 40 g	120	1	33	2	0
Fancy Apricots, 40 g	100	0	25	3	1
Pineapple Rings, 40 g	170	5	30	10	0
Tropical Fruit Mix, 40 g	130	1	32	4	2
Welch's					
Berry Medley, 40 g	135	0	32	1	1
Cranberries & Spiced Apples, 40 g	135	0	34	1	0
Dried Cherries, 40 g	140	0	32	1	1
• Dried Fruit Variety Packs, 26 g	90	0	20	1	0
Dried Mixed Fruit, 40 g	140	0	32	2	1

Fruits, Frozen & Fresh	Cal	Fat	Cbs	Fbr	Prtn
Cascadian Farm					
Blackberries, 140 g	80	1	22	7	1
Blueberries, 140 g	70	1	17	4	1
Sliced Peaches, 140 g	50	0	14	2	1
• Strawberries, 140 g	45	0	13	3	1
Sweet Cherries, 140 g	90	0	22	3	1
Dole					
Blackberries, 140 g	90	0	22	7	2
Blueberries, 140 g	70	1	17	4	0
• Dark Sweet Cherries, 140 g	90	4	22	3	2
Mango Chunks, 140 g	90	0	24	3	N/A
Mango Slices, 140 g	90	0	24	3	N/A
Mixed Berries, 140 g	70	0	17	5	N/A
Mixed Fruit, 140 g	60	0	16	2	0
Organics, 140 g	90	0	24	3	N/A
Raspberries, 140 g	70	0	16	5	N/A

(• = most healthy • = least healthy)   **POPULAR BRANDS • 455**

POPULAR BRANDS

FRUITS

Fruits, Frozen & Fresh (cont.)	Cal	Fat	Cbs	Fbr	Prtn
Dole (cont.)					
Whole Strawberries, 140 g	50	0	13	3	0
Wild Blueberries, 140 g	70	0	17	4	N/A

Fruits, Jarred	Cal	Fat	Cbs	Fbr	Prtn
Apple Time					
Natural Apple Sauce, 4 oz.	50	N/A	12	2	N/A

Fruits, Packaged Fresh	Cal	Fat	Cbs	Fbr	Prtn
Chiquita					
Bananas, 126 g	110	0	29	4	1
Cantaloupe, 134 g	50	0	12	1	1
Grapefruit, 154 g	60	0	16	6	1
Grapes, 138 g	90	1	24	1	1
Honeydew Melons, 134 g	50	0	13	1	1
Other Fruits and Vegetables					
Apples, 154 g	80	0	22	5	0
Apricots, 114 g	60	1	11	1	0
Avocados, 1.1 oz.	55	5	3	3	1
Cherries, 140 g	90	1	22	9	2
Kiwifruit, 148 g	100	1	24	4	2
Nectarines, 140 g	70	1	16	2	1
Peaches, 98 g	40	0	10	2	1
Pears, 166 g	100	1	25	4	1
Plums, 132 g	80	1	19	2	1
Tangerines, 109 g	50	1	15	3	1
Dole					
Apples, 154 g	80	0	22	5	0
Apricots, 114 g	60	1	11	1	0
Avocados, 30 g	55	5	3	3	1
Bananas, 126 g	110	0	29	4	1
Cantaloupe, 134	50	0	12	1	1
Cherries, 140 g	90	0	22	3	2
Coconuts, 50 g	180	17	8	5	2
Cranberries, 55 g	30	0	7	2	0
Goji Berries, 30 g	110	0	22	2	4
Grapes, 138 g	30	1	24	1	1
Honeydew Melons, 134 g	50	0	13	1	1
Mangoes, 104 g	70	0	17	1	0
Oranges, 154 g	70	0	21	7	1
Peaches, 98 g	40	0	10	2	1
Pears, 166 g	100	1	25	4	1
Pineapples, 112 g	60	0	16	1	1
• Plantains, 200 g	232	0	62	5	2
Plums, 66 g	40	0	10	1	0
Raspberries, 125 g	50	0	17	8	1
Strawberries, 147 g	45	0	12	4	1
Sunkist					
Grapefruit, 154 g	60	0	15	2	1
• Lemons, 58 g	15	0	5	2	0
Limes, 67 g	20	0	7	2	0
Oranges, 154 g	80	0	19	3	1

FRUITS

Fruits, Packaged Fresh (cont.)

	Cal	Fat	Cbs	Fbr	Prtn
Sunkist (cont.)					
Tangerines, 109 g	50	0	13	2	1

GRAINS, PASTA & BEANS

Canned Beans

	Cal	Fat	Cbs	Fbr	Prtn
Allens					
Baked Beans					
Barbeque Baked Beans, 128 g	150	1	29	5	6
Homestyle Baked Beans, 128 g	140	1	29	5	6
Maple Cured Bacon Baked Beans, 128 g	140	1	27	4	6
Onion Baked Beans, 128 g	140	2	25	4	5
Original Baked Beans, 129 g	150	1	29	8	6
Vegetarian Baked Beans, 128 g	140	0	28	4	6
Black Beans					
Black Beans, 128 g	100	1	19	8	6
Blackeyed Peas					
Blackeyed Peas with Bacon, 128 g	120	2	20	5	7
Blackeyed Peas with Snaps, 126 g	120	1	20	5	8
Blackeyed Peas, 126 g	120	1	21	6	7
Dry Blackeye Peas, 126 g	110	1	18	4	7
Butter Beans					
Baby Butter Beans, 129 g	120	1	22	6	7
Garbanzo Beans, 125 g	120	3	19	8	5
Large Butter Beans, 128 g	120	1	20	7	7
Kidney Beans					
Dark Red Kidney Beans, 128 g	130	1	22	8	8
Light Red Kidney Beans, 129 g	120	1	22	8	6
Lima Beans					
Green & White Lima Beans, 128 g	110	1	20	9	6
Medium Green Lima Beans, 128 g	120	0	23	8	7
Northern Beans					
Great Northern Beans, 128 g	100	1	19	7	6
Navy Beans, 129 g	110	1	19	6	6
Red Beans, 128 g	100	1	19	9	6
Pinto Beans					
Pinto Beans, 128 g	110	1	20	7	5
Refried Beans					
Refried Beans, 128 g	150	3	24	11	7
Refried Black Beans No Fat Added, 121 g	120	0	23	8	7
American Roland Food Corporation					
Beans, Black, 130 g	120	0	21	6	8
Beans, Garbanzo, 130 g	110	1	20	7	7
Beans, Red Kidney, 130 g	110	0	18	7	9
Beans, Spicy Black, 130 g	110	2	0	5	6
Campbell's Soups					
Bkd Beans Brwn Sugar & Bcn Flvrd Beans, 1/2 cup	160	3	30	8	5
Pork and Beans, 1/2 cup	140	2	25	7	6
Luck's					
Blackeye Peas, 1/2 cup	120	2	20	4	6
Fat Free Lima Beans, 1/2 cup	120	0	22	5	7
Fat Free Pinto Beans, 1/2 cup	110	0	21	6	7
Giant Lima Beans, 1/2 cup	130	2	22	5	7

(•= most healthy •= least healthy)

GRAINS, PASTA & BEANS

Canned Beans (cont.)	Cal	Fat	Cbs	Fbr	Prtn
Luck's (cont.)					
Great Northern Beans, 1/2 cup	130	2	20	6	7
Mixed Bean & Pork, 1/2 cup	130	2	21	7	7
Pinto Beans, 1/2 cup	130	2	21	6	7
Red Kidney, 1/2 cup	110	0	22	6	6
Progresso					
Beans Black, 130 g	100	1	17	5	6
Beans Cannellini, 130 g	110	0	20	6	8
Beans Chick Peas, 126 g	100	2	17	4	5
Beans Red Kidney, 130 g	110	0	20	6	8
Ranch Style					
Beans, 1/2 cup	130	3	20	6	6
Beans with Jalapeño, 1/2 cup	120	3	19	6	5
Beans with Onion, 1/2 cup	130	3	19	6	5
Black Beans, 1/2 cup	100	1	19	6	6
Jalapeño Beans, 1/2 cup	130	3	21	6	6
Kidney Beans, 1/2 cup	110	0	21	6	7
Original Beans, 1/2 cup	130	3	19	5	5
Rosarita					
Fat Free Refried Beans, 1/2 cup	100	0	19	6	7
Traditional Refried Beans, 1/2 cup	120	2	18	6	7
Vegetarian Refried Beans, 1/2 cup	120	2	19	7	7
Van Camp's					
Baked Beanee Weenees, 1 can	290	8	42	6	13
BBQ Beanee Weenees, 1 can	260	8	35	9	15
Beanee Weenees with Chili, 1 can	240	9	26	6	14
• Dark Red Beans, 1/2 cup	90	0	19	6	7
Hickory & Bacon Baked Beans, 1/2 cup	150	1	32	5	7
Homestyle Baked Beans, 1/2 cup	170	1	33	6	7
Original Baked Beans, 1/2 cup	140	1	30	6	7
• Original Beanee Weenees, 1 can	340	11	39	11	20

Dry Beans	Cal	Fat	Cbs	Fbr	Prtn
Bush's Beans					
Baked Beans					
Barbecue, 130 g	150	1	32	5	6
Bold & Spicy, 130 g	110	1	24	5	6
• Honey Baked, 130 g	160	1	32	6	6
Original, 130 g	140	1	29	5	6
Vegetarian, 130 g	130	0	29	5	6
Other Varieties of Beans					
Black Beans, 130 g	110	1	23	7	8
Blackeye Peas, 130 g	100	0	15	3	5
Butter Beans – Baby, 130 g	120	1	19	5	7
Chili Beans, 130 g	120	1	20	6	6
• Field Peas with Snaps, 130 g	80	0	16	2	5
Garbanzo Beans, 130 g	105	2	20	5	6
Great Northern Beans, 130 g	80	0	17	6	6
Kidney Beans – Dark Red, 130 g	105	0	22	8	7
Navy Beans, 130 g	80	0	17	7	6
Pinto Beans, 130 g	110	0	19	6	6
Purple Hull Peas, 130 g	90	0	19	5	6

GRAINS, PASTA & BEANS

Dry Beans (cont.)

	Cal	Fat	Cbs	Fbr	Prtp
Bush's Beans (cont.)					
Other Varieties of Beans (cont.)					
Red Beans, 130 g	110	1	19	6	6

Grains

	Cal	Fat	Cbs	Fbr	Prtn
Purity Foods					
Non-Organic Spelt Kernel, 46 g	130	1	32	8	7
Organic Spelt Kernel, 46 g	130	1	32	8	7
Organic Wheat Kernels (Berries), 47 g	160	1	34	7	6

Pasta

	Cal	Fat	Cbs	Fbr	Prtn
Purity Foods					
White Vita-Spelt Elbows, 2 oz.	210	1	42	2	9
White Vita-Spelt Lasagna, 2 oz.	210	1	42	2	9
White Vita-Spelt Spaghetti, 2 oz.	210	1	42	5	8
Whole Grain Vita-Spelt Elbows, 2 oz.	190	2	40	5	8
Whole Grain Vita-Spelt Lasagna, 2 oz.	190	2	40	5	8
Whole Grain Vita-Spelt Spaghetti, 2 oz.	190	2	40	5	8
Ronzoni Healthy Harvest					
7 Grain Pasta					
7 Grain Fussilli, 2 g	180	2	40	5	8
7 Grain Spaghetti, 2 g	180	2	40	5	8
Whole Wheat Blend Pasta					
Lasagna, 2 g	180	2	41	6	7
Linguine, 2 g	180	2	41	6	7
Penne Regate, 2 g	180	2	41	6	7
Rotini, 2 g	180	2	41	6	7
Spaghetti, 2 g	180	2	41	6	7

Rice

	Cal	Fat	Cbs	Fbr	Prtn
American Roland Food Corporation					
Basmati Rice, 50 g	180	2	37	4	5
Jasmine Rice, 100% Natural, 45 g	160	0	36	0	3
Sushi Rice - Calrose, 45 g	160	0	36	0	3
Wild Rice, 100% Natural, 45 g	170	0	35	2	6
Carolina Enriched Rice					
Brown Rice Whole Grain, 42 g	150	1	32	1	3
Gold (Parboiled), 47 g	160	0	37	1	3
Aromatic Rice					
Indian Basmati, 45 g	160	0	36	0	3
Thai Jasmine, 45 g	160	0	36	0	3
Goya Foods					
Brown, 98 g	108	1	22	2	3
Regular White, 79 g	103	0	22	0	2
Parboiled, 88 g	100	0	22	0	2
Precoocked White, 83 g	81	0	18	1	2
Mahatma Rice					
Aromatic Rice					
Indian Basmati, 45 g	160	0	36	0	3
Thai Jasmine, 45 g	160	0	36	0	3
Regular Rice					
Brown Rice (Whole Grain), 42 g	150	1	32	1	3
Gold (Parboiled), 47 g	160	0	37	1	3

(•= most healthy •= least healthy)

POPULAR BRANDS

GRAINS, PASTA & BEANS

Rice (cont.)

	Cal	Fat	Cbs	Fbr	Prtn
Mahatma Rice (cont.)					
Regular Rice (cont.)					
Valencia (Short Grain), 46 g	160	0	36	1	3
White Rice, 45 g	150	0	35	0	3
Minute Rice					
Boil-In-Bag, 50 g	180	0	41	1	4
Brown Rice, 43 g	150	2	34	2	3
Minute Ready To Serve Brown Rice, 125 g	170	5	28	2	3
Minute Ready To Serve Rice, 125 g	190	4	34	0	3
Minute Ready To Serve White Rice, 125 g	190	4	34	0	3
Premium White Rice, 50 g	190	0	41	0	5
White Rice, 55 g	200	0	45	0	5
Uncle Ben's					
White Rice					
Boil-In-Bag Rice, 58 g	190	1	44	1	4
Instant Rice, 52 g	190	1	43	1	3
Original Converted, 49 g	170	0	38	N/A	4
Whole Grain Brown Rice					
Fast & Natural™ Instant Brown Rice, 47 g	170	1	36	N/A	5
Natural Whole Grain Brown Rice, 47 g	170	2	35	N/A	5
• Ready Rice® Whole Grain Brown, 140 g	220	4	41	2	5

MEAT

Bacon

	Cal	Fat	Cbs	Fbr	Prtn
Butterball					
Original Bacon Style Turkey, 30 g	70	6	1	0	4
Salt Reduced Bacon Style Turkey, 30 g	70	6	1	0	4
Farmer John					
• Dry Salt Pork, 56 g	250	24	1	0	7
Premium Low Sodium Bacon, 16 g	80	7	0	0	6
Premium Regular Smoked Bacon, 16 g	70	5	0	0	6
Premium Thick Sliced Bacon, 12 g	60	4	0	0	5
Jimmy Dean					
• Hardwood Smoked Trky Premium Bacon, 14 g	25	2	0	0	2
Lower Sodium Premium Bacon, 10 g	50	4	0	0	4
Original Premium Bacon, 10 g	50	4	0	0	4
Thick Slice Premium Bacon, 14 g	80	6	0	0	5
Oscar Mayer					
Bacon Lower Sodium, 14 g	70	6	0	N/A	4
Bacon Natural Smoked Uncured, 15 g	60	5	0	N/A	7
Bacon Ready To Serve, 16 g	70	6	0	N/A	4
Tyson Chicken					
Fully Cooked Hickory Bacon, 15 g	90	7	0	0	5
Ready to Cook Hickory Bacon, 15 g	90	7	0	0	5
Ready To Cook Thick Cut Hickory Bacon, 24 g	140	11	0	0	8

Beef

	Cal	Fat	Cbs	Fbr	Prtn
Libby's					
• Corned Beef, 2 oz.	120	7	0	N/A	14
• Corned Beef Hash, 1 cup	420	24	33	3	19
Hawaiian Corned Beef, 2 oz.	120	7	0	N/A	14
Potted Meat, 1/4 cup	121	9	0	0	0

MEAT

Beef (cont.)	Cal	Fat	Cbs	Fbr	Prtn
Tyson Chicken					
Country Fried Steak, 90 g	310	23	15	1	10
Seasoned Beef Strips, 84 g	130	6	1	0	18
Steak Fingers, 71 g	250	18	14	1	8

Ham	Cal	Fat	Cbs	Fbr	Prtn
Farmer John					
Bone-In Ham					
Gold Trad Prem Brwn Sugar & Hny Half Ham, 56 g	70	1	3	0	11
Gold Trad Prem Original Smoked Half Ham, 56 g	110	7	3	0	9
Maple Ham Steak, 56 g	60	1	1	0	10
Original Ham Steak, 56 g	50	1	2	0	9
Premium Ham Sliced Ham Steaks, 84 g	160	11	4	0	13
Premium Spiral Sliced Whole Hams, 56 g	90	4	3	0	12
Whole Hams, 56 g	110	7	3	0	9
Sliced Ham					
Premium Black Forest Sliced Ham, 38 g	35	1	1	0	7
Premium Brown Sugar & Honey Sliced Ham, 38 g	45	1	2	0	7
Premium Sliced Ham, 57 g	50	2	1	0	10

Hot Dogs & Franks	Cal	Fat	Cbs	Fbr	Prtn
Ball Park Franks					
Ball Park Franks					
Ball Park Cheese Franks, 57 g	190	16	3	0	7
Ball Park Franks, 56 g	180	16	3	0	6
Better For You Franks					
Bun Size Smkd White Turkey Franks, 50 g	45	0	5	0	6
Fat Free Franks, 50 g	40	0	4	0	5
Lite Franks, 50 g	100	7	3	0	6
Bun Size Franks					
Bun Size Franks, 56 g	180	16	3	0	6
Bun Size Smkd White Turkey Franks, 50 g	45	0	5	0	6
Grillmaster®					
Deli Style Beef, 81 g	250	23	3	0	8
Hearty Beef Franks, 81 g	250	23	3	0	9
Butterball					
Biggies Turkey Smokies, 75 g	150	12	2	0	10
Turkey Franks, 56 g	120	8	5	0	6
Empire Kosher					
Chicken Franks, 57 g	100	7	0	0	6
Turkey Franks, 57 g	100	8	0	0	6
Farmer John					
Official Dodger Dogs®, 76 g	240	22	2	0	8
Premium Jumbo Meat Wieners, 57 g	170	17	0	0	7
Premium Quarter Pounder Beef Franks, 113 g	350	31	5	0	13
Premium Meat Wieners, 46 g	140	13	0	0	6
Hebrew National					
Beef Knockwurst, 2 oz.	180	17	0	0	6
Dinner Frank, 1 Frank	360	33	1	0	13
Franks in a Blanket, 5 Pieces	300	24	12	1	8
Light Bologna, 4 Slices	80	5	1	N/A	9
Light Salami, 4 Slices	90	5	0	N/A	9

(•= most healthy •= least healthy)

POPULAR BRANDS

MEAT

Hot Dogs & Franks (cont.)	Cal	Fat	Cbs	Fbr	Prtn
Oscar Mayer					
Beef Franks					
Jumbo, 57 g	170	15	1	N/A	7
Light, 45 g	90	6	2	N/A	5
Regular, 45 g	130	12	1	N/A	5
Fast Franks					
Beef, 96 g	300	8	21	1	10
Fast Franks, 96 g	290	19	21	1	10
Little Wieners Little Smokies					
Little Smokies Cheese, 57 g	190	17	2	N/A	7
Little Smokies, 57 g	170	15	1	N/A	7
Little Wieners, 57 g	180	17	1	N/A	6
Smokies					
Beef, 50 g	150	13	1	N/A	6
Sausage, 50 g	150	13	1	N/A	6
Wieners					
• 98% Fat Free, 50 g	40	0	3	N/A	5
Jumbo, 57 g	170	16	0	N/A	6
Light, 45 g	90	7	1	N/A	5
Regular, 45 g	130	12	1	N/A	5

Meat Alternatives	Cal	Fat	Cbs	Fbr	Prtn
Boca Meatless					
Boca In A Bun Chik'n & Swiss Sandwiches, 143 g	350	14	44	6	20
Bratwurst Sausage, 71 g	140	7	6	1	14
Breakfast Links, 45 g	70	3	5	2	8
Breakfast Patties Made w/ Organic Soy, 38 g	70	3	5	2	8
• Breakfast Patties, 38 g	60	3	5	2	7
Bruschetta Tomato Basil Parmesan Pattie, 71 g	70	2	9	4	10
Cheeseburger, 71 g	100	5	5	4	13
Garden Vegetable Burger, 71 g	130	3	9	4	15
Grilled Vegetable, 71 g	80	1	7	4	12
Original Chik'n Nuggets, 87 g	180	7	17	3	14
Savory Mushroom Mozzarella Pattie, 71 g	100	3	11	4	13
Spicy Chik'n Patties, 71 g	160	6	15	2	11
Gardenburger					
Black Bean Chipotle, 71 g	80	3	13	5	5
California Burger, 71 g	90	4	12	2	3
Flame Grilled, 71 g	90	4	5	4	11
Garden Vegan, 71 g	100	1	12	3	10
Portabella, 71 g	90	3	15	5	5
Sun-Dried Tomato Basil, 71 g	100	3	15	5	5
The Original, 71 g	100	4	14	5	5
Veggie Medley, 71 g	90	3	15	5	5
Morningstar Farms					
Veggie Bacon Strips, 16 g	60	5	2	1	2
Veggie Sausage Links, 45 g	80	3	3	2	9
Veggie Sausage Patties, 38 g	80	3	3	1	10
Burgers					
Grillers Prime® Veggie Burgers, 71 g	170	9	4	2	17
Grillers® Original, 64 g	130	6	5	2	15
Grillers® Vegan, 71 g	100	3	7	4	12

MEAT

Meat Alternatives (cont.)	Cal	Fat	Cbs	Fbr	Prtn
Morningstar Farms (cont.)					
Burgers (cont.)					
Philly Cheese Steak Burgers, 64 g	120	6	6	3	10
Chik'n					
Buffalo Wings Veggie Wings, 85 g	200	8	20	3	12
Chik'n Nuggets, 86 g	190	7	18	2	12
Chik'n Patties® Original, 71 g	150	6	16	2	9
Chik'n Patties® Parmesan Ranch, 71 g	170	7	17	2	10
Dogs					
America's Original Veggie Dog® Links, 57 g	80	1	6	1	11
Mini Veggie Corn Dogs, 76 g	160	5	21	1	11
Veggie Corn Dogs, 71 g	150	4	22	3	7
Meal Starters					
Meal Starters™ Chik'n Strips, 85 g	140	4	6	1	23
Meal Starters™ grillers® Recipe Crumbles, 55 g	80	3	4	3	10
Meal Starters™ Veggie Steak Strips, 85 g	150	4	8	1	22
Organic and Natural					
Breakfast Pattie, 38 g	80	3	4	1	8
Classic Burger, 64 g	150	6	9	3	14
Thai Burger, 67 g	100	4	7	3	10
Vegan Burger, 71 g	90	2	8	4	13
Veggie Corn Dogs, 71 g	170	5	22	1	8
Veggie Medley Burger, 67 g	120	4	11	2	11
Soy Boy					
Baked Tofu					
Smoked Tofu, 2 oz.	100	5	3	0	11
Tofu Lin, 2 oz.	100	5	4	0	11
Meat Alternatives					
Not Dogs, 43 g	95	3	10	1	7
Okara Courage Burger, 64 g	130	5	8	2	13
Vegetarian Franks, 43 g	65	2	2	1	11
SoyBoy Organic Tofu					
Organic Tofu Extra Firm, 3 oz.	110	6	1	N/A	12
Organic Tofu Firm, 3 oz.	90	5	1	N/A	10

Pork	Cal	Fat	Cbs	Fbr	Prtn
Farmer John					
California Natural Fresh Pork					
Boneless Pork Butt, 112 g	210	13	0	0	21
Boneless Pork Sirloin, 112 g	220	14	0	0	24
Extra Lean Ground Pork, 4 oz.	180	4	0	0	35
• Tenderloins, 112 g	120	3	0	0	24
Jimmy Dean					
Fully Cooked					
Original Sausage Links, 272 g	240	22	1	0	9
Original Sausage Patties, 34 g	240	23	1	0	9
Turkey Sausage Links, 272 g	120	7	1	0	13
Turkey Sausage Patties, 34 g	120	7	1	0	13
Heat N' Serve					
Sausage Links Hot, 55 g	230	22	2	2	6
Sausage Links Maple, 55 g	250	25	2	0	6
Sausage Links, 55 g	250	24	2	0	7

(•= most healthy •= least healthy)

Pork (cont.)	Cal	Fat	Cbs	Fbr	Prtn
Jimmy Dean (cont.)					
Heat N' Serve (cont.)					
Sausage Patties, 51 g	190	18	1	0	6
Links & Patties					
Maple Links, 56 g	170	14	2	0	7
Maple Patties, 53 g	170	14	2	0	7
Original Links, 53 g	170	14	1	0	7
Original Patties, 69 g	240	23	1	0	9
Tyson Chicken					
Fresh Boneless Loin Roast, 112 g	190	12	0	0	20
Fresh Loin Back Ribs, 112 g	250	20	0	0	17
Fresh Pork Chops, 112 g	200	13	0	0	20
Fresh Pork Roasts, 112 g	130	5	0	0	21
Fresh Sirloin Roast, 112 g	140	6	0	0	21
• Fresh Spareribs, 112 g	290	24	0	0	16
Fresh Tenderloin, 112 g	120	4	0	0	21

Sausage	Cal	Fat	Cbs	Fbr	Prtn
Butterball					
Bratwurst, 94 g	160	10	3	0	13
Hardwood Smoked, 94 g	160	10	4	0	13
Monterey Jack Cheese, 94 g	150	10	4	0	12
Spicy Chipotle Peppers, 94 g	170	10	6	0	13
Empire Kosher					
• Mushroom Garlic Sausages, 71 g	80	2	3	0	13
Sun Dried Tomato Basil Sausages, 71 g	80	2	3	0	13
Sweet Apple & Cinnamon Sausages, 71 g	80	2	3	0	13
Farmer John					
Breakfast Sausage					
Old-Fashioned Maple Skinless Links, 37 g	150	13	2	0	7
Original Skinless Links, 37 g	140	12	1	0	6
Premium Original Chorizo, 3 oz.	220	19	2	0	10
Premium Sausage Patties Lowfat, 39 g	110	8	1	0	7
Dinner Sausage					
Premium Beef Rope Sausage, 56 g	150	12	3	0	8
Premium Polish Sausage, 56 g	170	16	1	0	8
Premium Pork Rope Sausage, 56 g	160	14	0	0	8
Red Hots Ext Hot! Prem Smoked Sausage, 85 g	270	24	2	0	11
Hebrew National					
Polish Sausage, 1 link	240	22	2	0	11
Jimmy Dean					
All Natural Hot, 2 oz.	210	17	1	0	12
Premium Pork Italian, 16 oz.	190	17	1	N/A	8
Premium Pork Light, 12 oz.	140	11	1	0	9
Premium Pork Mild Country, 16 oz.	200	21	1	N/A	9
Premium Pork Regular, 2 oz.	180	16	1	0	8
Johnsonville					
Brats					
Cheddar Bratwurst Links, 85 g	170	22	3	N/A	15
Johnsonville Grilling Chorizo, 85 g	280	22	3	N/A	16
• Natural Casing Stadium Style Brats, 102 g	330	30	2	N/A	10
Original Bratwurst, 85 g	270	22	2	N/A	15

MEAT

Sausage (cont.)

	Cal	Fat	Cbs	Fbr	Prtn
Johnsonville (cont.)					
Brats (cont.)					
Smoked Brats, 76 g	240	21	2	N/A	9
Breakfast Sausage					
Brown Sugar & Honey Links, 55 g	170	13	4	N/A	8
Home-style Breakfast Patties, 43 g	140	11	0	N/A	8
Original Breakfast Links, 55 g	180	14	2	N/A	11
Original Breakfast Patties, 65 g	210	17	2	N/A	12
Italian Sausage					
All Natural Ground Mild Italian Sausage, 2 oz.	170	13	1	N/A	10
Heat & Serve Italian Sausage, 81 g	280	24	3	N/A	12
Mild Italian Links, 85 g	270	22	3	N/A	15
Smoked Sausage					
Beef Summer Sausage, 2 oz.	170	15	1	0	9
Hot Links, 76 g	230	20	2	N/A	9
New Orleans Brand Smoked Sausage, 76 g	230	20	2	N/A	9
Original Summer Sausage, 2 oz.	170	15	1	0	9
Polish Sausage, 76 g	240	21	2	N/A	9
Smoked Turkey Sausage, 64 g	110	6	4	N/A	10
Libby's					
BBQ Vienna Sausage, 3 Links	140	12	4	1	5
Oscar Mayer					
Beef Summer Sausage, 28 g	90	7	1	N/A	4
Hard Salami, 27 g	100	8	1	N/A	7
Summer Sausage, 46 g	140	12	0	0	7
Perdue Farms					
Lean Turkey Sausage Links, Sweet Italian, 91 g	150	8	4	N/A	15
Turkey Breakfast Sausage, 2 oz.	80	5	0	N/A	9
Turkey Breakfast Sausage, Sweet Italian, 2 oz.	90	5	2	N/A	9

POULTRY

Chicken

	Cal	Fat	Cbs	Fbr	Prtn
Bumblebee Tuna					
Prime Fillet® Chkn Brst w/ BBQ Sauce, 4 oz.	170	2	10	0	29
Prime Fillet® Chkn Brst w/ Garlic & Herbs, 4 oz.	110	2	1	0	24
Prime Fillet® Chkn Brst w/ S.W. Seasonings, 4 oz.	120	1	1	0	26
Empire Kosher					
Chicken Burgers, 112 g	150	9	1	0	18
Chicken Thighs, 112 g	220	16	0	0	19
Fresh Boneless Skinless Breasts, 112 g	180	9	0	0	23
Fresh Ground Chicken, 112 g	150	9	1	0	18
Fresh Leg Quarters, 113 g	210	14	0	0	20
Fresh Whole Broiler, 112 g	240	17	0	0	21
Roasters, 112 g	220	15	0	0	19
Rock Cornish Broiler, 112 g	165	10	0	0	19
Oscar Mayer					
Breast Cuts - Honey Roasted, 85 g	130	3	3	0	22
Breast Cuts Oven Roasted, 85 g	130	3	1	N/A	22
Breast Strips - Grilled, 84 g	110	3	1	N/A	19
Breast Strips - Italian, 84 g	110	3	1	N/A	19
Breast Strips- Breaded Restaurant Style, 84 g	170	6	14	N/A	15

(•= most healthy •= least healthy)

POULTRY

Chicken (cont.)	Cal	Fat	Cbs	Fbr	Prtn
Perdue Farms					
Cooked Chicken					
Carved Chicken Breast, 71 g	100	2	2	N/A	17
Carved Chicken Breast, Grilled, 71 g	90	2	1	N/A	16
Carved Chicken Breast, Original Roasted, 71 g	90	2	0	N/A	16
Fit & Easy® Chicken					
Boneless, Skinless Chkn Breast Tenderloins, 4 oz.	120	1	0	N/A	26
Boneless, Skinless Chicken Breasts, 4 oz.	110	1	0	N/A	26
Boneless, Skinless Chkn Thighs, 4 oz.	140	6	0	N/A	22
Fresh Baked Breaded Chicken					
Breast Cutlets, Homestyle, 3 oz.	160	7	12	N/A	12
Breast Pattie, 114 oz.	230	12	14	N/A	18
Breast Tenderloins, 3 oz.	170	7	15	N/A	12
Nuggets with Whole Grain Breading, 80 g	160	7	13	N/A	10
Fresh Breaded Chicken					
Chicken Breast Cutlets, Original, 3 oz.	210	12	13	N/A	10
Chicken Breast Nuggets, Dinosaur Shapes, 3 oz.	180	9	12	N/A	12
Chicken Breast Nuggets, Original, 3 oz.	200	12	14	N/A	10
Chicken Breast Strips, Original, 74 oz.	180	11	11	N/A	10
Fresh Chicken Parts					
• Boneless, Skinless Chkn Thighs, 3 oz.	70	9	0	N/A	23
Chicken Drumsticks, 2 oz.	110	6	0	N/A	14
Chicken Thighs, 3 oz.	240	19	0	N/A	17
Chicken Wings, 3 oz.	210	15	0	N/A	19
Frozen Breaded Chicken					
Breast Nuggets, 95 g	230	14	14	N/A	12
Breast Tenders, 99 oz.	240	14	14	N/A	12
Strips, Buffalo Style, 3 oz.	180	7	14	N/A	14
Strips, Homestyle, 3 oz.	230	9	21	N/A	15
Ground Chicken					
Fresh Ground Chkn Filet of Breast Meat, 4 oz.	100	1	0	N/A	24
Fresh Ground Chicken, 4 oz.	180	12	0	N/A	19
Ground Chicken Patties, 4 oz.	170	11	0	N/A	19
Perfect Portions® Chicken					
Boneless, Skinless Chicken Breasts, 5 oz.	130	2	0	N/A	29
Boneless, Skinless Chkn Brsts, All Natural, 5 oz.	140	2	0	N/A	32
Boneless, Skinless Chkn Brsts, Teriyaki, 5 oz.	160	2	7	N/A	28
Tyson Chicken					
Fresh Boneless, Skinless Chkn Brsts, 112 g	110	3	0	0	23
Fresh Chicken Breast Tenders, 112 g	100	1	0	0	22
Fresh Chicken Drumsticks, 112 g	150	9	0	0	18
Fresh Chicken Leg Quarters, 112 g	190	13	0	0	18
Fresh Chicken Thighs, 112 g	220	17	0	0	16
Fresh Family Roaster, 112 g	210	15	0	0	19
Fresh Split Chicken Breasts with Ribs, 112 g	170	10	0	0	21
• Fresh Young Chicken, 112 g	250	19	0	0	19

Turkey	Cal	Fat	Cbs	Fbr	Prtn
Butterball					
Roast 'n Slice Boneless Stuffed Turkey, 100 g	140	7	5	1	15
Fresh Whole Turkey					
Fresh - 5 to 7 kilos, 100 g	160	9	0	0	20

OULTRY

Turkey (cont.)

	Cal	Fat	Cbs	Fbr	Prtn
Butterball (cont.)					
Fresh Whole Turkey (cont.)					
Fresh - 7 to 9 kilos, 100 g	210	14	0	0	20
Fresh - Over 9 kilos, 100 g	190	12	0	0	20
Fresh- Under 5 kilos, 100 g	160	9	0	0	20
Frozen Specialty Roasts - Cook from Frozen					
Boneless Light & Dark Turkey Roast, 100 g	90	2	0	0	17
Boneless Stuffed Turkey Breast, 100 g	120	4	7	1	15
Boneless Turkey Breast, 100 g	80	1	0	0	19
Stuffed Turkey Breast with bone, 100 g	150	6	11	1	14
Turkey Breast with bone, 100 g	100	3	0	0	19
Frozen Whole Turkey - Plump & Juciy					
5 to 7 kilos, 100 g	120	5	0	0	19
7 to 9 kilos, 100 g	120	4	1	0	20
9 to 11 kilos, 100 g	220	17	1	0	16
Over 5 kilos, 100 g	160	9	2	0	18
Under 5 kilos, 100 g	150	8	1	0	19
Stuffed Whole Turkey					
Frozen- 5 to 7 kilos, 100 g	160	7	12	1	12
Frozen- 7 to 9 kilos, 100 g	170	10	9	2	13
Turkey Chicken Trio					
• Smoked Ham Style Turkey, 33 g	40	2	1	0	5
Smoked Turkey Breast, 33 g	30	1	1	0	6
Empire Kosher					
Fresh White Ground Turkey, 112 g	140	5	0	0	23
Fresh Whole Turkey Breast, 112 g	210	1	0	0	23
Fresh Whole Turkey, 112 g	180	9	0	0	23
• Frozen Ground Turkey, 112 g	230	17	0	0	19
Frozen Whole Breast, 112 g	160	7	0	0	22
Frozen Whole Turkey, 112 g	180	10	0	0	21
Turkey Burgers, 112 g	220	15	0	0	21
Turkey Tenders, 112 g	120	1	0	0	23
Perdue Farms					
Cooked Turkey					
Carved Turkey Breast, Oven Roasted, 71 g	90	1	2	N/A	20
FIT & EASY® Turkey					
Boneless, Skinless Tkey Brst Fillets, 4 oz.	120	1	0	N/A	27
Boneless, Skinless Tkey Brst Tendorloin, 4 oz.	120	1	0	N/A	27
Boneless, Skinless Tkey Brsts, Thin-Slice, 3 oz.	100	1	0	N/A	23
Ground Turkey					
Turkey Breast, 4 oz.	120	2	0	N/A	27
Turkey Patties, 4 oz.	160	8	0	N/A	21
Turkey, 4 oz.	230	17	0	N/A	18
Ground Turkey, 4 oz.	160	8	0	N/A	24
Turkey Parts					
Fresh Turkey Drumsticks, 3 oz.	130	5	0	N/A	22
Fresh Turkey Thighs, 3 oz.	190	12	0	N/A	20
Fresh Turkey Wings, 3 oz.	160	8	0	N/A	22
Fresh Whole Turkey Breast, 3 oz.	170	8	0	N/A	23
Whole Turkey					
Fresh Turkey (Roasted Dark Meat), 3 oz.	190	11	0	N/A	21
Fresh Turkey (Roasted White Meat), 3 oz.	150	7	0	N/A	23

(• = most healthy • = least healthy)

POPULAR BRANDS

PREPACKAGED MEALS & SIDES

Baby Food

	Cal	Fat	Cbs	Fbr	Prtn
Beech-Nut Baby Food					
DHA Plus					
Banana Supreme, 1 jar	110	0	25	1	1
• Carrots, 1 jar	45	0	10	3	1
• Whole Wheat Pasta Parmesan, 1 jar	230	5	37	3	10
New Beverages					
G.M. Chiquita Banana Juice w/Yogurt, 6 fl.oz.	110	1	25	2	1
Good Evening Veggie Delight Juice, 6 fl.oz.	130	1	27	3	4
Yogurt Blends w/ Juice-mixed Berry, 6 fl.oz.	90	1	20	2	1
Stage 2					
Apples & Bananas, 1 jar	70	0	16	1	0
Corn & Sweet Potatoes, 1 jar	90	0	18	1	1
Good Evening Turkey Tetrazzini, 1 jar	130	3	23	1	4
Wholesome New					
G.E. Whole Wheat Pasta In Tomato Sauce, 1 jar	100	2	19	2	3
G.E. Whole Wheat With Raisins Cereal, 15 g	50	0	10	1	2
Whole Wheat Pasta Parm, 1 jar	230	5	37	3	10

Boxed Salad Mixes

	Cal	Fat	Cbs	Fbr	Prtn
South Beach Living					
• Cranberry Walnut Chicken Salad Kit, 6 oz.	290	13	25	7	24
Santa Fe Style Chicken Salad Kit, 7 oz.	240	6	24	6	29
Tyson Chicken					
• Premium Chunk Chicken Salad Kit, 108 g	210	9	15	1	18

Canned Meals

	Cal	Fat	Cbs	Fbr	Prtn
Bush's Beans					
Bush Chunky Chili, 246 g	260	10	28	8	15
Bush Hot Chili, 246 g	250	10	26	7	14
Bush No Bean Chili, 246 g	240	14	16	3	13
Bush Original Chili, 246 g	250	10	26	7	14
Chef Boyardee					
2 Cheese Pizza, 1 cup	250	4	45	2	9
Beef Ravioli, 1 cup	250	8	32	3	9
Beefaroni, 1 cup	240	9	30	3	9
Big Beefaroni, 1 cup	260	9	32	4	12
Cheese Ravioli, 1 Bowl	200	5	31	2	8
Cheese Ravioli, 1 cup	240	7	32	3	9
Cheesy Burger Macaroni, 1 cup	200	5	30	3	9
Cheesy Burger Ravioli, 1 cup	250	6	38	3	11
Cheesy Nacho Twistaroni, 1 cup	220	7	32	2	8
Chili Mac, 1 cup	260	13	26	3	9
Fat Free Beef Ravioli, 1 cup	170	2	33	2	7
Mini Bites Beef Ravioli, 1 cup	280	13	31	3	10
Mini Bites Pasta Shells, 1 Bowl	210	8	27	2	8
Mini Bites Ravioli, 1 cup	250	9	35	3	8
Mini Bites Spaghetti & Meatballs, 1 cup	250	10	30	3	10
Overstuffed Beef Ravioli, 1 cup	270	6	42	3	11
Rice with Chicken, 1 Bowl	230	9	30	2	6
Rings with Meatballs, 1 cup	240	9	30	2	9
• Sauce with Meat, 1/2 cup	80	4	10	2	3
Tomato & Beef Twistaroni, 1 cup	230	5	38	2	8

REPACKAGED MEALS & SIDES

Canned Meals (cont.)

Canned Meals (cont.)	Cal	Fat	Cbs	Fbr	Prtn
Chef Boyardee (cont.)					
Twistaroni Chili Chesse Do, 1 cup	220	6	32	2	9
Dennison's					
Chili Con Carne, 1 cup	350	15	31	11	22
Chili Con Carne with Beans, 1 cup	360	14	38	11	20
Chunky Chili with Beans, 1 cup	300	10	32	9	20
Fat Free Chili with Beans, 1 cup	210	2	29	8	20
Hot Chili with Beans, 1 cup	350	14	11	2	21
Hot Chunky Chili with Beans, 1 cup	300	10	32	9	20
Turkey Chili, 1 cup	210	3	29	7	16
Vegetarian Chili, 1 cup	190	2	34	9	9
Luck's					
Chicken Dumplings, 1 cup	170	5	21	2	12

Dinner Mixes

Dinner Mixes	Cal	Fat	Cbs	Fbr	Prtn
Betty Crocker					
Chicken Helper Jambalaya, 45 g	150	2	30	1	6
Complete Meals Chkn & Buttermilk Biscuits, 155 g	280	11	37	2	9
Hamburger Helper Cheddar Cheese Melt, 36 g	130	1	26	1	4
Tuna Helper Tetrazzini, 40 g	140	1	29	1	4
Bumblebee Tuna					
Chunk Light Tuna in Water, 3 oz.	70	1	0	0	15
Fat Free Tuna Salad with Crackers, 3 oz.	70	0	10	0	7
Regular Keebler Crackers, 1 oz.	90	5	12	0	2
Sensations® EZ Pl Bowls Lmn & Crckd Pepper, 5 oz.	130	4	2	0	21
Sensations® EZ Pl Bowls Spicy Thai Chili, 5 oz.	190	8	11	1	17
Tuna Salad Original with Crackers, Crackers, 1 oz.	90	5	12	0	2
Tuna Salad Original with Crackers, Tuna Salad, 3 oz.	190	16	6	1	8

Lunch/Dinner Meals

Lunch/Dinner Meals	Cal	Fat	Cbs	Fbr	Prtn
Campbell's Soups					
Herb Chicken With Rice, 1/7 Box	160	2	33	1	4
Lemon Chicken With Herb Rice, 1/7 Box	160	2	34	1	3
Southwestern-style Chicken With Rice, 1/6 Box	150	1	32	2	4
Traditional Roast Chicken With Stuffing, 1/6 Box	160	3	29	2	5
Chef Boyardee					
Cheese Pizza Kit Single, 1/4 Package	260	5	45	2	10
Pepperoni Pizza Mix, 1/4 Package	290	8	44	2	11
Hamburger Helper					
Cheesy Baked Potato, 36 oz.	130	2	27	2	2
Cheesy Hashbrowns, 48 oz.	170	1	37	2	3
Crunchy Taco, 42 oz.	140	3	26	1	2
Double Cheese Quesadilla, 46 oz.	160	1	36	1	3
Lunchables					
Chicken Dunks - With 100% White Meat, 1 pk.	310	6	52	0	12
Cracker Stackers - Ham & Cheddar, 1 pk.	400	20	40	1	16
Cracker Stackers - Turkey & Cheddar, 1 pk.	400	13	59	0	12
Mini - Tacos Beef, 1 pk.	410	10	61	1	19
Mini Hot Dogs - Hot Dogs, 1 pk.	380	11	61	1	14
Pizza - Pizza & Treatza, 1 pk.	460	10	79	4	14
Starkist Tuna					
StarKist Lunch To-Go®, 1 Kit	210	9	27	2	20

(• = most healthy • = least healthy)

PREPACKAGED MEALS & SIDES

Lunch/Dinner Meals (cont.)	Cal	Fat	Cbs	Fbr	Prtn
Taco Bell Home Originals					
Soft Taco Dinner - Flour Tortillas & Sauce, 93 g	230	5	40	2	6
Taco Dinner - Cheesy Double Decker, 67 g	230	9	30	2	5
Taco Dinner - Sauce & Taco Shells, 60 g	250	5	20	2	2
Tyson Chicken					
Beef Chuck Roast Kit w/ Vegetables, 4 oz.	320	21	14	2	18
Beef Fajitas Meal Kit, 107 g	140	4	17	2	9
Beef Pot Roast in Gravy, 140 g	170	8	2	0	23
Beef Steak Quesadilla Kit, 1 Quesadilla	270	14	19	1	15
Beef Stew Kit with Vegetables, 194 g	240	13	20	3	13
Beef Tips in Gravy, 140 g	200	12	5	0	17
Pork Roast Kit with Vegetables, 4 oz.	190	4	18	2	21
Seasoned Beef Meatloaf, 140 g	320	23	16	0	14
Zatarain's					
Ready-to-Serve					
Blackened Chkn w/ Yellow Rice, 1 pkg	300	5	52	1	12
Dirty Rice with Pork, 1 cup	280	5	54	2	6
Red Beans & Rice with Sausage, 184 g	350	7	57	6	13
Sausage & Chicken Gumbo, 1 pkg	150	7	16	1	7

Microwave Meals	Cal	Fat	Cbs	Fbr	Prtn
Betty Crocker					
Bowl Appetit Cheddar Broccoli Rice, 74 g	290	7	51	2	8
Bowl Appetit Herb Chicken Vegetable Rice, 68 g	260	5	49	2	7
• Bowl Appetit Three-Cheese Rotini, 88 g	360	10	55	2	13
Campbell's Soups					
Campbell's® Microwavable Bowls					
Chicken Noodle Soup, 1 cup	70	2	10	1	4
Creamy Tomato Soup, 1 cup	160	5	25	3	3
Tomato Soup, 1 cup	110	0	24	3	3
Vegetable Beef Soup, 1 cup	80	1	15	3	5
Vegetable Soup, 1 cup	110	0	22	3	4
Campbell's® Chunky™ Microwavable Bowls					
Beef w/ Country Vegetables Soup, 1 cup	150	3	21	5	10
New England Clam Chowder, 1 cup	180	8	20	20	6
Sirloin Burger w/ Country Vegetables Soup, 1 cup	160	4	18	4	10
Campbell's® Healthy Request® Chunky™ Microwavable Bowls					
Classic Chicken Noodle Soup, 1 cup	110	3	15	1	7
Grilled Chicken & Sausage Gumbo, 1 cup	130	3	20	3	8
Campbell's® Healthy Request® Select™ Microwavable Bowls					
Italian Wedding Soup, 1 cup	120	3	15	2	7
Mexican Style Chicken Tortilla, 1 cup	130	3	19	3	8
Campbell's® Select™ Microwavable Bowls					
98% Fat Free New England Clam Chowder, 1 cup	110	2	16	3	6
Chicken with Egg Noodles Soup, 1 cup	90	2	12	2	8
Mexican Style Chicken Tortilla Soup, 1 cup	130	3	18	2	8
Minestrone Soup, 1 cup	100	1	19	4	4
Campbell's® Soup at Hand®					
• Chicken & Stars Soup, 1 container	60	2	10	2	3
Creamy Chicken Soup, 1 container	130	9	13	4	4
Creamy Tomato Soup, 1 container	190	4	34	23	4
Velvety Potato Soup, 1 container	161	7	21	4	2

REPACKAGED MEALS & SIDES

Microwave Meals (cont.)

	Cal	Fat	Cbs	Fbr	Prtn
Chef Boyardee					
Microwave Beef Ravioli Bowl, 1 cup	60	7	32	3	8
Microwave Beefaroni Bowl, 1 cup	250	9	31	3	10
Microwave Mini Beef Bowl, 1 cup	240	8	33	3	8
Healthy Choice					
Chicken Noodle Soup Microwaveable Bowl, 1 cup	110	2	17	3	8
Chicken w/ Rice Soup Microwaveable Bowl, 1 cup	90	0	13	2	6
Kraft Macaroni and Cheese					
Easy Mac Macaroni & Cheese					
Bacon Microwave cup, 58 g	220	5	38	1	7
Extreme Cheese Microwavable, 61 g	230	4	42	1	7
Original Microwavable, 61 g	230	4	42	1	7
Original Microwave cup, 2 oz.	220	3	39	1	6
Triple Cheese Microwave cup, 2 oz.	220	5	39	1	7
Luck's					
Microwave Chicken Dumpling, 1 Bowl	160	4	21	2	12
Progresso					
Beef Vegetable, 250 g	100	2	15	2	8
Chicken Noodle Soup, 240 g	80	2	10	1	6
Italian-Style Wedding Soup w/ Meatballs, 239 g	120	4	14	1	6
Lentil Soup, 241 g	130	3	21	3	7
Minestrone Soup, 240 g	90	2	17	4	4

Pasta Mixes

	Cal	Fat	Cbs	Fbr	Prtn
Betty Crocker					
Chicken Helper Creamy Chicken & Noodles, 28 g	90	1	19	1	3
Hamburger Helper Salisbury, 34 g	120	1	25	1	4
Tuna Helper Creamy Broccoli, 47 g	170	1	34	2	6
Chef Boyardee					
Lasagna Kit, 5 oz.	210	4	35	3	9
Hamburger Helper					
Bacon Cheeseburger, 49 oz.	190	3	34	1	5
Beef Pasta, 31 oz.	110	1	22	1	4
Cheddar Cheese Melt, 36 oz.	130	1	26	1	4
Cheeseburger Macaroni, 31 oz.	110	1	23	1	3
Double Cheeseburger Macaroni, 33 oz.	130	2	25	1	3
Four Cheese Lasagna, 38 oz.	130	1	28	1	4
Italian Sausage, 39 oz.	130	1	29	1	4
Hamburger Helper Lasagna, 35 oz.	120	1	26	1	3
Philly Cheesesteak, 37 oz.	140	4	24	1	4
Knorr-Lipton					
Fiesta Sides					
Beef Lo Mein, 62 g	230	4	14	8	9
Jalapeño Jack Pasta, 62 g	230	4	15	8	8
Nacho Pasta, 63 g	230	4	15	8	8
Teriyaki Noodles, 66 g	250	5	15	8	8
Thai Sesame Noodles, 62 g	230	5	14	8	8
Grain Sides					
Alfredo, 60 g	300	17	14	16	10
Chicken, 62 g	270	12	15	16	9
Pasta Sides					
Alfredo Broccoli, 63 g	250	9	13	4	9

(•= most healthy •= least healthy)

PREPACKAGED MEALS & SIDES

Pasta Mixes (cont.)

	Cal	Fat	Cbs	Fbr	Prtn
Knorr-Lipton (cont.)					
Pasta Sides (cont.)					
Alfredo, 62 g	240	9	13	4	8
Cheesy Cheddar, 59 g	220	3	14	4	8
Parmesan, 60 g	230	7	13	4	9
Stroganoff, 56 g	210	3	13	4	7
Kraft Macaroni and Cheese					
Bistro Deluxe - Creamy Portabello Mushroom, 98 g	310	11	40	3	12
Bistro Deluxe - Sundried Tomato Parmesan, 98 g	300	11	40	3	12
Bistro Deluxe - Three Cheese Italiano, 98 g	310	11	40	3	12
Mac & Chz Deluxe w/ Orig Cheddar Chz Sauce, 98 g	320	10	45	1	12
Mac & Chz Premium Thick 'N Creamy, 2 oz	250	2	50	2	9
Mac & Chz Dinner - The Cheesiest, 70 g	260	4	48	1	9
Rice-A-Roni and Pasta Roni					
Classic Favorites					
Angel Hair Pasta with Herbs, 2 oz.	190	3	38	2	7
Fettuccine Alfredo, 3 oz.	250	6	44	2	9
White Cheddar & Broccoli, 2 oz.	200	4	36	2	7
Nature's Way					
Creamy Parmesan, 2 oz.	200	3	38	2	7
Mushrooms in Cream Sauce, 2 oz.	200	3	37	2	8
Olive Oil & Italian Herb, 2 oz.	200	3	38	2	8
Soy Boy					
Original Tofu Ravioli, 100 g	180	3	31	0	10
Ravioli Rosa, 100 g	180	3	29	4	10
Velveeta					
• Rotini & Cheese - Broccoli, 126 g	400	16	49	2	15
Shells & Cheese - 2% Milk, 112 g	330	5	58	2	14
Shells & Cheese - Bacon, 112 g	360	14	45	1	14
Shells & Cheese - Original, 112 g	360	12	49	2	13
Zatarain's					
Alfredo Pasta Mix, 36 g	140	4	22	0	5
Gumbo Pasta Dinner Mix, 1 cup prepared	120	1	23	2	4
Scampi Pasta Dinner, 35 g	110	1	21	1	4

Potato Mixes

	Cal	Fat	Cbs	Fbr	Prtn
Betty Crocker					
• Potatoes Specialty Four Cheese Mashed, 25 g	80	0	19	1	2
Specialty Deluxe 3 Chz Mashed Potato Bake, 45 g	150	5	24	1	3
• Sweet Potato Casserole, 44 g	210	5	39	2	2
Campbell's Soups					
Cheesy Chicken with pasta, 1/7 box	150	3	24	1	5
Creamy Stroganoff Sauce with pasta, 1/6 box	190	4	33	1	6
Garlic Chicken with pasta, 1/7 box	190	2	36	2	8
Martha White					
Hush Puppy Mix, 1/4 cup	120	N/A	25	1	3
Spud Flakes, 1/3 cup	80	N/A	17	2	2
Simply Potatoes					
Country Style Mashed Potatoes, 141 g	110	2	20	3	3
Mashed Sweet Potatoes, 141 g	100	1	21	3	2
Sour Cream and Chive Mashed Potatoes, 141 g	130	5	18	3	3

POPULAR BRANDS

PREPACKAGED MEALS & SIDES

Potato Mixes (cont.)

	Cal	Fat	Cbs	Fbr	Prtn
Velveeta					
Cheesy Au Gratin, 58 g	180	6	26	2	5
Cheesy Bacon Scalloped, 60 g	190	7	26	2	6
Cheesy Mashed, 42 g	140	5	19	1	4
Zatarain's					
Hush Puppy Mix, 3 tbsp.	100	1	23	1	2

Rice Mixes

	Cal	Fat	Cbs	Fbr	Prtn
Carolina Enriched Rice					
Authentic Spanish, 2 oz.	180	0	42	1	4
Black Beans & Rice, 2 oz.	200	2	39	5	7
Broccoli & Cheese, 2 oz.	200	3	39	1	5
Chicken & Rice, 2 oz.	190	0	42	1	5
Classic Pilaf, 2 oz.	190	1	43	1	5
Long Grain & Wild, 2 oz.	200	1	43	2	5
Red Beans & Rice, 2 oz.	190	1	41	3	7
Saffron Yellow, 2 oz.	190	0	43	1	4
Spicy Yellow, 2 oz.	180	1	41	1	4
Knorr-Lipton					
Chicken Broccoli, 63 g	270	11	15	12	7
Chipotle Rice, 72 g	260	2	18	8	7
Mexican Rice, 68 g	250	2	17	8	7
Sesame Chicken, 70 g	300	14	17	12	7
Spanish Rice, 67 g	240	2	17	8	6
Taco Rice, 68 g	250	2	17	8	7
Asian Sides					
Chicken Fried Rice, 66 g	240	2	16	4	7
Teriyaki Rice, 65 g	240	2	17	4	6
Cajun Sides					
Dirty Rice, 68 g	250	2	17	8	8
Garlic Butter Rice, 67 g	260	6	16	4	7
New Orleans Style Chicken Rice, 67 g	240	2	17	8	7
Red Beans and Rice, 80 g	290	2	21	16	7
Rice Sides					
Chicken, 65 g	250	5	16	4	7
Creamy Chicken, 68 g	270	8	16	4	7
Mushroom, 67 g	240	2	17	4	7
Rice Medley, 62 g	230	3	15	4	7
Rice Pilaf, 61 g	220	2	15	4	6
Mahatma Rice					
Authentic Spanish, 2 oz.	180	0	42	1	4
Broccoli & Cheese, 2 oz.	230	4	43	1	6
Classic Pilaf, 2 oz.	190	1	43	1	5
Long Grain & Wild, 2 oz.	200	1	43	2	5
Saffron Yellow, 2 oz.	190	0	43	1	4
Minute Rice					
Ready To Serve					
Chicken Rice Mix, 125 g	190	4	35	1	3
Long Grain & Wild Rice Mix, 125 g	190	4	34	1	4
Yellow Rice Mix, 125 g	190	4	35	1	3

(● = most healthy ● = least healthy) **POPULAR BRANDS • 473**

Rice Mixes (cont.)	Cal	Fat	Cbs	Fbr	Prtn
Rice-A-Roni and Pasta Roni					
Classic Favorites					
Broccoli Au Gratin, 3 oz.	260	6	46	2	7
Chicken & Broccoli, 3 oz.	240	3	47	3	9
Long Grain & Wild Rice, 2 oz.	190	1	42	2	5
Nature's Way					
Italian Cheese & Herb, 3 oz.	270	6	50	1	6
Long Grain & Wild Rice, 2 oz.	190	1	43	1	5
Parmesan & Romano Cheese, 2 oz.	210	3	40	1	5
Savory Whole Grain Blends					
Chicken & Herb Classico, 2 oz.	190	2	41	4	6
Roasted Garlic Italiano, 2 oz.	210	3	41	3	6
Spanish, 2 oz.	200	2	42	3	5
Uncle Ben's					
Country Inn®					
Broccoli Rice Au Gratin, 57 g	200	2	43	1	4
Chicken & Broccoli Rice, 57 g	190	1	42	1	5
Chicken & Wild Rice, 57 g	200	1	42	1	5
Oriental Fried Rice, 57 g	200	1	42	1	6
Long Grain & Wild Rice					
Butter & Herb, 57 g	190	1	40	1	5
Roasted Garlic & Olive Oil, 54 g	180	1	39	3	5
Vegetable Pilaf, 57 g	180	1	40	3	5
Ready Rice					
Creamy Four Cheese Flavored, 160 g	230	4	44	2	6
Long Grain & Wild, 153 g	220	3	43	2	5
Rice Pilaf, 155 g	220	4	42	2	6
Spanish Style, 144 g	200	3	41	3	4
Ready Whole Grain Medley™					
Brown & Wild, 146 g	220	4	42	3	6
Santa Fe, 160 g	220	3	42	5	7
Vegetable Harvest, 153 g	220	3	44	5	5
Zatarain's					
Reduced Sodium					
Dirty Rice, 38 g	130	0	29	1	3
Jambalaya, 38 g	130	0	29	1	3
Red Beans & Rice, 57 g	190	0	40	5	8
Rice Mixes					
Caribbean Rice Mix, 45 g	160	2	34	1	3
Chicken Flavored Rice, 1 cup prepared	210	1	44	1	5
Dirty Rice Mix, 46 g	130	0	29	1	3
Long Grain & Wild Rice, 33 g	230	1	49	1	6
Red Beans & Rice, 28 g	190	0	40	5	8
Spanish Rice, 26 g	180	0	41	1	4
• Yellow Rice Mix, 1/2 cup prepared	110	0	23	N/A	3

Stuffing	Cal	Fat	Cbs	Fbr	Prtn
Butterball					
• Homestyle Stuffing, 75 g	190	9	25	1	3
Pepperidge Farm					
Cornbread Stuffing, 3/4c	170	2	33	2	4
Country Style Stuffing, 3/4c	140	1	27	2	5

PREPACKAGED MEALS & SIDES

Stuffing (cont.)

	Cal	Fat	Cbs	Fbr	Prtn
Pepperidge Farm (cont.)					
Herb Seasoned Stuffing, 3/4c	170	2	33	3	5
Sage & Onion Stuffing, 3/4c	140	1	26	3	5
Stove-Top					
Stuffing Mix - Chicken One Step, 28 g	150	3	20	1	3
Stuffing Mix - Traditional Sage, 28 g	110	1	21	1	3
Stuffing Mix - Turkey, 28 g	110	1	20	1	3
Zatarain's					
Cornbread Stuffing, 1/2 cup prepared	100	1	21	1	3
Creole Chicken Stuffing, 1/2 cup prepared	100	1	20	1	3
French Bread Stuffing, 1/2 cup prepared	100	1	20	1	3

SALAD DRESSING & TOPPINGS

Croutons & Toppings

	Cal	Fat	Cbs	Fbr	Prtn
Betty Crocker					
Bacos Bits, 7 g	30	2	2	N/A	3
Bacos Chips, 7 g	30	2	2	N/A	3
French's					
French Fried Onions, 7 g	45	4	3	0	0
McCormick					
Bac'n Pieces™ Bacon Flavored Bits, 7 g	30	2	2	N/A	3
Bac'n Pieces™ Bacon Flavored Chips, 7 g	30	2	2	N/A	3
Salad Toppins™ Garden Vegetable, 7 g	35	2	3	N/A	1
Salad Toppins™, 7 g	35	2	2	N/A	1
Pepperidge Farm					
• Classic Caesar Croutons, 6 croutons	30	1	5	0	1
Four Cheese and Garlic Croutons, 6 croutons	30	1	5	0	1
Seasoned Croutons, 6 croutons	30	1	5	0	1
Zesty Italian Croutons, 6 croutons	30	1	5	0	1
Sargento					
Potato Finishers					
All American, 39 g	130	9	3	0	8
Au Gratin, 39 g	130	9	5	0	5
Cheddar Broccoli, 39 g	140	10	2	0	8
Salad Finishers					
Bistro Chicken, 44 g	110	7	2	1	10
• Cheddar Bacon, 36 g	160	9	9	0	9
Cheddar Chicken, 53 g	150	8	9	0	11
Chicken Caesar, 41 g	100	4	6	0	9
Cranberry Pecan, 33 g	140	5	9	1	5

Dressing Mix

	Cal	Fat	Cbs	Fbr	Prtn
Good Seasons					
Cheese Garlic, 2 oz.	5	0	1	N/A	0
• Garlic & Herb, 2 oz.	5	0	1	N/A	0
• Gourmet Caesar, 4 oz.	15	0	2	N/A	0
Mild Italian, 4 oz.	10	0	2	N/A	0

Salad Dressings

	Cal	Fat	Cbs	Fbr	Prtn
Annie's Naturals					
Dressings					
Balsamic Vinaigrette, 29 g	100	10	3	N/A	0

Salad Dressings (cont.)	Cal	Fat	Cbs	Fbr	Prtn
Annie's Naturals (cont.)					
Dressings (cont.)					
Goddess Dressing, 31 g	130	13	2	N/A	1
• Strawberry & Balsamic Dressing, 15 ml.	10	0	2	0	0
Organic Dressings					
Buttermilk Dressing - Organic, 30 g	70	7	1	N/A	1
Caesar Dressing - Organic, 30 ml.	120	12	1	N/A	1
Red Wine & Olive Oil Vinaigrette, 29 g	160	17	1	N/A	0
Bernsteins					
Fat Free					
Cheese and Garlic Italian, 30 g	10	0	2	0	0
Light Fantastic					
Cheese Fantastico, 32 g	25	2	3	0	1
Parmesan Garlic Ranch, 32 g	50	3	6	0	1
Roasted Garlic Balsamic, 30 g	45	4	3	0	0
Regular					
Chunky Blue Cheese, 30 g	120	13	2	0	1
Creamy Caesar, 29 g	120	13	1	0	0
Italian Dressings & Marinade, 30 g	110	12	1	0	0
Betty Crocker					
Suddenly Salad Caesar, 47 g	170	1	34	1	6
Suddenly Salad Chipotle Ranch, 40 g	140	1	28	1	6
• Suddenly Salad Classic, 51 g	180	1	37	2	6
California Sun Dry					
Sun-Dried Tomato Salad Dressing, 2tbs	20	13	N/A	N/A	N/A
Good Seasons					
Asian Sesame With Ginger, 32 oz.	110	9	7	0	0
Clas Balsamic Vinaigrette w/ Ex Virgin Olive, 31 oz.	90	8	4	0	0
Creamy Caesar w/ Aged Parmesan, 30 oz.	100	9	3	0	1
Red Raspberry Vinaigrette w/ Poppyseed, 32 oz.	60	4	5	0	0
Kraft Salad Dressings					
Creamy Italian, 30 g	100	11	2	0	0
French Style Fat Free, 2 tbsp.	45	0	11	0	0
Honey Dijon Fat Free, 2 tbsp.	50	0	12	0	0
Italian Fat Free, 2 tbs.	20	0	4	0	0
Light Done Right Caesar, 2 tbsp.	60	5	3	0	1
Light Done Right Creamy French, 33 g	80	5	10	0	0
Ranch Garlic, 30 g	120	12	3	0	0
Special Collection Greek Vinaigrette, 30 g	110	12	2	0	0
Special Collection Parm Romano, 29 g	140	14	2	0	1
Marzetti					
1000 Island Dressing, 28 g	150	15	5	0	0
Buttermilk Ranch Dressing, 29 g	160	17	1	0	1
Caesar Dressing, 30 g	140	15	1	0	1
Ginger Mango Dressing, 32 g	120	9	8	0	0
Light Caesar Dressing, 31 g	70	7	2	0	1
Light Honey Dijon Dressing, 32 g	90	6	8	0	0
Lite Ranch Dressing, 31 g	80	8	2	0	1
Strawberry Chardonnay Dressing, 32 g	110	9	7	0	0
Sweet Italian Dressing, 31 g	150	14	8	0	0
Ultimate Blue Cheese Dressing, 31 g	160	17	1	0	1

SALAD DRESSING & TOPPINGS

Salad Dressings (cont.)

	Cal	Fat	Cbs	Fbr	Prtn
Paul Newman's Own					
Lighten Up					
Balsamic Vinaigrette Dressing, 30 g	45	4	2	0	0
Light Cranberry Walnut, 30 g	70	4	8	0	1
Lowfat Sesame Ginger Dressing, 30 g	135	2	5	0	0
Sun Dried Tomato Dressing, 30 g	60	4	5	0	0
Organic					
Organic Creamy Caesar Dressing, 30 g	170	18	1	0	0
Organic Light Balsamic Dressing, 30 g	45	4	3	0	0
Organic Lowfat Asian Dressing, 32 g	35	2	5	0	0
Organic Tuscan Italian Dressing, 30 g	100	11	1	0	0
Regular					
Balsamic Vinaigrette Dressing, 30 g	90	9	3	0	0
Caesar Dressing, 31 g	150	16	1	0	1
Family Recipe Italian Dressing, 30 g	120	13	1	0	1
Parme & Roasted Garlic Dressing, 29 g	110	11	2	0	0
Two Thousand Island Dressing, 30 g	140	14	4	0	0
Salad Mist					
Asian Sesame Natural Salad Mist, 8 ml.	10	1	1	0	0
Balsamic Natural Salad Mist, 8 ml.	15	1	2	0	0
Tuscan Italian Natural Salad Mist, 8 ml.	10	1	1	0	0
Seven Seas Salad Dressing					
Creamy Italian, 30 g	110	12	2	0	0
Green Goddess, 2 tbsp.	130	13	2	0	0
Red Wine Vinaigrette Fat Free, 32 g	15	0	3	0	0
Red Wine Vinaigrette, 2 tbsp.	90	9	2	0	0
Viva Italian, 30 g	90	9	2	0	0
Viva Italian Reduced Fat, 31g	45	4	2	0	0
South Beach Living					
Balsamic Vinaigrette Dressing, 32 g	50	4	4	0	0
Italian Dressing, 31 g	30	4	3	0	0
Ranch Dressing, 29 g	70	7	2	0	1

Vinegar

	Cal	Fat	Cbs	Fbr	Prtn
Progresso					
Vinegar Balsamic, 15 ml.	10	0	2	N/A	0

SAUCES & MARINADES

Barbecue Sauce

	Cal	Fat	Cbs	Fbr	Prtn
Annie's Naturals					
Annie's Original BBQ Sauce - Organic, 33 g	45	1	9	N/A	0
Consorzio BBQ Sauce, 35 g	45	0	11	0	1
Smokey Maple BBQ Sauce - Organic, 33 g	45	1	9	N/A	0
Cattleman's Sauces					
Cattlemen's Classic, 2 tbsp.	60	0	15	0	0
Cattlemen's Gold, 2 tbsp.	60	0	14	0	0
Cattlemen's Hot & Spicy, 2 tbsp.	45	0	11	0	0
Cattlemen's Original, 2 tbsp.	40	0	9	2	0
Cattlemen's Smoky, 2 tbsp.	40	0	9	0	0
Cattlemen's Sweet & Bold, 2 tbsp.	60	0	14	0	0
• Honey BBQ Sauce, 2 tbsp.	70	0	17	0	0

(•= most healthy •= least healthy)

SAUCES & MARINADES

Barbecue Sauce (cont.)

	Cal	Fat	Cbs	Fbr	Prtn
Texas Pete					
• Original BBQ Sauce, 4 g	5	0	0	N/A	0

Gravy & Glazes

	Cal	Fat	Cbs	Fbr	Prtn
Campbell's Soups					
Campbell's™ Gravies					
Beef Gravy, 1/4 cup	25	1	3	3	1
• Country Style Sausage Gravy, 1/4 cup	70	5	4	0	2
• Fat Free Beef Gravy, 1/4 cup	15	0	3	0	1
Turkey Gravy, 1/4 cup	25	1	3	0	1
Campbell's™ Microwavable Gravies					
Beef Gravy, 1/4 cup	25	1	3	0	1
Chicken Gravy, 1/4 cup	40	3	3	0	0
Turkey Gravy, 1/4 cup	25	1	3	0	1
Franco-American Gravies					
Fat Free Slow Roast Beef Gravy, 1/4 cup	20	0	3	0	1
Fat Free Slow Roast Chkn Gravy, 1/4 cup	20	0	4	0	1
Fat Free Slow Roast Tkey Gravy, 1/4 cup	20	0	4	0	1
Slow Roast Beef Gravy, 1/4 cup	25	1	3	0	1
Slow Roast Chicken Gravy, 1/4 cup	20	1	3	0	1
Slow Roast Turkey Gravy, 1/4 cup	25	0	4	0	1
McCormick					
Homestyle Gravy Mix, 6 g	25	1	4	N/A	0
Mushroom Gravy Mix, 5 g	20	1	2	N/A	0
Original Country Gravy Mix, 9 g	50	4	4	N/A	0
Peppered Country Gravy Mix, 9 g	45	3	4	N/A	0

Hot Sauce

	Cal	Fat	Cbs	Fbr	Prtn
Del Monte					
Chili Sauce, 18 g	20	0	5	0	0
Frank's Red Hot Sauces					
Buffalo Sandwich Sauce, 1 tbsp.	5	0	1	0	0
Buffalo Wing Sauce, 15 ml.	5	0	1	0	0
• Chile 'N Lime™ Hot Sauce, 1 tsp.	0	0	0	0	0
• Gold Fever™ Zing Sauce, 1 tbsp.	40	5	8	0	0
Original Cayenne Pepper Sauce, 1 tsp.	0	0	0	0	0
Xtra Hot Cayenne Pepper Sauce, 5 ml.	0	0	0	0	0
Taco Bell Home Originals					
Hot, 5 g	0	0	0	N/A	0
Mild, 5 g	0	0	0	N/A	0
Texas Pete					
Buffalo Style Chicken Wing BBQ Sauce, 36 g	30	1	5	N/A	1
Hot Sauce, 4 g	0	0	0	N/A	0

Marinades

	Cal	Fat	Cbs	Fbr	Prtn
Annie's Naturals					
Mango Cilantro Marinade - Organic, 15 g	20	1	3	0	0
Organic Steak Marinade, 30 g	50	4	5	N/A	1
• Smokey Tomato Marinade - Organic, 30 g	60	6	1	N/A	0
Lawry's					
Herb & Garlic, 15 ml.	10	0	2	N/A	0
• Mesquite, 15 ml.	5	0	1	0	0
Sesame Ginger, 15 ml.	30	0	7	0	0

SAUCES & MARINADES

Marinades (cont.)

	Cal	Fat	Cbs	Fbr	Prtn
Lawry's (cont.)					
Tequila Lime, 15 ml.	15	0	4	0	0
Teriyaki, 15 ml.	20	0	5	0	0
Paul Newman's Own					
Herb & Roasted Garlic Marinade, 15 ml.	20	1	3	0	0
Lemon Pepper Marinade, 15 ml.	15	0	3	0	0
Teriyaki Marinade, 15 ml.	25	0	6	0	0

Meat & Steak Sauce

	Cal	Fat	Cbs	Fbr	Prtn
A-1 Steak Sauce					
A1 Original Steak Sauce, 15 ml.	30	0	8	N/A	0
A1 Zesty Steak Sauce, 15 ml.	12	0	3	N/A	0
Del Monte					
Hickory Flavor, 69 g	60	0	14	0	1
Hickory Flavor, 69 g	60	0	14	0	1
Original Recipe, 67 g	50	0	11	0	1
Original Recipe, 67 g	50	0	11	0	1
French's					
• Worcestershire Sauce Tabletop, 1 tsp.	0	0	0	0	0
Manwich					
BBQ Sloppy Joe Sauce, 1/4 cup	50	0	13	1	1
• Bold Sloppy Joe Sauce, 1/4 cup	60	1	13	1	1
Original Sloppy Joe Sauce, 1/4 cup	30	0	7	1	1
Sloppy Joe Sauce, 1/4 cup	30	0	7	1	1
McCormick					
Beef					
Beef Stew Seasoning Mix, 5 g	15	0	2	N/A	0
Sloppy Joes Seasoning Mix, 5 g	20	0	3	N/A	0
Swedish Meatballs Seasoning & Sauce Mix, 11 g	45	1	4	N/A	0
Chicken					
Hickory BBQ Buffalo Wings Seasoning Mix, 8 g	25	0	5	N/A	0
Original Buffalo Wings Seasoning Mix, 8 g	30	0	5	N/A	0
Pace Foods					
Enchilada Sauce, 1/4 cup	25	0	5	1	1
Taco Sauce, 2 tbsp.	10	0	2	0	0
Paul Newman's Own					
All-Natural Steak Sauce, 17 g	20	1	4	0	0
Taco Bell Home Originals					
Taco Sauce - Medium, 31 g	10	0	2	0	0
Texas Pete					
Chili, 14 g	10	0	0	N/A	1
Chili No Beans, 283 g	340	13	22	7	23
Worcestershire Sauce, 4 g	5	0	0	N/A	0

Seafood Sauces

	Cal	Fat	Cbs	Fbr	Prtn
Del Monte					
Seafood Cocktail Sauce, 78 g	100	0	24	0	1
McCormick					
Cocktail & Tartar Sauces					
Fat Free Tartar Sauce for Seafood, 32 g	32	0	7	N/A	0
Original Cocktail Sauce for Seafood, 67 g	100	0	18	N/A	0
Original Tartar Sauce for Seafood, 28 g	160	15	3	N/A	0

(• = most healthy • = least healthy)

POPULAR BRANDS

SAUCES & MARINADES

Seafood Sauces (cont.)

	Cal	Fat	Cbs	Fbr	Prtn
McCormick (cont.)					
Seafood Sauces & Marinades					
Cajun Seafood Sauce, 32 g	15	0	3	N/A	0
Lemon Butter Dill Seafood Sauce, 29 g	100	9	4	N/A	0
Lemon Herb Seafood Sauce, 30 g	140	15	1	N/A	0
• Mediterranean Seafood Sauce, 32 g	20	0	4	N/A	0
• Scampi Seafood Sauce, 28 g	160	17	0	N/A	0
Texas Pete					
Seafood Cocktail, 60 g	50	1	11	N/A	0
Zatarain's					
Cocktail Sauce, 1/4 cup	70	0	17	0	1

Pasta Sauce

	Cal	Fat	Cbs	Fbr	Prtn
California Sun Dry					
Sun-Dried Tomato Pesto, 1/4 cup	130	13	N/A	N/A	N/A
Del Monte					
Italian Herb Chunky Spaghetti Sauce, 124 g	60	1	12	1	2
Spaghetti Sauce w/ Grn Pepper & Mshrms, 125 g	80	1	16	3	2
Spaghetti Sauce w/ Tomatoes & Basil, 125 g	70	1	16	3	2
Spaghetti Sauce with Meat, 125 g	60	1	14	3	3
Healthy Choice					
Garlic Herb Pasta Sauce, 1/2 cup	60	0	12	3	2
Traditional Pasta Sauce, 1/2 cup	60	0	13	3	2
Zesty Gumbo Soup, 1 cup	100	2	16	4	6
Hunt's					
Paste					
Tomato Paste Basil, Garlic and Oregano, 2 tbsp.	25	0	6	2	1
Tomato Paste No Salt Added, 2 tbsp.	30	0	6	2	1
Sauce					
Tom Sauce Basil, Garlic & Oregano Sauce, 1/4 cup	15	0	3	1	1
Tomato Sauce No Salt Added, 2 tbsp.	30	0	6	2	1
Tomato Sauce Roasted Garlic, 1/4 cup	15	0	3	1	1
McCormick					
Creamy Garlic Alfredo Sauce Mix, 18 g	90	6	4	N/A	3
Four Cheese Sauce Mix, 1 1/3 tbsp.	40	2	5	N/A	1
Italian-Style Spaghetti Sauce Mix, 11 g	35	0	7	N/A	0
• Pesto Sauce Mix, 4 g	10	0	1	N/A	1
Muir Glen					
Pasta Sauces					
Fire Roasted Tomato, 125 g	70	2	11	2	2
Four Cheese, 125 g	80	3	11	2	4
Garden Vegetable, 125 g	60	1	10	2	2
Portobello Mushroom, 125 g	50	0	10	2	2
Tomato Sauces, Pastes and Purees					
Chunky Tomato Sauce, 65 g	15	0	4	1	1
Pizza Sauce, 62 g	40	2	6	1	1
Tomato Paste, 33 g	30	0	6	1	1
Tomato Puree, 63 g	25	0	6	1	1
Paul Newman's Own					
Organic					
Marinara Sauce, 124 g	70	2	12	1	2
Tomato Basil Sauce, 124 g	91	5	12	1	2

SAUCES & MARINADES

Pasta Sauce (cont.)

	Cal	Fat	Cbs	Fbr	Prtn
Paul Newman's Own (cont.)					
Organic (cont.)					
Traditional Herb Sauce, 124 g	90	4	13	1	2
Original					
Bombolina Sauce, 125 g	40	5	13	1	2
Five Cheese Sauce, 124 g	80	3	10	1	3
Italian Sausage & Peppers Sauce, 126 g	90	4	11	1	4
Marinara Sauce, 125 g	70	2	12	1	2
Roasted Garlic & Peppers Sauce, 125 g	70	3	11	4	2
Sweet Onion & Roasted Garlic Pasta Sauce, 124 g	60	2	12	1	2
Vodka Sauce, 124 g	110	5	11	0	5
Prego Sauces					
Chunky Garden Italian Sauce					
Garden Combo, 1/2 cup	70	2	13	3	2
Mushroom Supreme, 1/2 cup	90	3	13	3	2
Tomato, Onion & Garlic, 1/2 cup	90	3	13	3	2
Classic Italian Sausage					
Flavored with Meat, 1/2 cup	130	5	19	3	2
Fresh Mushroom, 1/2 cup	90	3	14	3	2
Marinara, 1/2 cup	100	5	11	4	2
Mini Meatball, 1/2 cup	110	5	13	3	4
Onion & Garlic, 1/2 cup	100	5	12	3	2
Roasted Garlic & Herb, 1/2 cup	90	4	13	3	2
Roasted Garlic Parmesan, 1/2 cup	70	1	13	3	3
Tomato, Basil & Garlic, 1/2 cup	80	3	12	3	2
Traditional, 1/2 cup	80	3	13	3	2
Heart Smart Italian Sauces					
Mushroom Italian Sauce, 1/2 cup	100	3	15	3	2
Traditional Italian Sauce, 1/2 cup	90	3	13	3	2
Organic Italian Sauces					
Mushroom Italian Sauce, 1/2 cup	70	3	13	4	2
Tomato & Basil Italian Sauce, 1/2 cup	80	3	13	4	2
Progresso					
Pasta Sauce Red Clam, 125 g	60	1	8	1	4
• Pasta Sauce White Clam, 124 g	130	10	5	0	6
Tomato Puree, 63 g	25	0	5	1	1
Tomatoes Whole Peeled Italian with Basil, 121 g	20	0	4	1	1

Pizza Sauce

	Cal	Fat	Cbs	Fbr	Prtn
Boboli					
Sauces, 71 g	50	0	10	1	2
Chef Boyardee					
• Pizza Sauce, 1/8 package	280	7	440	2	11
Contadina					
• Four Cheese Pizza Sauce 15 oz., 63 g	30	0	3	1	1
Italian Bread Crumbs 10 oz., 28 g	100	2	19	1	3
Pizza Sauce-Original 8 oz., 63 g	30	0	6	1	1
Sweet & Sour Sauce 16 oz., 33 g	40	1	8		0

(•= most healthy •= least healthy)

SEAFOOD

Crab & Lobster	Cal	Fat	Cbs	Fbr	Prtn
Bumblebee Tuna					
Lump Crabmeat, 2 oz.	40	1	0	0	8
Pink Crabmeat, 2 oz.	35	1	0	0	7
White Crabmeat, 2 oz.	40	1	0	0	8
Chicken of the Sea					
Fancy Crabmeat, 6.00oz., 2 oz.	40	0	2	0	7
• Pink Crab Meat, 6.00oz., 2 oz.	30	0	1	0	7
Premium Imitation Crab Pouch, 3 oz.	40	0	6	1	3
White Crabmeat, 6.00oz., 2 oz.	30	0	1	N/A	7
Louis Kemp Seafood					
Crab Delight					
Crab Delights® Chunk Style, 85 g	70	0	10	1	7
Crab Delights® Easy Shreds, 85 g	80	0	12	1	7
• Crab Delights® Flake Style, 85 g	70	0	10	1	7
Lobster Delights					
Lobster Delights® Chunk Style, 85 g	70	0	10	1	7
Lobster Delights® Salad Style, 85 g	70	0	10	1	7

Fish	Cal	Fat	Cbs	Fbr	Prtn
Bumblebee Tuna					
Prime Fillet® Salmon Steaks					
Pink Salmon, 2 oz.	90	5	0	0	12
Red Salmon, 2 oz.	110	7	0	0	13
Teriyaki Salmon, 4 oz.	160	3	8	0	24
Sardine Mackerel					
Sardines in Hot Sauce, 160 g	170	12	1	0	15
Sardines in Oil, 75 g	130	9	0	0	13
Sardines in Water, 75 g	120	7	0	0	13
Tuna					
Coral® Chunk Light Tuna in Oil, 2 oz.	110	6	0	0	13
Coral® Chunk Light Tuna in Water, 2 oz.	60	1	0	0	13
Prime Fillet® Solid White Albacore in Water, 2 oz.	70	1	0	0	16
Sensations® EZ Peel Bowls Spicy Thai Chili, 5 oz.	190	8	11	1	17
Chicken of the Sea					
Albacore Tuna					
Genova Solid White Tuna in Olive Oil, 2 oz.	110	6	0	0	14
Genova Solid White Tuna in Water, 2 oz.	70	1	0	0	15
Solid White Albacore Tuna in Oil, 2 oz.	90	3	0	0	14
Solid White Albacore Tuna in Spring Water, 2 oz.	70	1	0	0	15
Light Tuna					
Chunk Light Tuna in Oil, 2 oz.	110	6	0	0	13
• Chunk Light Tuna in Spring Water, 2 oz.	60	1	0	0	13
Genova Tonno in Olive Oil, 2 oz.	130	8	0	0	14
Genova Tonno in Water, 2 oz.	70	1	0	0	14
Mackerel					
Jack Mackerel in Tomato Sauce, 1/4 cup	70	3	2	0	10
Jack Mackerel in Water, 1/3 cup	90	4	0	0	13
Salmon					
Prem Skinless & Boneless Pink Salmon Pouch, 2 oz.	60	2	0	0	10
Skinless & Boneless Pink Salmon, 2 oz.	60	2	0	0	10
Traditional Red Salmon, 1/4 cup	110	7	0	0	13

SEAFOOD

Fish (cont.)

	Cal	Fat	Cbs	Fbr	Prtn
Chicken of the Sea (cont.)					
Sardines					
Fish Steaks in Hot Sauce, 2 oz.	70	3	1	1	9
Sardines in Mustard Sauce, 1 can	150	8	2	2	17
Sardines in Tomato Sauce, 1 can	130	6	2	2	17
Sardines in Water, 1 can	100	4	2	0	13
Smoked Sardines in Oil, 1 can	190	14	2	0	12
Progresso					
Tuna Albacore in Olive Oil, 56 g	90	3	0	0	16
Tuna Light in Olive Oil, 56 g	120	6	0	0	15
Starkist Tuna					
Chunk Light Tuna, 2 oz.	60	5	0	0	13
Gourmet Choice Tuna Fillet, 2 oz.	60	1	0	0	13
Low Sodium Tuna, 2 oz.	60	5	0	0	13
Solid White Albacore Tuna, 2 oz.	70	1	0	0	15
StarKist Flavor Fresh Pouch®, 2 oz.	90	1	0	0	19
StarKist Select®, 2 oz.	60	1	0	0	13
StarKist Tuna Creations™, 2 oz.	60	1	0	0	13

Oysters, Clams & Scallops

	Cal	Fat	Cbs	Fbr	Prtn
Bumblebee Tuna					
Clam					
• Chopped Clams, 2 oz.	25	0	2	0	4
Fancy Whole Baby Clams, 2 oz.	50	1	2	0	9
Smoked Clams, 2 oz.	130	9	1	0	11
Oyster					
Smoked Oysters, 2 oz.	120	7	6	0	10
Whole Oysters, 2 oz.	70	3	3	0	7
Chicken of the Sea					
Clams					
Chopped Clams, 1/4 cup	30	0	2	0	5
Minced Clams, 1/4 cup	30	0	2	N/A	5
Premium Whole Baby Clams Pouch, 3 oz.	40	1	1	0	7
Oysters					
Oysters, 2 oz.	80	3	6	0	7
• Smoked Oysters in Oil, 1 can	170	8	8	0	10
Smoked Oysters in Water, 1 can	120	3	10	0	12

Shrimp & Prawns

	Cal	Fat	Cbs	Fbr	Prtn
Bumblebee Tuna					
• Deveined Medium Shrimp, 2 oz.	40	0	0	0	10
Regular Broken Shrimp, 2 oz.	40	0	0	0	10
Regular Medium Shrimp, 2 oz.	40	0	0	0	10
Chicken of the Sea					
Frozen Shrimp					
Premium Cooked, 3 oz.	80	1	0	0	18
Premium Raw, 4 oz.	120	2	1	0	23
• Ready to Cook Medium, 4 oz.	120	2	1	0	23
Ready to Eat Medium, 3 oz.	80	1	0	0	18
Shrimp					
Medium Deveined Shrimp, 2 oz.	45	1	1	0	10
Medium Shrimp, 2 oz.	45	1	1	0	10

(•= most healthy •= least healthy)

POPULAR BRANDS

SEAFOOD

Shrimp & Prawns (cont.)	Cal	Fat	Cbs	Fbr	Prtn
Chicken of the Sea (cont.)					
Shrimp (cont.)					
Premium Shrimp Pouch, 3 oz.	55	1	1	0	12
Tiny Shrimp, 2 oz.	45	1	1	0	10

SNACKS

Chips & Crisps	Cal	Fat	Cbs	Fbr	Prtn
100 Calorie Packs					
Toasted Chips - Baked Snack Crackers, 21 g	100	3	16	1	2
Toasted Chips - Ritz Minis Original, 22 g	100	3	17	0	2
Toasted Chips - Ritz Snack Mix, 22 g	100	3	16	1	2
Toasted Chips - Wheat Thins Minis Multi-grain 6 Ct, 22 g	100	3	16	1	2
Bugles					
Bugles Nacho Cheese, 30 g	160	9	18	1	1
Bugles Original, 30 g	160	9	18	1	1
Cheetos					
Asteroids® 100 Calorie Mini Bites Chz, 1 pkg	100	6	9	1	1
Baked! Crunchy 100 Calorie Mini Bites Chz, 1 pkg	100	4	14	0	2
Baked! Crunchy Cheese Flavored Snacks	130	5	19	0	2
Baked! Flamin' Hot® Cheese Flavored Snacks	130	5	19	1	3
Cracker Trax Chzy Cheddar, 30 g	140	5	21	1	3
Cracker Trax Spicy Cheddar, 30 g	140	5	21	1	3
• Crunchy Cheddar Jalapeño Flavored Snacks	170	11	15	1	2
Crunchy Cheese Flavored Snacks	160	10	15	1	2
Fantastixi Chili Chz, 1 pkg	130	5	19	1	2
Flamin' Hot® Cheese Flavored Snacks	170	11	15	1	2
Flamin' Hot® Limon Cheese Flavored Snacks	160	11	15	1	1
Jumbo Puffs Cheese Flavored Snacks	160	10	13	0	2
Jumbo Puffs Flamin' Hot Cheese Flavored Snacks	150	10	14	1	1
Mix & Move Cheese Flavored Snacks	160	11	14	1	2
Natural White Cheddar Puffs Chz	150	9	16	1	2
Puffs Cheese Flavored Snacks	160	10	15	1	2
Twisted Cheese Flavored Snacks	160	10	13	0	2
Xxtra Flamin' Hot Cheese Flavored Snacks	170	11	15	1	2
Flat Earth					
Apple Cinnamon Grove Fruit Crisps, 1 oz.	130	5	21	2	1
Farmland Cheddar Veggie Crisps, 1 oz.	130	5	19	2	2
Garlic & Herb Field Veggie Crisps, 1 oz.	130	5	19	2	2
Peach Mango Paradise Fruit Crisps, 1 oz.	130	5	21	1	1
Tangy Tomato Ranch Veggie Crisps, 1 oz.	130	5	19	2	2
Wild Berry Patch Flavored Baked Fruit Crisps, 1 oz.	130	5	21	1	1
Garden Harvest					
Apple Cinnamon, 28 g	120	3	22	3	2
Tomato Basil, 28 g	120	4	20	3	2
Vegetable Medly, 28 g	120	4	20	3	2
Lays					
Baked! Barbeque Flavored Potato Crisps, 1 oz.	120	3	22	2	2
Baked! Cheddar & Sour Cream Crisps, 1 oz.	120	4	21	2	2
Baked! Original Potato Crisps, 1 oz.	110	2	23	2	2
Classic Potato Chips, 1 oz.	150	10	15	1	2
Cracker Crisps Delightfully Crispy, 1 package	100	4	17	1	2
Hot 'N Spicy Barbeque Flavored Potato Chips, 1 oz.	160	10	15	1	2

Chips & Crisps (cont.)

	Cal	Fat	Cbs	Fbr	Prtn
Lays (cont.)					
Kettle Cooked Original Potato Chips, 1 oz.	150	8	18	1	2
Kettle Cooked Reduced Fat, 1 oz.	140	6	19	2	2
Light BBQ Flavored Potato Chips, 1 oz.	75	0	17	1	2
Light Original Potato Chips, 1 oz.	75	0	17	1	2
Sour Cream & Onion Potato Chips, 1 oz.	160	10	15	1	2
Wavy Ranch Flavored Potato Chips, 1 oz.	150	10	16	1	2
Wavy Regular Potato Chips, 1 oz.	150	10	15	1	2
Pringles					
Extreme					
Blazin' Buffalo Wing, 1 oz.	150	10	14	1	1
Kickin' Cheddar, 1 oz.	150	11	14	1	1
Flavors					
Original, 1 oz.	160	11	14	1	1
Sour Cream & Onion, 1 oz.	150	10	14	1	1
Select					
Cheddar Jack, 1 oz.	130	8	16	1	1
Cinnamon Sweet Potato, 1 oz.	150	9	16	1	1
Smart Snacking					
Fat Free Original, 1 oz.	70	0	15	1	1
Smart Flavors Original, 1 oz.	140	8	17	1	1
Stix					
Stix Pizza, 1 oz.	90	4	11	0	2
Snyder's of Hanover					
Baked Pita Chips Sundried Tomato & Herb, 28 g	140	5	17	3	4
Cheddar Baked Crunchies, 28 g	130	6	18	2	2
French Onion Sunflower Chips, 28 g	140	6	20	2	2
White Cheddar Puffs, 30 g	130	6	19	3	2
Chips					
BBQ Potato Chip, 1 oz.	150	6	20	4	2
Original Potato Chip, 1 oz.	150	7	19	3	2
Salt & Vinegar Potato Chip, 1 oz.	140	6	19	4	2
Sour Cream & Onion Potato Chip, 1 oz.	150	6	20	4	2
SunChips					
Cinnamon Flavor Multigrain Snacks, 1 oz.	130	6	18	2	2
French Onion Flavor Multigrain Snacks, 1 oz.	140	6	18	2	2
Garden Salsa Flavor Multigrain Snacks, 1 oz.	140	6	19	2	2
Original Flavor Multigrain Snacks, 1 oz.	140	6	18	2	2

Cookies

	Cal	Fat	Cbs	Fbr	Prtn
100 Calorie Packs					
Chewy Granola Bars - Nutter Butter, 28 g	100	2	21	2	2
Chewy Granola Bars - Oreo, 28 g	100	2	21	2	2

Crackers

	Cal	Fat	Cbs	Fbr	Prtn
100 Calorie Packs					
Cookie Crisps - Barnum's Animals Choco , 22 g	100	3	17	1	1
Cookie Crisps - Cheese Nips, 21 g	100	3	15	1	2
American Roland Food Corporation					
Rice Crackers - Nori Seaweed, 30 g	110	0	25	2	2
Rice Crackers - Original, 30 g	110	0	25	2	2
Rice Crackers - Wasabi, 30 g	110	0	25	2	2

(• = most healthy • = least healthy)

SNACKS

Crackers (cont.)	Cal	Fat	Cbs	Fbr	Prtn
Arrowroot					
• National Biscuit, 5 g	20	1	4	0	0
Barnum's Animal Crackers					
Animal Crackers, 2 oz.	120	4	22	1	2
Blue Diamond Almonds					
Nut Thins® Almond, 16 crackers	130	3	23	1	3
Nut Thins® Hazelnut, 16 crackers	130	3	23	1	2
Nut Thins® Pecan, 16 crackers	130	4	23	1	2
Cheese Nips					
Cheddar Reduced Fat, 30 g	150	6	1	1	3
Cheddar, 35 g	170	7	22	1	3
Crackers - Cheddar, 30 g	150	6	19	1	3
Four Cheese, 30 g	150	7	18	1	3
Flavor Originals					
Better Cheddars Baked, 31 g	160	8	18	1	3
Chicken In A Biskit, 31 g	160	8	19	1	2
Sociables Baked Savory Crackers, 14 g	70	4	9	0	1
Vegetable Thins Crackers, 30 g	150	7	20	1	2
Handi-Snacks					
Oreo Cookie Sticks 'N Creme, 28 g	140	7	20	1	1
Premium Breadsticks 'N Cheeez, 31 g	110	5	13	0	3
Ritz Crackers 'N Cheez, 27 g	100	6	10	0	2
Honey Maid					
Grahams Chocolate, 31 g	130	3	24	1	2
Grahams Cinnamon, 31 g	130	3	25	1	2
Grahams Honey, 31 g	130	4	24	1	2
Grahams Squares, 27 g	120	4	20	1	2
Keebler					
Club Crackers					
Club® & Cheddar Cracker, 36 g	190	10	23	1	4
Original, 14 g	70	3	9	1	1
Puffed Original, 30 g	140	6	20	1	2
Reduced Fat, 16 g	70	3	12	1	1
Snack Sticks Original, 29 g	130	6	19	1	1
Grahams					
Honey, 31 g	140	4	23	1	2
Lowfat Honey, 27 g	110	2	22	1	2
Original, 29 g	130	4	22	1	2
On The GO					
Animals Variety Pack, 28 g	180	6	30	1	2
Cinnamon Snack Pack, 28 g	120	4	20	1	2
Right Bites® Variety Pack, 28 g	100	4	17	1	1
Variety Snack Pack, 28 g	140	5	23	1	2
Sandwich Crackers					
Cheese & Peanut Butter, 39 g	200	10	23	1	4
Club® & Cheddar, 36 g	190	10	23	1	4
Toast & Peanut Butter, 39 g	200	10	23	1	4
Wheat & Cheddar, 36 g	190	10	23	1	3
Toasteds					
Buttercrisp, 16 g	80	4	10	1	1
Organic, 29 g	130	6	20	1	2
Wheat, 16 g	80	4	10	1	1

SNACKS

Crackers (cont.)

	Cal	Fat	Cbs	Fbr	Prtn
Keebler (cont.)					
Townhouse					
Original, 16 g	80	5	10	1	1
Reduced Fat, 15 g	60	2	11	1	1
Toppers Original, 14 g	70	3	9	0	1
Wheatables					
Multigrain, 30 g	140	6	20	1	2
Original Golden Wheat, 30 g	140	6	20	1	2
Reduced Fat, 31 g	140	4	22	1	2
Pepperidge Farm					
Baby Cheddar Goldfish, 89 pieces	140	5	20	1	4
Cinnamon Goldfish Graham Snacks, 1 pk	210	8	32	1	3
Original Goldfish, 55 pieces	150	6	20	1	3
Parmesan Goldfish, 60 pieces	130	4	20	1	4
Pizza Goldfish, 55 pieces	140	5	20	1	3
Premium					
Fat Free, 15 g	60	0	12	0	1
Low Sodium, 14 g	60	2	11	0	1
Multigrain, 14 g	60	2	10	0	1
Original, 15 g	60	2	11	0	1
Toasted Onion, 15 g	60	2	11	1	1
Purity Foods					
Cajun Spelt Sesame Sticks, 28 g	150	9	15	1	3
Garlic Spelt Sesame Sticks, 28 g	150	9	15	2	3
Whole Grain Spelt Sesame Sticks, 28 g	150	9	14	2	3
Wild Rice Spelt Sesame Sticks, 28 g	140	0	17	1	3
Ritz					
Real Cheese, 39 oz.	200	12	22	1	2
Low Sodium, 16 oz.	80	4	10	0	1
Peanut Butter, 39 oz.	190	9	24	1	4
Sargento					
Cheese Dip & Cheddar Sticks , 28 g	100	6	11	0	2
Cheese Dip & Crackers , 27 g	100	5	10	0	2
Social Tea					
Biscuits, 31 g	140	4	24	1	2
Stauffer's					
All Natural Animal Crackers					
Chocolate, 1 oz.	130	3	23	1	2
Original & Chocolate, 1 oz.	120	3	25	1	2
Original, 1 oz.	120	2	24	1	2
Animal Crackers					
Chocolate, 1 oz.	120	3	23	1	2
Chocolate Graham Crackers, 1 oz.	120	3	23	1	2
Cinnamon, 1 oz.	110	2	21	1	2
Cinnamon Graham Crackers, 1 oz.	110	2	21	1	2
Original, 1 oz.	120	2	24	1	2
Assorted Crackers					
Cheese, 1 oz.	140	7	17	1	3
Chicken Flavored, 1 oz.	150	8	19	1	2
Stauffer's Oyster, 1 oz.	120	3	22	1	3
Whales Baked, 2 oz.	210	9	27	1	4

(●= most healthy ●= least healthy)

SNACKS

Crackers (cont.)

	Cal	Fat	Cbs	Fbr	Prtn
Sunridge Farms					
Organic Japanese Rice Crackers, 30 g	110	0	26	0	2
Teddy Grahams					
Chocolate, 30 g	130	5	22	2	2
Cinnamon, 35 g	150	5	26	1	2
Honey, 30 g	130	4	23	1	2
Oatmeal, 30 g	130	4	23	1	2
Triscuit					
Baked Whole Grain Deli-style Rye, 28 g	120	5	19	3	3
Baked Whole Grain Thin Crisps, 30 g	130	5	21	3	3
Wheat Thins					
Low Sodium, 31 g	150	6	22	1	2
Multi-Grain, 30 g	140	5	22	2	2
Original, 31 g	140	6	21	1	2
Ranch, 29 g	130	6	20	1	2
Reduced Fat, 29 g	130	4	21	1	2
Zwieback					
Stay Fresh Crackers, 8 g	35	1	6	0	1

Fruit Snacks

	Cal	Fat	Cbs	Fbr	Prtn
Betty Crocker					
Fruit By The Foot Tropical Tango, 21 g	80	1	17	N/A	0
• Fruit Gushers Watermelon Blast, 25 g	90	1	20	0	0
• Fruit Roll-Ups Strawberry, 14 g	50	1	12	N/A	0
Tropicana Juice					
Cherry, 19 g	70	0	17	1	0
Strawberry, 19 g	70	0	17	1	0

Jerky

	Cal	Fat	Cbs	Fbr	Prtn
Pemmican					
Natural Hickory Smoked Beef Jerky, 1 bag	140	2	6	1	24
Natural Sweet & Hot Beef Jerky, 1 bag	150	2	9	1	24
• Original Beef Jerky, 1 bag	70	1	4	1	12
Original Steak Tips, 1 oz.	70	2	5	0	9
Shredded Peppered Beef Jerky, 1 oz.	80	2	3	1	12
Teriyaki Shredded Beef Jerky, 1 oz.	80	2	3	1	12
Slim Jim					
Beef Jerky Canister, 7 pcs	130	8	3	0	11
• Classic Handipack, 1 box	210	19	3	1	8
Giant Jerk, 1 pkg	80	5	2	0	6
Giant Jerk Caddy, 1 pkg	80	5	2	0	6
Giant Pepperoni Caddy, 1 pkg	150	13	3	0	6
Mild Canister, 4 pcs	170	15	2	1	6
Natural Peppered Beef Jerky, 1 oz.	80	2	4	0	12
Original Canister, 4 pcs	170	15	2	1	6
Pepperoni Canister, 4 pcs	170	15	2	1	6

Nuts & Trail Mix

	Cal	Fat	Cbs	Fbr	Prtn
American Almond					
Almonds, 1 oz.	167	15	6	3	6
Hazelnuts, 1 oz.	179	19	4	2	4
Macadamias, 1 oz.	199	21	4	3	2
Peanuts (Unsalted), 1 oz.	166	14	6	2	7

SNACKS

Nuts & Trail Mix (cont.)

	Cal	Fat	Cbs	Fbr	Prtn
American Almond (cont.)					
Pecans, 1 oz.	189	19	5	2	2
Walnuts, 1 oz.	182	18	5	1	4
Blue Diamond Almonds					
Honey Roast Almonds, 28	170	14	8	3	5
Jordan Almonds, 40	180	8	28	2	3
Oven Roasted No Salt, 1 oz.	170	15	5	3	6
Chex					
Mix Bold Party Blend, 30 g	140	6	20	1	3
Mix Cheddar, 30 g	130	4	22	1	2
Mix Hot 'n Spicy, 30 g	130	4	20	1	2
Mix Peanut Lovers, 30 g	140	5	19	1	3
Mix Select - Chocolate PB, 33 g	150	5	24	1	3
Mix Select - Chocolate Turtle, 33 g	150	5	24	1	2
Mix Select - Dark Chocolate, 30 g	140	5	23	1	2
Mix Sweet 'n Salty Caramel Crunch, 30 g	130	4	23	1	2
Mix Sweet 'n Salty Honey Nut, 30 g	130	4	22	1	2
Mix Sweet 'n Salty Trail Mix, 32 g	140	5	22	1	2
Mix Traditional, 30 g	130	4	22	1	2
Simply Chex Cheddar, 30 g	130	4	22	1	3
Corn Nuts					
Barbecue, 48 g	220	8	34	4	4
Chile Picante, 48 g	210	8	33	4	1
Nacho Cheese, 28 g	130	5	19	2	3
Original, 28 g	120	5	20	2	3
Ranch, 48 g	220	8	33	4	8
Salsa Jalisco, 48 g	220	8	34	4	4
David Seeds					
BBQ Sunflower Seed Kernels, 1/4 cup	190	15	5	3	8
• In Shell Sunflower Seeds, 1/4 cup	260	21	7	6	12
Jalapeño & Hot Salsa In Shll Snflwr Seeds, 1/4 cup	180	14	6	2	8
Nacho In Shell Snflwr Seeds, 1/4 cup w/o Shell	170	14	5	2	7
Pumpkin Seeds, 1/4 cup	160	12	4	1	9
Red Sodium Snflwr Seeds, 1/4 cup w/o Shell	190	14	7	3	9
Sunflower Seeds, 1/4 cup	190	15	4	5	9
Fisher Nuts					
Almonds, 1 oz.	170	14	6	3	7
Butter Toffe Peanuts, 1 oz.	130	6	17	1	3
Dry Roasted Peanuts, 1 oz.	170	14	6	2	7
Honey Roasted Peanuts, 1 oz.	170	13	7	2	7
Jumbo Cashews, 1 oz.	170	15	8	1	5
Mixed Nuts, 1 oz.	180	16	5	2	6
Oil Roasted Peanuts, 1 oz.	170	15	5	2	7
Pecans, 1 oz.	200	20	4	2	3
Walnuts, 1 oz.	200	20	3	3	5
Mauna Loa					
Mauna Loa Macadamias					
Honey Roasted, 28 g	180	16	9	2	2
Maui Onion & Garlic, 14 g	100	11	2	1	1
Salted Dry Roasted, 28 g	230	24	4	2	2
Unsalted Dry Roasted, 28 g	230	24	4	2	2

(• = most healthy • = least healthy)　　　**POPULAR BRANDS • 489**

SNACKS

Nuts & Trail Mix (cont.)	Cal	Fat	Cbs	Fbr	Prtn
Mauna Loa (cont.)					
Mauna Loa Mix					
Island Nut & Fruit, 30 g	150	10	16	2	2
Macadamias & Almonds, 28 g	180	17	4	3	6
Mixers					
Snack Mix - Cheddar, 28 g	130	5	19	1	2
Snack Mix - Traditional, 30 g	130	5	21	1	2
Nature Valley					
Trail Mix Bars Apple Cinnamon, 35 g	140	4	25	1	2
Trail Mix Bars Fruit & Nut, 35 g	140	4	25	1	3
Trail Mix Bars Mixed Berry, 35 g	140	4	26	1	2
Planters					
Cashew Halves & Pieces					
Lightly Salted, 28 g	170	14	8	1	5
Regular, 28 g	170	14	8	1	5
Chocolate Covered Almonds					
Chocolate Lovers, 41 g	220	17	18	3	4
Deluxe & Select Mixed Nuts,					
Deluxe Regular, 28 g	170	15	6	2	5
Select Cashew, Almond & Pecan, 28 g	170	16	6	2	5
Select Macadamia, Cashew & Almond, 28 g	180	17	6	2	4
Cocktail Peanuts					
Honey Roasted, 28 g	160	13	8	2	6
Lightly Salted, 28 g	170	15	5	2	7
Regular, 28 g	170	14	6	2	7
Unsalted, 28 g	170	14	6	2	7
Dry Roasted Peanuts					
Honey Roasted, 28 g	150	12	7	2	6
Lightly Salted, 28 g	160	14	5	2	7
Regular, 28 g	170	14	5	2	8
Unsalted, 28 g	170	14	5	2	8
Fruit & Raisin Mixes					
Fruit & Nut, 28 g	140	9	14	2	4
Mixed Nuts & Raisins, 29 g	150	11	10	2	5
Nuts, Seeds & Raisins, 31 g	160	12	11	2	6
Lovers' Mixes					
Cashew, 28 g	180	17	6	2	4
Macadamia, 28 g	190	19	4	3	3
Pecan, 28 g	180	17	6	2	4
Pistachio, 28 g	160	13	7	3	6
Mixed Nuts					
Honey Roasted, 28 g	160	12	9	2	5
Lightly Salted, 28 g	170	15	5	2	6
Regular, 28 g	170	15	5	2	6
Unsalted, 28 g	170	15	5	2	6
More Cashews					
Chocolate Lovers, 42 g	230	16	20	1	5
Dry Roasted, 19 g	160	12	9	1	5
Jumbo, 28 g	171	14	8	1	2

SNACKS

Nuts & Trail Mix (cont.)

	Cal	Fat	Cbs	Fbr	Prtn
Planters (cont.)					
Other Nuts (cont.)					
Nutrition Salted, 28 g	170	15	6	3	6
Nutrition Smoked, 28 g	170	15	6	3	6
Spanish Peanuts, 28 g	180	14	5	2	8
Sweet n' Crunchy Peanuts, 28 g	140	7	16	2	4
Sweet & Salty Mixes					
Energy Mix, 42 g	240	19	14	3	6
Honey Nut Medley, 32 g	160	10	16	1	4
Nut & Chocolate, 33 g	160	10	16	2	4
Sweet & Nutty, 30 g	150	10	14	2	4
Whole Cashews					
Honey Roasted, 28 g	150	12	11	1	4
Lightly Salted, 28 g	170	14	8	1	5
Regular, 28 g	170	14	8	1	2
Poppycock					
Cashew Lovers, 30 g	140	6	21	1	2
Original, 31 g	160	8	20	1	2
Pecan Delight, 30 g	150	8	20	0	1
Sunridge Farms					
Organic Cranberry Harvest, 30 g	140	9	13	2	4
• Oriental Cracker Mix, 30 g	110	0	27	0	2
Oriental Party Mix, 30 g	160	11	12	2	5
Sesame Sticks, 30 g	170	12	14	1	3
Super Deluxe Trail Mix, 30 g	150	11	11	2	5
Tropical Trail Mix, 30 g	140	9	13	3	4
Wasabi Peas, 30 g	120	1	20	2	7
Nuts and Seeds					
Almonds, Roasted, No Salt, 30 g	180	15	6	3	6
California Almonds Supreme, 30 g	190	15	5	4	8
Fancy Mixed Nuts, 30 g	180	15	5	3	7
Honey Mixed Nuts, 30 g	170	14	9	1	5
Natural Pumpkin Seeds, 30 g	160	14	5	1	7
Natural Sunflower Seeds, 30 g	170	14	6	2	6
Pecan Halves, 30 g	220	20	4	2	5
Walnut Halves, 30 g	200	21	4	1	4

Popcorn

	Cal	Fat	Cbs	Fbr	Prtn
Act II Microwave Popcorn					
94% Fat Free Butter Popcorn, 3 tbsp.	130	3	28	5	1
Butter Lovers Popcorn, 2 tbsp.	170	12	16	3	2
Butter Popcorn, 2 tbsp.	160	10	18	3	3
Extreme Butter Popcorn, 2 tbsp.	180	13	15	3	2
Movie Theater Butter Popcorn, 2 tbsp.	170	12	16	3	2
Healthy Choice					
Butter Popcorn, 3 tbsp.	130	3	28	5	4
Natural Popcorn, 3 tbsp.	130	3	28	5	4
Jiffy Pop					
Butter Popcorn, 2 tbsp.	140	7	19	0	3
Orville Redenbacher's					
Movie Theater					
Butter Light Popcorn, 2 tbsp.	120	5	19	3	3

SNACKS

Popcorn (cont.)

	Cal	Fat	Cbs	Fbr	Prtn
Orville Redenbacher's (cont.)					
Movie Theater (cont.)					
Butter Popcorn, 2 tbsp.	170	12	16	3	2
Popcorn					
• Butter Popcorn, 2 tbsp.	210	14	20	4	3
Light Butter Popcorn, 2 tbsp.	120	5	19	3	3
Popcorn Cakes					
• Caramel Popcorn Cakes, 1 Cake	45	0	11	N/A	1
White Cheddar Popcorn Cakes, 2 Cakes	60	1	14	2	2
Smart Pop					
Movie Theater Butter Popcorn, 2 tbsp.	130	3	28	5	4
Popcorn, 1 Bag	110	2	240	4	3
Paul Newman's Own					
94% Fat Free Microwave Popcorn, 30 g	110	2	20	4	3
Butter Microwave Popcorn, 30 g	130	5	18	3	3
Light Butter Microwave Popcorn, 30 g	120	4	19	4	3
White Kernel Popcorn, 30 g	130	5	18	3	2
Pop Secret					
1-Step Cheddar, 3 tbsp.	180	13	17	3	2
94% Fat Free Butter, 30 g	120	2	26	4	4
Butter, 3 tbsp.	180	12	17	3	3
Extra Butter, 3 tbsp.	180	13	17	3	2
Homestyle, 3 tbsp.	170	12	17	3	3
Kettle Corn, 3 tbsp.	180	13	15	3	2
Light Butter, 23 g	140	5	24	4	3
Smart Balance					
Light Butter Popcorn, 28 g	120	5	18	4	3
Smart 'n Healthy Popcorn, 31 g	120	2	24	5	4
Smart Movie Style Popcorn, 32 g	170	11	16	3	3

Pretzels

	Cal	Fat	Cbs	Fbr	Prtn
Gardetto's					
Deli-Style Mustard Pretzel Mix, 30 g	130	2	24	1	3
Italian Cheese Blend, 30 g	140	5	20	1	3
Original, 30 g	150	6	20	1	3
Reduced Fat Original, 30 g	130	4	20	1	3
Roasted Garlic Rye Chips, 30 g	160	10	16	1	2
Purity Foods					
Spelt Pretzels, 1 oz.	110	2	21	1	4
Vita Spelt Low Sodium Pretzels, 1 oz.	110	2	21	1	4
Vita Spelt Organic Sourdough Pretzels, 1 oz.	110	1	23	3	3
Snyder's of Hanover					
Multigrain					
Honey Mustard & Onion Nibblers, 30 g	140	5	20	3	3
Lightly Salted Pretzel Sticks, 30 g	120	2	23	3	3
Olde Tyme Pretzel Twists, 30 g	120	2	22	2	3
Pretzel Crackers					
Butter Sesame Pretzel Crackers, 30 g	120	3	23	1	3
Original Pretzel Crackers, 30 g	120	3	23	2	2
Pumpernickel & Onion Pretzel Crackers, 28 g	120	3	22	3	3
Pretzels					
Garlic Bread Nibblers, 1 oz.	130	3	24	1	2

SNACKS

Pretzels (cont.)

	Cal	Fat	Cbs	Fbr	Prtn
Snyder's of Hanover (cont.)					
Pretzels (cont.)					
Homestyle Pretzels, 1 oz.	120	1	25	1	3
Honey Mustard & Onion Nibblers, 1 oz.	130	3	23	1	3
Honey Wheat Sticks, 1 oz.	120	2	24	2	3
Mini Pretzels, 1 oz.	110	1	25	1	3
Thins, 1 oz.	100	0	23	1	3
Sunridge Farms					
Yogurt Pretzels, 40 g	190	7	29	0	2

Snack Bars

	Cal	Fat	Cbs	Fbr	Prtn
100 Calorie Packs					
Chewy Granola Bars - Chips Ahoy!, 28 g	100	2	22	2	2
Balance Bar					
Balance 100 Calories					
Chocolate Carmel Crisp, 28 g	100	4	14	5	6
Peanut Butter Crisp, 28 g	100	5	14	5	6
Vanila Crisp, 28 g	100	4	15	5	5
Balance Bar Original					
Almond Brownie, 50 g	200	6	22	2	14
Chocolate, 50 g	200	6	23	1	14
Peanut Butter, 50 g	200	6	22	1	14
Balance Carbwell					
Carmel N Chocolate, 50 g	190	7	23	1	14
Chocolate Fudge, 50 g	190	6	23	2	14
Chocolate Peanut Butter, 50 g	200	8	22	1	14
Balance Gold					
Chewy Chocolate Chip, 20 g	210	7	25	0	13
Cookies N Crème Crunch, 50 g	210	6	22	1	15
Triple Chocolate Chaos, 50 g	210	7	24	1	13
Balance Organic					
Apricot Mango Crisp, 45 g	180	7	23	5	10
Canberry Pomegranate Crisp, 45 g	180	7	23	5	10
Cherry Almond Crisp, 45 g	180	7	23	5	10
Cascadian Farm					
Chewy Granola Bars Chocolate Chip, 35 g	140	3	25	1	2
Chewy Granola Bars Fruit & Nut, 35 g	140	4	24	1	2
Chewy Granola Bars Harvest Berries, 35 g	130	2	27	1	2
Chewy Granola Bars Multi Grain, 35 g	130	2	27	1	2
Clif Products					
Clif Bar					
Apricot, 68 g	230	3	45	5	10
Carrot Cake, 68 g	240	4	46	5	10
Chocolate Almond Fudge, 68 g	250	5	44	5	10
Oatmeal Raisin Walnut, 68 g	240	5	43	5	10
Clif Builders					
Chocolate, 68 g	270	8	30	4	20
• Chocolate Mint, 68 g	270	8	31	4	20
Cookies N Cream, 68 g	270	8	30	4	20
Clif Kid Twisted Fruit					
• Grape, 20 g	70	0	16	1	0
Pineapple, 20 g	70	0	16	1	0

(•= most healthy •= least healthy)

SNACKS

❯ Snack Bars (cont.)	Cal	Fat	Cbs	Fbr	Prtn
Clif Products (cont.)					
Clif Kid Twisted Fruit (cont.)					
Luna, 20 g	70	0	16	1	0
Sour Apple, 20 g	70	0	16	1	0
Clif Kid Zbar					
Apple Cinnamon, 36 g	120	2	23	3	3
Blueberry, 36 g	120	3	23	3	3
Honey Graham, 36 g	130	2	26	3	3
Peanut Butter, 36 g	140	5	20	3	3
Clif Minis					
Mini Chocolate Brownie, 28 g	100	2	18	2	4
Mini Chocolate Chip, 28 g	100	2	18	2	4
Mini Crunchy Peanut Butter, 28 g	100	3	17	2	5
Clif Mojo					
Fruit Nut Crunch, 45 g	190	7	24	3	9
Honey Roasted Peanut, 45 g	200	10	20	2	10
Mixed Nuts, 45 g	210	11	19	2	10
Peanut Butter Pretzel, 45 g	200	9	21	2	10
Clif Mojo Dipped					
Chocolate Peanut, 45 g	210	10	22	2	9
Fruit & Nut, 45 g	200	8	24	3	8
Peanut Butter and Jelly, 45 g	220	11	21	2	9
Clif Nectar					
Apple Cinnamon, 45 g	160	6	30	6	2
Cherry Pomegranate, 45 g	150	5	29	7	3
Cranberry Apricot Almond, 45 g	170	6	29	4	3
Lemon Vanilla Cashew, 45 g	160	6	27	6	4
Clif Nectar Cacao					
Dark Chocolate Mocha, 45 g	160	6	27	5	3
Dark Chocolate Raspberry, 45 g	150	5	29	7	3
Dark Chocolate Walnut, 45 g	160	6	27	6	3
Clif Shot Bloks					
Black Cherry, 30 g	100	0	24	0	0
Cola, 30 g	100	0	24	0	0
Piña Colada, 30 g	100	0	24	0	0
Strawberry, 30 g	100	0	24	0	0
Luna Bar					
Berry Almond, 48 g	180	4	27	3	9
Chai Tea, 48 g	180	5	25	3	10
Cookies N Cream Delight, 48 g	180	5	26	3	10
Peanut Butter Cookie, 48 g	180	6	23	3	10
Luna Sport					
Blueberry Moons Energy Chews, 30 g	100	0	24	0	0
Dark Chocolate Recovery Smoothie, 1 oz.	120	N/A	21	1	8
Strawberry Banana Recovery Smothie, 1 oz.	120	N/A	21	1	8
Luna Sunrise					
Apple Cinnamon, 48 g	180	5	27	5	8
Blueberry Bliss, 48 g	170	5	26	5	8
Strawberry Crumble, 48 g	170	5	26	5	8
Vanilla Almond, 48 g	180	5	29	5	8
Luna Teacakes					
Berry Pomegranate, 40 g	140	2	30	2	2

NACKS

Snack Bars (cont.)

	Cal	Fat	Cbs	Fbr	Prtn
Clif Products (cont.)					
Luna Teacakes (cont.)					
Mint Chocolate, 40 g	130	3	25	3	3
Orange Blossom, 40 g	130	2	30	3	2
Vanilla Macadamia, 40 g	150	4	28	3	2
Honey Maid					
Snack Bars - Oatmeal, 34 g	150	6	24	1	2
Snack Bars Oatmeal Raisin, 34 g	150	6	24	1	2
Nature Valley					
Chwy Granola Bars Blueberry Yogurt, 35 g	140	4	26	1	2
Granola Bars Apple Crisp, 42 g	180	6	29	2	4
Granola Bars Vanilla Nut, 42 g	190	7	28	2	4
Healthy Heart Granola Bars Honey Nut, 40 g	160	4	28	3	3
Roasted Nut Bars - Almond Crunch, 35 g	200	14	11	2	7
Nutri-Grain					
Fruit & Nut Bars - Berry & Almond, 32 g	120	4	22	3	3
Fruit & Nut Bars - Cranberry, Raisin & Peanut, 32 g	120	4	22	3	3
Yogurt Bars - Strawberry, 37 g	140	4	25	2	2
Yogurt Bars - Vanilla, 37 g	140	4	26	2	2
Philadelphia Cream Cheese					
Snack Bars - Classic Cheesecake, 42 g	190	11	20	0	2
Snack Bars - Marble Brownie, 42 g	170	9	20	1	3
Snack Bars - Strawberry Cheesecake, 42 g	180	9	22	0	2
Snack Bites - Chocolate Covered Strawberry, 28 g	130	7	15	0	1
Pop-Tarts					
Go-Tarts!™ Frstd Bwn Sugr Cinn Snack Bars, 35 g	140	4	24	1	1
Go-Tarts!™ Frstd Chocolate Chip Snack Bars, 35 g	140	5	24	1	1
Go-Tarts!™ Frstd Choco Fudge Snack Bars, 35 g	140	4	24	1	1
Go-Tarts!™ Frstd Strawberry Snack Bars, 35 g	140	4	25	1	1
Rice Krispies					
Treats® Chocolatey Peanut Butter bars, 22 g	100	4	15	1	1
Treats® Mini-Squares, 44 g	180	5	34	0	1
Treats® Original, 22 g	90	3	17	0	1
Treats® Rainbow, 22 g	90	3	17	0	1
Solo GI					
Berry Bliss Bar, 50 g	200	6	25	3	11
Chocolate Charger Bar, 50 g	200	7	26	4	11
Mint Mania Bar, 50 g	200	7	26	4	11
Peanut Power, 50 g	200	8	23	3	11
South Beach Living					
Caramel Peanut Crispy Meal Bar, 60 g	210	7	26	5	19
Chocolate Caramel Meal Bar, 50 g	180	5	22	4	15
Chocolate Crispy Meal Bar, 60 g	210	6	26	5	19
Chocolate Mint Snack Bar Delights, 28 g	100	4	15	5	6
Nut Medley Sweet Nut Creations, 35 g	150	7	18	3	6
Peanut Butter Snack Bar Delights, 28 g	100	4	14	5	6
Roasted Pnut Sweet Nut Creations, 35 g	150	7	18	3	6
Vanilla Crème Crispy Meal Bar, 60 g	220	7	26	5	19
Special K					
Bar Chocolatey Drizzle, 22 g	90	2	17	1	1
Bar Strawberry, 23 g	90	2	18	1	1
Bliss™ Bar Orange, 22 g	90	2	17	1	1

(• = most healthy • = least healthy)

SNACKS

Snack Bars (cont.)	Cal	Fat	Cbs	Fbr	Prtn
Special K (cont.)					
Bliss™ Bar Raspberry, 22 g	90	2	17	1	1
Protein™ Meal Bar Double Choco, 45 g	180	5	25	5	10
Protein™ Meal Bar Strawberry, 45 g	180	5	24	5	10
Protein™ Snack Bar Chocolate Peanut, 26 g	110	4	15	1	4

Snack Dips & Spreads	Cal	Fat	Cbs	Fbr	Prtn
California Sun Dry					
Sun-Dried Tomato Salsa, 2 tbsp.	20	3	N/A	N/A	N/A
Country Fresh					
French Onion Dip, 30 g	80	8	3	0	1
Veggie Dip, 31 g	60	6	2	0	1
Dean's					
French Onion Dip, 30 g	80	8	3	0	1
Veggie Dip, 31 g	60	6	2	0	1
McCormick					
Ranch Dip Mix, 2 g	5	0	0	N/A	0
Spinach Dip Mix, 2 g	10	0	1	N/A	0
Vegetable Dip Mix, 2 g	5	0	0	N/A	0
Muir Glen					
Salsa Black Bean & Corn Medium, 31 g	20	0	4	1	1
Salsa Medium, 31 g	10	0	3	0	0
Salsa Mild, 31 g	10	0	3	0	0
Pace Foods					
• Mexican Four Cheese Salsa con Queso, 2 tbsp.	90	7	5	0	2
Picante Sauce, 2 tbsp.	10	0	2	1	0
Pico De Gallo, 2 tbsp.	10	0	3	0	0
Salsa Verde, 2 tbsp.	15	1	2	0	0
Tequila Lime Salsa, 2 tbsp.	15	0	3	0	0
Thick & Chunky Salsa, 2 tbsp.	10	0	2	1	0
Paul Newman's Own					
All-Natural Bandito Chunky Salsa Peach, 32 g	25	0	6	1	0
All-Natural Bandito Salsa Mild, 32 g	10	0	2	1	0
• All-Natural Bandito Salsa Tequila Lime, 31 g	15	0	3	2	N/A
Farmer's Garden Salsa, 32 g	15	0	4	0	1
Mango Salsa, 32 g	20	0	5	2	1
Organic Chunky Medium Salsa, 31 g	10	0	3	0	0
Snyder's of Hanover					
Fire Roasted Salsa, 1 oz.	150	6	20	4	2
Garden Style Sweet Salsa, 2 tbsp.	20	0	5	0	0
Salsa Con Queso, 2 tbsp.	35	2	4	0	0
Tres Bean Dip, 2 tbsp.	25	0	5	1	1
Taco Bell Home Originals					
Bean Con Queso - Home Originals, 31 g	35	2	2	1	1
Chili Con Queso - Home Originals With Meat, 31 g	40	2	3	0	2
Salsa - Thick 'N Chunky Medium, 31 g	15	0	3	0	1
Salsa - Thick 'N Chunky Mild, 31 g	15	0	3	0	1

Tortilla/Corn Chips	Cal	Fat	Cbs	Fbr	Prtn
Azteca Foods					
Chips					
Fried White Corn Tortilla Chips, 1 oz.	140	6	19	4	2

SNACKS

Tortilla/Corn Chips (cont.)

	Cal	Fat	Cbs	Fbr	Prtn
Azteca Foods (cont.)					
Chips (cont.)					
Fried Yellow Corn Tortilla Chips, 1 oz.	140	6	19	4	2
Unfried Corn Tortilla Chips, 1 oz.	80	1	15	1	2
Salad Shells					
Salad Shells, 59 g	280	16	29	1	4
Tortillas					
Pressed Flour Tortillas, 51 g	153	3	27	1	4
White Corn Tortillas, 1 oz.	75	1	15	1	2
Yellow Corn Tortillas, 1 oz.	75	1	15	1	2
Doritos					
Baked! Nacho Cheese® Flavored Chips, 1 oz.	120	4	21	2	2
Cool Ranch® Flavored Chips, 1 oz.	140	7	18	1	2
Fiery Habanero Flavored Chips, 1 oz.	130	7	16	1	2
Light Nacho Cheese® Flavored Chips, 1 oz.	100	2	19	2	2
Nacho Cheese® Flavored Chips, 1 oz.	140	8	17	1	2
Salsa Verde Flavored Chips, 1 oz.	140	7	19	1	2
Smokin' Cheddar BBQ Flavored Chips, 1 oz.	150	8	17	1	2
Spicy Nacho Flavored Chips, 1 oz.	140	7	18	1	2
Toasted Corn Chips, 1 oz.	140	7	18	1	2
Fritos					
BBQ Flavored Corn Chips, 1 oz.	150	10	16	1	2
Chili Cheese Flavored Corn Chips, 1 oz.	160	10	15	1	2
Original Corn Chips, 1 oz.	160	10	15	1	2
SCOOPS!® Corn Chips, 1 oz.	160	10	16	1	2
Tangy Roasted Corn Flavored Corn Chips, 1 oz.	160	1	16	1	2
Snyder's of Hanover					
Restaurant Style Tortillas, 1 oz.	130	5	20	4	2
Savory Blue Tortillas, 28 g	140	7	17	3	2
White Corn Tortillas, 1 oz.	140	5	23	2	0
Yellow Corn Tortillas, 1 oz.	140	5	23	2	2
Tostitos					
Baked! Scoops!® Tortilla Chips, 1 oz.	120	3	22	2	2
Flour Tortilla Chips, 1 oz.	140	7	19	1	2
Light Restaurant Style Tortilla Chips, 1 oz.	90	1	20	1	2
Multigrain Tortilla Chips, 1 oz.	150	8	18	2	2
Restaurant Style Tortilla Chips, 1 oz.	140	7	19	1	2
Scoops!® Tortilla Chips, 1 oz.	140	7	18	1	2

SOUPS & BROTHS

Bouillon/Broths

	Cal	Fat	Cbs	Fbr	Prtn
Allens					
Allens Chicken Broth, 225 g	10	0	0	0	1
Campbell's Soups					
Beef Broth, 1/2 cup	15	0	1	0	3
Chicken Broth, 1 cup	25	1	1	0	4
• Scotch Broth, 1/2 cup	70	2	9	2	3
College Inn					
Beef Broth					
Beef Broth, 240 ml.	25	1	0	0	4
French Onion, 240 ml.	15	0	0	0	4

(•= most healthy •= least healthy)

SOUPS & BROTHS

Bouillon/Broths (cont.)	Cal	Fat	Cbs	Fbr	Prtn
College Inn (cont.)					
Chicken Broth					
Chicken Broth, 240 ml.	15	1	0	0	1
• Chicken Fat Free, 240 ml.	5	0	0	0	1
Chicken Light, 240 ml.	15	1	0	0	1
Lemon Herb, 240 ml.	15	1	0	0	1
Roasted Garlic, 240 ml.	20	0	3	0	1
Roasted Veggies and Herb, 240 ml.	20	0	3	0	1
Garden Vegetable Broth					
Garden Veg, 243 ml.	25	0	6	0	0
Turkey Broth					
Turkey Broth, 240 ml.	20	0	0	0	1
Swanson Broth					
Beef Broth, 1 cup	15	0	1	0	2
Certified Organic Beef Broth, 1 cup	15	1	1	0	2
Certified Organic Chicken Broth, 1 cup	15	1	1	0	1
Chicken Broth, 1 cup	10	1	1	0	1
Seasoned Beef Broth, 1 cup	20	1	2	0	2
Seasoned Chicken Broth w/ Roasted Garlic, 1 cup	20	1	2	0	1
Vegetable Broth, 1 cup	15	0	3	0	0

Canned Soup	Cal	Fat	Cbs	Fbr	Prtn
Campbell's Soups					
Beef Noodle Soup, 1/2 cup	70	2	8	1	4
Cream of Broccoli Soup, 1/2 cup	90	4	12	1	2
Cream of Onion Soup, 1/2 cup	100	6	10	3	1
French Onion Soup, 1/2 cup	45	2	6	1	2
Tomato Soup, 1/2 cup	90	0	20	1	2
Vegetable Beef Soup, 1/2 cup	90	1	15	3	5
Chunky™ Soups					
Hearty Beef Barley Soup, 1 cup	170	3	26	4	10
Hearty Chicken with Vegetables Soup, 1 cup	90	2	13	2	7
Hold the Beans Chili, 1 cup	240	10	20	5	10
New England Clam Chowder, 1 cup	210	9	25	5	7
Chunky™ Fully Loaded Soups					
Beef Stew Soup, 1 cup	160	4	20	3	10
Rigatoni & Meatballs Soup, 1 cup	220	8	24	6	13
• Stroganoff-Style Beef Soup, 1 cup	250	14	18	4	12
Turkey Pot Pie Soup, 1 cup	200	8	21	4	11
Healthy Request® Chunky™ Soups					
Beef Barley Soup, 1 cup	140	2	21	5	9
Chicken Noodle Soup, 1 cup	120	3	15	1	7
Old Fashioned Veggie Beef Soup, 1 cup	110	2	17	3	7
Healthy Request® Condensed Soups					
Chicken Noodle Soup, 1/2 cup	60	2	8	1	3
Tomato Soup, 1/2 cup	90	2	17	1	2
Vegetable Soup, 1/2 cup	100	1	19	3	4
Healthy Request® Select™ Soups					
Chicken with Egg Noodles, 1 cup	100	3	13	2	7
Italian-Style Wedding, 1 cup	120	3	15	2	7
Mexican Style Chicken Tortilla, 1 cup	130	3	20	3	8
Savory Chicken and Long Grain Rice, 1 cup	110	2	18	2	7

SOUPS & BROTHS

Canned Soup (cont.)

	Cal	Fat	Cbs	Fbr	Prtn
Campbell's Soups (cont.)					
Low Sodium Soups					
Chicken with Noodles Soup, 1 can	160	5	17	2	12
Cream of Mushroom Soup, 1 can	160	8	19	3	4
Select™ Gold Label Soup					
Creamy Tomato Parmesan, 1 cup	200	9	25	4	5
Italian Tomato with Basil & Garlic, 1 cup	90	0	19	3	3
Southwestern Corn Soup, 1 cup	190	8	26	4	3
Select™ Soups					
98% Fat Free New England Clam Chowder, 1 cup	110	2	18	2	5
Creamy Chicken Alfredo Soup, 1 cup	180	7	18	2	10
New England Clam Chowder, 1 cup	160	8	15	2	6
Potato Broccoli Cheese Soup, 1 cup	120	4	18	4	3
Healthy Choice					
Bean & Ham Soup, 1 cup	180	2	29	10	11
Chicken & Dumplings Soup, 1 cup	140	3	21	3	9
Chicken Noodle Soup, 1 cup	100	2	13	2	9
Chicken Rice Soup, 1 cup	110	2	17	3	7
Country Vegetables Soup, 1 cup	110	1	19	4	5
Hearty Chicken Soup, 1 cup	130	2	20	3	9
New England Clam Chowder, 1 cup	110	1	19	2	5
Split Pea & Ham, 1 cup	140	2	22	3	9
Vegetable Beef Soup, 1 cup	130	1	22	4	9
Muir Glen					
Classic Minestrone, 245 g	110	2	19	5	4
Creamy Tomato, 253 g	170	6	26	4	4
Garden Vegetable, 246 g	80	1	16	3	3
Hearty Tomato, 250 g	130	2	25	2	5
Homestyle Split Pea, 248 g	170	1	35	5	10
Progresso					
Low-Fat/Low-Carb					
Light Homestyle Vegetable and Rice, 242 g	60	0	14	4	2
Light Italian-Style Vegetable, 242 g	60	0	14	4	2
Light Savory Vegetable Barley, 243 g	60	0	14	4	2
Light Southwestern-Style Vegetable, 242 g	60	0	12	4	3
Healthy Favorites 50% Less Sodium					
Chicken Gumbo, 248 g	110	2	18	2	7
Chicken Noodle, 240 g	90	2	12	1	7
Garden Vegetable, 250 g	100	0	22	3	3
Minestrone, 252 g	120	2	24	4	5
Rich & Hearty					
Chicken & Homestyle Noodles, 246 g	110	2	14	1	8
Chicken Corn Chowder, 255 g	210	9	23	2	7
Chicken Pot Pie Style, 245 g	170	6	21	2	8
Creamy Chicken Wild Rice, 245 g	150	8	13	1	6
New England Clam Chowder, 240 g	190	9	22	2	6
Savory Beef Barley Vegetable, 245 g	130	1	22	3	9
Slow Cooked Vegetable Beef, 246 g	120	1	20	3	8
Steak & Roasted Russet Potatoes, 246 g	140	2	23	2	8
Traditional					
Carb Monitor Chicken Cheese Enchilada, 235 g	170	12	8	1	8
Manhattan Clam Chowder, 239 g	100	2	17	2	3

(• = most healthy • = least healthy)

POPULAR BRANDS

SOUPS & BROTHS

Canned Soup (cont.)

	Cal	Fat	Cbs	Fbr	Prtn
Progresso (cont.)					
Traditional (cont.)					
Chicken Noodle, 237 g	100	3	12	1	7
Chicken Sausage Gumbo, 249 g	130	4	18	1	6
Minestrone with Chicken, 236 g	120	4	16	3	6
New England Clam Chowder, 240 g	190	10	20	2	6
Potato Broccoli & Cheese Chowder, 252 g	180	10	18	2	5
Soup Turkey Noodle, 238 g	80	2	12	1	5
Vegetable Classics					
99% Fat Free Minestrone, 236 g	100	1	19	4	4
Creamy Mushroom, 230 g	130	10	9	1	2
French Onion, 230 g	50	2	8	1	1
Green Split Pea with Bacon, 244 g	170	1	28	5	9
Hearty Penne in Chicken Broth, 238 g	80	1	14	1	4
Lentil, 241 g	150	2	28	5	9
Macaroni & Bean, 246 g	160	4	25	6	7
Tomato Basil, 244 g	160	3	30	1	2

Soup Mix

	Cal	Fat	Cbs	Fbr	Prtn
Campbell's Soups					
Onion Soup Mix, 1 tbsp.	15	0	4	0	0
Top Ramen					
Beef, 100 g	83	4	11	N/A	2
Chicken, 100 g	83	4	11	N/A	2
Oriental, 100 g	83	4	11	N/A	2
Pork, 100 g	83	4	11	N/A	2
Uncle Ben's					
Hearty Soup Broccoli Chz & Rice, 28 g	110	2	43	1	3

SYRUP, JAMS, NUT BUTTERS

Fruit Spreads

	Cal	Fat	Cbs	Fbr	Prtn
Apple Time					
Apple Butter, 1 tbsp.	30	N/A	8	N/A	N/A
Brummel & Brown					
Simply Strawberry® Creamy, 12 g	50	4	3	N/A	0
Cascadian Farm					
Apricot, 19 g	40	0	10	N/A	0
Blackberry, 19 g	45	0	11	N/A	0
Blueberry, 19 g	45	0	11	N/A	0
Strawberry, 19 g	40	0	10	N/A	0
Knott's Berry Farm					
Light Strawberry Jam, 1 tbsp.	20	0	5	N/A	0
Strawberry Jam, 1 tbsp.	50	0	13	N/A	0
Lucky Leaf					
Lucky Leaf Apple Butter, 1 tbsp.	30	N/A	8	N/A	N/A
Smuckers					
Fruit Butter					
Cider Apple Butter, 19 g	45	0	11	N/A	0
Spiced Apple Butter, 19 g	45	0	11	N/A	0
Jam					
Blackberry, 20 g	50	0	13	N/A	0
Concord Grape, 20 g	51	0	13	N/A	0

SYRUP, JAMS, NUT BUTTERS

Fruit Spreads (cont.)	Cal	Fat	Cbs	Fbr	Prtn
Smuckers (cont.)					
Jam (cont.)					
Raspberry, 20 g	50	0	13	N/A	0
Jelly					
Apple, 20 g	50	0	13	N/A	0
Blackberry, 20 g	50	0	13	N/A	0
Mixed Fruit, 20 g	50	0	13	N/A	0
Low Sugar					
Apricot, 17 g	21	0	6	N/A	0
Strawberry, 17 g	25	0	6	N/A	0
Sweet Orange Marmalade, 17 g	25	0	2	N/A	0
Preserves					
Boysenberry, 20 g	50	0	13	N/A	0
Cherry, 20 g	50	0	13	N/A	0
Peach, 20 g	50	0	13	N/A	0
Simply Fruit					
Black Cherry, 19 g	40	0	10	N/A	0
Blueberry, 19 g	40	0	10	N/A	0
Red Raspberry, 19 g	40	0	10	N/A	0
Sugar Free					
Boysenberry Preserves with Splenda, 17 g	10	0	5	N/A	0
Concord Grape Jam with Splenda, 17 g	10	0	5	N/A	0
Strawberry with NutraSweet, 17 g	10	0	5	N/A	0
Welch's					
Jelly, Jam & Spread Jars, 20 g	50	0	13	N/A	0

Nut Butter	Cal	Fat	Cbs	Fbr	Prtn
Jif					
Reduced Fat Jif Creamy, 36 g	190	12	15	1	8
Reduced Fat Jif Crunchy, 36 g	190	12	15	1	8
Regular Jif Creamy, 32 g	190	16	7	2	8
Regular Jif Extra Crunchy, 32 g	190	16	7	2	8
Nutella					
Hazelnut Spread w/ Skim Milk & Cocoa, 37 g	200	11	23	2	2
Peter Pan					
Creamy Peanut Butter, 2 tbsp.	190	17	6	2	7
Crunchy Peanut Butter, 2 tbsp.	190	16	6	3	8
• Whipped Creamy Peanut Butter, 2 tbsp.	140	12	5	2	6
Skippy Peanut Butter					
Creamy, 32 g	190	16	7	2	7
Natural, 32 g	180	17	6	2	7
Reduced Fat Creamy, 36 g	180	12	15	2	7
Reduced Fat Super Chunk, 35 g	180	12	15	2	7
Roasted Honey Nut Creamy, 32 g	190	16	7	2	7
Roasted Honey Nut Super Chunk, 32 g	190	16	6	2	7
Super Chunk®, 32 g	190	16	7	2	7
Smart Balance					
Chunky, 32 g	200	17	6	2	7
Creamy, 32 g	200	17	6	2	7
Smuckers					
Goober PB & J					
• Grape, 53 g	240	13	24	2	7

(• = most healthy • = least healthy)

SYRUP, JAMS, HONEY, NUT BUTTERS

Nut Butter (cont.)	Cal	Fat	Cbs	Fbr	Prtn
Smuckers (cont.)					
Goober PB & J (cont.)					
Strawberry, 53 g	240	13	24	2	7
Natural Peanut Butter					
Chunky, 32 g	210	16	6	2	8
Creamy, 32 g	210	16	6	2	8
Honey, 33 g	200	16	9	2	7

Syrup	Cal	Fat	Cbs	Fbr	Prtn
Aunt Jemima					
Lite, 1/4 cup	100	0	26	1	0
Original, 1/4 cup	210	0	52	N/A	0
Eggo					
Butter Pecan Syrup, 60 ml.	220	0	55	N/A	0
Buttery Syrup, 60 ml.	160	0	41	N/A	0
Lite Syrup, 60 ml.	110	0	27	N/A	0
Original Syrup, 60 ml.	240	0	60	N/A	0
Karo Syrup					
Dark Corn Syrup, 30 ml.	120	0	31	N/A	0
Light Corn Syrup, 30 ml.	120	0	31	N/A	0
• Pancake Syrup, 60 ml.	240	0	63	N/A	0
Knott's Berry Farm					
Blueberry Syrup, 1/4 cup	210	0	52	N/A	0
Boysenberry Syrup, 1/4 cup	210	0	52	N/A	0
Mrs. Butterworth's					
Original Syrup	220	0	55	N/A	0
Smuckers					
Blackberry, 60 ml.	210	0	52	N/A	0
Blueberry, 60 ml.	210	0	52	N/A	0
Red Raspberry, 60 ml.	210	0	52	N/A	0
Strawberry, 60 ml.	210	0	52	N/A	0
Sugar Free Breakfast Syrup, 60 ml.	20	0	8	N/A	0
Sorbee					
Blueberry Syrup, 60 ml.	10	0	4	N/A	0
Chocolate Syrup, 32 g	15	0	4	N/A	0
• Strawberry Syrup, 31 g	5	0	2	N/A	0

VEGETABLES

Vegetables, Canned	Cal	Fat	Cbs	Fbr	Prtn
Allens					
Carrots					
Tiny Sliced Carrots, 127 g	35	0	8	3	0
Green Beans					
Cut Green Beans, 120 g	30	0	6	3	0
French Style Green Beans, 119 g	25	0	4	2	1
Green Bean Casserole, 120 g	40	1	6	1	2
Green Beans No Salt, 120 g	15	0	3	2	0
Whole Green Beans, 124 g	30	0	6	3	1
Greens					
Collard Greens No Salt, 116 g	30	1	5	3	1
Kale Greens No Salt, 116 g	30	1	3	2	2
Mixed Greens No Salt, 121 g	30	1	8	4	1

VEGETABLES

Vegetables, Canned (cont.)	Cal	Fat	Cbs	Fbr	Prtn
Allens (cont.)					
Greens (cont.)					
Mustard Greens No Salt, 118 g	30	1	5	3	1
Seasoned Collard Greens, 118 g	35	1	5	1	3
Seasoned Kale Greens, 118 g	35	1	5	1	3
Seasoned Mixed Greens, 118 g	45	1	6	1	4
Seasoned Mustard Greens, 118 g	45	1	6	1	4
Seasoned Turnip Greens w/Diced Turnips, 118 g	35	1	5	1	4
Seasoned Turnip Greens, 118 g	35	1	5	2	4
Turnip Greens No Salt, 121 g	25	1	3	2	2
Turnip Greens w/ Diced Turnip No Salt, 119 g	30	1	5	3	1
Hominy					
Golden Hominy, 128 g	120	1	27	4	2
Pepi Golden Hominy, 128 g	120	1	27	4	2
White Hominy, 127 g	100	1	22	4	2
Okra					
Cut Okra & Tomatoes, 114 g	30	0	5	3	1
Cut Okra, 124 g	30	0	6	3	1
Cut Okra, Tomatoes & Corn, 117 g	30	0	6	4	1
Peas					
Allens Field Peas with Snaps, 128 g	120	1	21	6	6
Crowder Peas, 127 g	110	1	19	8	6
Purple Hull Peas, 126 g	120	1	21	6	7
American Roland Food Corporation					
Artichokes					
Bottoms, 130 g	50	0	10	5	2
Hearts, Marinated, 30 g	20	2	2	1	1
Hearts, Small, 126 g	35	0	6	4	2
Asparagus					
Spears, Green, 130 g	20	0	3	2	2
Spears, White, 135 g	30	0	5	1	2
Bamboo Shoots					
Sliced, 130 g	25	0	3	2	1
Strips, 130 g	25	0	3	2	1
Carrots					
Baby Carrots, 120 g	35	0	7	3	1
Julienne Strips, 120 g	45	0	9	3	1
Peas & Carrots, 120 g	90	0	17	4	4
Celery					
Hearts, 120 g	15	0	2	1	1
Knob Strips, 120 g	45	0	10	3	1
Chestnuts					
Cream - Creme de Marrons, 30 g	80	0	18	2	0
In Water - Marrons, 30 g	30	0	7	1	0
Natural Chestnuts - Marrons, 30 g	50	0	11	2	0
Corn					
Baby Corn, Cut, 130 g	25	0	4	2	2
Baby Corn, Medium Whole, 130 g	25	0	4	2	2
White Corn, Organic, 100 g	110	1	23	4	2
Eggplant					
Eggplant Appetizer, 142 g	140	10	11	7	2
Stuffed Eggplants, 101 g	80	4	11	4	1

(•= most healthy •= least healthy)

VEGETABLES

Vegetables, Canned (cont.)	Cal	Fat	Cbs	Fbr	Prt
American Roland Food Corporation (cont.)					
Mushrooms					
Mushrooms, Whole, 120 g	25	0	4	2	1
Mushrooms, Wild Forest, 120 g	85	0	1	1	1
Shiitake, Dried, 9 g	30	0	5	2	2
Onions					
Baby Whole, 130 g	24	0	5	2	1
Cocktail, 14 g	0	0	0	0	0
• Whole, 130 g	25	0	5	2	1
Peas					
Peas & Carrots, 120 g	90	0	17	4	4
Peas, Green Extra Fine, 120 g	120	0	21	6	7
Peas, Pigeon, 130 g	80	0	15	4	4
Sundried Tomatoes					
Sundried Tomatoes, 5 g	15	0	3	1	1
Sundried Tomato Strips w/ Herbs, 15 g	35	1	6	0	0
Sundried Tomatoes in Olive Oil, 8 g	25	2	3	1	1
• Sweet Dried Tomatoes, 40 g	130	0	31	3	1
Bush's Beans					
Greens					
Chopped Collard Greens, 130 g	30	0	4	2	2
Chopped Kale Greens, 130 g	30	0	4	2	2
Chopped Mixed Greens, 130 g	25	0	3	2	2
Chopped Mustard Greens, 130 g	25	0	3	2	2
Chopped Turnip Greens, 130 g	25	0	3	2	2
Hominy					
Golden Hominy, 130 g	60	0	13	3	1
White Hominy, 130 g	70	1	14	4	1
California Sun Dry					
Julienne Cut Sun-Dried Tomatoes in Oil, 10 g	45	3	N/A	N/A	N/A
Sun-Dried Tomato Garlic, 2tbs	90	7	N/A	N/A	N/A
Sun-Dried Tomato Halves in Oil, 10 g	45	3	N/A	N/A	N/A
Sun-Dried Tomato Sun-Cups, 1 oz.	15	0	N/A	N/A	N/A
Contadina					
Recipe Ready Tomatoes					
Crushed Tomatoes 28 oz, 61 g	20	0	4	1	1
Crushed Tomatoes w/ Italian Herbs 28 oz, 61 g	20	0	3	1	1
Crushed Tomatoes w/ Roasted Garlic 28 oz, 61 g	20	0	3	1	1
Diced Tomatoes - Marinara 15 oz, 122 g	70	2	13	2	1
Diced Tomatoes 15 oz, 122 g	30	0	6	1	1
Diced Tomatoes with Italian Herbs 15 oz, 122 g	45	0	10	1	1
Stewed Tomatoes					
Italian Style Stewed Tomatoes 15 oz, 122 g	35	0	8	1	1
Stewed Tomatoes 15 oz, 122 g	35	0	9	1	1
Tomato Paste					
Tomato Paste 6 oz, 33 g	30	0	6	1	1
Italian Paste w/ Italian Seasonings 6 oz, 33 g	35	1	7	1	1
Tomato Paste 12 oz, 33 g	30	0	6	1	2
Tomato Puree					
Tomato Puree 15 oz, 63 g	20	0	4	1	1
Tomato Sauce					
Tomato Sauce 8 oz, 61 g	15	0	3	1	1

Vegetables, Canned (cont.)	Cal	Fat	Cbs	Fbr	Prtn
Contadina (cont.)					
Tomato Sauce (cont.)					
Extra Thick and Zesty Tomato Sauce 15 oz, 62 g	20	0	3	1	1
Garlic & Onion Tomato Sauce 15 oz, 61 g	20	0	4	1	1
Tomato Sauce 29 oz, 61 g	15	0	3	1	1
Del Monte					
Asparagus					
Asparagus Cuts & Tips, 124 g	20	0	3	1	2
Asparagus Spears, 124 g	20	0	3	1	2
Extra Long Asparagus Spears, 124 g	20	0	3	1	2
Beans					
Lima Beans, 126 g	80	0	15	4	4
Wax Beans, 121 g	20	0	4	2	1
Carrots					
Honey Glazed Carrots, 130 g	70	0	18	1	1
Peas & Carrots, 128 g	60	0	11	2	2
Sliced Carrots, 123 g	35	0	8	3	0
Corn					
Corn in Butter Sauce, 126 g	90	3	14	1	2
Sweet Corn Cream Style, 125 g	60	1	14	2	1
White Corn, 125 g	60	1	11	3	2
White Corn Cream Style, 125 g	100	1	21	2	2
Diced Tomatoes					
Diced Tomatoes, No Salt Added, 126 g	25	0	6	2	1
Diced with Basil, Garlic and Oregano, 126 g	50	0	11	1	2
Diced with Green Pepper and Onion, 126 g	40	0	9	2	1
Diced with Mushroom and Garlic, 126 g	45	0	10	1	1
Green Beans					
Cut Green Beans, 121 g	20	0	4	2	1
Cut Italian Beans, 121 g	30	0	6	3	1
French Style Green Beans, 121 g	20	0	4	2	1
Whole Green Beans, 121 g	20	0	4	2	1
Mixed Vegetables					
Homestyle Vegetable Medley, 120 g	70	3	11	2	1
Mixed Vegetables, 124 g	40	0	8	2	2
Peas & Carrots, 128 g	60	0	11	2	2
Peas					
Peas & Carrots, 128 g	60	0	11	2	2
Sweet Peas, 125 g	60	0	13	4	3
Very Young Small Sweet Peas, 125 g	60	0	10	4	3
Petite Cut Diced Tomatoes					
Diced Tomatoes, 126 g	25	0	6	2	1
With Garlic and Olive Oil, 126 g	45	1	10	1	1
With Zesty Jalapeños, 126 g	30	0	6	1	1
Potatoes					
Diced New Potatoes, 122 g	45	0	11	1	1
Mixed Vegetables with Potatoes, 125 g	45	0	10	2	2
Potatoes Au Gratin, 124 g	80	3	13	1	2
Whole New Potatoes, 158 g	60	0	13	2	1
Sauerkraut					
Sauerkraut, 30 g	0	0	0	1	0
Bavarian Sauerkraut, 30 g	15	0	4	0	0

(• = most healthy • = least healthy)

VEGETABLES

Vegetables, Canned (cont.)	Cal	Fat	Cbs	Fbr	Prtn
Del Monte (cont.)					
Spinach					
Chopped Spinach, 115 g	30	0	4	2	2
Whole Leaf Spinach, 115 g	30	0	4	2	2
Stewed Tomatoes					
Italian Recipe, 126 g	30	0	8	2	1
Mexican Recipe, 126 g	35	0	9	2	1
Original Recipe, 126 g	35	0	9	2	1
Wedges					
Tomato Wedges, 126 g	35	0	9	2	1
Zucchini					
Zucchini with Tomato Sauce, 121 g	30	0	7	1	1
Green Giant					
Asparagus, 123 g	20	0	3	1	2
Cream Style Sweet Corn, 127 g	90	1	19	1	2
Cut Green Beans, 120 g	20	0	4	1	1
Mushrooms Whole, 120 g	25	0	4	1	2
Sweet Peas, 122 g	60	0	12	3	4
Whole Kernel Sweet Corn, 124 g	60	1	11	2	2
Hunt's					
Diced					
Original Tomatoes, 1/2 cup	20	0	5	1	1
Tomatoes in Sauce, 1/2 cup	30	0	7	1	1
Tomatoes with Roasted Garlic, 1/2 cup	30	0	6	1	1
Tomatoes with Sweet Onions, 1/2 cup	45	0	10	1	1
Stewed					
Tomatoes, 1/2 cup	30	0	7	1	1
Tomatoes No Salt Added, 1/2 cup	40	0	9	1	1
Whole					
Tomatoes No Salt Added, 1/2 cup	20	0	4	1	1
Tomatoes, 1/2 cup	20	0	4	1	1
Libby's Pumpkin					
Libby's 100% Pure Pumpkin, 1/2 cup	40	1	9	5	2
Muir Glen					
Crushed Tomatoes with Basil, 65 g	25	0	5	1	1
Ground Peeled Tomatoes, 65 g	20	0	4	1	1
Stewed Tomatoes, 128 g	30	0	6	1	1
Whole Peeled Tomatoes, 122 g	25	0	5	1	1
Progresso					
Artichoke Hearts Marinated, 32 g	60	5	2	0	0
Artichoke Hearts, 130 g	30	0	7	2	1
Ro*Tel					
Chunky Tomatoes with Green Chilis, 1/2 cup	20	0	4	1	1
Diced Tomatoes, 1/2 cup	25	0	5	1	1
Hot Diced Tomatoes, 1/2 cup	20	0	4	1	1
Italian Diced Tomatoes, 1/2 cup	30	0	6	1	1
Mexican Fiesta Diced Tomatoes, 1/2 cup	30	0	6	1	1
Tomatoes with Green Chilis, 1/2 cup	20	0	4	1	1

Vegetables, Dried	Cal	Fat	Cbs	Fbr	Prtn
California Sun Dry					
Sun-Dried Tomato Cello Bags, 1 oz.	15	0	N/A	N/A	N/A

Vegetables, Frozen & Fresh	Cal	Fat	Cbs	Fbr	Prtn
Cascadian Farm					
Gourmet Boxed					
Broccoli Florets, 85 g	25	0	4	2	2
Cut Spinach, 85 g	25	0	3	1	2
French Green Beans w/ Almonds, 105 g	70	3	8	2	3
Winter Squash, 130 g	70	0	19	2	2
Premium Bagged					
Broccoli Florets, 85 g	20	0	4	2	2
Peas & Carrots, 85 g	50	0	10	3	2
Sweet Corn, 85 g	90	1	19	2	3
Sweet Peas, 85 g	70	0	12	4	4
Premium Blends					
California-Style Blend, 85 g	25	0	5	2	1
Chinese Stirfry, 85 g	25	0	6	2	2
Gardener's Blend, 85 g	50	0	11	3	2
Mixed Vegetables, 85 g	60	0	12	2	2
Thai Stirfry, 85 g	25	0	5	2	1
Green Giant					
Corn On The Cob					
Extra Sweet, 62 g	60	1	11	1	2
Nibblers, 61 g	70	1	14	1	2
Bagged					
Broccoli & Carrots With Garlic Herbs, 112 g	40	1	7	2	2
Garden Vegetable Medley, 120 g	70	1	14	2	2
Plain Chopped Broccoli, 79 g	25	0	4	2	1
Plain Mixed Vegetables, 84 g	50	0	11	2	2
Plain Sweet Peas, 89 g	70	0	12	4	5
Select Sugar Snap Peas, 79 g	40	0	9	2	2
Select Whole Green Beans, 83 g	30	0	5	2	1
Boxed - Simply Steam					
Baby Veggie Medley Seasoned, 103 g	40	1	9	2	1
Broccoli and Carrots, 131 g	60	3	8	3	2
Garden Vegetable Medley, 99 g	50	1	11	1	2
No Sauce Asparagus Cuts, 86 g	20	0	3	1	2
• No Sauce Baby Lima Beans, 76 g	80	0	15	3	4

Vegetables, Packaged Fresh	Cal	Fat	Cbs	Fbr	Prtn
Chiquita					
Bell Peppers, 148 g	30	0	7	2	1
Cucumbers, 99 g	15	0	3	1	1
Tomatoes, 48 g	35	1	7	1	1
Dole					
Fresh Vegetables					
Artichokes, 56 g	25	0	6	3	2
Asparagus, 93 g	25	0	4	2	2
Broccoli, 148 g	45	0	8	5	4
Brussels Sprouts, 84 g	40	0	6	3	2
Butter Lettuce, 85 g	10	N/A	N/A	N/A	N/A
Carrots, 78 g	35	0	8	2	1
Cauliflower, 99 g	25	0	5	2	2
Celery, 110 g	20	0	5	2	1
Green Cabbage, 92 g	20	N/A	N/A	N/A	N/A

VEGETABLES

Vegetables, Packaged Fresh (cont.)	Cal	Fat	Cbs	Fbr	Prtn
Dole (cont.)					
Fresh Vegetables (cont.)					
Green Leaf Lettuce, 90 g	15	N/A	3	1	1
Iceberg Lettuce, 89 g	15	0	3	1	1
• Mushrooms, 35 g	9	0	1	0	1
Romaine Lettuce, 85 g	20	0	3	1	1
Packaged Salads					
Baby Spinach, 85 g	20	0	3	2	2
Butter & Red Leaf, 85 g	10	0	3	1	1
Classic Cole Slaw, 85 g	25	0	5	2	1
European, 85 g	15	0	3	1	1
Field Greens, 100 g	150	11	10	N/A	2
Italian, 85 g	15	0	3	1	1
Leafy Romaine, 85 g	15	0	3	1	1
Light Caesar Kit, 85 g	15	0	3	1	1
Mediterranean, 85 g	100	7	8	1	3
Romano Kit, 85 g	15	0	3	2	1
Shredded Carrots, 85 g	40	0	9	2	1
Spinach, 85 g	150	12	9	2	3
Fresh Express					
Complete Salad Kits					
Caesar Lite, 10 oz.	100	7	8	2	2
• Caesar Supreme, 8 oz.	170	14	8	2	3
Caesar, 8 oz.	150	13	8	2	2
Crispy Lettuces					
Green & Crisp w/ Double Carrots, 85 g	20	0	4	1	1
Original Iceberg Garden Salad, 85 g	15	0	3	4	1
Premium Romaine, 85 g	15	0	3	2	1
Flavorful Whole Baby Blends					
Baby Spinach, 85 g	20	0	0	2	2
Sweet Baby Greens, 85 g	10	0	2	1	1
Veggie Spring Mix, 85 g	20	0	5	2	1
Organics					
Baby Spinach, 85 g	35	0	9	4	2
Hearts of Romaine, 85 g	15	0	2	1	1
Italian, 85 g	15	0	3	1	1
Tender Lettuce Mixes					
Fancy Field Greens™, 85 oz.	20	0	3	2	1
Hearts of Romaine, 85 oz.	15	0	3	2	1
Italian, 85 oz.	15	0	2	1	1
Veggie Lovers Salad, 85 oz.	20	0	4	1	1
River Ranch					
Cut Vegetables					
Broccoli Florets, 85 g	25	0	4	3	3
Broccoli Stir Fry, 85 g	30	0	5	2	2
Cauliflower Florets, 85 g	20	0	4	2	1
Vegetable Medley Blend, 85 g	25	0	6	2	2
Salads					
Caesar Salad Kit, 100 g	150	12	7	2	3
Chopped Romaine, 85 g	10	0	2	1	1
Cole Slaw Mix, 85 g	25	0	5	2	1
European Salad Blend, 85 g	10	0	2	1	1

Vegetables, Packaged Fresh (cont.)	Cal	Fat	Cbs	Fbr	Prtn
River Ranch (cont.)					
Salads (cont.)					
Garden Salad, 85 g	15	0	3	1	1
Italian Salad Blend, 85 g	15	0	2	1	1
Raspberry Vinaigrette Salad Kit, 100 g	130	8	13	2	2
Shredded Carrots, 85 g	35	0	9	3	1
Soy Boy					
Organic 5 Grain Tempeh, 3 oz.	130	3	15	2	11
Organic Soy Tempeh's, 3 oz.	160	6	9	2	17

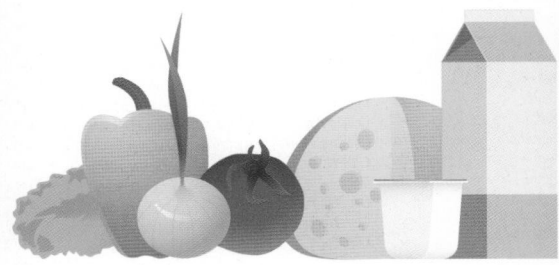

FOOD INDEX OF POPULAR BRANDS

FOOD INDEX OF POPULAR BRANDS

FOOD INDEX OF POPULAR BRANDS

Other Health & Fitness Books
By Alex A. Lluch

I WILL LOSE WEIGHT THIS TIME! DIET JOURNAL

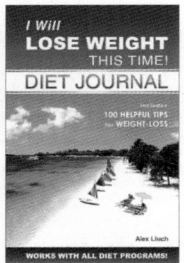

THE ULTIMATE POCKET DIET JOURNAL

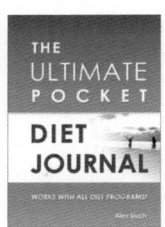

THE ULTIMATE POCKET WORKOUT JOURNAL

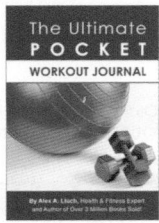

I WILL GET FIT THIS TIME! WORKOUT JOURNAL

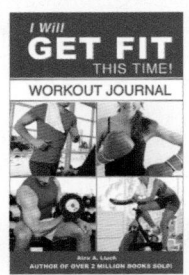

SIMPLE PRINCIPLES TO GET FIT

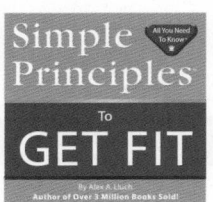

SIMPLE PRINCIPLES TO EAT SMART AND LOSE WEIGHT

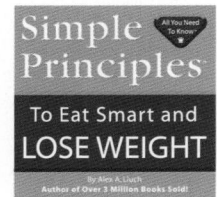

Visit www.WSPublishingGroup.com for more information.

Other Health & Fitness Books
By Alex A. Lluch

**DAILY PLANNER
WORKOUT JOURNAL**

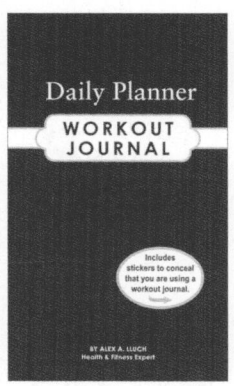

**DAILY PLANNER
DIET JOURNAL**

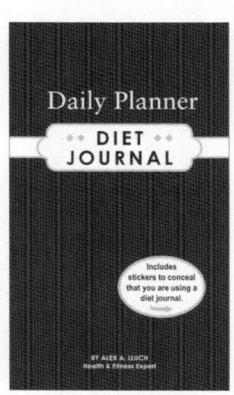

**EASY FAT, CARB &
CALORIE COUNTER**

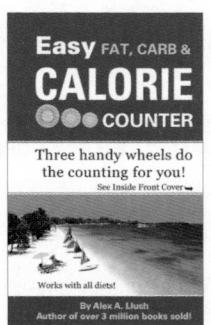

**LOSE WEIGHT NOW!
DIET JOURNAL & ORGANIZER**

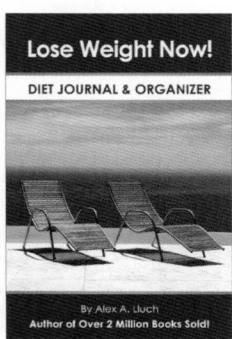

Visit www.WSPublishingGroup.com for more information.